AN INTRODUCTION TO FACIAL COSMETIC AND RECONSTRUCTIVE SURGERY

Dr. Shreya Das

ALLIED HEALTH PRESS

An Introduction to Facial Cosmetic and Reconstructive Surgery

Author: **Dr. Shreya Das**

Allied Health Press
4164 Lakeshore Road
Burlington ON L7L 1A4
Canada
www.alliedhealthpress.com
Email: orders@arclereducation.com

ISBN: 978-1-77956-818-2

ABOUT THE AUTHOR

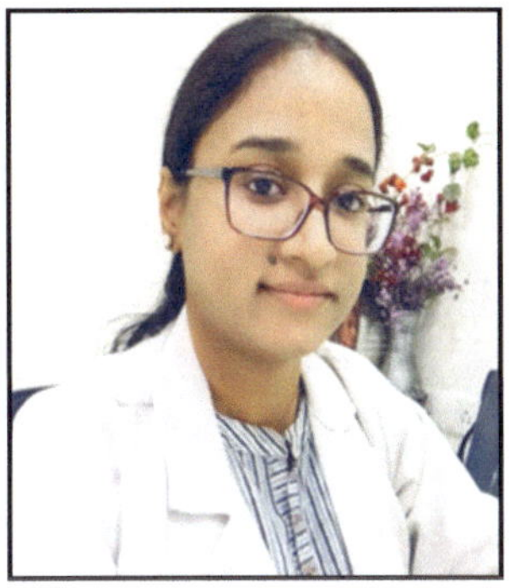

Dr. Shreya Das is an Oral and Maxillofacial Surgeon with specialized training and clinical experience in facial cosmetic surgery and aesthetic medicine. A university gold medalist, she completed her MDS in Oral and Maxillofacial Surgery and has since worked across reputed hospitals and wellness organizations. With a strong interest in facial aesthetics, her work bridges surgical precision and minimally invasive cosmetic procedures. She is passionate about advancing evidence-based practices in facial cosmetic and reconstructive surgery and contributing to the education of clinicians in this evolving field.

Brief Table of Contents

1. Introduction to Facial Anatomy and Aesthetics 1
2. Principles of Cosmetic and Reconstructive Surgery 37
3. Patient Assessment and Surgical Planning in Cosmetic Facial 73
4. Blepharoplasty (Eyelid Surgery) in Facial Cosmetic 107
5. Rhytidectomy (Facelift) and Neck Lift 141
6. Rhinoplasty (Nose Surgery) 175
7. Brow Lift and Forehead Rejuvenation in Facial Cosmetic 211
8. Facial Implants and Contouring: Chin, Cheek, and Jaw Implants; Fat Grafting and Liposculpture 243
9. Botulinum Toxin and Dermal Fillers in Facial Cosmetic 273
10. Skin Resurfacing and Laser Treatments 305
11. Principles of Facial Reconstruction 337
12. Trauma Reconstruction in Facial Cosmetic 369
13. Congenital and Developmental Deformities in Facial Cosmetic 401
14. Oncologic and Post-Tumor Reconstruction in Facial Cosmetic 433
15. Advances, Technologies, and Practice Management in Facial Cosmetic 465

Index 499

Getting Started with This Book

Chapter Openers

A list of Chapter Outline is presented providing a brief Introduction to what will be covered in the chapter.

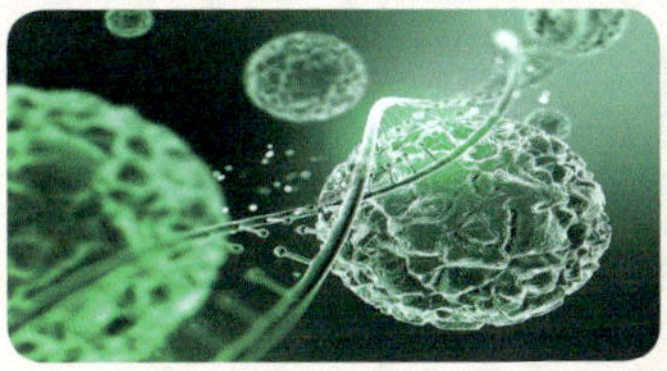

Introduction

Often referred to as the science of life, biology is a broad field of study aimed at comprehending the several kinds of life on Earth, from tiny creatures to sophisticated multicellular entities. Comprising several subfields, including molecular biology, ecology, and evolutionary biology, each of which advances our knowledge of living systems, this field clarifies the mechanisms controlling life events, including development, reproduction, and interaction with the surroundings, which is the central goal of biology. Moreover, biology fills in the void between the natural sciences and medicine by offering a necessary understanding of health, illness, and the interactions between organisms and their environments. Dealing with urgent global issues such as climate change, biodiversity loss, and new diseases depends on an awareness of these complex biological interactions, therefore highlighting the critical part biology plays in modern civilization. Fundamentally, biology explores and tests ideas about the living world using the scientific method. Through methodical observation and experimentation,

LEARNING OBJECTIVES

After studying this chapter, you will be able to:

1. Discuss the scientific method in biology;
2. Explain the cell theory;
3. Discuss the genetics and heredity;
4. Evolution and natural selection;
5. Focus on ecology and ecosystems;
6. Learn about human biology;
7. Evaluate the plant biology;
8. Explain the microbiology;
9. Focus on current trends in biology.

1.1. The Scientific Method in Biology

Learning Outcome

1. Describe the steps of the scientific method;
2. Focus on hypothesis formation;
3. Learn about experimental design.

Learning Outcomes

The beginning of each section of every chapter contains a set of Learning Outcomes that inform students of concepts they should understand. These outcomes help students understand what they should be able to do if they have mastered the material in that section.

Test Your Knowledge

Throughout each chapter, Test Your Knowledge cues you to note which topics have been covered and to self-test your understanding of the material presented.

Test Your Knowledge

1. Explain why correlation does not imply causation in scientific experiments.
2. How does the scientific method help reduce the influence of personal opinions in research?

Chapter Summary

The Summary Section appear at the end of each chapter and summarize main concepts covered throughout the chapter. These points provide key concepts in an engaging and meaningful way.

Summary

The investigation of biological principles highlights the importance of a comprehensive view of life by reflecting the intricate interactions that occur within living systems. The complexity of biology goes beyond individual species or systems, as this essay highlights; it also includes the interactions that mold ecosystems and affect biodiversity. Researchers can conduct in-depth analyses of metabolomic data using sophisticated technologies like MetaboAnalyst, which offer insights into the molecular mechanisms underlying these interactions. As demonstrated by the developments in MetaboAnalyst, for example, the integration of diverse omics data promotes a thorough understanding of metabolic pathways and helps identify important biological markers necessary for research on development and disease (Chong et al., 2018). Additionally, the phenomenon of ecological invasions is a key component of biological research and a vital field of study. The introduction of non-native species into unfamiliar habitats has significant ramifications and calls for multidisciplinary management strategies. Examining the origins and effects of these biological incursions, invasion science has become a crucial field that highlights the need to comprehend ecological dynamics and community interactions. As interest in biological invasions increases, new findings are emerging that put conventional ecological theories and practices to the test. The importance of incorporating various scientific viewpoints is shown by this developing discipline, which also highlights how invasive species shape ecosystems and advances our knowledge of ecological resilience (David et al., 2013). When taken as a whole, these discoveries from invasion science and metabolomics highlight the value of multidisciplinary biology research. Fostering cross-disciplinary collaboration and utilizing technological breakthroughs to improve our comprehension of intricate biological interactions are crucial as we look to the future of biological research. In addition to deepening our understanding of the complexities of life, this method lays the groundwork for tackling urgent environmental issues. Future studies can ensure the continued relevance of biology in a world that is constantly changing by acknowledging the interconnection of biological systems and opening the door to creative solutions that support sustainability and biodiversity conservation. We might imagine a thorough comprehension of life that serves both academia and society at large through ongoing investigation and integration of scientific knowledge.

Knowledge Assessment

The chapter includes material designed to review and reinforce each content. It includes Critical Thinking Questions to help test of your understanding of information presented in the chapter and Short answer Questions to review your understanding of the key concepts presented in the chapter.

Critical Thinking Questions

1. **Who is known as the "Father of Modern Biology"?**
   a. Aristotle
   b. Charles Darwin
   c. Gregor Mendel
   d. Louis Pasteur
2. **What is the basic unit of life?**
   a. Atom
   b. Molecule
   c. Cell
   d. Organism
3. **Which branch of biology studies the interaction of organisms with their environment?**
   a. Genetics
   b. Ecology
   c. Physiology
   d. Botany
4. **Which macromolecule is the main source of energy for living organisms?**
   a. Proteins
   b. Lipids
   c. Carbohydrates
   d. Nucleic acids
5. **DNA is primarily responsible for which function in living organisms?**
   a. Energy production
   b. Protein synthesis
   c. Storing genetic information
   d. Regulating body temperature

Short Answer Questions

1. What is biology, and why is it important to study biology?
2. What are the three main domains of life, and how are they different from one another?
3. Define homeostasis and give an example of how it works in living organisms.
4. What is the cell theory, and why is it fundamental to biology?
5. How do autotrophs and heterotrophs differ in the way they obtain energy?
6. What is the scientific method, and how is it applied in biological research?
7. Discuss how biology helps address global challenges such as climate change, disease, and food security.
8. Explain the levels of biological organization from the smallest unit to the largest. Provide examples at each level.
9. Describe the relationship between structure and function in biology, giving specific examples from cells or organs
10. How has the discovery of genetics shaped our understanding of inheritance and variation among organisms?

Supplementary Materials

Key Terms: A list of key terms is given for quick reference

KEY TERMS FROM THIS CHAPTER

Annotation enrichment analysis
Cell theory
Ecosystems
Microbiology
Plant biology
Biological structure
Cellular structure
Genetics
Natural selection
Cell
Ecology
Human biology
Organism

Further Resources: Recommendations for additional readings, websites, and multimedia resources.

References

1. Argelaguet, R., Velten, B., Arnol, D., Dietrich, S., Zenz, T., Marioni, J. C., Buettner, F., et al. (2018). Multi-omics factor analysis—A framework for unsupervised integration of multi-omics data sets. *Molecular Systems Biology, 14*. https://doi.org/10.15252/msb.20178124.
2. Bacher, S., Blackburn, T. M., Essl, F., & Genovesi, P. (2017). *Socio-Economic Impact Classification of Alien Taxa (SEICAT).* https://core.ac.uk/download/286567949.pdf (accessed on 8th March 2025).
3. Barnett, R., Brace, S., Cucchi, T., & Dobney, K. (2013). *Divergent Evolutionary Processes Associated with Colonization of Offshore Islands.* https://core.ac.uk/download/20664364.pdf (accessed on 8th March 2025).

Detailed Table of Contents

List of Figures *xvii*
Preface *xxv*

CHAPTER 1

Introduction to Facial Anatomy and Aesthetics 1

Introduction **1**
1.1. The Skeletal Framework of the Face **5**
1.1.1. Key Bones Involved in Facial Structure 6
1.1.2. The Role of the Skull in Aesthetic Appearance 7
1.1.3. Common Facial Skeletal Disorders 7
1.2. Muscles of Facial Expression **9**
1.2.1. Major Muscles and Their Functions 10
1.2.2. The Impact of Muscle Tone on Aesthetics 11
1.2.3. Techniques for Assessing Muscle Function 12
1.3. Skin and Its Role in Facial Aesthetics **13**
1.3.1. Layers of the Skin and Their Functions 14
1.3.2. Factors Affecting Skin Health and Appearance 15
1.3.3. Common Skin Conditions and Treatments 16
1.4. The Importance of Facial Proportions **17**
1.4.1. Historical Perspectives on Facial Proportions 18
1.4.2. Modern Standards of Beauty and Aesthetics 19
1.4.3. Tools for Measuring Facial Proportions 20
1.5. Aesthetic Procedures and Treatments **22**
1.5.1. Overview of Non-Surgical Treatments 22
1.5.2. Surgical Options for Facial Enhancement 23
1.5.3. Risks and Benefits of Aesthetic Procedures 24
1.6. Psychological Aspects of Facial Aesthetics **25**
1.6.1. The Connection Between Facial Appearance and Self-Esteem 26
1.6.2. Cultural Influences on Perceptions of Beauty 27
1.6.3. The Role of Social Media in Shaping Aesthetic Standards 28
Summary **30**
References **33**

CHAPTER 2

Principles of Cosmetic and Reconstructive Surgery 37

Introduction **37**
2.1. Historical Background **41**
2.1.1. Origins of Cosmetic Surgery 41
2.1.2. Development of Reconstructive Techniques 42
2.1.3. Milestones in Surgical Advancements 43
2.2. Ethical Considerations **45**
2.2.1. Patient Consent and Autonomy 45
2.2.2. Psychological Impacts of Surgery 46
2.2.3. Ethical Dilemmas in Cosmetic Procedures 47
2.3. Surgical Techniques **49**
2.3.1. Common Cosmetic Procedures 50
2.3.2. Reconstructive Surgery Techniques 50
2.3.3. Innovations in Surgical Technology 51
2.4. Patient Selection Criteria **53**
2.4.1. Assessing Medical History 54

2.4.2. Psychological Evaluation 54
2.4.3. Setting Realistic Expectations 55
2.5. Risks and Complications **56**
2.5.1. Common Risks Associated with Surgery 57
2.5.2. Long-term Complications 58
2.5.3. Managing Patient Safety 59
2.6. Postoperative Care **60**
2.6.1. Importance of Follow-up Appointments 61
2.6.2. Recovery Process and Timeline 62
2.6.3. Addressing Complications and Concerns 63
Summary **65**
References **68**

CHAPTER 3

Patient Assessment and Surgical Planning in Cosmetic Facial **73**

Introduction **73**
3.1. The Role of Patient History **77**
3.1.1. Gathering Comprehensive Medical History 78
3.1.2. Understanding Psychological Factors 78
3.1.3. Assessing Previous Surgical Experiences 79
3.2. Physical Examination Techniques **81**
3.2.1. Visual Assessment of Facial Features 82
3.2.2. Palpation and Functional Assessment 83
3.2.3. Documentation of Findings 83
3.3. Patient Expectations and Goals **84**
3.3.1. Discussing Desired Outcomes 85
3.3.2. Managing Unrealistic Expectations 86
3.3.3. Importance of Clear Communication 87
3.4. Risk Assessment and Management **88**
3.4.1. Identifying Potential Surgical Risks 89
3.4.2. Evaluating Patient Health Status 90
3.4.3. Developing a Risk Mitigation Plan 90
3.5. Surgical Planning Strategies **92**
3.5.1. Creating a Tailored Surgical Plan 93
3.5.2. Selecting Appropriate Surgical Techniques 93
3.5.3. Considering Postoperative Care 94
3.6. Ethical Considerations in Cosmetic Surgery **96**
3.6.1. Informed Consent Process 97
3.6.2. Addressing Ethical Dilemmas 97
3.6.3. Importance of Patient Autonomy 98
Summary **100**
References **103**

CHAPTER 4

Blepharoplasty (Eyelid Surgery) in Facial Cosmetic **107**

Introduction **107**
4.1. Types of Blepharoplasty **111**
4.1.1. Upper Eyelid Blepharoplasty 112
4.1.2. Lower Eyelid Blepharoplasty 113
4.1.3. Transconjunctival Blepharoplasty 114
4.2. Indications for Blepharoplasty **115**
4.2.1. Cosmetic Reasons for Eyelid Surgery 115
4.2.2. Functional Implications of Eyelid Conditions 116
4.2.3. Age-Related Changes and Their Impact 117
4.3. The Surgical Procedure **118**
4.3.1. Preoperative Consultation and Assessment 119
4.3.2. Surgical Techniques and Approaches 120
4.3.3. Anesthesia Options and Patient Comfort 120
4.4. Risks and Complications **122**
4.4.1. Common Risks Associated with Blepharoplasty 123
4.4.2. Potential Complications and Their Management 124
4.4.3. Importance of Choosing a Qualified Surgeon 125
4.5. Recovery Process **126**
4.5.1. Immediate Postoperative Care 127
4.5.2. Timeline for Healing and Activity Resumption 128
4.5.3. Long-Term Care and Follow-Up 129
4.6. Psychological and Social Impacts **130**
4.6.1. Effects on Self-Image and Confidence 131
4.6.2. Social Perceptions of Aesthetic Surgery 132
4.6.3. Patient Satisfaction and Quality of Life 133

Summary 135

References 138

CHAPTER 5

Rhytidectomy (Facelift) and Neck Lift 141

Introduction 141

5.1. Historical Background 144

5.1.1. Evolution of Facelift Techniques 145

5.1.2. Key Figures in Cosmetic Surgery 145

5.1.3. Milestones in Rhytidectomy Development 146

5.2. Types of Facelift Procedures 148

5.2.1. Traditional Facelift 148

5.2.2. Mini Facelift 149

5.2.3. Non-Surgical Facelift Options 150

5.3. Neck Lift Procedures 152

5.3.1. Definition and Purpose of Neck Lift 153

5.3.2. Techniques Used in Neck Lifts 153

5.3.3. Differences Between Neck Lift and Facelift 154

5.4. Indications for Surgery 155

5.4.1. Age-Related Changes in the Face and Neck 156

5.4.2. Genetic Factors Influencing Skin Elasticity 157

5.4.3. Psychological Motivations for Undergoing Surgery 158

5.5. Risks and Complications 159

5.5.1. Common Surgical Risks 160

5.5.2. Potential Complications Specific to Rhytidectomy 161

5.5.3. Importance of Choosing a Qualified Surgeon 161

5.6. Recovery and Aftercare 163

5.6.1. Typical Recovery Timeline 164

5.6.2. Post-Operative Care Instructions 164

5.6.3. Long-Term Maintenance of Results 165

Summary 167

References 170

CHAPTER 6

Rhinoplasty (Nose Surgery) 175

Introduction 175

6.1. Types of Rhinoplasty 179

6.1.1. Primary vs. Secondary Rhinoplasty 180

6.1.2. Open vs. Closed Rhinoplasty Techniques 180

6.1.3. Cosmetic vs. Functional Rhinoplasty 181

6.2. Indications for Rhinoplasty 182

6.2.1. Aesthetic Concerns and Personal Preferences 183

6.2.2. Medical Reasons, Such as Breathing Difficulties 184

6.2.3. Trauma or Injury to the Nose 185

6.3. The Rhinoplasty Procedure 187

6.3.1. Pre-Operative Consultation and Assessment 187

6.3.2. Surgical Techniques and Anesthesia Options 188

6.3.3. Post-Operative Care and Recovery Process 189

6.4. Risks and Complications 190

6.4.1. Common Risks Associated with Surgery 191

6.4.2. Potential Complications Specific to Rhinoplasty 192

6.4.3. Importance of Choosing a Qualified Surgeon 193

6.5. Psychological Impact of Rhinoplasty 194

6.5.1. Effects on Self-Esteem and Body Image 195

6.5.2. Patient Expectations and Satisfaction Rates 196

6.5.3. Role Of Counseling in the Decision-Making Process 197

6.6. Cultural Perspectives on Rhinoplasty 198

6.6.1. Rhinoplasty Trends in Different Cultures 199

6.6.2. Societal Pressures and Beauty Standards 200

6.6.3. Ethical Considerations in Cosmetic Surgery 201

Summary 203

References 206

CHAPTER 7

Brow Lift and Forehead Rejuvenation in Facial Cosmetic 211

Introduction 211
7.1. Historical Background 214
7.1.1. Evolution of Cosmetic Surgery Techniques 215
7.1.2. Milestones in Brow Lift Procedures 215
7.1.3. Cultural Perceptions of Beauty and Aging 217
7.2. Anatomy of the Forehead and Brow Area 218
7.2.1. Key Facial Muscles Involved in Expression 219
7.2.2. Skin Structure and Aging Effects 220
7.2.3. Importance of Understanding Anatomy for Surgical Outcomes 221
7.3. Indications for Brow Lift and Forehead Rejuvenation 222
7.3.1. Common Aesthetic Concerns Addressed 223
7.3.2. Psychological Impact of Aging on Self-Esteem 224
7.3.3. Patient Demographics and Trends 225
7.4. Surgical Techniques 226
7.4.1. Traditional vs. Endoscopic Brow Lift Methods 227
7.4.2. Anesthesia Options and Considerations 228
7.4.3. Post-Operative Care and Recovery 229
7.5. Risks and Complications 230
7.5.1. Common Surgical Risks Associated with Brow Lifts 231
7.5.2. Long-Term Effects and Potential Complications 231
7.5.3. Importance of Choosing a Qualified Surgeon 232
7.6. Non-Surgical Alternatives 234
7.6.1. Botox and Fillers for Brow and Forehead Rejuvenation 234
7.6.2. Laser Treatments and Their Effectiveness 235
7.6.3. Comparison of Non-Surgical vs. Surgical Options 236
Summary 238
References 241

CHAPTER 8

Facial Implants and Contouring: Chin, Cheek, and Jaw Implants; Fat Grafting and Liposculpture 243

Introduction 243
8.1. Types of Facial Implants 246
8.1.1. Chin Implants 247
8.1.2. Cheek Implants 248
8.1.3. Jaw Implants 248
8.2. Benefits of Facial Implants 250
8.2.1. Enhanced Facial Symmetry 251
8.2.2. Improved Self-Esteem and Confidence 251
8.2.3. Long-Lasting Results Compared to Non-Surgical Options 252
8.3. Risks and Considerations 254
8.3.1. Potential Complications and Side Effects 255
8.3.2. Importance of Choosing a Qualified Surgeon 255
8.3.3. Psychological Considerations before Undergoing Surgery 256
8.4. Fat Grafting 257
8.4.1. Definition and Process of Fat Grafting 258
8.4.2. Advantages of Using Body Fat for Contouring 259
8.4.3. Areas Commonly Treated with Fat Grafting 260
8.5. Liposculpture 261
8.5.1. Definition and Techniques of Liposculpture 262
8.5.2. Differences Between Liposuction and Liposculpture 263
8.5.3. Ideal Candidates for Liposculpture 264
8.6. Combining Procedures 265
8.6.1. Benefits of Combining Implants with Fat Grafting 266
8.6.2. Case Studies of Successful Combined Procedures 267
8.6.3. Considerations for Recovery and Aftercare 267
Summary 269
References 272

CHAPTER 9

Botulinum Toxin and Dermal Fillers in Facial Cosmetic 273

Introduction 273
9.1. History of Botulinum Toxin in Aesthetics 277
9.1.1. Discovery and Medical Uses 278
9.1.2. Introduction to Cosmetic Applications 279
9.1.3. Evolution of Public Perception 280
9.2. Mechanism of Action of Botulinum Toxin 281
9.2.1. Neuromuscular Blockade 282
9.2.2. Effects on Facial Muscles 282
9.2.3. Duration of Results 283
9.3. Types of Dermal Fillers 284
9.3.1. Hyaluronic Acid Fillers 285
9.3.2. Collagen-based Fillers 286
9.3.3. Synthetic Fillers 287
9.4. Comparison of Botulinum Toxin and Dermal Fillers 288
9.4.1. Treatment Areas 289
9.4.2. Results and Longevity 290
9.4.3. Side Effects and Risks 291
9.5. Safety and Regulatory Aspects 292
9.5.1. Food and Drug Administration (FDA) Approval Process 292
9.5.2. Common Adverse Effects 293
9.5.3. Importance of Qualified Practitioners 294
9.6. Trends in Facial Cosmetic Procedures 295
9.6.1. Increasing Popularity Among Different Age Groups 296
9.6.2. Cultural Influences on Cosmetic Choices 297
9.6.3. Innovations in Techniques and Products 298
Summary 300
References 303

CHAPTER 10

Skin Resurfacing and Laser Treatments 305

Introduction 305
10.1. Types of Skin Resurfacing Techniques 309
10.1.1. Chemical Peels 310
10.1.2. Microdermabrasion 311
10.1.3. Laser Resurfacing 312
10.2. Understanding Laser Treatments 313
10.2.1. Types of Lasers Used in Dermatology 314
10.2.2. Mechanism of Action of Laser Treatments 315
10.2.3. Comparison of Ablative and Non-Ablative Lasers 315
10.3. Benefits of Skin Resurfacing and Laser Treatments 317
10.3.1. Improvement in Skin Texture and Tone 317
10.3.2. Reduction of Fine Lines and Wrinkles 318
10.3.3. Treatment of Acne Scars and Pigmentation Issues 319
10.4. Risks and Side Effects 320
10.4.1. Common Side Effects of Laser Treatments 321
10.4.2. Potential Complications and Long-Term Effects 322
10.4.3. Importance of Professional Consultation 323
10.5. Pre-Treatment Considerations 324
10.5.1. Skin Assessment and Consultation 325
10.5.2. Preparing the Skin for Treatment 326
10.5.3. Setting Realistic Expectations 327
10.6. Post-Treatment Care 328
10.6.1. Immediate Aftercare Instructions 328
10.6.2. Long-term Skincare Regimen 329
10.6.3. Monitoring for Adverse Reactions 330
Summary 331
References 334

CHAPTER 11

Principles of Facial Reconstruction 337

Introduction 337
11.1. The Science of Facial Reconstruction 340
11.1.1. Anatomy of the Human Face 341
11.1.2. Role of Forensic Science in Reconstruction 342
11.1.3. Techniques Used in Facial Reconstruction 342
11.2. Methods of Facial Reconstruction 344
11.2.1. 2D Reconstruction Techniques 344

11.2.2. 3D Modeling and Printing 345
11.2.3. Traditional Sculpting Methods 346
11.3. Applications of Facial Reconstruction 347
11.3.1. Forensic Investigations 348
11.3.2. Medical Applications in Reconstructive Surgery 349
11.3.3. Historical and Archaeological Reconstructions 350
11.4. Ethical Considerations 351
11.4.1. Consent and Privacy Issues 352
11.4.2. Cultural Sensitivity in Reconstruction 353
11.4.3. Implications of Misrepresentation 354
11.5. Challenges in Facial Reconstruction 355
11.5.1. Limitations of Available Data 356
11.5.2. Variability in Human Features 356
11.5.3. Technological Constraints 357
11.6. Future Directions in Facial Reconstruction 359
11.6.1. Advances in Technology and Software 359
11.6.2. Integration of Artificial Intelligence (AI) 360
11.6.3. Potential for Virtual Reality (VR) Applications 361
Summary 363
References 366

CHAPTER 12

Trauma Reconstruction in Facial Cosmetic 369

Introduction 369
12.1. Types of Facial Trauma 372
12.1.1. Common Causes of Facial Injuries 373
12.1.2. Classification of Facial Trauma 374
12.1.3. Impact of Trauma on Facial Structure 375
12.2. Psychological Effects of Facial Trauma 376
12.2.1. Emotional and Mental Health Implications 376
12.2.2. Social Stigma and Its Effects on Recovery 377
12.2.3. Role of Self-image in Psychological Healing 378
12.3. Surgical Techniques in Facial Reconstruction 379
12.3.1. Overview of Surgical Options Available 380
12.3.2. Innovations in Surgical Technology 381
12.3.3. Importance of Personalized Treatment Plans 382
12.4. Role of Cosmetic Procedures in Reconstruction 383
12.4.1. Integration of Cosmetic Techniques in Trauma Recovery 384
12.4.2. Non-Surgical Options for Facial Enhancement 385
12.4.3. Patient Satisfaction and Quality of Life Improvements 386
12.5. Multidisciplinary Approach to Treatment 387
12.5.1. Collaboration Between Surgeons, Psychologists, and Therapists 388
12.5.2. Importance of a Holistic Treatment Plan 389
12.5.3. Case Studies Demonstrating Successful Multidisciplinary Outcomes 389
12.6. Ethical Considerations in Facial Reconstruction 391
12.6.1. Informed Consent and Patient Autonomy 391
12.6.2. Balancing Aesthetic Desires with Medical Needs 392
12.6.3. Addressing Disparities in Access to Care 393
Summary 395
Short Answer Questions 397
References 398

CHAPTER 13

Congenital and Developmental Deformities in Facial Cosmetic 401

Introduction 401
13.1. Types of Congenital Deformities 404
13.1.1. Cleft Lip and Palate 405
13.1.2. Craniosynostosis 406
13.1.3. Hemifacial Microsomia (HFM) 407
13.2. Types of Developmental Deformities 408
13.2.1. Facial Asymmetry 409
13.2.2. Acquired Deformities Due to Trauma 409
13.2.3. Deformities Resulting from Medical Conditions 410
13.3. Causes of Congenital Deformities 411
13.3.1. Genetic Factors 412
13.3.2. Environmental Influences 413
13.3.3. Maternal Health During Pregnancy 413

13.4. Psychological Impact of Facial Deformities **415**
13.4.1. Self-esteem and Body Image Issues 416
13.4.2. Social Stigma and Discrimination 416
13.4.3. Mental Health Implications 417
13.5. Treatment Options for Facial Deformities **419**
13.5.1. Surgical Interventions 420
13.5.2. Orthodontic Treatments 421
13.5.3. Psychological Support and Counseling 421
13.6. Advances in Facial Aesthetic Procedures **423**
13.6.1. Innovations in Surgical Techniques 424
13.6.2. Role of 3D Imaging and Modeling 424
13.6.3. Non-Surgical Aesthetic Enhancements 425
Summary **427**
References **430**

CHAPTER 14

Oncologic and Post-Tumor Reconstruction in Facial Cosmetic 433

Introduction **433**
14.1. Understanding Oncologic Surgery **437**
14.1.1. Types of Cancers Affecting the Facial Region 438
14.1.2. Surgical Techniques Used in Oncologic Procedures 439
14.1.3. Goals of Oncologic Surgery in Facial Aesthetics 439
14.2. The Role of Reconstruction in Facial Cosmetic Surgery **441**
14.2.1. Definition and Purpose of Reconstructive Surgery 442
14.2.2. Techniques Used in Facial Reconstruction 442
14.2.3. Psychological Impact of Facial Reconstruction on Patients 443
14.3. Preoperative Considerations **445**
14.3.1. Patient Assessment and Evaluation 445
14.3.2. Importance of Multidisciplinary Teams 446
14.3.3. Planning for Aesthetic Outcomes 447
14.4. Surgical Techniques in Reconstruction **449**
14.4.1. Flap Techniques and Their Applications 450
14.4.2. Grafting Methods in Facial Reconstruction 450
14.4.3. Innovations in Surgical Technology 451
14.5. Postoperative Care and Recovery **452**
14.5.1. Importance of Follow-up Care 453
14.5.2. Managing Complications and Risks 453
14.5.3. Rehabilitation And Support For Patients 454
14.6. Ethical Considerations in Oncologic and Reconstructive Surgery **455**
14.6.1. Informed Consent and Patient Autonomy 456
14.6.2. Balancing Aesthetics with Medical Necessity 457
14.6.3. Addressing Disparities in Access to Care 458
Summary **459**
References **462**

CHAPTER 15

Advances, Technologies, and Practice Management in Facial Cosmetic 465

Introduction **465**
15.1. Historical Context of Facial Cosmetics **469**
15.1.1. Evolution of Cosmetic Practices 470
15.1.2. Key Milestones in Cosmetic Technology 471
15.1.3. Cultural Influences on Cosmetic Use 471
15.2. Current Technologies in Facial Cosmetics **473**
15.2.1. Innovations in Cosmetic Formulations 474
15.2.2. Advances in Application Techniques 474
15.2.3. Role of Digital Technology in Cosmetic Design 475
15.3. Non-Surgical Cosmetic Procedures **477**
15.3.1. Overview of Popular Non-Surgical Treatments 478
15.3.2. Safety and Efficacy of Non-Surgical Options 479
15.3.3. Patient Satisfaction and Outcomes 479
15.4. Surgical Advances in Facial Cosmetics **480**
15.4.1. Latest Techniques in Facial Surgery 481
15.4.2. Minimally Invasive Surgical Options 482
15.4.3. Ethical Considerations in Surgical Practices 483
15.5. Practice Management in Cosmetic Clinics **484**
15.5.1. Importance of Effective Management Strategies 485
15.5.2. Staff Training and Development 486

15.5.3. Patient Relationship Management 487
15.6. Regulatory and Ethical Considerations 488
15.6.1. Overview of Regulations Governing Cosmetic Practices 489
15.6.2. Ethical Dilemmas in Cosmetic Procedures 489
15.6.3. Impact of Regulations on Practice Management 490
Summary 492
References 495
Index 499

LIST OF FIGURES

Figure 1.1. Importance of facial anatomy
Figure 1.2. The intricate structure of facial anatomy serves essential functions in aesthetics
Figure 1.3. The skeletal framework of the face
Figure 1.4. The facial skeleton comprises several key bones that provide structure and support to the face
Figure 1.5. Common facial skeletal disorder
Figure 1.6. The muscles of facial expression represent a complex system integral to human communication
Figure 1.7. The major muscles and their functions
Figure 1.8. The impact of muscle tone on aesthetics
Figure 1.9. Skin and its role in facial aesthetics
Figure 1.10. The layers of the skin are essential for anyone studying facial anatomy and aesthetics
Figure 1.11. Common skin conditions and treatments
Figure 1.12. The concept of facial proportions plays a pivotal role in the realm of aesthetics
Figure 1.13. The evolution of modern standards of beauty and aesthetics
Figure 1.14. The tools for measuring facial proportions
Figure 1.15. Surgical options for facial enhancement
Figure 1.16. The intricate interplay between psychological aspects and facial aesthetics
Figure 1.17. The concept of beauty is significantly shaped by cultural influences that dictate societal standards of attractiveness
Figure 2.1. Cosmetic surgery encompasses a subfield of medical practice
Figure 2.2. Reconstructive surgery occupies a critical place in the medical field
Figure 2.3. The origins of cosmetic surgery
Figure 2.4. Development of reconstructive techniques
Figure 2.5. Milestones in surgical advancements
Figure 2.6. Patient consent and autonomy
Figure 2.7. The psychological impacts of surgery
Figure 2.8. The ethical dilemmas surrounding cosmetic procedures
Figure 2.9. The realm of cosmetic and reconstructive surgery
Figure 2.10. Common cosmetic procedures
Figure 2.11. Reconstructive surgery encompasses a variety of techniques

Figure 2.12. Innovations in surgical technology
Figure 2.13. Patient selection criteria
Figure 2.14. Psychological evaluation serves as a critical component in the context of cosmetic and reconstructive surgery
Figure 2.15. The field of cosmetic and reconstructive surgery
Figure 2.16. Long-term complications
Figure 2.17. Managing patient safety in cosmetic and reconstructive surgery
Figure 2.18. Effective postoperative care is critical in the realm of cosmetic and reconstructive surgery
Figure 2.19. The role of follow-up appointments in the realm of cosmetic and reconstructive surgery
Figure 3.1. Cosmetic facial surgery
Figure 3.2. The surgical planning process in cosmetic facial surgery
Figure 3.3. The accurate assessment of patient history
Figure 3.4. Gathering a comprehensive medical history
Figure 3.5. The psychological factors influencing patient assessment
Figure 3.6. The physical examination techniques utilized in cosmetic facial surgery
Figure 3.7. The visual assessment of facial features
Figure 3.8. Patient expectations and goals
Figure 3.9. Managing unrealistic expectations
Figure 3.10. The identification of potential surgical risks
Figure 3.11. Developing a risk mitigation plan
Figure 3.12. In cosmetic facial surgery, meticulous surgical planning
Figure 3.13. Considering postoperative care
Figure 3.14. Ethical considerations in cosmetic surgery
Figure 3.15. The importance of patient autonomy in cosmetic facial surgery cannot be overstated
Figure 4.1. Blepharoplasty, commonly referred to as eyelid surgery
Figure 4.2. An overview of eyelid surgery
Figure 4.3. The blepharoplasty serves multiple purposes
Figure 4.4. Upper eyelid blepharoplasty, a surgical procedure designed to rejuvenate the eyelids
Figure 4.5. As a pivotal procedure in facial aesthetics, lower eyelid blepharoplasty addresses aesthetic and functional concerns related to the lower eyelids
Figure 4.6. Cosmetic reasons for eyelid surgery
Figure 4.7. The aging process brings about a myriad of changes that significantly impact facial aesthetics
Figure 4.8. A comprehensive preoperative consultation and assessment
Figure 4.9. The selection of appropriate anesthesia options is critical in achieving patient comfort during blepharoplasty
Figure 4.10. Common risks associated with blepharoplasty

Figure 4.11. Importance of choosing a qualified surgeon
Figure 4.12. The recovery process following blepharoplasty
Figure 4.13. The immediate postoperative care following blepharoplasty
Figure 4.14. Psychological and social impacts
Figure 4.15. The effects of blepharoplasty on self-image are profound
Figure 4.16. The social perceptions surrounding aesthetic surgery
Figure 4.17. Patient satisfaction and quality of life
Figure 5.1. The term rhytidectomy
Figure 5.2. Facial aesthetics play a critical role in human interactions
Figure 5.3. The evolution of facelift techniques reflects a broader shift
Figure 5.4. Key figures in cosmetic surgery
Figure 5.5. The landscape of facelift procedures has evolved significantly over the years
Figure 5.6. The traditional facelift
Figure 5.7. Mini facelift
Figure 5.8. Non-surgical facelift options
Figure 5.9. Neck lift procedures
Figure 5.10. The techniques employed in neck lifts
Figure 5.11. The decision to pursue rhytidectomy, commonly referred to as a facelift, hinges on several clinical and aesthetic indications
Figure 5.12. The genetic factors influencing skin elasticity
Figure 5.13. The incidence of surgical risks during rhytidectomy
Figure 5.14. Importance of choosing a qualified surgeon
Figure 5.15. The recovery phase following a rhytidectomy
Figure 5.16. The post-operative care instructions are essential for patients undergoing rhytidectomy (facelift) and neck lift procedures
Figure 6.1. The rhinoplasty, commonly referred to as nose surgery
Figure 6.2. Importance of rhinoplasty in modern medicine
Figure 6.3. Rhinoplasty encompasses a variety of surgical techniques
Figure 6.4. The distinctions between primary and secondary rhinoplasty
Figure 6.5. Cosmetic vs. functional rhinoplasty
Figure 6.6. The decision to undergo rhinoplasty
Figure 6.7. Medical reasons for rhinoplasty extend beyond aesthetic improvements
Figure 6.8. Trauma or injury to the nose
Figure 6.9. The rhinoplasty procedure
Figure 6.10. Surgical techniques and anesthesia options
Figure 6.11. Common risks associated with surgery
Figure 6.12. Importance of choosing a qualified surgeon

Figure 6.13. Psychological impact of rhinoplasty
Figure 6.14. Patient expectations and satisfaction rates in cosmetic
Figure 6.15. Rhinoplasty, a surgical procedure primarily focused on altering the shape and function of the nose
Figure 6.16. Societal pressures regarding beauty standards
Figure 6.17. Ethical considerations in cosmetic
Figure 7.1. The brow lift and forehead rejuvenation
Figure 7.2. Importance of facial aesthetics in modern society
Figure 7.3. The evolution of cosmetic surgery techniques
Figure 7.4. Milestones in brow lift procedures
Figure 7.5. Cultural perceptions of beauty and aging
Figure 7.6. The anatomy of the forehead and brow area encompasses a complex interplay of tissues
Figure 7.7. Skin structure and aging effects
Figure 7.8. Indications for brow lift and forehead rejuvenation
Figure 7.9. Psychological impact of aging on self-esteem
Figure 7.10. The evolution of surgical techniques in facial rejuvenation
Figure 7.11. The brow lift is a critical procedure in facial cosmetic surgery
Figure 7.12. Post-operative care and recovery
Figure 7.13. Importance of choosing a qualified surgeon
Figure 7.14. Botox and fillers for brow and forehead rejuvenation
Figure 7.15. Laser treatments and their effectiveness
Figure 8.1. The concept of facial implants and contouring
Figure 8.2. The significance of facial aesthetics in modern society
Figure 8.3. Types of facial implants
Figure 8.4. Chin implants
Figure 8.5. The utilization of jaw implants as a form of facial contouring
Figure 8.6. Facial implants have gained considerable traction in aesthetic surgery
Figure 8.7. The pursuit of enhanced facial symmetry
Figure 8.8. Improved self-esteem and confidence
Figure 8.9. The pursuit of facial beauty through implants and contouring procedures
Figure 8.10. Potential complications and side effects
Figure 8.11. The choice of a qualified surgeon is paramount when considering facial implants and contouring procedures
Figure 8.12. Fat grafting, also known as autologous fat transfer
Figure 8.13. Fat grafting is a dual-process cosmetic procedure
Figure 8.14. Liposculpture represents an advanced evolution of traditional liposuction

Figure 8.15. The distinctions between liposuction and liposculpture hold significant relevance in contemporary cosmetic surgery
Figure 9.1. Botulinum toxin
Figure 9.2. The dermal fillers treatment areas
Figure 9.3. The contemporary landscape of facial cosmetics
Figure 9.4. The historical journey of botulinum toxin in aesthetics
Figure 9.5. Introduction to cosmetic applications
Figure 9.6. Mechanism of action of botulinum toxin
Figure 9.7. Neuromuscular blockade
Figure 9.8. The variety of dermal fillers available has expanded significantly
Figure 9.9. The emergence of hyaluronic acid fillers
Figure 9.10. Collagen-based fillers
Figure 9.11. The synthetic fillers have emerged as essential components in cosmetic procedures
Figure 9.12. Treatment areas
Figure 9.13. Safety and regulatory aspects in cosmetics
Figure 9.14. Importance of qualified practitioners
Figure 9.15.
Figure 9.16. Cultural influences on cosmetic choices
Figure 10.1. Skin resurfacing encompasses a variety of cosmetic procedures
Figure 10.2. An overview of laser treatments
Figure 10.3. Importance of skin health and aesthetics
Figure 10.4. Skin resurfacing techniques have evolved significantly
Figure 10.5. Chemical peels constitute a significant segment of skin resurfacing techniques
Figure 10.6. Microdermabrasion
Figure 10.7. Laser resurfacing
Figure 10.8. Types of lasers used in dermatology
Figure 10.9. Comparison of ablative and non-ablative lasers
Figure 10.10. Improvement in skin texture and tone
Figure 10.12. Treatment of acne scars and pigmentation issues
Figure 10.13. Common side effects of laser treatments
Figure 10.14. The significance of professional consultation
Figure 10.15. Skin assessment and consultation
Figure 10.16. The significance of post-treatment care
Figure 11.1. Facial reconstruction
Figure 11.2. Science of facial reconstruction
Figure 11.3. Anatomy of the human face

Figure 11.4. Facial reconstruction techniques
Figure 11.5. Methods of facial reconstruction
Figure 11.6. 2D reconstruction techniques
Figure 11.7. 3D modeling and printing of facial reconstruction
Figure 11.8. Multifaceted applications of facial reconstruction
Figure 11.9. Medical applications in reconstructive surgery
Figure 11.10. Historical and archaeological reconstructions
Figure 11.11. Cultural sensitivity in facial reconstruction
Figure 11.12. Facial-reconstruction-in-colour-with-eyes
Figure 11.13. Human facial variability
Figure 11.14. Evolution of facial reconstruction technological constraints that ultimately shape their effectiveness and reliability
Figure 11.15. Exploration of virtual reality (VR) applications
Figure 12.1. Trauma reconstruction
Figure 12.2. Importance of facial aesthetics in psychological recovery
Figure 12.3. Facial trauma
Figure 12.4. Facial injuries
Figure 12.5. Trauma on facial structure
Figure 12.6. Psychological effects of facial trauma
Figure 12.7. Emotional and mental health implications of facial cosmetic procedures
Figure 12.8. Role of self-image in psychological healing
Figure 12.9. Surgical techniques in facial reconstruction
Figure 12.10. Surgical options for trauma reconstruction
Figure 12.11. Innovations in surgical technology
Figure 12.12. Importance of personalized treatment plans
Figure 12.13. Cosmetic procedures
Figure 12.14. Non-surgical options for facial enhancement
Figure 12.15. Patient satisfaction and quality
Figure 13.1. Congenital and developmental deformities
Figure 13.2. Facial aesthetics in social interactions
Figure 13.3. Congenital deformities manifest
Figure 13.4. Cleft lip and palate
Figure 13.5. Craniosynostosis
Figure 13.6. Hemifacial microsomia (HFM)
Figure 13.7. Types of developmental deformities
Figure 13.8. Facial asymmetry
Figure 13.9. Causes of congenital deformities

Figure 13.10. Maternal health during pregnancy influences a child's autism
Figure 13.11. Psychological impact of facial deformities
Figure 13.12. Self-esteem and body image issues
Figure 13.13. Social stigma and discrimination
Figure 13.14. Treatment options for facial deformities
Figure 13.15. Surgical interventions play a pivotal role in addressing congenital and developmental deformities in facial aesthetics
Figure 13.16. Orthodontic treatments
Figure 13.17. Facial aesthetics
Figure 14.1. Oncologic surgery
Figure 14.2. Facial cosmetic surgery
Figure 14.3. Oncologic surgery represents a critical intersection between cancer management and reconstructive techniques
Figure 14.4. Cancers affecting the facial region
Figure 14.5. Surgical techniques used in oncologic procedures
Figure 14.6. Goals of oncologic surgery in facial aesthetics
Figure 14.7. Role of reconstruction in facial cosmetic surgery
Figure 14.8. Purpose of reconstructive surgery
Figure 14.9. Techniques used in facial reconstruction
Figure 14.10. Psychological impact of facial reconstruction on patients
Figure 14.11. Oncologic and post-tumor reconstruction in facial cosmetic surgery
Figure 14.12. Patient assessment and evaluation
Figure 14.13. Importance of multidisciplinary teams
Figure 14.14. Planning for aesthetic outcomes
Figure 14.15. Surgical techniques in reconstruction
Figure 15.1. Woman getting an injection in her face at plastic surgery
Figure 15.2. Evolution of technology in reshaping the landscape of facial cosmetics
Figure 15.3. Historical evolution of facial cosmetics
Figure 15.4. Cosmetic practices
Figure 15.5. Cosmetic technology
Figure 15.6. Cultural influences on cosmetic use
Figure 15.7. Current technologies in facial cosmetics
Figure 15.8. Cosmetic formulations
Figure 15.9. Application techniques in facial cosmetics
Figure 15.10. Role of digital technology in cosmetic design
Figure 15.11. Non-surgical cosmetic procedures

Figure 15.12. Popular non-surgical treatments
Figure 15.13. Safety and efficacy of non-surgical options
Figure 15.14. Surgical advances in facial cosmetics
Figure 15.15. Advances in facial surgery
Figure 15.16. Minimally invasive surgical options
Figure 15.17. Practice management in cosmetic clinics

PREFACE

Facial reconstructive and cosmetic surgery is a specialty where scientific accuracy meets artistic sense. To create outcomes that are both safe and in keeping with each individual's traits, an understanding of the complex framework of muscle, nerve, and vessel buried beneath the skin is required. Surgeons must combine precise anatomical information with an appreciation of proportional balance to restore function, remove deformity, or enhance form. Whether addressing age-related changes or congenital differences, the goal remains the same: to help patients feel more confident and to improve their quality of life through surgical intervention.

Over the past century, advances in surgical instruments, imaging modalities, and biomaterials have transformed what is possible on the operating table. Techniques once reserved for the most specialized centers are now part of standard practice worldwide. At the same time, patients expect naturally occurring outcomes with a short downtime. Such an active environment demands practitioners to be up to date on newer methods, safety protocols, and postoperative technique skills. Continuing education and skills training ensure that surgeons possess the capability to apply the optimal method for each patient's unique anatomy and goal.

The book, *An Introduction to Facial Cosmetic and Reconstructive Surgery*, combines fundamental principles, practice guidelines, and experiential knowledge in one master reference. It aims to guide readers through theoretical principles and step-by-step techniques of everyday as well as challenging procedures. Evidence-based recommendations and everyday case examples form the foundation of decision-making for every step from consultation to long-term follow-up.

Chapter 1 presents the fundamental anatomy of the face, encompassing bony landmarks, soft tissue planes, and neurovascular structures. In addition to the anatomy, the chapter delves into the aesthetic proportion principle and how such concepts as the golden ratio and facial thirds influence perception. Basic diagrams and surface markings enable structures to be precisely localized.

Chapter 2 deals with the principles that regulate both reconstructive and cosmetic surgery. Topics covered include tissue management, stages of wound healing, care of scars, and the ethical considerations particular to elective rather than medically indicated surgery. The reader establishes a paradigm for balancing patient expectations with results that can be attained.

Chapter 3 outlines the patient examination process and operating room planning. The process of history-taking, physical examination techniques, photographic protocols, and the use of imaging tools like three-dimensional simulation are addressed. Decision trees and checklists facilitate the process of performing complete assessments of medical, psychological, and aesthetic aspects before proceeding to the operating room.

Blepharoplasty or eyelid surgery is described in complete detail in Chapter 4. Operating indications, incision site, and upper and lower lid surgical techniques are described, including suggestions on how to manage fat pads, muscle laxity, and tear trough deformities. Postoperative maneuvers are designed to minimize bruising and maximize recovery.

Chapter 5 addresses rhytidectomy (facelift) and neck lift. The chapter compares deep plane, SMAS, and minimal-access techniques, with patient selection criteria and complications presented. Illustrations show vector planning and skin redraping maneuvers to produce natural contour renewal.

Chapter 6 covers rhinoplasty, with open and closed approaches being reported. Anatomical dissection of nasal morphology determines intervention on the bony vault, cartilaginous dorsum, and tip complex. Cartilage grafting techniques and approaches to maintain nasal airway integrity are highlighted.

Chapter 7 covers brow lift and forehead rejuvenation. Endoscopic and coronal technique methods are outlined, with attention to eyebrow shape, muscle alteration, and scalp incision placement. The text explains how ptosis is addressed and smooth forehead lines are removed with preservation of sensitivity.

Chapter 8 discusses facial contouring and implants. Chin, cheek, and jaw implant options are compared, , such as custom implant planning and intraoperative shaping. Fat grafting is also discussed as a secondary or alternate approach to soft tissue augmentation.

Chapter 9 discusses non-surgical injectable treatments, including botulinum toxin and dermal fillers. Action mechanisms, product type, dosing protocol, and injection technique are discussed. Safety considerations like vascular anatomy and managing complications are emphasized.

Chapter 10 addresses skin resurfacing and laser procedures. Ablative versus non-ablative procedures are compared, with methods of chemical peels, fractional lasers, and energy devices provided. Patient selection, pre-treatment preparation, and combined therapy techniques are addressed.

Chapter 11 introduces the principles of facial reconstruction, including tissue transfer procedures, flap design, and graft selection. The chapter covers local, regional, and free flap options, and how to choose donor tissue attributes to meet facial subunit requirements.

Chapter 12 deals with trauma reconstruction, including handling lacerations of soft tissue, orbital and nasal fractures, and mandibular or midfacial injuries. Stages of emergency stabilization, staged repairs, and long-term rehabilitation are classified with regard to functional restoration and aesthetic outcomes.

Chapter 13 highlights congenital and developmental abnormalities , such as cleft lip and palate, hemifacial microsomia, and craniofacial syndromes. Multidisciplinary treatment models, intervention timing, and growth factors are discussed to promote facial symmetry and optimal psychosocial development.

Chapter 14 deals with oncologic and post-tumor reconstruction. Oncologic resection principles are blended with reconstructive procedures utilizing local flaps, free tissue transfer, and prosthetic material. Rehabilitation needs and surveillance protocols for cancer patients are also discussed in the chapter.

Chapter 15 highlights the current trends, new technologies, and management issues of practice. Trends , such as three-dimensional printing, augmented reality planning, and robotic support are introduced. Advice on patient communication, regulatory compliance, and practice organization will help practitioners build sustainable, patient-centered services.

This book is written for plastic and reconstructive surgery residents and fellows, otolaryngology residents, maxillofacial surgery residents, and practicing surgeons seeking a complete yet brief reference. It will also be beneficial to dermatologists, physician assistants, and nurse practitioners who are delivering aesthetic and reconstructive treatment.

INTRODUCTION TO FACIAL ANATOMY AND AESTHETICS

1

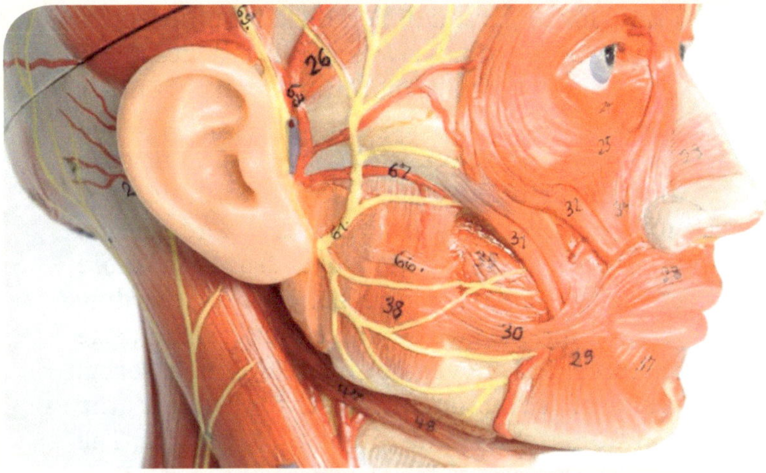

LEARNING OBJECTIVES

After studying this chapter, you will be able to:

1. Describe the facial skeletal architecture;
2. Describe the facial expression muscles;
3. Highlight skin and its role in facial aesthetics;
4. Appreciate the importance of facial proportions;
5. Understand aesthetic treatments and procedures;
6. Understand psychological concepts in facial aesthetics.

Introduction

Anatomical learning of the face involves a thorough understanding of the structural components that comprise the human face. These include both the skeletal and muscular systems, which work harmoniously together to facilitate facial expression, communication, and visual presentation. The facial skeleton consists of several bones, including the zygomatic bones, maxilla, and mandible, which determine the shape of the face and offer support. Some muscles, including the zygomaticus major and orbicularis oris, are important in supporting facial movement to enable expressions that are used in communicating a range of feelings. Understanding these anatomical structures is not only crucial for doctors but also for the practitioners of aesthetic procedures, where knowledge of internal structures can lead to successful intervention and improvement of facial appearance. Secondly, the incorporation of the psychological theory of face perception and attractiveness is a significant contribution towards understanding facial anatomy's aesthetic perspective. Research has established that some facial characteristics and ratios are globally recognized as beautiful and influence social interactions and individuals' self-perceptions. This intersection of anatomy and psychology provokes practitioners to examine the role of facial structures in defining societal beauty ideals. By studying such phenomena as the kot-mi-nam phenomenon, whereby Korean cultural norms shape perceptions of attractiveness, we can see that facial beauty is as much a function of biology as it is culturally conditioned (Kim et al., 2013). Both their biological and cultural components have led to the identification of the necessity for an integrative understanding of facial anatomy, one in which both their physical and cultural elements are acknowledged. The increase in facial modeling technology also shows the significance of anatomical proficiency in aesthetic treatment. The development of new devices, such as the Bezier curve-based 3D facial customization system, allows for precise impressions of facial features, opening the way for the expansion of the discipline of plastic surgery as well as cosmetic treatments. As one has seen in non-surgical aesthetics studies, systematic training in such technologies is required so that practitioners are able to offer proper and safe intervention (Kumar, 2021). Through the study of the biological origin of the face as well as embracing technological advancement, one acquires a more cohesive understanding of facial anatomy. This overview emphasizes the intersection of anatomy, aesthetics, and cultural attitudes, providing a rich context for clinicians who want to improve facial beauty in a manner respectful to natural structure and individual identity.

Definition and Importance of Facial Anatomy

Facial anatomy knowledge is significant to many fields, including medicine, dental care, and aesthetics. Facial anatomy essentially constitutes the shape and arrangement of the facial region, such as the bones, muscles, nerves, and skin, all of which contribute their part towards the overall appearance and functionality of the face. Facial anatomy awareness facilitates proper diagnosis and intervention of varied medical and cosmetic issues, ranging from reconstructive surgery to cosmetic enhancement. For instance, having a good idea about the underlying musculature allows practitioners to predict how facial expressions become apparent and how facial expressions can be manipulated using clinical methods. In addition, anatomical awareness is useful for understanding individual differences, which is particularly critical for aesthetic surgery to obtain a natural and harmonious outcome. Besides surgical application, facial anatomy is vital in maximizing communication and social interaction. Facial expressions of non-verbal communications are fundamental to social communication and are likely more efficient compared to verbal forms. According to descriptions given by research, facial muscle gestures and movement express a non-verbal form of communication that reflects the emotional state and intent of a person. The subtle nuances of facial expression, grounded in face awareness of facial anatomy, hold immense power over social interaction and can be recognized universally across cultures. Underlying anatomical structures that enable such expressions and render this knowledge necessary are what make anatomy not just a part of beauty appreciation but of human interpersonal relations as well (Hugill et al., 2010). In the field of aesthetics, accurate facial analysis is necessary to achieve the desired outcome from cosmetic treatments. Determination of reliable anatomical landmarks is crucial during the planning of procedures because these landmarks guide the practitioner in sculpting and lifting facial features to maintain balance and proportion. Recent studies indicate that some facial landmarks, such as in the regions around the nose and mouth, are consistently more precise than others when compared across imaging modalities, reinforcing the useful benefits of highly precise anatomical knowledge

(Payne, 2013). In addition, successful utilization of facial anatomy enhances the accuracy of treatment as well as patient satisfaction since individuals are looking for results that reflect their own beauty ideals. Thus, the knowledge of facial anatomy not only improves clinical efficacy but also forms the basis of the broader cultural and aesthetic values of facial beauty, and hence is a crucial component of medical as well as artistic practice (Figure 1.1).

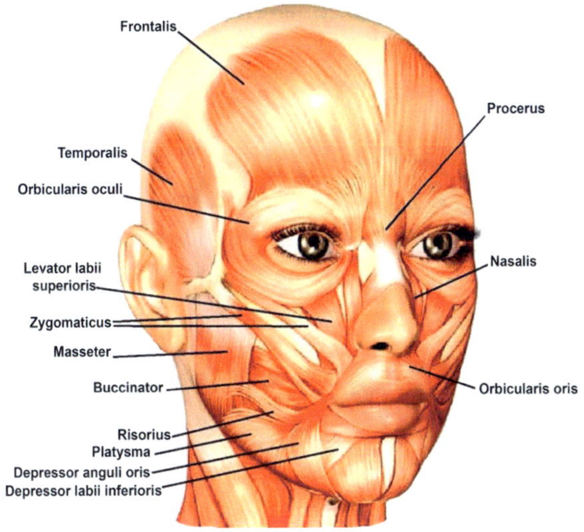

Figure 1.1. Importance of facial anatomy.

Source: https://hair-and-makeup-artist.com/wp-content/uploads/2012/06/facial-muscles-1.jpg.

Major Structures of the Face

To grasp the large structures of the face, one must first take into account the facial anatomy's layered constitution, which is bone, muscle, fat, and skin. The facial skeleton is made up mainly of 14 bones, which are the mandible, maxilla, and zygomatic bones, providing the foundation for the face. Not only do these bones establish the shape and form, but they also bear the weight of soft tissue. The relationship between these bony structures and the musculature that covers them is crucial to expressive movement. Muscles, such as orbicularis oris and zygomaticus major, are responsible for enabling a range of facial expressions. The superficial relationship between these forms acts as the foundation of aesthetic issues, where proportion, together with balance, is necessary to achieve a pleasing face. Such knowledge assists in aesthetic surgery and cosmetic procedures aimed at enhancing facial harmony. Soft facial tissues like adipose tissue and muscles also contribute to facial aesthetic features. Deposits of fat supply volume and form and contribute to shaping the appearance of facial youthfulness and vitality. Fat redistribution due to aging or heredity can drastically alter the facial look and make some features stand out at the cost of others. The muscles of the face also allow movement and expression, with intricate intertwining that allows voluntary regulation of a subtle movement, such as a smile or a frown. This dynamic architecture accommodates numerous aesthetic procedures, such as fillers and botulinum toxin, whose goals are to restore or improve facial volume and muscle function. The intricate relationship between these structures is critical to understanding the changes related to aging, given that the young face is defined by certain proportions that progressively alter as one gets older, calling for further investigation of rejuvenation methods. Cultural influences also play a tremendous role in perception and beauty standards in the face, as seen in variations of aesthetic ideals across various societies. Anatomical structure of the face must be learned with regard to sociocultural influence on beauty norms, emphasizing the extent to which assessments of beauty can differ significantly across cultures. For instance, the "kot-mi-nam" phenomenon of Korean culture is a culturally desired ideal that merges gender fluidity with some aesthetic properties, which may not be universally desirable. The phenomenon embodies the concurrency of anatomy, psychology, and culture in facial aesthetics, reflecting the need for a multi-dimensional perspective to the study of the face. Identification of these cultural significations improves facial anatomy comprehension not just as a physical construct but also as it influences the look and application of cosmetic enhancements. This information enriches the aesthetics discourse of the face, reminding us of the importance of situating anatomical studies within their cultural frame of reference (Kim et al., 2013; Reiter et al., 2015).

Functions of Facial Anatomy in Aesthetics

The complex anatomy of the face plays vital roles in aesthetics and greatly influences one's looks and emotional state. Different elements, including the underlying skeletal system, musculature, and soft tissues, collaborate to produce unique facial features. The zygomatic bones, for example, are vital in determining cheek prominence, a characteristic usually related to youth and beauty. Similarly, the ratio and contours of the jawline can influence how one is seen as strong and with character. The integration of these anatomical structures not only creates an attractive face but also enables numerous expressions that are crucial in non-verbal communication. Hence, facial aesthetics is founded on structural stability and concordance of anatomical structures that collectively convey beauty and emotional status and, ultimately, influence social interactions and self-esteem. Aesthetic enhancements, whether surgical or otherwise, generally address these major anatomical structures to achieve desired outcomes. Surgical procedures, such as rhinoplasty, facelifts, or fillers, are strategically aimed at the enhancement of specific facial zones to adapt to modern beauty ideals. All of these have to respect the harmony and proportion of facial forms as defined by underlying anatomy. This is especially important in a bid to create results that not only beautify but also maintain facial movement functions, such as speaking and expressing emotions. To this end, advances in materials and techniques have enabled the practitioner to achieve outcomes that appear natural and pleasing to the eye. Such a variation in facial appearance can lead to greater confidence on the part of the individual, allowing him/her to engage fully in occupational and social life, demonstrating the close relationship between facial anatomy and aesthetics. The study of facial beauty points out that anatomical and perceptual elements both contribute significantly to the assessment of attractiveness. Recent studies indicate symmetry to be significant in perceived beauty, but one should bear in mind that beauty is not simply decided upon using mathematical principles of proportion.

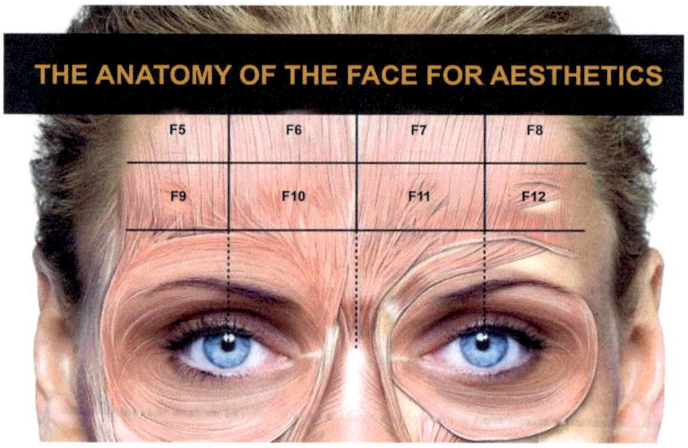

Figure 1.2. The intricate structure of facial anatomy serves essential functions in aesthetics.

Source: https://l1p.co.uk/wp-content/uploads/2020/05/aesthetics-anatomy-of-the-face.jpg.

Beauty also lies in the eyes of the beholders and in cultural standards. According to recent research, while observer biases affect identity judgments of facial appearances, there is a critical input of the owner's faces' inherent properties, including asymmetry and proportion, to attractiveness ratings (Chen et al., 1997). This interplay between perception and anatomy directs attention to the multidimensional nature of facial beauty, where biological elements interact with social perception, emphasizing the importance of omnitemporal knowledge of facial anatomy in aesthetic interventions.

These observations validate the complex, interdependent relationship between appearance and anatomical form in the context of beauty (Figure 1.2).

1.1. The Skeletal Framework of the Face

Learning Outcome

1. Discuss Key Bones Involved in Facial Structure
2. Explain The Role of the Skull in Aesthetic Appearance
3. Focus on Common Facial Skeletal Disorders

The skeletal structure of the face is key to deciding not only the anatomical structure but also the beauty of the person. It is made up of important bones like the maxilla, zygomatic, mandible, and nasal bones and is the framework onto which the muscles controlling the expression and movement are attached. These bones serve as support upon which the delicate nuances of the face are built. They form a canvas on which emotional and social information is conveyed. Understanding this framework is extremely worthwhile in the fields of plastic surgery, orthodontics, and aesthetic facial rejuvenation, where practitioners work to enhance or restore facial structures without sacrificing balance and proportion. The size and shape of facial bones play an important role in beauty and health perceptions due to the fact that they determine proportions, which are typically culturally defined. For example, jaw length or cheekboneness among facial shape features have been found to be linked directly to societal standards of attractiveness. Moreover, variations in these skeletal features impact the respiratory well-being of people, something that was understood in research taking into account conformational disorders of conformation, such as Brachycephalic Obstructive Airway Syndrome (BOAS). Even though facial beauty complexities are more than just skeletal composition, the connection between skeleton anatomy and conceptions of beauty is central, given that they construct our definition of beauty through a biological and cultural lens. In addition, how the bony framework cooperates with soft tissue has significant implications for facial aesthetics. The facial skeleton provides support for many muscles, fascia, and skin, and they all work to build the face we present to the world. Non-verbal communication, particularly facial expression, relies on the exact motion facilitated by this skeletal system. Research indicates that facial expressions convey significant information about emotion and intention, further signifying the significance of the skeletal system to human communication. Therefore, a complete examination of the facial anatomy calls for an exploration of how the underlying skeleton and covering tissues combine to form the expressive functions needed to make our social lives work, thus revealing the rich tapestry of human facial beauty (Hugill et al., 2010; Reiter et al., 2015) (Figure 1.3).

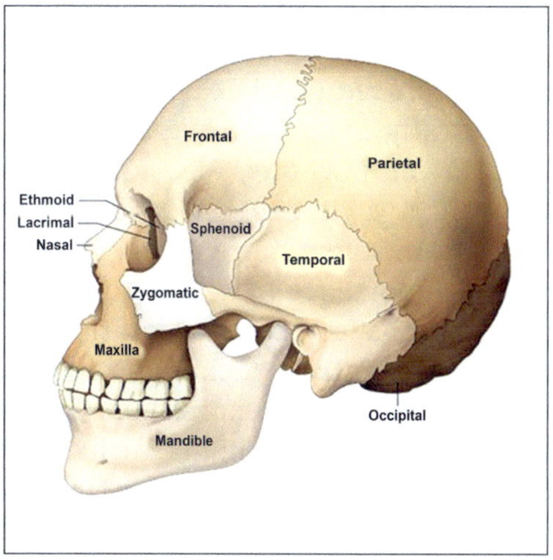

Figure 1.3. The skeletal framework of the face.

Source: https://images.ctfassets.net/u2qv1tdtdbbu/1TpiCif7Rohxr3UqQhrL2K/46cfaf39edf4f916825327e783bd2225/ce500-fig01-skull-lateral.jpg.

1.1.1. Key Bones Involved in Facial Structure

The facial skeleton is made up of some significant bones that provide the face with structure and support to both form and function. Among them, the upper jawbone or maxilla is significant in the case of facial symmetry as well as midface integrity. It houses the upper teeth and forms part of the nasal cavity, providing necessary support to the surrounding soft tissues. The zygomatic bones, simply referred to as cheekbones, are also important in the sense that they belong to the facial contour and play a vital role in defining the rim of the orbit. Temporal bone changes, e.g., resorption processes that occur with aging, can cause profound alterations in facial appearance, including deep nasolabial folds and decreased midface volume (Berg et al., 2024). An understanding of the anatomy and function of these bones takes precedence when face aesthetics and intervention techniques are on the table. Joining the facial structure are nasal bones, which not only outline the bridge of the nose but also greatly influence facial balance and proportion. The area of the nose becomes a focal point in aesthetic procedures because changes here will significantly change the overall appearance. Also, the lower jawbone, also known as the mandible, plays a vital role in facial movement and expression, once more highlighting bone structure's importance in aesthetic evaluation. The harmonious coexistence of the maxilla and mandible controls facial functions, such as chewing, speech, and expression. Therefore, alterations to these bones in the form of surgery or fillers require them to be handled with a considerate understanding of their interrelated functions. Ethnic differences in bone structure must be addressed by individualized aesthetic methods to attain a balanced and natural outcome (Lim et al., 2024). Finally, one cannot overstate the importance of respecting the association of the cranial bases with facial bones. The cranial base is tasked with providing fundamental support and orientation of the facial skeleton, and interference in its structure will carry significant aesthetic and functional consequences. Complications arising from cosmetic facial procedures aimed at improving facial beauty can arise when bony anatomy is not adequately assessed. For instance, risk areas during injection are those close to large vascular and nervous pathways along the facial bones' course, and therefore, there must be proper knowledge for intervention without damaging the tissues (Berg et al., 2024).

Without this level of understanding, practitioners run the risk of creating such conditions as Facial Overfilled Syndrome (FOS), where excessive use of fillers distorts the intended aesthetic proportion, particularly in complex areas, such as the cheeks and chin (Lim et al., 2024). Increased awareness of the underlying foundational bones of the face is essential in order to achieve intended aesthetic outcomes without compromising function and safety (Figure 1.4).

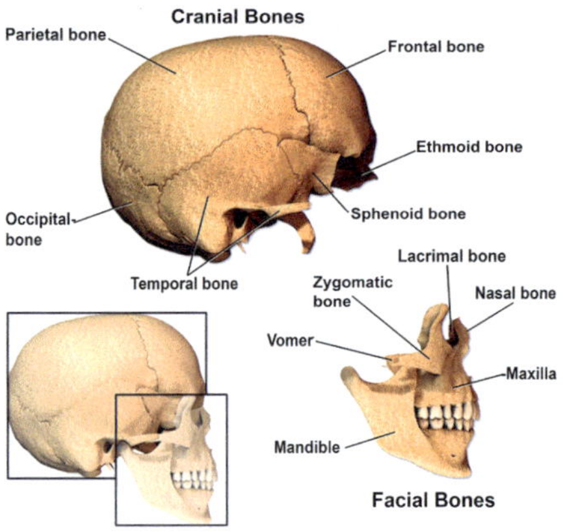

Figure 1.4. The facial skeleton comprises several key bones that provide structure and support to the face.

Source: https://biologydictionary.net/wp-content/uploads/2020/09/labeledfacialbones.png.

1.1.2. The Role of the Skull in Aesthetic Appearance

The aesthetic look of the face largely relies on the skeletal structure underlying it, the skull here. Being the face's structure, the skull influences chief features, such as contour, symmetry, and proportion, features that significantly contribute to perceived beauty and desirability. The degree of facial symmetry, for example, is often correlated with social judgments of beauty; balanced, symmetrical faces are perceived to be more beautiful. Further, studies have shown that variations in skull structure have been the cause of considerable facial aesthetic differences that not only affect physical appearance but also the self-esteem of individuals involved. For instance, patients with craniosynostosis, which is a disorder characterized by premature sagittal craniosynostosis, may develop challenges related to facial asymmetry with subsequent long-term psychological implications (Anesi et al., 2014). Secondly, the progress in surgical techniques like osteotomy and craniofacial surgery accentuates the importance of the aesthetics of the skull in reconstruction and augmentation. The introduction of ultrasonic osteotomes, cited as referenced in recent studies, has been promising in inducing greater healing since they are capable of cutting mineralized bone more precisely without damaging the surrounding tissue. These technologies enable a more accurate technique in craniofacial operations, which subsequently results in improved cosmetic outcomes. Osteotomy device choice affects not just the procedure but also the final outcome of facial and skull structure, showing the significance of the correlation between surgical method, skull structure, and aesthetic results (Anesi et al., 2014). Psychological assessments of the patient undergoing craniofacial surgery show that there is complexity in the relationship between surgical result and self-perceived esteem. Research has indicated that although patients may feel physical improvement post-operatively, the psychological impact of facial asymmetry is generally long-lasting. Patients who have a history of conditions, such as sagittal or metopic synostosis, experience that despite achieving a certain amount of symmetry through surgery, self-esteem measures remain comparable with those of controls. This points out that while physical appearance is unquestionably influenced by skull structure and cosmetic surgery, psychological dimensions related to body image remain a key factor in determining the overall effectiveness of aesthetic procedures (Svalina, 2024). Thus, the role of the skull in aesthetic appearances is not restricted to mere physical characteristics, but it is linked to psychological health and social perception.

1.1.3. Common Facial Skeletal Disorders

Facial skeletal disorders comprise a continuum of conditions that can have a significant effect on aesthetic appearance and functional ability. Some of the most common disorders are craniosynostosis, where premature closure of skull sutures prevents normal development of the skull, and facial asymmetry, which can result from genetics or developmental anomalies. The effects of these disorders are not merely cosmetic, as they often lead to psychological trauma for the individual. Apart from this, malocclusion is produced by disorders , such as maxillary hypoplasia or mandibular hyperplasia and will influence both the chewing and speech functions. Greater knowledge about facial anatomy has facilitated improved diagnostic techniques that allow earlier intervention, which is advantageous in treating these conditions effectively. Surgical remedies, such as orthognathic surgery, provide a means for improving function while also improving facial appearance. Treatment of typical facial skeletal disorders has also become better over time, thanks to developments in surgical techniques and technology. Piezosurgery is one such innovation that has been embraced, which uses ultrasonic osteotomes to cut through bone. Research indicates that the process is able to achieve smoother bone surfaces and minimizes trauma to the supportive tissues, thereby achieving better healing outcomes compared to traditional instruments (Anesi et al., 2014). Selective cutting through mineralized tissues without compromising the adjacent soft tissues enhances the effectiveness of craniofacial procedures.

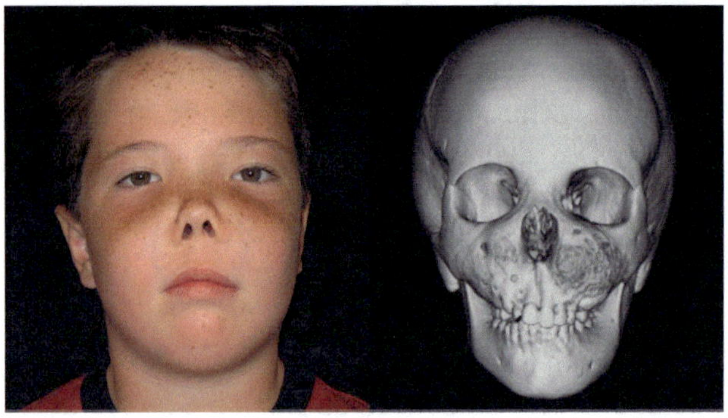

Figure 1.5. Common facial skeletal disorder.

Source: https://external-content.duckduckgo.com/iu/?u=https%3A%2F%2Fwww.chop.edu%2Fsites%2Fdefault%2Ffiles%2Ffibdispl-causian-boy-front-view-780x439.jpg&f=1&nofb=1&ipt=58aaf63bca0539321f4374c7e90b787a70cf01cd0b4b08af5cf43937cd40723e.

This technique is a perfect example of how the incorporation of technology into surgical procedures can influence treatment directions for facial skeletal disorders. With each evolving procedure and adaptation, the potential for enhancing patient outcomes in aesthetics and function becomes a reality. New modalities, such as stem cell therapy and tissue engineering, offer significant hope for treating craniofacial skeletal disorders.

Even at the experimental stage, such modalities utilize the regenerative potential of the stem cell to promote healing and restoration of craniofacial structures (Hughes & Song, 2016). The new technique would not only repair the bone abnormality but also restore the integrity of the soft tissues around affected areas. The growing volume of publications indicates various sources of stem cells and scaffold biomaterials, again stimulating research into the most optimal solutions for craniofacial tissue regeneration. Despite all existing hurdles in clinical applications, craniofacial reconstruction can look forward to revolutionary breakthroughs, upgrading the quality of life of patients suffering from skeletal diseases. All these innovations suggest that there is a need for further research and collaboration in the field of facial anatomy and esthetics (Figure 1.5).

Test Your Knowledge

1. Which bones constitute the primary skeletal framework of the face and what are their key roles?
2. How does the skull influence overall facial aesthetics and proportions?
3. What are some common facial skeletal disorders, and how can they affect appearance and function?

1.2. Muscles of Facial Expression

Learning Outcome

1. Discuss Major Muscles and Their Functions
2. Impact of Muscle Tone on Aesthetics
3. Explain the Techniques for Assessing Muscle Function

Facial expression muscles are a highly developed system that is involved in human communication and are crucial for nonverbal communication, emotional expression, and social interaction. Facial expression muscles are found in the superficial layer of the face and are primarily responsible for actions, such as smiling, frowning, and eyebrow movements, which are crucial to the expression of emotions and social information. The facial musculature is innervated by the facial nerve (cranial nerve VII), highlighting its singular function in the nervous system and enhancing the interconnectedness of anatomy and behavioral expression. By virtue of their fundamental function in expressing emotions, the muscles are examined to an extent of applicability beyond mere aesthetics, also in psychological usage, highlighting the ingrained relationship between physical expression and human emotion. In aesthetics, knowledge of facial expression muscles is key to practitioners who aspire to enhance or restore youthful appearances. Shattering breakthroughs in non-surgical treatments, such as botulinum neurotoxin type A (BoNTA), highlight the need for full knowledge of facial expression muscles. The success of BoNTA in treating dynamic wrinkles caused by muscle contractions relies on skillful application methods and extensive facial anatomy knowledge. As reiterated in the present guidelines laid out by expert panels, like South Korean ones, the practitioners need to stay current with recommended injection sites and amounts to get maximum effects with minimal complications in treatments of facial expression muscles (Rho et al., 2025). This attention to detail in anatomical knowledge is the signpost of the comingling of art and science of facial aesthetics. Moreover, new pedagogical strategies, such as clay modeling, have been found effective in mastering the intricate anatomy of facial expression muscles, particularly under the constraints of resource shortage in traditional anatomy education (Chiappini et al., 2025). Through clay modeling, students can experience active learning and collaboration to enhance their understanding of anatomical structures and functions.

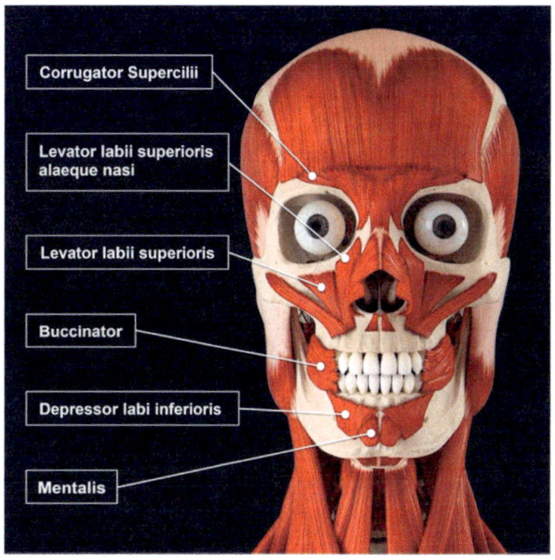

Figure 1.6. The muscles of facial expression represent a complex system integral to human communication.

Source: https://external-content.duckduckgo.com/iu/?u=https%3A%2F%2Fcdn.completeanatomy.cn%2Fwebsite%2Fblog%2Ffacial-expression%2Ffacial-expression2.jpg&f=1&nofb=1&ipt=e7db03babf1a680058ff46bb37ecf9224f23da0dbff3845d278879957ebb182a.

Student feedback from students undertaking such activities is that there is a positive correlation with learning, leading to increased motivation and enjoyment. This focus highlights the need for flexibility in anatomy education, particularly in terms of aesthetic improvements.

Through incorporating creative learning approaches, teaching professionals can well bridge learning knowledge with practice in the area of facial anatomy so that there is a complete learning experience for the next generation of practitioners in this discipline (Figure 1.6).

1.2.1. Major Muscles and Their Functions

Information regarding primary muscles and their functions is extremely relevant in analyzing the aesthetics of facial anatomy. The human face has a host of muscles, which are largely categorized into two groups: the superficial facial muscles of expression and the deep masticatory muscles. The facial muscles, such as the orbicularis oris and the zygomaticus, have essential roles in communicating feelings and emotions through movements. For instance, the zygomaticus major enables smiling, which has significant social roles in human interpersonal communications. Additionally, facial muscles have certain anatomical structures that allow them to move smoothly and quickly, thus enabling humans to visually communicate a range of different emotions. This multiplicity of expression is not only intrinsic to social interaction but is of paramount significance in such fields as aesthetics and plastic surgery, where the sensitive dissection of muscle function is the key to fruitful results. The deeper muscles, the masseter and temporalis, are more involved with mastication, or chewing. These muscles work in concert to allow efficient grinding and food processing, emphasizing an aesthetic aspect of facial structure that intersects with function.

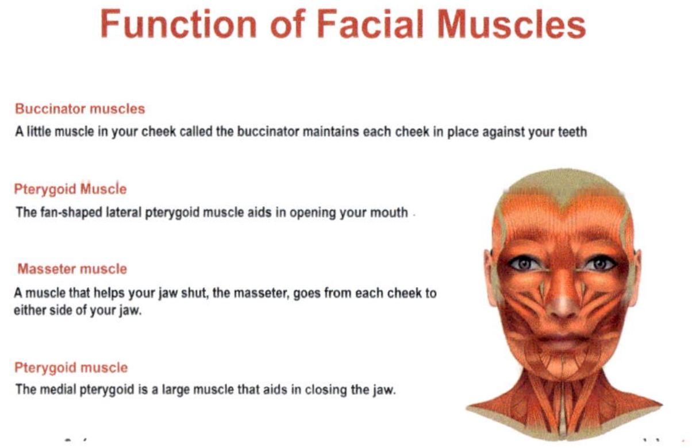

Figure 1.7. The major muscles and their functions.

Source: https://assets.lybrate.com/imgs/tic/enadp/function-of-facial-muscles.webp.

The external appearance of the face shifts over time due to soft tissue dynamics during mastication, as TMJ and associated musculature can affect overall facial symmetry and structure. Research into the biomechanics of these facial muscles has helped in developing new surgical methods and aesthetic procedures aimed at enhancing their functionality as well as maintaining a natural appearance. The research continues to better our understanding of facial movement mechanical properties, hence the facial aesthetics field as a whole that considers appearance and functionality. In addition, cultural facial aesthetics are usually an indication of the understanding of muscles and their function. As observed in recent studies, some facial features and expressions are usually highly valued in some societies, determining standards of beauty. For example, analysis of the kot-mi-nam phenomenon in Korean society proves within the intersection of anatomy and beauty are complexities, showing facial customization efforts are inextricably linked to physiological traits as well as cultural narrative (Kim et al., 2013). Further, the application of sophisticated modeling techniques to model and control facial features is a demonstration of how the anatomy of muscles can enable more efficient control of appearance change. As the discipline progresses, it is increasingly important that scientists consider not only the anatomical and functional aspects of facial muscles but also the way in which they are embedded in wider aesthetic ideals within diverse sociocultural contexts (Hannam et al., 2008) (Figure 1.7).

1.2.2. The Impact of Muscle Tone on Aesthetics

The interplay between muscle tone and the aesthetics of the face is a fundamental aspect of understanding how physical qualities add to perceptions of beauty. Muscle tone, or the continuous, passive contraction of muscles, is a significant factor in defining the contours and overall form of the face. This resting tension creates a structural framework that influences facial feature shaping and support. The aesthetic outcome is frequently a combination of both genetic and lifestyle elements, and well-developed facial muscles contribute to a youthful, vibrant appearance. In contrast, low muscle tone may result in sagging skin and a tired appearance, and the significance of muscle dynamics in facial aesthetics. Besides, the re-creation or restoration of muscle tone through intervention has a remarkable impact on physical appearance and self-image, providing a choice for aesthetic enhancement in those who wish to optimize facial features. Furthermore, the integration of muscle tone in clinical practice indicates its role in aesthetic therapy. Advances in surgical and non-surgical aesthetics have also drawn attention towards maximizing muscle tone as a key component of facial rejuvenation. Treatments, such as botulinum toxin injections and facial fillers, directly target the inhibition of muscle contractions and, in the process, alter facial expression dynamics with an overall boost in aesthetic value. Design and development of these treatments are not only based on imagination but also on well-researched knowledge of facial anatomy, as is evidenced by research that determines the relationship between aesthetics and muscle function. As a case in point, the strategic reintroduction of tonicity specifically works on facial symmetry and contouring and allows for a more balanced appearance.

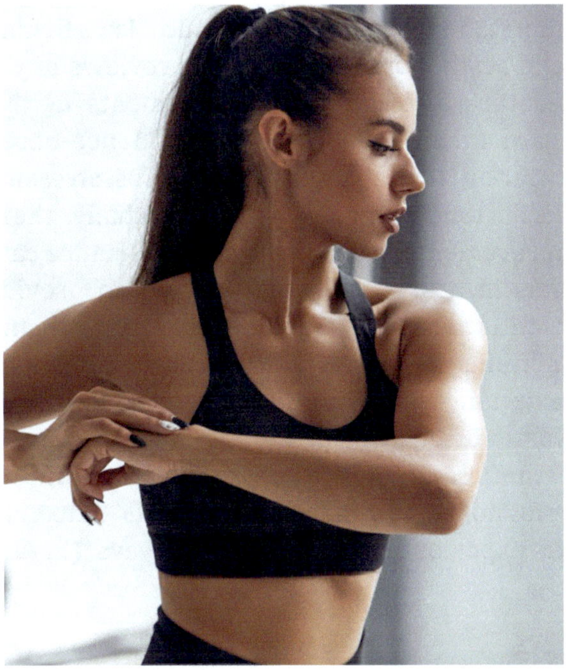

Figure 1.8. The impact of muscle tone on aesthetics.

Source: https://external-content.duckduckgo.com/iu/?u=https%3A%2F%2Fwestcoastwellnessandaesthetics.com%2Fwp-content%2Fuploads%2F2022%2F02%2FMuscle-Tone-872x1024.jpg&f=1&nofb=1&ipt=6051fe3206889e6735260388793b409e6151642cac7cc3e202e4b64b14fd1809.

This approach is consonant with the growing trend in aesthetic medicine that aims for natural results with the emphasis on maximum muscle tone as a significant variable in the pursuit of facial beauty (Hernández-Gómez et al., 2019). The importance of evidence-based learning in aesthetics, and by extension, muscle tone management, is increasing recognition in curricular models. Recent advances have aimed at establishing formal postgraduate programs to deliver the nuances of non-surgical aesthetic procedures and the interlinking between facial aesthetics and muscle tone.

Fostering critical reflection and inquiry-based learning, such programs advance a deeper understanding of the biomechanical laws behind facial aesthetics. The systematic reviews of the literature and the needs assessments in this regard further described the evidence-based education of non-surgical procedures, stressing muscle tone (Kumar, 2021). Eventually, these improvements in education aim to enhance care levels in aesthetic clinics in order to provide practitioners with adequate anatomical and functional information involved in achieving maximum aesthetic outcomes. Through these efforts, discussion of muscle tone and facial aesthetics not only changes but also allows professionals to enhance their clients' outcomes and experiences in meaningful ways (Figure 1.8).

1.2.3. Techniques for Assessing Muscle Function

In facial aesthetics, the assessment of muscle function is the essence of successful treatment planning and aesthetically successful results. Various testing techniques of muscle function provide useful information to the clinician about muscular dynamics in the face. Manual muscle testing is one of the important methods, which involves testing the strength of some muscle groups through resisted movement. This technique can identify areas of weakness or imbalance, and this can then be followed by direct aesthetic interventions. Furthermore, functional movement tests, often conducted through dynamic simulations measuring facial expression interaction, reveal a comprehensive understanding of muscle coordination. By incorporating these tests, practitioners can more precisely identify functional muscle behaviors required for effective aesthetic medicine so that treatments become harmonious with the unique anatomical structure of the patient, as evident by ongoing controversy concerning the need for standardized training in non-surgical aesthetics (Kumar, 2021).

The other important approach is through the application of imaging modalities, such as ultrasound and electromyography (EMG), which provide objective data regarding muscle function and activity. Ultrasonography allows clinicians to visualize muscle structure and assess changes in muscle thickness and quality, gaining information that manual testing may not be able to fully obtain.

EMG, on the other hand, picks up electrical activity generated from muscle contraction and provides immediate feedback of muscle function during various facial expressions. Such advanced imaging techniques not only enhance the understanding of muscle activity but also direct the intervention planning, such as botulinum toxin injections. Through explanations of the nuances of facial muscular movement, such methods aid in minimizing risks for aesthetic interventions, highlighting the necessity of precision in injection procedures to avoid complications identified by recent studies on botulinum neurotoxin therapies (Kąpa et al., 2025). Moreover, the inclusion of subjective measures, such as patient self-reports of effect and satisfaction surveys, is essential in arriving at an interdisciplinary understanding of the function of muscles in aesthetics. Subjective measures allow practitioners to capture patients' impressions and experiences of their facial appearance and function following treatment. By combining qualitative data with quantitative measures, a robust evidence base can be obtained for treatment efficacy and patient satisfaction. Ultimately, using multiple methods of assessment will not only give a more precise measurement of the function of muscles but also lead to the development of treatment plans that are tailored to each individual. With the constantly evolving discipline of non-surgical aesthetics, the integrated approach to the assessment of muscle function continues to be of utmost importance in ensuring optimal aesthetic results, as well as in creating a culture of safer practice (Kumar, 2021).

Test Your Knowledge

1. What are the major muscles of facial expression and their primary functions?
2. How does muscle tone influence facial aesthetics and expression?
3. What techniques are used to assess the function and integrity of facial muscles?

1.3. Skin and Its Role in Facial Aesthetics

Learning Outcome

1. Explain Layers of the Skin and Their Functions
2. Discuss Factors Affecting Skin Health and Appearance
3. Focus on Common Skin Conditions and Treatments

Skin is a complex organ serving not only to cover and protect the body but also to play a multifunctional role in facial aesthetics. Its make-up consists of multiple layers, including the epidermis, dermis, and subcutaneous tissue, each contributing different features that build the look and feel of the skin. The outer layer, epidermis, is important for performing as barriers to environmental harm, while the dermis holds essential ingredients, such as collagen and elastin, which provide elasticity and firmness to the skin. The interactions between these layers and health directly affect facial appearance, e.g., controlling the texture, tone, and overall youthful appearance. The disintegration of collagen during aging, for instance, can lead to wrinkles and loose skin, hence altering one's face shape and attractiveness, placing significant emphasis on the role played by the integrity of the skin in facial beauty. In aesthetic medicine, it is of paramount importance in skin pathology and aesthetic treatment to understand the intricacies so that optimal results can be obtained. Utilization of minimally invasive treatments, such as botulinum toxin injection for dynamic wrinkles, has evolved the face of facial aesthetics. The use of abobotulinumtoxin A for aesthetic purposes as seen in a systematic review emphasizes safety and patient satisfaction in these treatments. Not only do these treatments enhance external beauty but they also have a positive effect on patients psychosocial well-being, confirming the interdependence of aesthetics and mental health. By addressing dynamic motions that produce static lines, these treatments illustrate the manner in which targeted aesthetic interventions may enhance the visible signs of aging while simultaneously influencing the disposition of people, illustrating high stakes in skin health and self-perception. Moreover, craniofacial disorders, such as craniofacial microsomia, provide important insight into the challenges of reconstructive surgery and how they impact patient satisfaction. Extreme ear developmental abnormalities have been shown to lead to increased surgical interventions and a negative influence on esthetic outcomes, particularly those with psychosocial considerations.

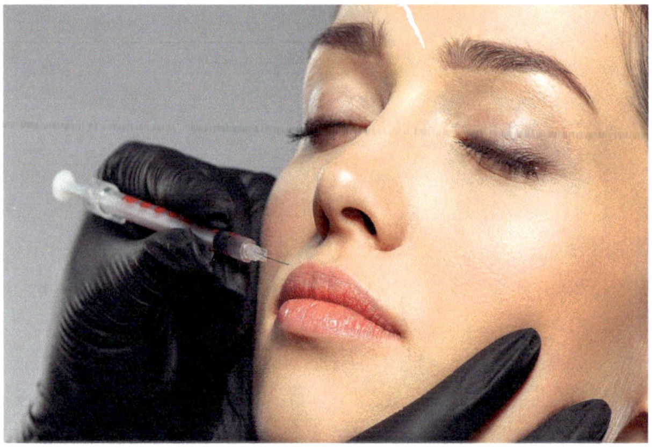

Figure 1.9. Skin and its role in facial aesthetics.

Source: https://external-content.duckduckgo.com/iu/?u=https%3A%2F%2Fwww.crowncliniclondon.com%2Fwp-content%2Fuploads%2F2023%2F06%2Ffacial-aesthetics-botox-crown-clinic-london.jpg&f=1&nofb=1&ipt=34400dc9d826c15b0b4ef39428d5c5fb01f87fe0156042f4c33c253fb10400e5.

For instance, in the case of microtia patients, not only is successful reconstruction an issue of achieving aesthetic harmony, but also restoring auditory function and overall quality of life. Interestingly, studies have demonstrated that restoration of hearing loss in such patients is significantly correlated with improved psychosocial outcomes, emphasizing the multifaceted role of the skin and its aesthetic impact. These findings reinforce the importance of mastering facial anatomy and aesthetics, emphasizing the important role skin and other anatomical structures play in physical appearance and psychological resilience (Figure 1.9).

1.3.1. Layers of the Skin and Their Functions

Understanding the skin layers is important for those studying facial anatomy and aesthetics since each of the layers plays distinct but complementary functions in keeping the skin healthy and looking good. Three primary layers comprise the skin: epidermis, dermis, and hypodermis, each playing an essential function in the overall performance of the skin. The outermost layer, the epidermis, is primarily responsible for protecting against external hazards, such as pathogens and toxic UV radiation. It contains melanocytes, which produce melanin, giving it pigmentation and protecting it to a certain extent against the damage from the sun. Furthermore, this layer constantly renews itself, allowing it to remove dead skin cells as well as allow new cells to grow, hence a youthful appearance. Beneath the epidermis is the dermis, which is thicker and more robust than the epidermis and offers structural and nourishment support to the epidermis. Comprising dense connective tissue, the dermis holds vital components like blood vessels, lymph vessels, hair roots, and sebaceous glands. These components work in perfect sync to keep the skin moist and elastic, which are vital for a young look. The dermal layer contains collagen and elastin fibers, which provide tensile strength and elasticity, respectively, to maintain healthy and supple skin. Many sensory receptors within the dermis are also responsible for the sensation of touch, pain, and temperature, as well as calling attention to the dermis role as protector and communicator. Finally, the hypodermis, or subcutaneous tissue, plays a support role by insulating the body and affixing the skin to underlying tissues, such as muscles and bones.

The hypodermis consists largely of fat and connective tissue that is not only a shock absorber but also stores energy and provides insulation. Hypodermal adipose tissue influences the overall facial shape and attractiveness of the face. Changes in the distribution of fat within this layer are linked with aging and may result in sagging skin and loss of volume, thereby affecting individual aesthetics. Understanding of these three different layers and how they work is critical to practitioners in aesthetic clinics since it has a direct bearing on treatment modalities and techniques in facial rejuvenation and upkeep (Heng et al., 2021; Marin et al., 2023) (Figure 1.10).

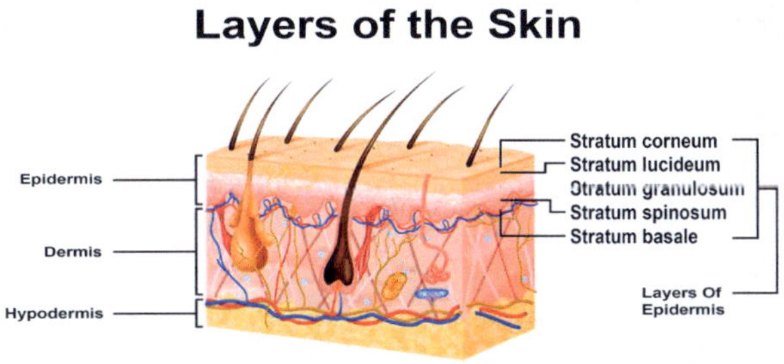

Figure 1.10. The layers of the skin is essential for anyone studying facial anatomy and aesthetics.

Source: https://external-content.duckduckgo.com/iu/?u=https%3A%2F%2Fmedia.geeksforgeeks.org%2Fwp-content%2Fuploads%2F20230316174511%2FLayers-of-Skin.png&f=1&nofb=1&ipt=49abaa48e2e4bb9a825c3cf9fa6045afe55d483a6401fdd20d1b3b095676e59c.

1.3.2. Factors Affecting Skin Health and Appearance

The health and appearance of skin are determined by many factors, which can be classified broadly into intrinsic and extrinsic factors. Intrinsic factors are genetic predispositions and biological processes, like aging, which lead to the natural slowing down of collagen production and skin elasticity. For example, mutations in genes may influence the production of melanin, altering skin color and sensitivity to environmental stress. In addition, intrinsic variables can be augmented by hormonal imbalances, which can accelerate conditions, such as acne or color alterations. It is important to comprehend these variables to create individualized skincare programs and aesthetic treatments that fit unique skin types and genetic profiles. Thus, professionals should note these inherent characteristics in treating skin wellness and aesthetic concerns, realizing that all patients' skin reflects a unique mix of genetic inheritance and physiological change due to aging. Besides intrinsic factors, extrinsic forces also play an important role in determining skin wellness and appearance. Extrinsic forces through UV radiation exposure, pollution, and lifestyle contribute immensely to the integrity of the skin. Prolonged exposure to sunlight results in photoaging, which appears as wrinkles, fine lines, and discoloration through the breakdown of collagen and elastin fibers. In the same way, environmental toxins can produce free radicals, promoting the acceleration of skin aging and making it lose its barrier function. Lifestyle, such as diet, stress, smoking, and hydration, also has an impact on skin resilience and appearance. A diet rich in antioxidants, for example, helps combat oxidative stress, while adequate hydration maintains the elasticity of skin. The synergy of these extrinsic factors necessitates an integrated process of aesthetic therapy and skincare, emphasizing environmental awareness and lifestyle modification as keystones in attaining the best skin health. Advances in technology have also revolutionized access and efficiency of skin examination methods and treatment equipment. Of these, the use of 3D printing technology in cosmetic dermatology presents a particular opportunity for customization of aesthetic treatments. As argued in recent works, 3D printing has made it possible to create personalized-fitted devices that are able to offer goal-directed treatments, thus improving patient results (Narongdej et al., 2024). Additionally, wearable technology has been developed to monitor skin conditions in real-time, allowing for the early identification of changes and timely treatments (Minaoglou et al., 2024). This kind of technological advancement allows practitioners to provide more precise and tailored treatment, once again decreasing the gap between cosmetic aspiration and achievable results. Using the newest technologies alongside the understanding of the multifactorial cause of skin health, professionals are better equipped to address the evolving needs of clients who need aesthetic enhancement.

1.3.3. Common Skin Conditions and Treatments

The human skin is susceptible to a variety of conditions that compromise aesthetic look and overall health. Acne, eczema, and psoriasis are among the most common skin conditions. Acne, as represented by the presence of pimples, blackheads, and cysts, is predominantly brought on by hormonal shifts and sebum overproduction, and is typically exacerbated by food and stress considerations. The patients then receive treatments that can range from over-the-counter topical preparations containing benzoyl peroxide to prescription drugs in the form of retinoids and antibiotics. In tandem, proper skincare regimens that include gentle cleansers and moisturizers are important in the treatment of acne. Similarly, eczema is irritated, itchy skin that can potentially impact one's quality of life greatly. Corticosteroids and moisturizers are usual treatments for eczema, though a change in lifestyle is significant in chronic management and flare avoidance. Aside from such normal conditions as acne and eczema, skin cancer is a serious condition for the majority of people. There are three main types of skin cancer: basal cell carcinoma, squamous cell carcinoma, and melanoma, all of which require early diagnosis for successful treatment. UV light overexposure, as well as genetic predisposition, raises the chance of developing skin cancer. Avoidance strategies in the form of sunscreen application and protective clothing, along with regular dermatological check-ups, are essential to curtail this risk. Treatment after diagnosis may involve removal of malignant tumors, cryosurgery, or topical chemotherapy, depending on the nature and severity of the cancers. Appropriate education of the patient regarding surveillance of the skin and high awareness is essential to initiate anticipatory healthcare practice, significantly improving outcomes as well as prognosis of skin cancer.

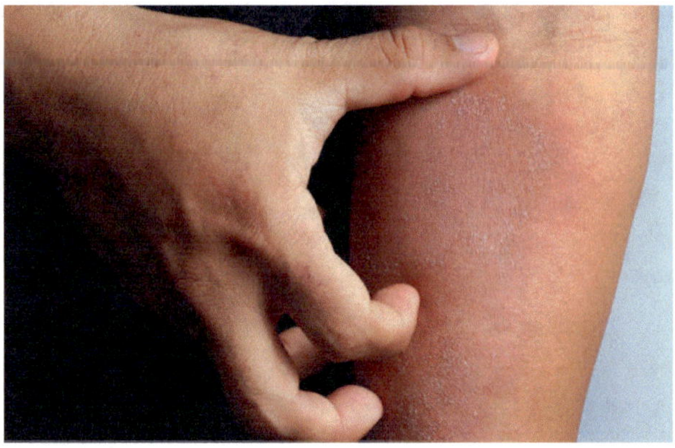

Figure 1.11. Common skin conditions and treatments.

Source: https://external-content.duckduckgo.com/iu/?u=https%3A%2F%2Fparmanandhospital.com%2Fwp-content%2Fuploads%2F2023%2F08%2Fimage.png&f=1&nofb=1&ipt=13ab9402fca3532fbf38a22615371de717fe3498b51b56550ff2846fd6ea3941.

More complex diseases, such as rosacea and psoriasis, typically require more subtle approaches due to their unpredictable nature and chronicity. Rosacea, which manifests as facial redness, visible blood vessels, and possibly papules and pustules in some cases, typically needs a treatment regimen that involves both topical and oral treatments to reduce inflammation and exacerbation. Lifestyle changes may also benefit patients by helping them avoid and discover provoking factors that may be dietary or environmental. Conversely, psoriasis, an autoimmune condition that manifests as red scaling patches of skin, frequently requires treatments like phototherapy or systemic medication for severe cases. New treatments, like biologics, demonstrate the rapid expansion of dermatologic treatment, which meets the unique complexities of skin disease. With the advancement of treatment modalities, a better understanding of the pathophysiology underlying these conditions will lead to more personalized and effective care programs for patients with common skin diseases (Anesi et al., 2014; Hughes & Song, 2016) (Figure 1.11).

Test Your Knowledge

1. What are the layers of the skin, and how does each contribute to facial aesthetics?
2. Which factors most significantly affect skin health and overall appearance?
3. What are common skin conditions affecting facial aesthetics, and what treatment options are available?

1.4. The Importance of Facial Proportions

Learning Outcome

1. Discuss Historical Perspectives on Facial Proportions
2. Explain Modern Standards of Beauty and Aesthetics
3. Focus on Tools for Measuring Facial Proportions

Facial proportion theory is at the core of aesthetics, dictating concepts of beauty throughout cultures and historical periods. Aesthetic laws would generally be founded on facial balance and symmetry because these elements play a significant role in the allure of a human face. Various studies have revealed that some of the measurements, such as in what proportion the face width relates to the height of the face, are fundamental to deciding beauty and attractiveness, making the use of a systematic method imperative for facial anatomy study. This systematic method can make individuals consciously more aware of face aesthetics and can be influential in applications ranging from cosmetic interventions to art and design. Thus, knowing the fundamental rules of facial proportions is a fundamental aspect of aesthetics learning. Recent studies emphasize the reliability of certain soft tissue landmarks in measuring facial proportions. As an example, studies aiming to develop a low-cost facial image capture system highlighted the reliable detection of the major landmarks, principally the facial areas around the mouth and nose, which were very consistent on frontal and sagittal images (Payne, 2013). This consistency is crucial for both aesthetic analysis and clinical purposes, for instance, orthodontia, where accurate measurements significantly control the success of treatment. Secondly, the study revealed variation in landmark effectiveness based on where they are located, which suggests that there must be a complex comprehension of such markers in order to offer complete facial analysis. Thus, working with facial proportions within a methodologically sound framework equips us to analyze facial symmetry and notions of beauty more effectively. Where science and beauty meet is clearer when examining facial proportions and their use across industries. Since research into beauty perception indicates consensus across some aspects of beauty, there has been a shift towards objective beauty measures.

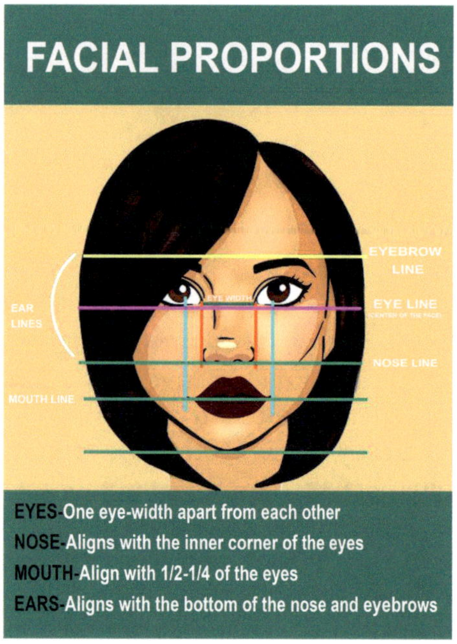

Figure 1.12. The concept of facial proportions plays a pivotal role in the realm of aesthetics.

Source: https://external-content.duckduckgo.com/iu/?u=https%3A%2F%2Fi.pinimg.com%2Foriginals%2F4d%2F08%2Fbc%2F4d08bcc6ccf075c1366618fd6da01366.jpg&f=1&nofb=1&ipt=1c4fd1a5579366daf74ae2730dc7414d67d6378e9b1c595c3f36fef13dab06ce.

From learning classifiers based on mean human ratings of facial attractiveness, researchers have devised tools with which to measure beauty systematically (Gunes et al., 2006). These mechanical systems have potential applications across various domains, including entertainment, cosmetics, and even plastic surgery, providing a paradigm for practices that are more effective and targeted. The analysis of facial proportions not only improves the aesthetic knowledge but also results in more sensitive and accountable practice in industries directly suffering from these aesthetic requirements. This underscores the relevance of facial proportions as a recurring topic both in scientific research and practical application within aesthetics (Figure 1.12).

1.4.1. Historical Perspectives on Facial Proportions

The facial proportions have a rich tapestry of beauty concepts that have stretched over the course of centuries. In ancient Greece, for example, beauty was pursued in terms of mathematics promoted by thinkers like Pythagoras, and later on, during Renaissance painting, by Leonardo da Vinci. Da Vinci's own work, specifically the Vitruvian Man, summed up the idea that beauty is mathematically visible, conforming to ordered ratios that establish perfect human proportions. These notions formed the basis for later explorations in both art and science into the facial structure, further establishing the idea of beauty as something measurable and codifiable. This idea persisted through the centuries, influencing not only the artistic process but also cultural attitudes towards beauty. With changing aesthetic treatments, the shift in the understanding of facial proportions began to involve anatomical and functional concerns along with solely aesthetic ones. The development of orofacial harmonization techniques is an outcome of this change, as it aimed at harmonizing aesthetics and biomechanical function. Modern facial aesthetics considers treatments not just related to visual appeal, but also internal mechanics of facial anatomy. This dual emphasis on maximizing the beauty of smiles, representative of appearance and sociability, functions to emphasize the integral relationship between form and function in facial beauty. These observations underscore a deeper aesthetic knowing that is beyond what lies on the surface, created through functionality as well as appearance, something that still persists today. With recent advancements, the training model of facial aesthetics has now turned increasingly formalized with the requirement of formal education in non-surgical aesthetic procedures. Recent studies have highlighted the importance of an evidence-based education with the inclusion of critical thinking and practical competency necessary for effective practice in non-surgical aesthetics and bridging the gap between the ideals of yesteryears and the present application. This system, informed by systematic reviews and Delphi studies, is a holistic comprehension of facial proportions merging cosmetic desire with scientific understanding of facial movements. It aims to equip practitioners with the information needed to navigate the complexity of facial beauty, finally ensuring that modalities of treatment preserve both aesthetic and functional integrity of facial structures and patient welfare (Kumar, 2021; Paschoalotto et al., 2023).

1.4.2. Modern Standards of Beauty and Aesthetics

The past of modern norms of beauty and aesthetics is closely tied to the progress of the knowledge of facial anatomy. As social attitudes towards what is considered beautiful evolve, the norms of beauty have increasingly relied on quantifiable parameters derived from biological and psychological science. Research indicates that averageness and symmetry of the face lie at the root of today's concept of beauty, since such features are always associated with genetic health and fertility fitness. Incorporating such scientific perspectives into beauty standards erodes conventional concepts rooted primarily in cultural and artistic representations, as found in ancient paintings. Beauty then increasingly depends on anatomical traits testifying to excellent health and genetic superiority, putting the study of facial aesthetics in the mainstream of observing contemporary standards of beauty. Moreover, the adoption of non-surgical cosmetic procedures has had a direct impact on the notion and chase of beauty in today's society. These procedures, which are typically performed in private clinics, are highly sought after because they provide individuals with the opportunity to beautify their features without the invasive nature of surgery. The implementation of a postgraduate program in non-surgical aesthetics, as detailed in recent research, indicates the popularity of systemized training in the field. This course is designed to address the knowledge gaps in training practitioners in how to enhance aesthetic results while preserving patient safety. The intricate relationship between facial anatomy and the application of such non-surgical interventions reflects how modern beauty standards are more and more being validated and refined through scientific evidence and professional education (Kumar, 2021). Finally, the scientific method brought to bear on beauty standards, whether symmetry and averageness of the face, reveals a fascinating confluence between art and evolutionary biology. Contemporary research in fields, such as neuro-aesthetics examines how aspects of attractiveness can be broken down into concrete elements, including pleasant facial expressions and youth, and thereby inform social expectations. The portrayal of beauty by the eye of art history shows how these ideals have been replicated and indulged throughout the ages, reflecting changing cultural values. With the changing standards of beauty, the underlying assumptions based on both anatomical research and psychological speculation will, in turn, define future concepts of aesthetic beauty. This integrative approach marks a revolutionary age where beauty is no longer just the outcome of cultural construction but is also a sign of biological needs (Suárez et al., 2016) (Figure 1.13).

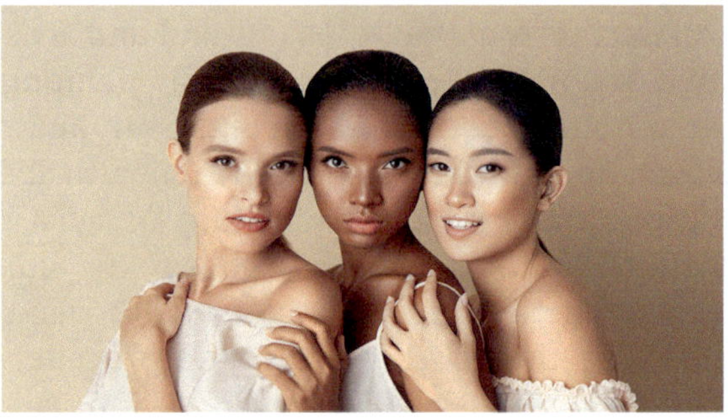

Figure 1.13. The evolution of modern standards of beauty and aesthetics.

Source: https://external-content.duckduckgo.com/iu/?u=https%3A%2F%2Fcdn.shedefined.com.au%2Fwp-content%2Fuploads%2F2021%2F02%2F26094221%2FHow-unrealistic-beauty-standards-profit-from-womens-insecurities-HERO.jpg&f=1&nofb=1&ipt=080c1297bae0847c10ccf691040a8715068012879d45fafa0e6321dc953f0e34.

1.4.3. Tools for Measuring Facial Proportions

Measurement of facial proportion is at the core of facial anatomy and beauty, providing essential information for both clinical application and artistic expression. There are numerous instruments being used in this endeavor, each of which offers unique advantages to accomplish certain requirements of measurement. For instance, calipers take precise measurements of facial features, such as nose width or lip height, to allow for quantitative assessment that can be utilized to guide surgery, particularly in reconstructive and aesthetic surgery. Anthropometric landmarks also serve as points of reference so that measurement may be carried out standardly among numerous populations.

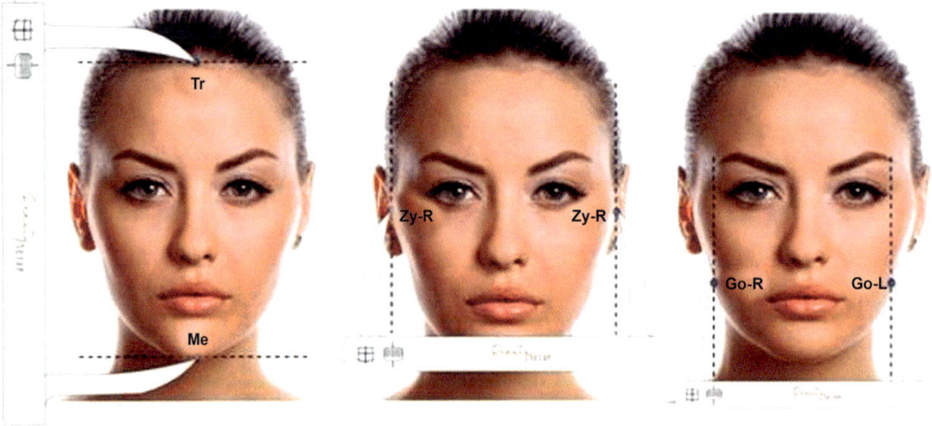

Figure 1.14. The tools for measuring facial proportions.

Source: https://www.mathewsopenaccess.com/userfiles/images/Fig%204%20facial%20heigh.jpg.

Reliability of data gathered with these instruments is important, with the requirement for practitioners employing proper measuring instruments and techniques to match the particular anatomical variation occurring in different ethnic populations, stressed by current anthropometric studies among Malays, Chinese, and Indians (Durairajanayagam, 2011). Over the past few years, discussion on non-surgical aesthetic (NSA) procedures has been increasingly in focus, affecting facial proportion measurement from being generally surgical to more varied aesthetic purposes. Education in NSA procedures has become indispensable, and hence, the establishment of a systematic educational model for practitioners is imperative. This involves methods that utilize measurement tools for dissecting and assessing facial aesthetics optimally. The evidence-based nature of a postgraduate curriculum underscores the significance of standard and measurement protocols in NSA. Effective understanding of facial proportions derived from such means not only enhances aesthetic outcomes but also instills critical sensitivity and informed decision-making in practitioners, allowing for more meaningful engagement with the aesthetics and harmony of facial anatomy (Kumar, 2021). Ultimately, the integration of various facial ratio tools into surgical and non-surgical aesthetics proves a meaningful contribution towards greater facial anatomical understanding. As more attention is given to personalized techniques in aesthetic procedures, practitioners need access to accurate and uniform measuring techniques. By establishing unique morphological criteria based on anthropometric data, specialists can modify their approach to the unique characteristics of different ethnic populations. As illustrated in studies to quantify individual facial morphology in Malaysian populations, the results of these studies not only supply a normative reference but also serve as working guidelines for reconstructive facial surgeons dealing with facial disfigurements (Durairajanayagam, 2011). Indeed, precise measurement of facial proportions not only enhances aesthetic outcomes but also enables one to inform ethical aesthetics, the union of science and art (Figure 1.14).

Test Your Knowledge

1. How did ancient civilizations such as the Greeks and Egyptians contribute to the early understanding of ideal facial proportions?
2. How do contemporary aesthetic guidelines differ from traditional or classical facial proportion norms?
3. What are the commonly used clinical tools for measuring facial proportions in aesthetic practice?

1.5. Aesthetic Procedures and Treatments

Learning Outcome

1. Give an Overview of Non-Surgical Treatments
2. Focus on Surgical Options for Facial Enhancement
3. Explain Risks and Benefits of Aesthetic Procedures

The realm of aesthetic procedures and treatments has dramatically changed, motivated by access to new technology as well as society's greater emphasis on body appearance. These treatments often augment facial elements or reduce the impact of aging in a number of methods, including injectables, laser, and surgical procedures. Understanding of the underlying facial anatomy is crucial to both practitioners and patients in order to ensure optimal results as well as safety. Knowledge of the vascular anatomy of the face, for instance, can be employed to minimize risks associated with procedures, such as dermal fillers or botulinum toxin. As a result, accurate knowledge of facial anatomy is increasingly regarded as a fundamental component of aesthetic practice, in the response to the ongoing shifts in regulating attitudes and standards of education within the specialty. Safety is most important when performing aesthetic treatments, and much controversy surrounds the necessity for education and proficiency in anatomical structures. A systematic review assessing the aesthetic use of abobotulinumtoxinA highlights the necessity to detect subtle reactions in varying populations and implies that competent practitioners with adequate knowledge can maximize patient satisfaction while minimizing risks (Cohen & Scuderi, 2017). Such a foundation is crucial because it equips aesthetic practitioners with the tools to make their way through the intricate facial topography, thereby avoiding unwanted complications. In addition, continued education and incorporation of new research findings into training schemes can ensure that practitioners are competent to apply new methods and technologies effectively and safely. Having aesthetic treatments underpinned by scientific evidence not only creates a culture of safety but also ensures good patient outcomes in a competitive market. Recent studies have established consensus on fundamental anatomical features that endorse the requirement of a core curriculum in aesthetic training. The implementation of a "Core Syllabus" based on peer-reviewed expert consensus would significantly improve practitioners' knowledge of major facial characteristics and thereby prevent calamitous complications secondary to nonsurgical therapies (Bland et al., 2018). Such consensus-driven education ensures that aesthetic practitioners are extremely proficient in the facial anatomy necessary for safe and proper application of aesthetic treatments. As these standards evolve further, they will facilitate continued refinement of practice guidelines, strengthen the foundations of aesthetic medical education, and ultimately lead to enhanced patient care across the aesthetics industry. By highlighting anatomical expertise, practitioners can enhance their proficiency and gain patient confidence with individuals who seek to take advantage of aesthetic enhancement.

1.5.1. Overview of Non-Surgical Treatments

Non-surgical treatments have revolutionized facial aesthetics, allowing patients to opt for less invasive methods of beauty enhancement. Procedures, such as Botox and dermal fillers, have been widely praised for how effective they are with minimal recovery time. Dermal fillers are used to replace volume and fill out wrinkles, while neuromodulators target muscle activity to reduce the appearance of fine lines. These treatments cater to a diverse client base who want aesthetic improvement without surgical risks. Furthermore, development in injectable techniques further refines these non-surgical treatments to address particular facial anatomy, ultimately improving a more natural and balanced appearance in facial structures, thus aiding the goals of current aesthetic medicine as outlined in facial plastic surgery (Bottino et al., 2012). The landscape of non-surgical aesthetic concerns is more extensive than injectables and includes treatments involving chemical peels, laser skin resurfacing, and microneedling. These are treatments designed to address skin texture, tone, and quality. Chemical peels utilize varying acidic solutions to peel the skin, revealing a brighter layer underneath, while laser resurfacing employs concentrated light to target and trigger skin rejuvenation. Microneedling, on the other hand, causes precise micro-trauma to initiate collagen production, leading to increased skin elasticity and tautness. Both techniques have a corresponding set of indications, benefits, and complications, requiring an adequate understanding of facial anatomy and the physiology of the skin. As the demand for non-surgical interventions continues to grow, thorough training and standardized curricula for therapists are now paramount in ensuring safe and effective delivery of these aesthetic treatments, a situation highlighted in recent studies (Kumar, 2021). As non-surgical treatments continue to gain popularity, so does the practice of formal education and training of practitioners in this field. Adding evidence-based courses to postgraduate education in non-surgical aesthetic training places additional importance on medical practitioners' staying abreast of the newer protocols and methods of safety. This structured process not only elevates the practitioner's proficiency level but also progresses patient care through the guarantee that aesthetic treatments are carried out at the highest level of knowledge. Besides, using models of critical thinking and enquiry-based learning has an extensive effect on mastering practical techniques and facial anatomy principles. Having integrated training programs, as argued in recent literature, offers a strategy for elevating standards within non-surgical aesthetics and addressing the demand for trained practitioners (Kumar, 2021).

1.5.2. Surgical Options for Facial Enhancement

Facial enhancement has made significant progress with improvements in surgical techniques and a greater understanding of facial anatomy. Facelifts are among the most effective surgical treatments, which attempt to retard signs of aging by tightening up the skin and facial support tissues. With facelifts, one can regain a youthful appearance by tightening sagging skin, deep lines, and jowls. Thanks to improved surgical techniques, such as the SMAS facelift, patients experience more lasting results and shorter recovery times. And the utilization of minimally invasive technology, such as endoscopic facelifts, has become increasingly popular, providing patients with excellent cosmetic outcomes while eliminating the usual noticeable scars associated with more invasive surgical procedures. Another key surgical procedure in facial rejuvenation is blepharoplasty, or what is generally known as eyelid surgery. Blepharoplasty specifically addresses sagging skin and fat on and around the eyelids, which can make one look tired and result in impaired vision. Removing or relocating these tissues, blepharoplasty improves both form and function, thus reviving the facial expression overall. Aside from traditional approaches, the creation of less invasive alternatives, such as laser blepharoplasty, offers clients options with shorter recovery periods and lower rates of complications. These new procedures are part of the broader trend toward embracing less invasive methods that aim to satisfy aesthetic needs by patients at the cost of compromising patient comfort and security, highlighting the necessity of uniting surgical alternatives with broader dermatological advancement in facial enhancement (Portilla et al., 2024). Innovation in cranio-facial surgery, with subsequent impacts on facial enhancement outcomes, comes in the form of ultrasonic osteotomes, such as Piezosurgery®, which has been developed. Research indicates that such equipment allows selective cutting of mineralized tissues while keeping the surrounding soft tissue structures intact, which is a critical factor in facial surgeries. The ability to achieve precise osteotomies with less invasiveness enhances improved results in healing and reossification, thus enhancing the general quality of facial aesthetic surgery (Anesi et al., 2014).

With surgeons adopting such advanced technologies, the importance of facial enhancement techniques is considerable, allowing for more intricate operations with less trauma to the surrounding tissues. Accordingly, the area of surgical operations for facial enlargement remains dynamic with ongoing investigation and development of technology, keeping the effectiveness in relation to safety for the patient (Figure 1.15).

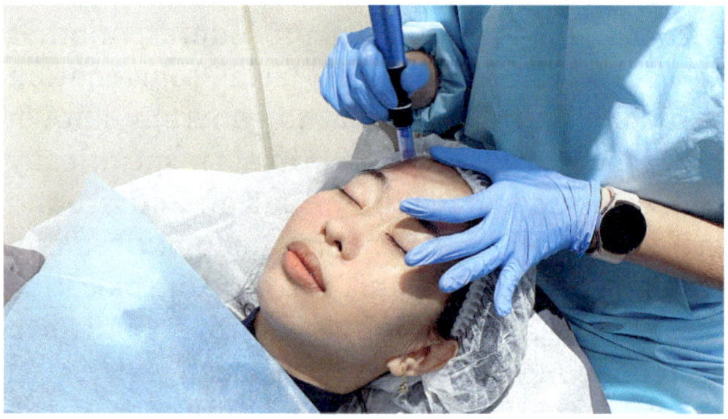

Figure 1.15. Surgical options for facial enhancement.

Source: https://external-content.duckduckgo.com/iu/?u=https%3A%2F%2Fskinpluseuromedica.ph%2Fwp-content%2Fuploads%2F2023%2F01%2FTREATMENT-FACE-ENHANCEMENT-TREATMENT-FACE-ENHANCEMENT-Salmon-DNA-Vital-1.jpg&f=1&nofb=1&ipt=8a518cc2cd2b35b644666742325e4369bf5ace5d64841a781da04a595d1c1c7b.

1.5.3. Risks and Benefits of Aesthetic Procedures

The growing popularity of aesthetic treatments is a reflection of the shifting cultural perception of the significance of physical looks, particularly facial aesthetics. Even though aesthetic treatments are normally desired to make one more beautiful as well as boost self-esteem, they also pose risks. Surgical interventions , such as facelift and nose surgery, have the potential to lead to complications of poor outcome, infection, and scarring, which actually exacerbate the psychological burden rather than ease it. Further, even less invasive techniques, such as fillers and botulinum toxin injection, are not free from risk with complications of allergic reactions and distorted skin texture.

Thus, an all-encompassing vision of both the possible advantages and disadvantages is most critical for those on the brink of such enhancements, as educated choice is required in facing the intricacies of cosmetic treatments. Aside from the physical complications, cosmetic treatments may interlink with psychological effects that need to be given the utmost consideration. Though most people go into these treatments anticipating increased self-esteem and better body image, outcomes can greatly differ. Some research shows that although the majority report a short-term boost of confidence, these findings do not necessarily translate to long-term satisfaction or happiness.

The possibility of surgery addiction can then emerge in some cases, where one constantly resorts to additional procedures with hopes of attaining an idealized body, thus representing an unhealthy correlation between self-worth and looks. The entwined dynamic between social norms of beauty, individual expectations, and the psychological effects of aesthetic treatments mirrors broader arguments concerning identity and self-expression within aesthetics as exemplified in plastic surgery discourse (Edmonds, 2014). The application of technology in aesthetic treatments is a double-edged sword that both improves and unveils new challenges. Technological advancements, such as the application of cone-beam computed tomography and minimally invasive procedures, have improved the precision and security of all manner of aesthetic treatments. For instance, these tools can assist in detailed assessments and more accurate treatment planning and significantly minimize risks of the treatment (Bosio et al., 2011). However, once available, the technology can also potentially become over-commodified in the form of procedures, where profit comes at the cost of patient care. The resulting proliferation of aesthetic suppliers can produce a situation with variable levels of qualifications and practices and therefore variable levels of standards of care. As the boundaries of aesthetic procedures are pushed, an important debate on ethical concerns and safety for the patient is necessary to ensure that the worth of innovation is not greater than the risk taken in the practices.

Test Your Knowledge

1. How do non-surgical procedures improve facial appearance without altering underlying structures?
2. What preoperative assessments are required before planning a facial aesthetic surgery?
3. How do the benefits of facial aesthetic procedures influence patient satisfaction and psychological well-being?

1.6. Psychological Aspects of Facial Aesthetics

Learning Outcome

1. Explain The Connection Between Facial Appearance and Self-Esteem
2. Focus on Cultural Influences on Perceptions of Beauty
3. Discuss The Role of Social Media in Shaping Aesthetic Standards

The intricate interaction between psychological aspects and facial beauty plays a central role in people's judgments of beauty and self-concept. Facial aesthetics, generally conceived relative to the social and cultural environment, have a deep influence on individuals' perception of their self-esteem and integration into society. Seeking facial harmony is an aesthetic but highly psychological pursuit, reflecting individuals' desires for societal integration and self-verification. This phenomenon is particularly relevant within the context of non-surgical aesthetic procedures that have increased in demand, as indicated by the recent reforms in education towards the standardization of training in the industry. A curriculum of evidence-based learning in non-surgical aesthetics seeks to address gaps in knowledge regarding the psychological impacts of aesthetic choices, thereby preparing practitioners to manage the mental health implications entailed with patient needs and wishes (Kumar, 2021). Moreover, ethnic identity also emerges as an important determinant of body perception and decision-making in cosmetic procedures. Especially for populations, such as African-American women, who may be required to navigate complex cultural concepts of beauty and social expectations, it would be expected that a strong ethnic identity would be positively correlated with body control and personal agency in desiring aesthetic change. When individuals become attuned to their cultural selves, they may feel more self-governing of their bodies, something that can lead to an empowered approach to cosmetic alteration. For such individuals, the desire to change their looks can be a process of aligning both individual values and overall societal pressures (Powell-Hicks et al., 2013).

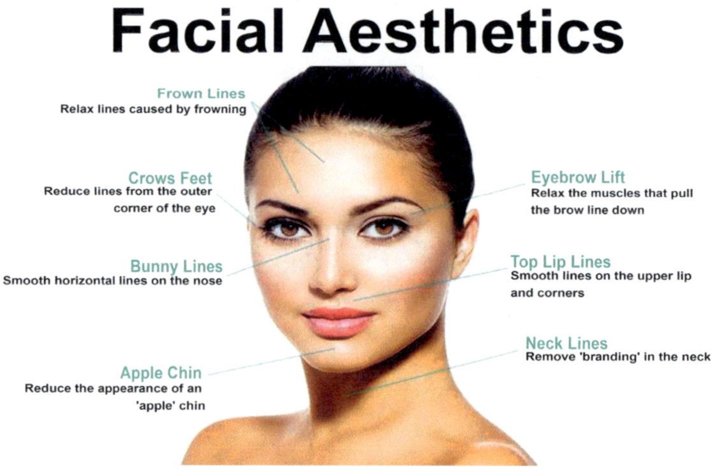

Figure 1.16. The intricate interplay between psychological aspects and facial aesthetics.

Source: https://drprasantakbanerjee.com/wp-content/uploads/2022/06/R82129954_g.jpg.

Therefore, it is important to realize ethnic identity's complex relationship with psychological factors in offering an integrated perspective of facial beauty and how it affects well-being. Lastly, the mental effects of aesthetic discontent can result in increased emotional distress and more chances of seeking cosmetic treatment. Individuals tend to have low self-esteem and body dissatisfaction when they experience difficulties adjusting between their present state and idealized standards. This detachment induces a psychological urge to achieve a desirable appearance, usually by surgical or non-surgical means. Professionals must take note of these issues not only to provide appropriate aesthetic remedies but also to meet the patients' deeper psychological wants. A profound comprehension of facial aesthetics, combined with sensitivity towards the psychological dimensions of such aesthetic expectations, can inform better practices both in aesthetic procedures as well as in patient care (Kumar, 2021). Thus, the psychological dimensions of facial aesthetics underscore the importance of an aware, empathic approach towards facilitating increased well-being in regard to facial beauty (Figure 1.16).

1.6.1. The Connection Between Facial Appearance and Self-Esteem

The interrelation of facial appearance and self-esteem is a complex and multifaceted process that largely relies on the psychological health of a person. Facial beauty tends to be associated with social judgments, which can form profound implications for self-esteem. A good face can evoke good treatment in society, work, and school, leading to a positive self-concept. Conversely, being viewed as lacking facial beauty has drawn negative peer judgments and is ultimately responsible for knocking down one's self-esteem. This emphasis on physical beauty from culture, endorsed by media portrayals, pressures one to conform to specific beauty standards. De-chronologized life course, for example, that which is studied regarding plastic surgery is a new frontier of managing self-esteem regarding aging and beauty. In this, individuals take interventions like cosmetic surgery as a means of not just physical enhancement but also mental enhancement, directly impacting their self-concept and social acceptance.

This paradox regarding aging and beauty intervention, however, can make female identity more complex because women face societal expectations while struggling with their self-concepts, which contributes to their overall level of mental health and self-concept. New facial prosthetic and reconstructive technologies highlight the evolving field of facial aesthetics and their contribution to self-esteem. Digital advancements enable the creation of facial prostheses that restore the appearances of patients with facial defects or disfigurements as a result of trauma or illness in a sequential process. These technologies enhance physical appearance as well as mental well-being. Research detailing the successful implementation of digital scanning and 3D printing identifies the ability of these methods to improve the quality of life for patients who cannot undergo traditional surgical reconstruction due to complications. Hence, such developments illustrate a significant juncture between facial form, cosmetic alterations, and self-esteem, demonstrating the way the restoration of one's appearance by technology could bring major psychological returns whilst establishing a new sense of self and self-worth in individuals suffering the challenges of facial disfigurement (Edmonds, 2014; Ciocca et al., 2023).

1.6.2. Cultural Influences on Perceptions of Beauty

The concept of beauty largely draws on cultural aspects that dictate social benchmarks of attractiveness. Within different cultures, the benchmarks of beauty can also be widely variant, from facial symmetry to color and even body shape. Such benchmarks hold historical and socio-economic undertones, further placing emphasis on the concept of beauty. For instance, in some societies, a more rounded figure is indicative of wealth and fertility, while in others, thinness is appreciated as ideal. Adhering to such cultural differences is essential in seeing standards of beauty shift, demonstrating that what is deemed attractive is not a matter of choice but rather collective constructs that reflect cultural values and ideals. Hence, it is crucial to comprehend the fluidity and multiplicity of beauty principles to perceive the richness of human aesthetics across various cultural realms. One cannot overestimate the significance of nonverbal communication in the beauty-perception realm. Cultural expectations shape not only ideals of physical appearance but also the means through which individuals communicate such ideals through body movement and posture. Research brings to the fore that attractiveness judgments are typically formed on the basis of dynamic cues, such as dance and walk. These facial cues are significant in judgments of mate quality and desirability and convey underlying cultural cues that influence beauty communication. Research on body movement as a basic element of human aesthetics acquaints us with the complexity of attraction and that the beauty story contains more than static qualities. This lends further support to the idea that cultural influences play a significant role in what we find beautiful and how we explain these perceptions to others (Ahuja et al., 2010). In addition, dance as a form of nonverbal communication is a wonderful example of how forms of cultural expression create perceptions of beauty and attraction. Dance, in the majority of cultures, is a primary form of courtship and provides visual and kinesthetic cues to the health, energy, and overall attractiveness of an individual. This aspect is crucial while attempting to understand how cultural models condition aesthetic judgments. As dance movements vary so widely across cultures, they retain their own meanings and values depending on the culture from which they originate. This shows that there is a global recognition of some rhythm of movement with accompanying culturally unique meanings for the movements, even further complicating the complexity of beauty. Hence, the acknowledgment of the interconnection among physical expressions and cultural norms validates the importance of observing beauty in multidimensional views (Hugill et al., 2010) (Figure 1.17).

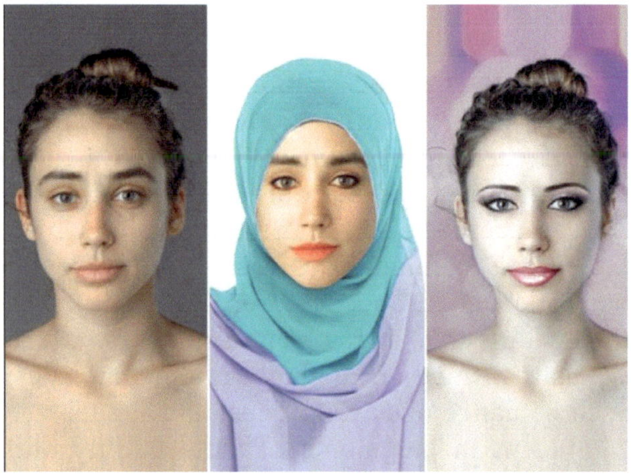

Figure 1.17. The concept of beauty is significantly shaped by cultural influences that dictate societal standards of attractiveness.

Source: https://www.drsunaina.com/wp-content/uploads/2021/04/How-Culture-Influences-Beauty.jpg.

1.6.3. The Role of Social Media in Shaping Aesthetic Standards

The role of social media in aesthetic standards is immense, considering that social media serves as a predominant channel for visual culture and personal representation. As people develop and personalize their online presence, they commit to and disseminate certain perceptions of beauty, leading to the rapid dissemination of aesthetic norms.

This trend has a deep impact on the way individuals conceive of their own body and other bodies because trending attributes on platforms like Instagram and TikTok are utilized to market particular facial features, body types, and styles in accordance with contemporary definitions of beauty. The consistent reinforcement of those ideals will then create a standard that individuals believe is a requirement to which they need to adhere, shaping their self-concept and beauty ideals. In this vein, the social media function is not merely an aesthetic expression enabler but also a beauty norm regulator that creates cultural expectations and individual behavior.

Furthermore, exposure to various aesthetic representations on social media can have bivalent effects on self-esteem and body satisfaction. While on the positive side, individuals can be empowered through representation as influencers highlight qualities that deviate from the traditional Western definition of beauty. This has the potential to provide a more tolerant and inclusive environment towards diverse ethnic identities and body forms. However, research shows that the extensive coverage of idealized images also heightens sentiments of inadequacy and objectification of the body, particularly among marginalized groups. For instance, the relationship between ethnic identity and body perception in African-American women indicates that lower endorsement of ethnic identity can be correlated with a higher probable tendency to pursue cosmetic treatments because individuals negotiate such complex aesthetic landscapes to meet common standards (Powell-Hicks et al., 2013). Thus, even though social media makes beauty discourses more democratic, it also has the potential to uphold harmful comparisons and a restricted understanding of beauty. Aesthetic education and training must address this evolving landscape driven by social media. As aesthetic standards continually get redefined through the world of digital media, medical and cosmetic professionals must quickly understand how these trends affect patients' experiences and expectations. Curriculum education for practitioners in non-surgical aesthetic (NSA) procedures has become a requirement in addressing best practices aligning with contemporary societal demands, hence enhancing patient care and informed choice making (Kumar, 2021). The educational process should emphasize critical thinking as well as identifying the impact of social media interaction on aesthetic expectations. Therefore, through the cultivation of an understanding of societal influences, practitioners are better equipped to engage with individuals seeking aesthetic enhancements and walk the narrow, tightrope between individual expression and societal ideals of beauty.

Test Your Knowledge

1. How does an individual's perception of their facial appearance influence their overall self-esteem and emotional well-being?
2. How do cultural norms and traditions shape what is considered attractive in different societies?
3. What psychological effects can social media filters and edited images have on individuals' self-perception?

SUMMARY

Summary of an exploration of facial anatomy and aesthetics assists in pulling out salient points garnered from throughout the discussion. Understanding of the intricate facial anatomy, including muscles, nerves, and blood supply, is essential for both aesthetic practitioners and clinical practitioners. By having expertise in facial anatomy, practitioners can better evaluate and enhance the facial elements of their patients, as well as maintain health and function. This foundational understanding enables the practitioner to make educated decisions about esthetic treatments, creating results that combine patient desires and anatomical realities for a harmonious blending of art and science in pursuit of beauty. Additionally, the interdisciplinary treatment approach towards facial aesthetics via the methodology outlined in the scholarly research highlights the team effort involved in effective therapeutic treatment strategies. As discussed in literature, such as the management of open gingival embrasures, orthodontists and specialists must work together to optimize outcomes. Treatments that address not only dental aesthetics but also harmony within the face exemplify the complexity of facial anatomy (Bosio et al., 2008). Hence, clinicians should foster holistic treatment planning of all facial anatomy, both enhancing function and aesthetics. Furthermore, technological advancement in facial analysis techniques, combined with emerging trends in facial imaging capture, points to the importance of accuracy both in research and scientific studies as well as clinical practice. The findings regarding the reliability of some soft tissue landmarks further highlight the significance of meticulous assessment in facial evaluation (Payne, 2013). This emphasis on a careful and systematic method of facial analysis enhances the reliability of aesthetic treatments, ultimately translating into improved patient outcomes. As the discipline continues to develop, education in emerging techniques and research becomes integral to those in the profession in order to be able to deliver aesthetically pleasing yet scientifically accurate results in facial aesthetics.

Facial anatomy encompasses a variety of disparate structures, which collectively provide the appearance and expression of an individual. Facial anatomy is an essential consideration not only in reconstructive surgery but also in cosmetic surgery, where balance between features is desired. An aesthetically pleasing balance can, in most instances, be attained by careful attention to proportions and relations between facial landmarks. Using advanced techniques, such as 3D imaging systems, surgeons can model anticipated outcomes based on anatomical variations. These systems can emphasize the need for measurement and assessment in defining standards of beauty, forming the cornerstone for making wise decisions in surgery that will be acceptable to patient expectations. The crossing of anatomy and aesthetics emphasizes the need for precision, as the outcome directly affects patient satisfaction and self-esteem. The role of facial features in non-verbal communication itself highlights the need for an extensive understanding of facial anatomy. It has been found through studies that a large portion of our social interaction is guided by subtle cues transmitted via gestures and facial expressions that are deeply embedded in our evolutionary history. These non-verbal tools are not only employed to transmit information but also to convey an individual's emotional state and intentions. Facial expressions, for instance, which are typically associated with hard-wired biological mechanisms, can express underlying personality and influence social dynamics. Thus, facial aesthetics as a science is more than a matter of appearance and addresses the psychological undertones in the ways individuals see and engage with one another. Integrating aesthetics and communication is paramount for practitioners who aim to optimize patient experience within aesthetic as well as reconstructive procedures. Integrating new technologies within studying and applying facial anatomy also extends the discourse of aesthetic outcomes. Systems that create 3D visualizations of potential surgical results have been set up in order to further facilitate decision-making for both surgeons and patients. The efficiency of such systems is seen in their ability to offer personalized simulations that respect one's very own anatomical form and provide aesthetically pleasing results of changes. Such technology increases the predictability and reliability of surgery, which ultimately results in greater rates of patient satisfaction. As facial aesthetics continues to advance, it is necessary to appreciate the need to blend scientific growth with knowledge of human behavior, developing an environment where both anatomical studies and principles of aesthetics meet to redefine beauty in modern society (Bottino et al., 2012; Hugill et al., 2010).

KEY TERMS FROM THIS CHAPTER

- Epidermis
- Dermis
- Hypodermis
- Orbicularis oculi
- Orbicularis oris
- Frontalis muscle
- Zygomaticus major
- Masseter muscle
- Buccal fat pad
- Zygomatic arch
- Mandibular angle
- Nasolabial fold
- Marionette lines
- Philtrum

CRITICAL THINKING QUESTIONS

1. **Which layer of the face contains most of the neurovascular structures?**
   a. Epidermis
   b. Dermis
   c. Subcutaneous tissue (SMAS layer)
   d. Periosteum
2. **The SMAS (Superficial Musculo aponeurotic System) is best described as:**
   a. A deep fascial layer covering the skull
   b. A fibromuscular layer that connects facial muscles to the skin
   c. A layer of fat above the dermis
   d. A ligament connecting the zygoma to the mandible
3. **Which artery is the main blood supply to the midface?**
   a. Facial artery
   b. Maxillary artery
   c. Superficial temporal artery
   d. Ophthalmic artery
4. **The zygomaticus major muscle is primarily responsible for:**
   a. Raising the eyebrows
   b. Frowning
   c. Smiling
   d. Puffing the cheeks
5. **The primary structural support of the face comes from:**
   a. Skin only
   b. Fat compartments
   c. Facial bones
   d. Ligaments only

Short Answer Questions

1. What is the SMAS, and why is it important in facial aesthetics?
2. Describe the three facial aesthetic thirds used for proportional analysis.
3. What are retaining ligaments of the face, and how do they influence aging changes?
4. Which nerve supplies the muscles of facial expression, and why is it important for cosmetic procedures?
5. Explain the concept of the "aesthetic ideal" in facial proportions.

Answers to Critical Thinking Questions

1. (c) 2. (b) 3. (a) 4. (c) 5. (c)

REFERENCES

1. Ahuja, A., Ahuja, A., Assad, M., Barnhart, C., Bodin, M., Borndörfer, R., Brännlund, U., et al. (2010). *Integrating body movement into attractiveness research*. https://core.ac.uk/download/pdf/41071694.pdf (accessed on 14th July 2025).
2. Anesi, A., Cavani, F., Chiarini, L., Ferretti, L., et al. (2014). *Preliminary findings of a potentiated piezosurgical device at the rabbit skull*. https://core.ac.uk/download/80171725.pdf (accessed on 14th July 2025).
3. Ciocca, L.; Emiliani, N.; Artuso, G.; Breschi, L.; Marcelli, E.; Cercenelli, L. An Update of Eyeglasses-Supported Nasal–Facial Prosthetic Rehabilitation of Cancer Patients with Post-Surgical Complications: A Case Report. *Appl. Sci.* **2023**, *13*, 4944. https://doi.org/10.3390/app13084944(accessed on 14th July 2025).
4. Kąpa, M., Szepietowski, B., Szustak, J., Wijata, M., Wijata, A. M., Przybyłek-Stępień, Z. A., ... Pasek, P. (2025). Complications and Anatomical Considerations in Botulinum Neurotoxin Type A Injections for Upper Face Rejuvenation: A Systematic Review. *Quality in Sport*, *39*, 58445. https://doi.org/10.12775/QS.2025.39.58445 (accessed on 14th July 2025).
5. Bland, J., Braz, A., Carruthers, J., Cotofana, S., Cottam, H., de Maio, M., Estai, M., et al. (2018). *Development of "core syllabus" for facial anatomy teaching to aesthetic physicians: A Delphi consensus*. https://core.ac.uk/download/157582889.pdf (accessed on 14th July 2025).
6. Bosio, J. A., Bradley, T. G., & Hefti, A. F. (2011). *Moving an incisor across the midline: A treatment alternative in an adolescent patient*. https://core.ac.uk/download/213089332.pdf (accessed on 14th July 2025).
7. Bosio, J. A., Furquim, B. D'Aurea, Maruo, H., Pascotto, R. C., et al. (2008). *The dilemma of the open gingival embrasure between maxillary central incisors*. https://core.ac.uk/download/213084039.pdf (accessed on 14th July 2025).
8. Bottino, A. G., De Simone, M., Laurentini, A., Sforza, C., et al. (2012). *A new 3D tool for planning plastic surgery*. https://core.ac.uk/download/pdf/11429366.pdf (accessed on 14th July 2025).
9. Bradley, J. P., Dubina, E., Ishiyama, A., Lee, M., et al. (2017). *Evaluation of 4 outcomes measures in microtia treatment: Exposures, infections, aesthetics, and psychosocial ramifications*. https://core.ac.uk/download/323076393.pdf (accessed on 14th July 2025).
10. Brauner, E., Ciolfi, A., Di Carlo, S., Guarino, A., et al. (2016). *Pleomorphic adenoma rehabilitative treatment in growing up patient: A 20-years follow-up*. https://core.ac.uk/download/80314602.pdf (accessed on 14th July 2025).
11. Portilla, A. S. P., Portilla, C. S. P., Palacios, G. S. G., Rodríguez, B. S. P., Castillo, S. G. A., Espin, N. E. P., & Pita, G. P. M. (2024). The integration of surgical and dermatological techniques in the treatment of cutaneous aging: multidisciplinary approaches and clinical outcomes - a comprehensive systematic review of current literature. *International Journal of Research in Medical Sciences*, *12*(5), 1659–1667. https://doi.org/10.18203/2320-6012.ijrms20240943(accessed on 14th July 2025).
12. Chen, A. C., German, C., & Zaidel, D. W. (1997). *Brain asymmetry and facial attractiveness: Facial beauty is not simply in the eye of the beholder*. https://core.ac.uk/download/pdf/84385.pdf (accessed on 14th July 2025).

13. Chiappini, T., Correia, J., Taylor, A. M., Van der Merwe, J., & Wessels, Q. (2025). Sculpting the science: Teaching anatomy of the facial muscles to medical students. *International Journal of Medical Students*. https://www.semanticscholar.org/paper/6304896a66c6d62a1a291267 0363cd92a76d6cc3 (accessed on 14th July 2025).

14. Cohen, J. L., & Scuderi, N. (2017). Safety and Patient Satisfaction of AbobotulinumtoxinA for Aesthetic Use: A Systematic Review. *Aesthetic surgery journal, 37*(suppl_1), S32–S44. https://doi.org/10.1093/asj/sjx010(accessed on 14th July 2025).

15. Durairajanayagam, S. (2011). *Anthropometric measurement of the lip-nose complex among young adults in Kuala Lumpur, Malaysia*. https://core.ac.uk/download/143644123.pdf (accessed on 14th July 2025).

16. Edmonds, A. (2014). *Surgery-for-life: Aging, sexual fitness and self-management in Brazil*. Anthropology & Aging Quarterly 2014: 34 (4). https://core.ac.uk/download/28979727.pdf (accessed on 14th July 2025).

17. Hugill, N., Fink, B., & Neave, N. (2010). The role of human body movements in mate selection. *Evolutionary psychology : an international journal of evolutionary approaches to psychology and behavior, 8*(1), 66–89. https://doi.org/10.1177/147470491000800107 (accessed on 14th July 2025).

18. Gunes, H., & Piccardi, M. (2006). *Assessing facial beauty through proportion analysis by image processing and supervised learning*. https://opus.lib.uts.edu.au/bitstream/10453/4141/1/2006005299.pdf (accessed on 14th July 2025).

19. Hannam, A. G., Stavness, I., Lloyd, J. E., & Fels, S. (2008). *Towards predicting biomechanical consequences of jaw reconstruction*. https://core.ac.uk/download/pdf/21747557.pdf (accessed on 14th July 2025).

20. Heng, W., Solomon, S. A., & Gao, W. (2021). Flexible electronics and devices as human–machine interfaces for medical robotics. *Advanced Materials, 34*. https://doi.org/10.1002/adma.202107902 (accessed on 14th July 2025).

21. Hernández-Gómez, J. J., Martínez-Sáez, L., Romero-Ángeles, B., Torres-San-Miguel, A., et al. (2019). *Design and manufacture of a customized temporomandibular prosthesis*. https://core.ac.uk/download/220112110.pdf (accessed on 14th July 2025).

22. Hughes, D., & Song, B. (2016). Dental and Nondental Stem Cell Based Regeneration of the Craniofacial Region: A Tissue Based Approach. *Stem cells international, 2016*, 8307195. https://doi.org/10.1155/2016/8307195(accessed on 14th July 2025).

23. Kim, L. (2013). *Analysis and construction of engaging facial forms and expressions: Interdisciplinary approaches from art, anatomy, engineering, cultural studies, and psychology*. https://core.ac.uk/download/51291628.pdf (accessed on 14th July 2025).

24. Kumar, N. (2021). *Design, development and implementation framework for a postgraduate non-surgical aesthetics curriculum*. A dissertation submitted in partial fulfilment of the requirements for the degree of Doctor of Philosophy of University College London. https://core.ac.uk/download/480391006.pdf (accessed on 14th July 2025).

25. Lim, T. S., Wanitphakdeedecha, R., & Yi, K. H. (2024). Exploring facial overfilled syndrome from the perspective of anatomy and the mismatched delivery of fillers. *Journal of Cosmetic Dermatology, 23*, 1964–1968. https://doi.org/10.1111/jocd.16244 (accessed on 14th July 2025).

26. Marin, E., & Lanzutti, A. (2023). Biomedical applications of titanium alloys: A comprehensive review. *Materials, 17*, 114–114. https://doi.org/10.3390/ma17010114 (accessed on 14th July 2025).

27. Minaoglou, P., Efkolidis, N., Manavis, A., & Kyratsis, P. (2024). A review on wearable product design and applications. *Machines, 12*, 62–62. https://doi.org/10.3390/machines12010062 (accessed on 14th July 2025).

28. Narongdej, P., Hassanpour, M., Alterman, N., Rawlins-Buchanan, F., & Barjasteh, E. (2024). Advancements in clear aligner fabrication: A comprehensive review of direct-3D printing technologies. *Polymers, 16*, 371–371. https://doi.org/10.3390/polym16030371 (accessed on 14th July 2025).

29. Paschoalotto, I. G., Santos, A. R. S., & Tessarin, G. W. L. (2023). *State of the art of orofacial harmonization: A review*. https://core.ac.uk/download/622811968.pdf (accessed on 14th July 2025).

30. Payne, Michael G., "The Reliability Of Facial Soft Tissue Landmarks With Photogrammetry" (2013). Master's Theses (2009 -). Paper 198. http://epublications.marquette.edu/theses_open/198 (accessed on 14th July 2025).

31. Powell-Hicks, A. (2013). *Body objectification, ethnic identity and cosmetic surgery in African-American women*. https://core.ac.uk/download/151738592.pdf (accessed on 14th July 2025).

32. Reiter, A., Yucel, A., Drake, A. G., Hendricks, A., Noller, C., Ambrósio, C. E., Knecht, C. D., et al. (2015). *Impact of facial conformation on canine health: Brachycephalic obstructive airway syndrome*. https://core.ac.uk/download/36778815.pdf (accessed on 14th July 2025).

33. Rho, N. K., Bae, G. Y., Choi, M. S., Chung, W. K., Kim, H. Y., Kim, H. M., Lee, H. K., et al. (2025). Consensus on the cosmetic use of a novel botulinum neurotoxin type A product (NEWLUX®) for facial expression muscles: 2024 guidelines and discussions by Korean experts. *Toxins, 17*. https://www.semanticscholar.org/paper/c621233f309ca09408d238f6d7d0987a5342a251 (accessed on 14th July 2025).

34. Svalina, A. (2024). *Long-Term Treatment Results of Craniosynostosis*. https://core.ac.uk/download/628875143.pdf (accessed on 14th July 2025).

35. Vasconcelos-Berg, R., Desyatnikova, S., Bonavia, P., Chammas, M. C., Navarini, A. A., & Sigrist, R. (2024). Best practices for the use of high-frequency ultrasound to guide aesthetic filler injections—Part 2: Middle third of the face, nose, and tear troughs. *Diagnostics, 14*, 2544–2544. https://doi.org/10.3390/diagnostics14222544 (accessed on 14th July 2025).

PRINCIPLES OF COSMETIC AND RECONSTRUCTIVE SURGERY

2

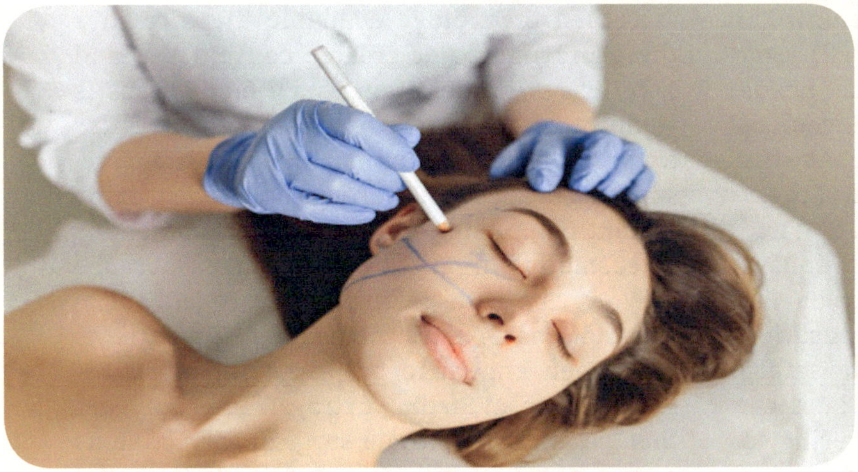

LEARNING OBJECTIVES

After studying this chapter, you will be able to:

1. Define the background history;
2. Identify ethical concerns;
3. Focus on surgical techniques;
4. Define the patient selection criteria;
5. Define the complications and risks;
6. Be familiar with postoperative management.

Introduction

Cosmetic and reconstructive surgery is an evolving specialty that incorporates art and science to improve aesthetic appearance and functional capability. This subspecialty includes a wide range of patient needs from elective cosmetic procedures for appearance enhancement to reconstructive surgery aimed at restoring form and function following trauma, disease, or congenital deformity. The principles behind these surgical endeavors are grounded in an understanding of human anatomy, the psychodynamics of patients, and an ethical obligation to improve patients' quality of life. With advancements in surgical technology and methodology, surgery always attempts to strike the appropriate balance between innovation, safety, and satisfaction for the patients, building the foundations for sophisticated surgical practice to improve function as well as appearance. Furthermore, with the integration of the latest cutting-edge technologies such as regenerative medicine and minimally invasive surgery, cosmetic and reconstructive surgery has been transformed in its scope. They not only enhance surgical outcomes but also reduce recovery times and improve patient satisfaction. For instance, adipose-derived stromal cells (ADSCs) described in recent literature constitute a new avenue for regenerative operations in reconstructive surgery with the potential of enormous therapy in various conditions (Bora & Majumdar, 2017). The interdisciplinary aspect of this field encourages dialogues between surgeons, scientists, and other medical professionals to create an integrated system for the treatment of patients. The teamwork ensures that the techniques used are efficient, safe, and tailored to meet the individual needs of patients in need of cosmetic enhancement as well as reconstructive surgery. As the climate of cosmetic and reconstructive surgery evolves, harmonization of practice with updated clinical guidelines and ethical considerations is important. Modern guidelines emphasize the importance of informed consent, education of the patient, and adherence to safety protocols to minimize the risk of surgical interventions. The importance of adhering to evidence-based practice is evidenced by the current controversies between professional organizations to achieve the optimum quality of care. Also, as in surgical guidelines for the treatment of conditions intersecting with surgical interventions, consideration of patient quality of life and an integral strategy to treatment have become increasingly vital (Speiser et al., 2018). Emphasizing these values not only improves the surgery process but also enables a degree of trust amongst patients and practitioners, affirming the dedication to excellence in the field of cosmetic and reconstructive surgery.

Definition of Cosmetic Surgery

Cosmetic surgery encompasses a subfield of medical practice dedicated to enhancing an individual's aesthetic appearance through surgical and non-surgical procedures. Unlike reconstructive surgery, which focuses on correcting deformities or restoring functionality to the body, cosmetic surgery primarily aims to improve aesthetic attributes, reflecting societal standards of beauty and individual desires for self-improvement. Procedures such as rhinoplasty, breast augmentation, and liposuction are representative of the range of options available, each being tailored to specific patient goals and needs. The growing trend toward cosmetic procedures can be attributed to various reasons, including increased exposure in the media, shifting beauty standards, and increased technology available that provides these procedures at greater convenience and with less risk. Identifying such motivations is significant for medical professionals in order to provide ethical and compassionate care, stressing the need for thorough assessment of the patient before surgery. Sociocultural functions of cosmetic surgery are high-stakes because they overlap with personal identity and social expectations of physical beauty. The patients have been known to grapple with pressures stemming from media portrayals of beauty and then go ahead to pursue surgical correction as a form of conforming to these ideals. Also, the pursuit of beauty through cosmetic procedures raises ethical concerns, particularly about mental health and self-perception. Alteration to appearance is an empowering experience to some but comes with body dysmorphic disorder or unrealistic expectation risks. Here, professionals need to tread the tightrope between enabling desire for enhancement in a patient and safeguarding their mental health. Thus, ethical cosmetic surgery practice demands extensive pre-operative counseling, balancing patient expectations with what can be achieved and emphasizing the necessity of putting mental health at the forefront of decision-making. Taking stock of the ethics that govern cosmetic surgery makes ethical practice central. Surgeons, in addition to the physical alteration of their patients, possess the awareness of the psychological effects of such alterations as a responsibility. Synthesizing evidence-based guidelines and patient-centered care can ensure desirable outcomes, as highlighted in recent clinical practice guidelines for various medical treatments (Speiser et al., 2018). Moreover, the commitment to long-term patient care, as suggested through in-depth studies of issues like disorders of sex development, suggests ongoing discussion and advice following the procedure (Cools et al., 2018). Overall, the phrase cosmetic surgery goes beyond mere enhancement; it is a complex blending of medical ability, ethical consideration, and knowledge of societal influence on personal identity. As the practice evolves, ethical models and patient welfare will become the focus to ensure the integrity of cosmetic surgery procedures (Figure 2.1).

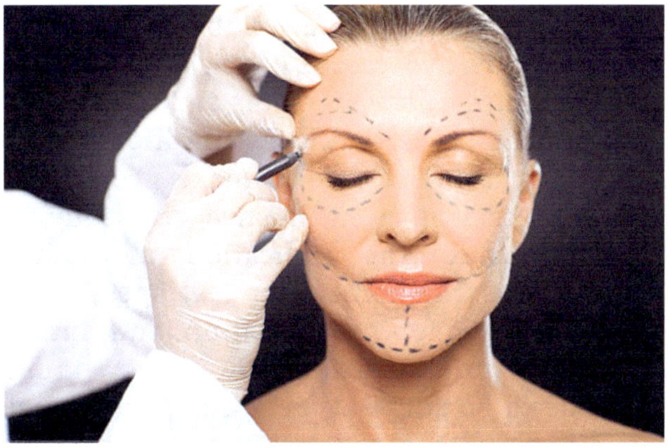

Figure 2.1. Cosmetic surgery encompasses a subfield of medical practice.

Source: https://drvinodvij.com/wp-content/uploads/2024/03/Cosmetic-surgery.png.

Definition of Reconstructive Surgery

Reconstructive surgery plays a pivotal role in the world of medicine, where it is applied mainly to restore function and shape following traumatic injury, congenital deformity, or disease. Unlike cosmetic surgery, whose only interest is in enhancing looks, typically for emotional wellness, reconstructive surgery is therapeutic in nature, treating medical conditions that impair one's functional capability. It encompasses a range of operations, including but not limited to tissue grafting, scar revisions, and major reconstructions following mastectomy or severe burns. This critical distinction emphasizes the role of reconstructive surgery not merely to improve external appearances, but also to facilitate the return of a patient to the pre-condition state quality of life, which in turn aligns with the general ideals of health restoration and wellness. The ethical importance inherent in reconstructive surgery emphasizes its role in policing against the backdrop of modern societal expectations regarding physical appearance. With its medical necessity, reconstructive surgery works to eliminate the perception of surgery as cosmetic. This line is important when considering the endemic culture that supports beauty ideals because military, trauma, and disease wounds always need reconstructive surgery. Where doctors are working, they must balance the need to heal with the potential role of societal pressure as a complicating agent for their clinical judgment. Hence, the ethical basis of reconstructive surgery can be multifariously determined by the same ideals tending to drive the demand for cosmetic enhancements, posing basic questions about the motivations behind surgical interventions and the position of medical professionals within this complex dynamic. Further analysis of reconstructive surgery substantiates the necessity of strict criteria for choosing to ensure well-supported practice. According to research, it is said that medical advisers apply specific preoperative criteria in approving requests for procedures like breast reduction and otoplasty, such criteria maintain the validity of reconstructive activity. For example, statistically significant results show that certain anatomical measurements and age consideration are most critical to determine if or not surgery is indicated (Sonnenfeld et al., 2016). This evidence highlights the importance of entrenched procedures that fortify the basis of equity and medical necessity within reconstructive surgery. These guidelines act to pre-empt grievances about overlap with cosmetics procedures, effectively safeguarding the standards of patient care as a response to the complex interplay of health, function, and societal norms within the context of surgical intervention (Figure 2.2).

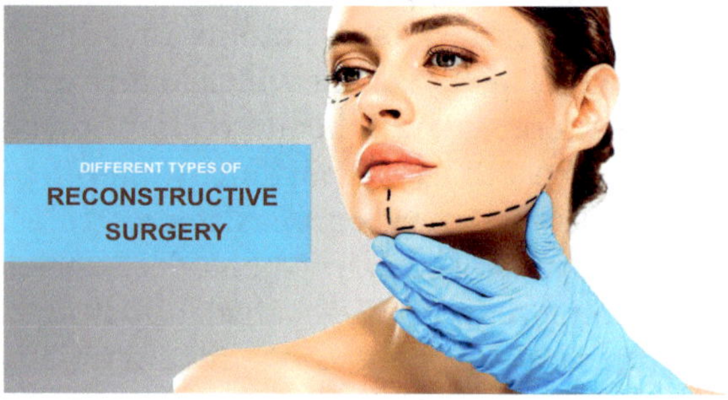

Figure 2.2. Reconstructive surgery occupies a critical place in the medical field.

Source: https://external-content.duckduckgo.com/iu/?u=https%3A%2F%2Fblogger.googleusercontent.com%2Fimg%2Fb%2FR29vZ2xl%2FAVvXsEhhAR-77OEtXDKY8kz7h1EeuYNrPHaJBTpN-bmlRfWYZCefoxXTkQ3AG7z6dnLSsj-NSFceWHwNX5vqQ2M61PYKOFUof7ALP-rnf4SQL3APVfdKsHVMqB2PmWAKt3c-ZWNQYMzzw-7XlVKdq1yAErFjRoOqI2iytyKuG4mDI95Kqjp1A6z-DL3fPbWb%2Fw1200-h630-p-k-no-nu%2FScreenshot%2520(98).png&f=1&nofb=1&ipt=ea48b96ed5c03d249b61d65b297a6265bf9e1e5d3381e1bf8d787a6c7d8dd988.

Importance of Understanding Both Fields

The field of cosmetic and reconstructive surgery is where art meets medical science, and therefore, the importance of knowledge in both disciplines. Aesthetic outcomes, which are the essence of cosmetic surgery, have their foundation in anatomical precision and surgical skill, which are the essence of reconstructive practice. Surgeons who have been trained in both disciplines are best able to utilize the subtleties of human anatomy together with new techniques to provide the most natural-looking outcomes, thereby optimizing patient satisfaction. Dual training allows better use of the reconstructive ideas to be modified for cosmetic treatments and gives the patient a one-stop solution for aesthetic enhancement and restoration of function. Finally, the role of integrating knowledge in both specialties places care in a greater plane, enabling surgeons to better handle the sophisticated needs of individuals who desire both aesthetic appeal and medical improvement. The inclusion of fresh advancements in surgical technology further underscores the necessity of an integral understanding of cosmetic and reconstructive surgery. Innovations such as robot-assisted surgery have revolutionized surgical technique, allowing for more precision and less recovery time, particularly useful in both cosmetic and rehabilitative cases. Physicians with an understanding of the strengths and limitations of the technologies and their application among specialties are best able to make productive use of the machines in practice. As Reddy et al. (2023) state, the applications of robotic surgery cross numerous surgical specialties, emphasizing ongoing education and inter-specialty collaboration. Surgeons must continue to be adept at integrating traditional techniques with cutting-edge methods in an effort to maximize patient satisfaction and outcomes, producing a tradition of ongoing learning and adaptation in an evolving discipline. Also included is the integration of allied medical advances' techniques, such as 3D printing, which helps further validate skill mastery of both reconstructive and cosmetic procedures. Precise pre-operative planning and the creation of individualized custom surgical guides become feasible with this state-of-the-art technology, again enhancing accuracy and success in surgery. With the progression of 3D printing, practitioners are now in a better position to visualize and understand patient-specific anatomy, resulting in patient-tailored interventions that precisely satisfy individual needs. As Meyer-Szary et al. (2022) have seen, this adaptability is especially vital in challenging surgical conditions, enabling informed decision-making and simulation of complex procedures. Emphasizing a keen understanding of both specialties ensures that surgeons are able to make more effective use of these revolutionary advances, ultimately leading to improved patient care and procedural outcomes in an increasingly personalized medicine-oriented environment.

2.1. Historical Background

Learning Outcome

1. Discuss the Origins of Cosmetic Surgery
2. Focus on Development of Reconstructive Techniques
3. Explain Milestones in Surgical Advancements

The history of cosmetic and reconstructive surgery traces its roots back to ancient civilizations, where early surgeons relied on simple techniques to repair damage and imperfections. Historical records indicate that as far back as 600 BC, Indian physician Sushruta performed reconstructive nose and ear repairs employing techniques that laid the basis for modern-day surgical methods. Sushruta's treatise, according to the Sushruta Samhita, highlighted principles of surgical anatomy and the requirement for aseptic technique and thus paved the way for the ethical and practical standards still utilized in surgery today. This early recognition of the potential benefits of surgery is the consistent push to improve body appearances and restore function, a cross-cultural and cross-temporal dedication to caring for the patient. The transition to more sophisticated methods arrived during the Renaissance when anatomical studies revolutionized medical knowledge. Surgeons soon discovered more about the human body's anatomy, and thus, surgery began to shift from the realm of superstition and experiment to one of scientific observation and empirical study. Central figures such as Andreas Vesalius pushed against traditional notions by advocating for direct observation via dissection, which improved surgical accuracy and success. This period laid the foundation for reconstructive surgical techniques that would become a reality in later centuries with the advent of anesthesia and antisepsis during the 19th century. These innovations permitted more extensive operations to be performed safely, resulting in enormous advances in cosmetic and reconstructive procedures. The 20th century was the turning point for the history of reconstructive and cosmetic surgery, as World Wars propelled the field to new levels. The need to repair widespread facial injuries to soldiers encouraged breakthroughs introduced by pioneers like Sir Harold Gillies, who is sometimes referred to as the father of modern plastic surgery. His innovative approaches to rebuilding facial frameworks addressed not only the physical war wounds of the body but also prioritized the psychological requirements of the patient and rehabilitation, encouraging the return of normalcy of appearance. His focus on holistic treatment revolutionized the model of surgical intervention, blending functionality with aesthetic considerations. As the specialty expands, the historical context is a reminder of the ethical obligations and dedication to patients' welfare that must continue in cosmetic and reconstructive surgery practice today.

2.1.1. Origins of Cosmetic Surgery

The ancient cultures find their roots in the history of cosmetic surgery, where the desire to change physical looks was often associated with religion and cultural beliefs. In India, for example, there is evidence that surgical procedures intended to change features trace back to approximately 600 B.C. In the ancient texts, such as the Sushruta Samhita, there are procedures like rhinoplasty and facial injury reconstruction, which demonstrate an advanced understanding of surgical principles resonating through contemporary practices. These initial procedures were as much about social status and allure as they were about restoring form, suggesting that cosmetic motivations are not a modern-day phenomenon but have roots going back centuries. Such treatments underscore a persistent human desire to improve oneself and look better, paving the way for the developing specialty of cosmetic surgery that would come in subsequent centuries. With the evolution of the art and science of medicine through the Middle Ages and Renaissance periods, cosmetic surgery developed from an amateurish undertaking into a more formalized area of practice. Surgeons in those days, having read the classical literature, started making procedures standardized, both with the aim of reconstructive as well as aesthetic outcomes. The Barbers Guild, which had played such a central role in surgery in the 16th century, began to differentiate between healing and cosmetic practice. Better understanding of anatomy and surgical methods, prompted by figures such as Ambroise Paré, widened the range of procedures available and increased still further the esteem in which possibilities for surgery to mend and to enhance were held. During this time, cultural definitions of beauty also started to evolve, becoming more and more linked with perceptions of morality and character, thus setting the stage for contemporary cosmetic practice. The 19th century was a watershed moment in the history of cosmetic surgery as developments in anesthesia and antisepsis altered surgical safety and possibilities. The work of pioneers like Sir Harold Gillies in World War I, who pioneered ways of facial reconstruction of war-injured soldiers, underscored the importance of cosmetic surgery to reinstate dignity and identity. With the line blurring between reconstructive and sheerly cosmetic surgery, the specialty gained acceptance more among the medical profession and the public. The growing interest in physical appearance, the emergence of a cult celebrity culture, and the growth of media that mirrored ideals of beauty propelled cosmetic surgery into the mainstream. These nascent developments reflect a convergence of technological innovation and sociocultural evolution that universally influenced the principles that guide both cosmetic and reconstructive surgery today (Figure 2.3).

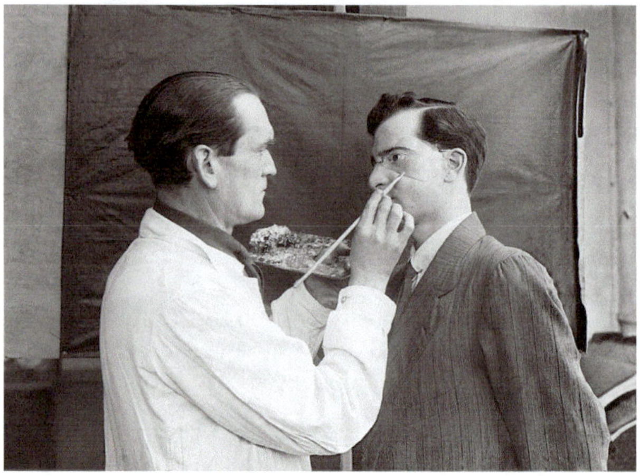

Figure 2.3. The origins of cosmetic surgery.

Source: https://external-content.duckduckgo.com/iu/?u=https%3A%2F%2Fwww.warhistoryonline.com%2Fwp-content%2Fuploads%2F2019%2F03%2F800px-the_development_of_reconstructive_plastic_surgery_during_the_first_world_war_q30457.jpg&f=1&nofb=1&ipt=3d6fcce5857d4765441b46df712298c4340da4bc6c40ead7bb06230a189657fa.

2.1.2. Development of Reconstructive Techniques

The history of reconstructive techniques, particularly for oncoplastic surgery, has had a significant role in influencing present practice in cosmetic and reconstructive surgery. Historically, the emphasis was placed on the functional need of patients for breast cancer operations. Once improvements in surgical technique started to evolve, the emphasis shifted towards not only preserving but also enhancing aesthetic outcomes. Growing realization of the psychological impact of unsatisfactory aesthetic results has placed surgeons in a position to strive higher for more favorable cosmetic forms following surgery. This change reflects a more universal realization of the double-pronged focus on beauty and health in surgical treatment, accentuating the multidisciplinary process involved in contemporary reconstructive surgery. The integration of advanced methods has now turned into a necessity in the alleviation of psychological pain, most frequently associated with malignancies and their treatment (Citgez et al., 2022). The incorporation of oncoplastic techniques is the best illustration of the integration of oncology principles and an aesthetic vision in enhancing the quality of care being imparted to breast cancer patients. Surgeons now employ methods such as therapeutic mammoplasty and fibroglandular flap advancement to correct extensive tumor excisions while preserving, to the extent possible, the outside attractiveness of the breast. These methods have not only resulted in improved cosmetic outcomes but have also reduced mastectomy requirements in most individuals. By enabling surgeons to undertake wide local excisions with exquisite cosmetic outcomes, these methods contribute to enhancing women's overall well-being and body image. In the case of breast reconstruction, advances in autologous and implant reconstruction have also led the way to new frontiers of reconstructing with immediate and delayed reconstructions, presenting possibilities for managing the diverse needs of patients (Citgez et al., 2022). Along with this, the advent of acellular dermal matrix (ADM) as well as improved liposuction technology has transformed the practice of reconstructive surgery. The ADM application has minimized donor site morbidity but expanded the reconstructive options, leading to patient satisfaction. Liposuction and incorporation into the lipo-modelling procedure are other examples of technology enhancing cosmetic outcomes from procedures. Surgeons now possess a greater arsenal at their disposal, with the end result being a refined technique to manage complicated reconstructive cases. With such advancements, oncoplastic surgery has developed, leading to an increased demand from patients towards aesthetically satisfactory results as well as effective therapeutic procedures. Such growth calls attention to the contribution of advancements in reconstructive techniques to the larger context of principles of cosmetic and reconstructive surgery, symbolizing a commitment to better functioning as well as appearance (Carmichael et al., 2016) (Figure 2.4).

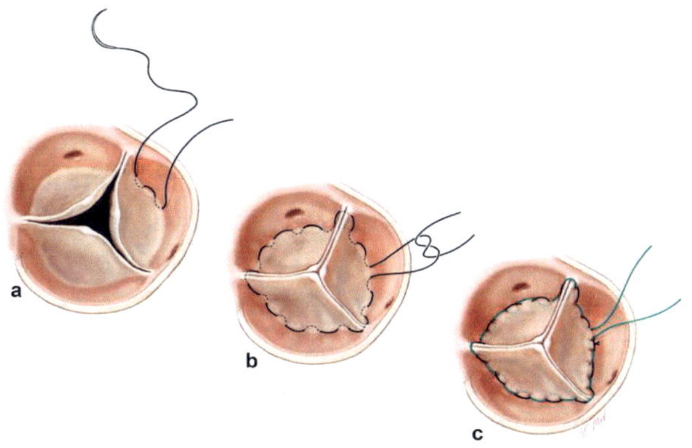

Figure 2.4. Development of reconstructive techniques.

Source: https://external-content.duckduckgo.com/iu/?u=https%3A%2F%2Fstorage.googleapis.com%2Fdl.dentistrykey.com%2Fclinical%2FReconstructiveTechniques%2F0_3s20B9780721691688500253.jpg&f=1&nofb=1&ipt=082b6877dbe7b772ab85aa815f24f233c1ca2652a67503d2542a2e0a5a1f662a.

2.1.3. Milestones in Surgical Advancements

Cosmetic and reconstructive surgery history has been marked by dramatic turning points in the development of these fields, both in terms of technique and patient outcome. Among the landmarks in this development is the use of 3D bioprinting technology, a combination of additive manufacturing and biology to create complex tissue architecture. This new approach not only supports reproducibility in tissue engineering but also answers the imperative need for personalized medicine. Although there is a growing call for treatments that are suited to the patient, researchers as well as industry players are being drawn towards 3D bioprinting, which is promising to exert its disruptive impact on surgery. Biologic tissue and organ reproductive ability can revolutionize preoperative planning and postoperative recovery, enhancing cosmetic and reconstructive patient care standards (Santoni et al., 2021). Another such game-changer in surgical technology is prepectoral breast reconstruction, which is also increasingly popular due to its benefit of maintaining pectoralis major muscle anatomy and function. This approach eliminates some of the drawbacks of traditional approaches, such as muscle damage and prolonged recovery. A retrospective audit of 1,450 procedures has provided extensive evidence, verifying the safety and efficacy of this technique and controlling potential complications like capsular contracture and implant loss. The substantial evidence of this multicenter work has contributed considerably to the understanding of prepectoral breast reconstruction and hence paved the way for more informed patient selection and customized management of postoperative care. Such milestones in research point out the importance of evidence-based approaches in surgical development and how these guide modern reconstructive practice (Masià, 2020). In addition, advances in technology and surgical techniques have ushered in an era of new safety and efficacy in cosmetic and reconstructive surgery. Enhanced recovery protocols and minimally invasive surgical procedures have not only improved the outcomes of surgery but also minimized the pain of patients and recovery times. Procedures are being performed with precision and less trauma, which is most crucial in the cosmetic sector where looks matter the most. Moreover, greater integration of artificial intelligence and machine learning in surgical planning and execution indicates a step towards more sophisticated surgical methods. This meeting of technology and surgery is a part of a greater tendency towards patient-focused care, which is still the crux of the principles of reconstructive and cosmetic surgery. The adoption of such pioneering developments ensures that surgical approaches stay at the forefront, responding to the evolving needs and requirements of patients in the quest for life-transforming outcomes (Figure 2.5).

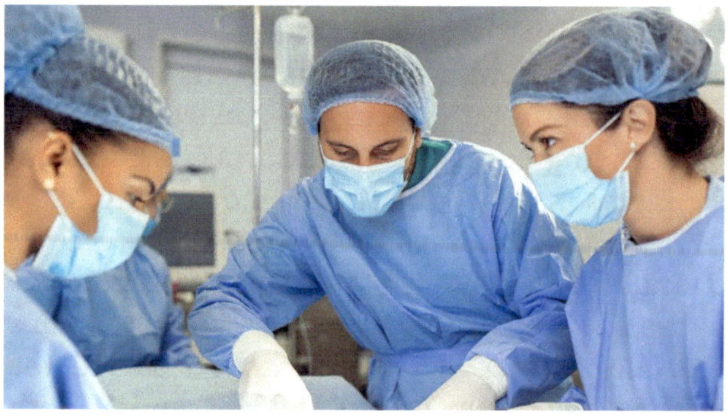

Figure 2.5. Milestones in surgical advancements.

Source: https://external-content.duckduckgo.com/iu/?u=https%3A%2F%2Flirp.cdn-website.com%2F9c17b0aa%2Fdms3rep%2Fmulti%2Fopt%2Ftheatre%2Bnurses%2Btalking-1920w.webp&f=1&nofb=1&ipt=92e9ab6bc9c6d908eb1c048002c580aca1f1e885f633d0f5029c6986c2cab4a7.

Test Your Knowledge

1. Which historical documents provide evidence of early cosmetic procedures such as rhinoplasty?
2. How did the introduction of anesthesia and antisepsis transform reconstructive surgery?
3. What technological innovation marked a turning point in minimally invasive surgical procedures?

2.2. Ethical Considerations

Learning Outcome

1. Discuss Patient Consent and Autonomy
2. Explain the Psychological Impacts of Surgery
3. Focus on Ethical Dilemmas in Cosmetic Procedures

Cosmetic and reconstructive surgery is driven by ethical concerns, which are the prime mover of practitioner actions in offering accountable and patient-centered care. Surgeons must deal with the consequences of their procedures, particularly in cosmetic surgery, where motivations may often extend beyond medical necessity to encompass desires for personal appearance. The challenge is how to balance ethically patient satisfaction with potential psychological impact. Surgeons must assure patients that they have correct expectations and a complete understanding of risks. This care responsibility is also according to the ethical principles of beneficence and non-maleficence, which test practitioners to prioritize patients' welfare while avoiding harm. With the increasing popularity of cosmetic surgery, ethical observation becomes essential to maintain professional standards and protect patients with the protection of their welfare. Further, new technologies applied in cosmetic and reconstructive surgery call for constant ethical scrutiny. The introduction of robot-assisted surgery and advanced methods such as 3D printing has reshaped surgical practice, ensuring unprecedented precision and customization of patient care. While such innovations pose challenges of access, equity, and informed consent, the same must be established on certain bases. For instance, since robotic surgery is associated with improved outcomes, the cost and technical feasibility may limit its provision to a specific subgroup of the population, hence sustaining health inequities. Similarly, with technologies like 3D printing making it possible for customized surgical methods and patient-specific anatomy modeling, practitioners have to tread the line between innovation and ethical regulation in a manner that prevents progress at the cost of patient safety or access equity. Resolving these challenges is important to ensuring that the development of surgical practice continues to be aligned with the core principles of medical ethics. In addition to these functional issues, the psychological implications of cosmetic and reconstructive surgery must be properly addressed ethically. Evidence indicates that patients seeking cosmetic procedures often have psychological issues, thus bringing into question the validity of certain interventions. Ethical practicing surgeons are required to conduct thorough psychological evaluations to identify a patient's motivations and verify whether interventions will address ingrained pathologies or simply fulfill selfish desires. Besides, informed consent is not merely a discussion of the benefits and risks but also an evaluation of the patients' psychological readiness for surgery and possible post-surgery outcomes. Thus, the interplay between surgical practice and psychological health must be outlined in the ethical practice of reconstructive and cosmetic surgery. Through vigilant attention to these ethical issues, practitioners can establish a more ethical and responsible practice of patient care, aligning their practices with the ultimate goals of health and well-being.

2.2.1. Patient Consent and Autonomy

The morality of cosmetic and reconstructive surgery is closely related to concepts of patient consent and autonomy. Patient consent in medical ethics is most crucial because it enables people to be capable of making decisions regarding their bodies and treatments. Surgeons must provide clear, understandable information on the risks, benefits, and probabilities of proposed procedures. Transparency leads to a condition where patients can practice autonomy, which means participation in decisions that are best suited to their own values and desires. Enhancing the process of decision-making means recognizing that patients will have varying degrees of comprehension and providing individualized educational materials to ensure that they are fully empowered in their consent process. Moreover, the evolving nature of medical technology with technological advances such as robotic surgery merely compounds the challenge of the dynamic of patient autonomy and consent. With these innovative techniques offering newer avenues for more efficient and safer procedures, they also pose ethical concerns regarding informed consent. The patients must be informed not just of the advantages of such technology but also of the limitations, potential complications, as well as the surgeon's skill with the device. Introduction of robotic systems in surgery is just one of the ways medical innovations are intricate in nature and call for extensive discussions on risks versus benefits, which have to be presented to allow the patient to make decisions that are reflective of their will and autonomy in the context of their surgical experience (Reddy et al., 2023). Extensive care must also be exerted while caring for complicated medical ailments that necessitate high-impact surgeries affecting the patient quality of life. As emphasized by new recommendations such as those for congenital adrenal hyperplasia, an integrated approach that includes patient safety, informed consent, and quality of life is a requirement in surgical practice (Speiser et al., 2018). The process of acquiring consent is not a legal ceremony, but an ethical necessity that reaffirms the partnership between patient and healthcare provider. Having patients engaged in discussion about their intended outcomes of health and treatment preferences should be a cornerstone, ensuring they are respected in their autonomy. Promoting this team atmosphere is useful in enhancing patient trust and satisfaction and, ultimately, the success of cosmetic and reconstructive surgical procedures in general (Figure 2.6).

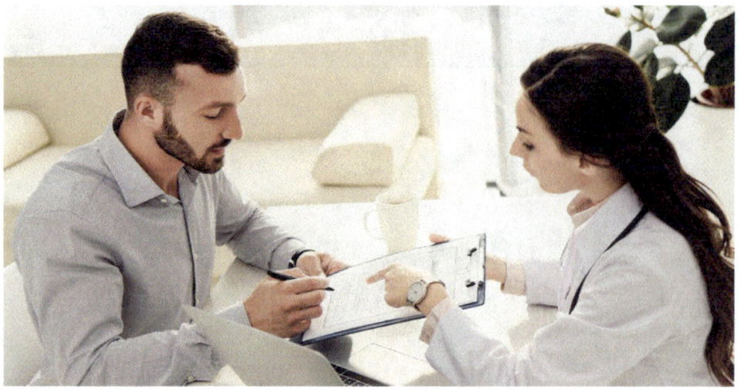

Figure 2.6. Patient consent and autonomy.

Source: https://external-content.duckduckgo.com/iu/?u=https%3A%2F%2Fmedia.post.rvohealth.io%2Fwp-content%2Fuploads%2F2019%2F10%2FPatient_Doctor_Signing_1200x628-facebook.jpg&f=1&nofb=1&ipt=3809627b61e2e53acf768fcaf8a4ce2a6518d2cc2739a8a918679652701d24ed.

2.2.2. Psychological Impacts of Surgery

The psychological impact of surgery, particularly in reconstructive and cosmetic surgery, is now widely recognized as a vital part of patient management. The patient arrives for surgery with an array of emotions, such as fear, depression, and an alteration in body image. These reactions can be associated with a variety of factors, including the invasive nature of the procedures, uncertainty of results, and social pressure for physical appearance. The fact that surgery anxiety exists is an argument for preoperative psychological assessments to become the rule and not the exception. In this manner, the emotional aftermaths of the surgeries are adequately prepared for by the patients, and finally, there is greater satisfaction with the outcome of the surgeries (Bülent Çıtgez et al., 2022). Moreover, their psychological aspects can be treated in order to avoid complications and make the surgical practice more integrative into the health frameworks. The advent of oncoplastic surgery has provided new avenues for reducing psychological upset among breast cancer patients. Traditional surgical methods like mastectomy, although life-saving, leave the patient grappling with severe body image issues and a compromised sense of femininity. In contrast, oncoplastic surgery is focused not only on excising the cancer but also on restoring form, thereby improving psychological well-being and overall life quality. As mentioned, these novel techniques have been demonstrated to provide great cosmetic results with equal survival rates, boosting patients' confidence after surgery (Bülent Çıtgez et al., 2022). Through placement of emphasis on aesthetic factors in reconstructive surgery, practitioners can profoundly influence patients' emotional recovery, indicating that there may be a high degree of correlation between good surgical results and good mental health.

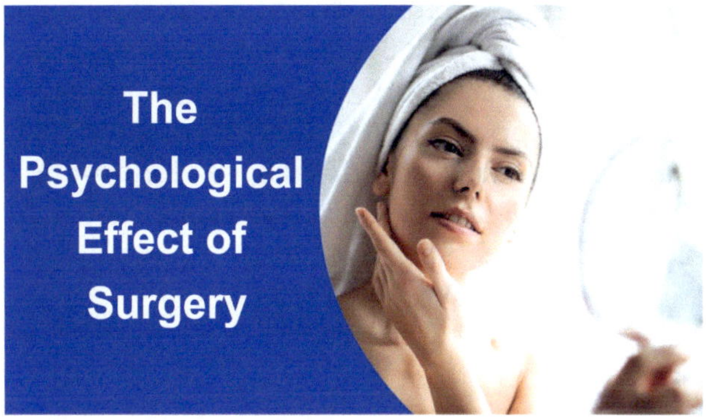

Figure 2.7. The psychological impacts of surgery.

Source: https://external-content.duckduckgo.com/iu/?u=https%3A%2F%2Fi.ytimg.com%2Fvi%2FXWnzCMfvGeE%2Fmaxresdefault.jpg&f=1&nofb=1&ipt=0ce2e227b4905a71bd3df5e02bb2708266aeaf92fdd9992aa6217eb7e0fd3e5e.

Additionally, the new social dynamics that developed as a result of the COVID-19 pandemic have brought the issue of the need for psychological counseling in the domain of cosmetic surgery to the forefront. With the advent of virtual interactions via video conferencing, it has made many people very self-conscious of their own faces, often causing increased dissatisfaction and body dysmorphic problems. These trends highlight the importance of giving consideration to psychological factors during cosmetic consultation and surgical planning. Surgeons must be attuned to such altered social pressures and include mental health screening and support systems in their practice. This anticipation is critical in prepping patients for surgery's life-altering processes and offering a safer and more supportive environment that tames the complex interplay between physical appearance and emotional health (Figure 2.7).

2.2.3. Ethical Dilemmas in Cosmetic Procedures

The ethical concerns of cosmetic procedures stem from the intersection of patient autonomy and the duty of medical providers. Because the procedures are generally voluntary and not for health purposes, the simplest question is whether or not the informed consent process works. Patients seeking enhancements are also under societal pressure and unrealistic standards of appearance perpetuated by the media, which undermine their autonomy of choice. Doctors need to overcome the hurdle of keeping patients well-informed of potential risks, psychological impacts, and realistic outcomes of cosmetic treatments. This ethical conflict is meant to highlight the importance of finding a balance between patients' desires and the duty of physicians to notify and safeguard their health, hence the importance of ongoing debate on ethical practice in cosmetic surgery (Pressman et al., 2024). Lack of standardization of training and practices among professionals is also an imperative one in aesthetic medicine. Most individuals involved in cosmetic procedures have various levels of education, and that leads to a disparity in the ethical levels and skills. An unevenness exists that makes individuals doubt the safety of the patients and the integrity of the procedure performed. As contemplated, the ethical implications of aesthetic treatments can further be intertwined with society's perspective in the wake of social media towards beauty, where being attractive and successful is commonly equated with youthful appearance (da Prato et al., 2024). The arrival of non-medically trained individuals performing such procedures outside of the controlled environment aggravates the ethical concerns since the patients may be treated sub-optimally or develop complications from incompetent operators. The intersection of technological advancement and cosmetic surgery adds new ethical dilemmas. With the growing use of artificial intelligence and big language models in surgery, there are three prominent ethical concerns: bias, confidentiality of patients, and the correctness of information provided by these models (Pressman et al., 2024). While they can enhance surgical performance and patient satisfaction, they raise concerns of ownership of data and liability in case of complications. While professionals strive to uphold the principles of beneficence and nonmaleficence, the need for robust ethical frameworks is imperative. Interdisciplinary collaboration in establishing ethical guidelines in cosmetic procedures will strive to ensure not just patient well-being but also to validate aesthetic medicine as a science for safety, confidentiality, and artistic integrity in changing appearance (da Prato et al., 2024) (Figure 2.8).

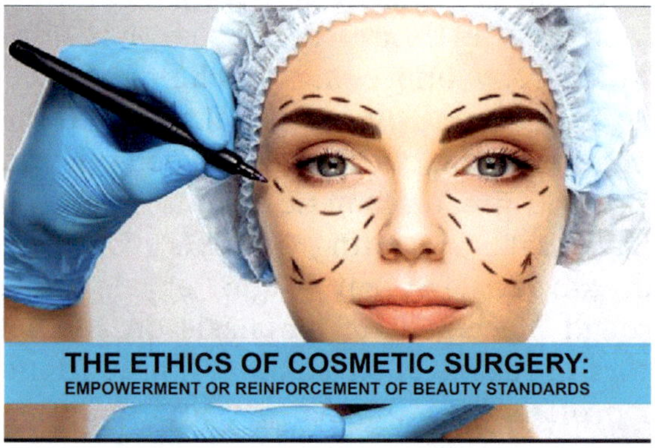

Figure 2.8. The ethical dilemmas surrounding cosmetic procedures.

Source: https://external-content.duckduckgo.com/iu/?u=https%3A%2F%2Faemagazine.pk%2Fposts%2Fthe_ethics_of_cosmetic_surgery_empowerment_or_reinforcement_of_beauty_standards.png&f=1&nofb=1&ipt=c89740ba3326218aa79fb92ad29fc02cc251fa40223713ff0a2baa7f579d7576.

Test Your Knowledge

1. What key elements must be included for informed consent to be considered valid in cosmetic surgery?
2. How can body dysmorphic disorder (BDD) affect the outcomes and ethics of cosmetic surgery?
3. What ethical challenges occur when patients request procedures that may be medically unnecessary or risky?

2.3. Surgical Techniques

Learning Outcome

1. Discuss the Common Cosmetic Procedures
2. Explain Reconstructive Surgery Techniques
3. Focus on Innovations in Surgical Technology

In the realm of reconstructive and cosmetic surgery, the adoption of advanced surgical techniques is a key factor in enhancing patient outcomes and aesthetic results. Techniques such as microsurgery and flap reconstruction have revolutionized the field, allowing surgeons to reconstruct complicated deficits while maintaining donor site morbidity to a bare minimum. For instance, microsurgical techniques enable the transplant of vascularized tissue from one site to another, a function crucial in reconstructive surgery following trauma or oncologic resections. The great level of attention to detail in these techniques, combined with enhanced imaging and preoperative planning, enables surgeons to reestablish function while achieving more aesthetic results, demonstrating that mastery of surgical technique is a necessity to the principles of effective cosmetic and reconstructive surgery. Oncoplastic surgery, a new technique integrating oncological and plastic surgery, is the other significant advance in the area. Oncoplastic surgery allows for massive resection of the tumor with concurrent restoration of breast form to reduce the psychological impact of cancer treatment. Oncoplastic procedures involve meticulous planning and consideration of many parameters, such as breast volume, tumor location, and amount of tissue lost. The synthesis of oncoplastic principles not only provides improved cosmetic outcomes but also enhances quality of life for patients, aligned with the universal intent of reconstructive surgery to reestablish form and function. Further evolution of these surgical procedures is designed to minimize mastectomy rates with no loss of local and long-term survival rates, thereby becoming the centerpiece of reconstructive practice today (Çıtgez et al., 2022). Further, the emphasis on evidence-based practice within plastic and reconstructive surgery emphasizes requirements for level evidence clinical research in order to establish surgical techniques. The attempt to grade presented evidence for strength within plastic surgery literature illustrates a need to enhance the quality of care provided to patients. By grading studies based on evidence, professionals can better assess the evidence-based validity of different surgical procedures and make informed decisions for their implementation. Evidence-based practice ensures maximum patient outcomes because it ensures the implementation of methods proven to work based on high-quality evidence (Sullivan et al., 2021). As the specialty continues to develop, the continued interaction between surgical innovation and empirical evidence will remain essential to the pursuit of excellence in cosmetic and reconstructive surgery (Figure 2.9).

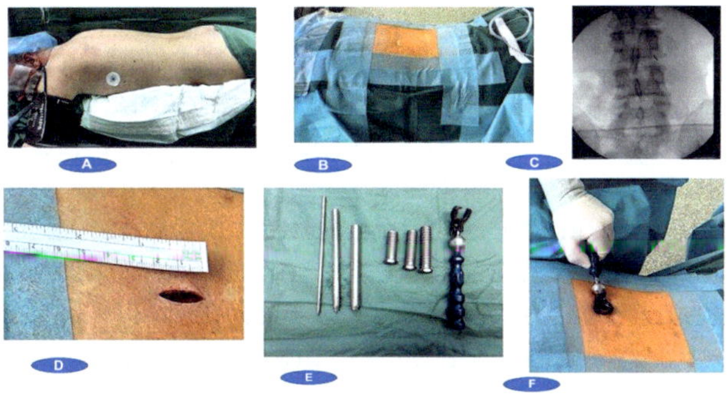

Figure 2.9. The realm of cosmetic and reconstructive surgery.

Source: https://external-content.duckduckgo.com/iu/?u=https%3A%2F%2Fwww.researchgate.net%2Fpublication%2F349870445%2Ffigure%2Ffig3%2FAS%3A11431281084468239%401663206885281%2FStep-by-step-explanation-of-the-surgical-technique-part-1.jpg&f=1&nofb=1&ipt=ddd757d4e63107f49191b37b370f38a423fbe6cc5254fe1677f4c55d7fa0a1f2.

2.3.1. Common Cosmetic Procedures

Recent years have seen common cosmetic procedures achieve broad popularity, an indicator of the social trend toward optimizing personal appearance. Rhinoplasty, breast augmentation, and liposuction are three of the most frequently requested procedures. Both a cosmetic and functional enhancement is carried out in rhinoplasty by reshaping the nose to improve its appearance as well as potentially treat obstructive airway issues. Such dual purpose is evidence of the principle of reconciling function and form, a pillar tenet in plastic surgery protocols. Furthermore, augmentation of the breasts through implantation or fat grafting meets the desire for increased breast volume and shape. Such changes not only change physical appearance but also very much affect self-esteem, highlighting the psychological implications that should always go with cosmetic procedures (Speiser et al., 2018). Liposuction, another very common cosmetic procedure, works mostly on localized fat deposits, allowing for body shaping for those who might not get to a preferred look based on diet and exercise. The technique involves the use of several modalities, including tumescent, ultrasound-guided, and laser modalities, each with its own strengths appropriate to patient goals. The options are reflected in the importance of individualized surgical treatments based on specific needs, which conforms to the principles of plastic surgery emphasizing accurate planning and action (Rohrich et al., 2017). Moreover, it reflects awareness of patient anatomy and the intended outcome to prove that surgical treatment has respect for body contours and achieves maximum aesthetic value. Thus, these common procedures are reflective of the union of art and science of cosmetic surgery. Moreover, non-surgical cosmetic treatments such as Botox and dermal fillers have also gained widespread popularity, offering patients a facial rejuvenation alternative that is less time-consuming and less costly than that of surgical procedures. Botox, being a neurotoxin, works by temporarily paralyzing specified muscles to minimize the appearance of wrinkles and fine lines. Dermal fillers, however, restore the lost volume due to aging by filling the nasolabial folds, cheeks, and lips. Dermal fillers are low-risk interventions, as the principles of cosmetic surgery mandate, aimed at safety, patient satisfaction, and the necessity to achieve a natural result that improves one without visible change (Speiser et al., 2018). As cosmetic surgery continues to move forward, it keeps patient-centered practice and ethical practice in check, ensuring ubiquitous procedures effectively treat the aesthetic outcomes and emotional health of individuals who choose to enhance themselves (Figure 2.10).

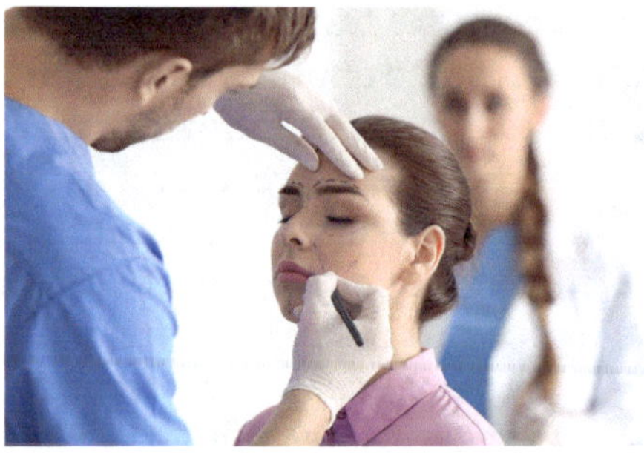

Figure 2.10. Common cosmetic procedures.

Source: https://external-content.duckduckgo.com/iu/?u=https%3A%2F%2Fwww.beastbeauty.co.uk%2Fwp-content%2Fuploads%2F2022%2F07%2FMost-Common-Plastic-Surgery-Procedures.jpg&f=1&nofb=1&ipt=1159e20cedda5709db4a487af45f6b9afcd5385dc4f6aa34fcf245e9579c7f40.

2.3.2. Reconstructive Surgery Techniques

Reconstructive surgery encompasses a range of techniques that help restore function and aesthetics to compromised or altered body structures. This field is founded on the practice of evidence-based medicine, which demands high-quality, science-driven practices. Techniques such as microsurgery, in which nerves and vessels are repaired, have revolutionized the treatment of traumatic injuries. A second mainstay of reconstruction, skin grafting, is widely applied to resurface defects caused by cancer resections, burns, and trauma. These strategies demonstrate an integrated approach to the restoration of not only the physical appearance but also the psychological well-being of patients, as effective reconstructive surgery has the potential to facilitate significant quality-of-life improvements. Continuing enhancements in surgical technique and technology ensure that reconstructive surgery remains a dynamic, ongoing field, responsive to the needs of diverse patient populations (Sullivan et al., 2021). Tissue engineering and regenerative medicine represent the future of reconstructive surgery with innovative solutions for complex clinical challenges. Through biomaterials and bioactive factors, surgeons are able to initiate the body's internal healing mechanisms and stimulate tissue regeneration. Techniques such as three-dimensional bioprinting are being established to create scaffolds for tissue replacement, which can improve the results of reconstructive surgery. This union of engineering science and practice of medicine is not only possible for the betterment of existing methodologies but also for the development of new modalities. Additionally, such technological advances necessitate ongoing research and rigorous examination to ascertain their safety and efficacy, further highlighting the importance of evidence-based principles in surgical practice (Rohrich et al., 2020). As these technologies become more advanced, they contain revolutionary power in the realm of reconstructive surgery that brings about procedures previously not possible. Multidisciplinary collaboration is paramount in this area of reconstructive surgery, as sophisticated cases require input from various specialties. Plastic surgeons, orthopedists, oncologists, and rehabilitation experts must be able to work well together in creating holistic treatment plans tailored specifically to individual patients. This team practice enhances the surgical result and minimizes the risk of complications, leading to better postoperative healing. Furthermore, the inclusion of patient-centered care within reconstructive practice allows for better communication and understanding of patient expectations, thereby enhancing the relationship between the surgical team and the patient. Through the inclusion of multidisciplinary teams and adherence to advancing techniques, not only is bodily restoration enhanced by reconstructive surgery, but overall well-being is also catered to, which demonstrates the nature of principles surrounding this life-saving specialty (Sullivan et al., 2021) (Figure 2.11).

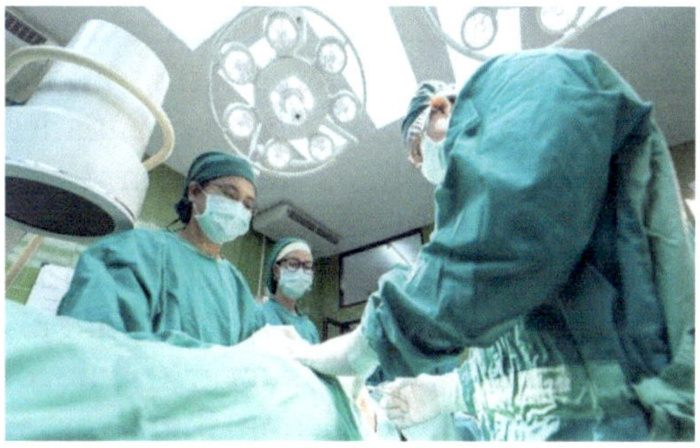

Figure 2.11. Reconstructive surgery encompasses a variety of techniques.

Source: https://www.rgcirc.org//wp-content/uploads/2020/02/Reconstructive-surgery.jpg.

2.3.3. Innovations in Surgical Technology

Advancements in surgical technology have revolutionized the field of cosmetic and reconstructive surgery, enabling more precise, less invasive procedures. One of the most significant innovations is the integration of artificial intelligence (AI) into surgical practices. This technology enhances diagnostic accuracy, treatment planning, and outcome predictions, leading to improved patient care. As noted in recent literature, AI applications have increased in orthodontics, facilitating tasks such as dental diagnostics and cephalometric evaluations, which align closely with reconstructive surgical planning. The careful implementation of AI underscores its potential to assist surgeons in making informed decisions while navigating complex anatomical structures. However, despite its efficacy, the inherent complexity and unpredictability of AI algorithms necessitate manual validation and a cautious approach in clinical settings, emphasizing the need for ongoing scrutiny and refinement in the integration of AI-driven solutions in surgery (Kazimierczak et al., 2024). Robotic surgery represents another groundbreaking innovation that has transformed various surgical specialties, including cosmetic and reconstructive surgery. These robotic systems offer enhanced precision, control, and visualization, which are crucial for delicate procedures. By facilitating minimally invasive techniques, robotic surgery significantly reduces recovery times and complications while enhancing the overall patient experience. According to current research, the applications of robotic systems extend across numerous surgical domains such as general surgery, gynecology, and orthopedics, highlighting their versatility and effectiveness. As the integration of these technologies becomes more widespread, the potential for personalized medicine increases, allowing for tailored surgical interventions that address individual patient needs. However, the successful adoption of robotic surgery involves overcoming challenges, including high costs and the necessity for specialized training, which remain pivotal for maximizing its benefits (Reddy et al., 2023). In addition to robotics and AI, other innovative technologies, such as augmented reality (AR) and 3D printing, have emerged, further advancing surgical techniques and outcomes. AR provides surgeons with enhanced visualization tools, overlaying critical data during procedures that improve spatial understanding and surgical accuracy. This technology can be especially beneficial in reconstructive surgery, where precise anatomical alignment is vital. Moreover, 3D printing has the potential to revolutionize preoperative planning and intraoperative practices by allowing surgeons to create patient-specific anatomical models. These innovations facilitate more effective communication with patients regarding their surgical options and outcomes, fostering a collaborative approach to care. Collectively, these advancements signify a transformative shift in cosmetic and reconstructive surgery, emphasizing the critical role of technology in enhancing procedural efficacy and patient safety. As the future unfolds, continuous integration and ethical governance of these innovations will be essential to ensuring their successful application in surgical practice (Figure 2.12).

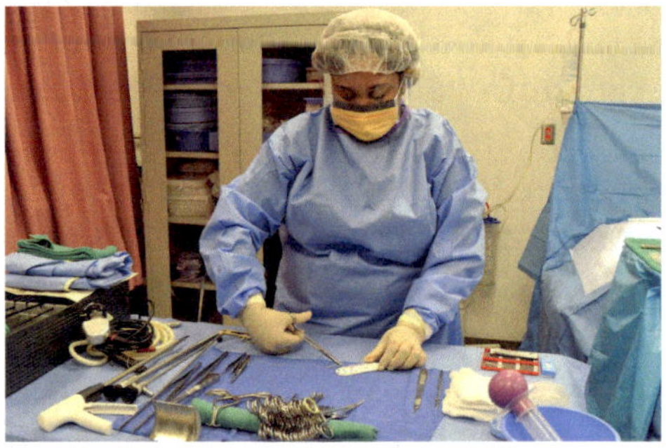

Figure 2.12. Innovations in surgical technology.

Source: https://mgccc.edu/wp-content/uploads/2019/08/GRD3438.jpg.

Test Your Knowledge

1. How do minimally invasive cosmetic techniques differ from traditional surgical approaches?
2. What principles guide the choice between skin grafts and local or free flaps in reconstructive surgery?
3. How are 3D imaging and computer-assisted planning transforming preoperative assessment and surgical accuracy?

2.4. Patient Selection Criteria

Learning Outcome

1. Discuss the Assessing Medical History
2. Explain the Psychological Evaluation
3. How to Setting Realistic Expectations

In the realm of cosmetic and reconstructive surgery, patient selection criteria serve as a foundational pillar that significantly influences surgical outcomes and patient satisfaction. Candidates for procedures must meet certain physical and psychological prerequisites to ensure both safety and efficacy. These criteria typically include factors such as age, overall health, and realistic expectations regarding surgical results. Patients who are too young may lack the psychological maturity required to comprehend the implications of surgery, while individuals with chronic health issues may face increased surgical risks. Moreover, surgeons assess the psychological readiness of candidates to navigate the emotional aspects of surgical transformations, which underscores the importance of a comprehensive evaluation before any intervention. A deeper analysis of patient selection criteria reveals that the decision-making process is often complex, especially in the context of cosmetic surgery. Many potential candidates are influenced by societal standards and external perceptions, particularly as social media plays a pivotal role in shaping their expectations and desires. Studies indicate that a significant proportion of plastic surgery patients rely on social media as a credible resource for information and guidance, further complicating the selection process. Scarcella et al. (2022) highlight that individuals with negative self-images frequently seek cosmetic enhancements and may pursue surgery based solely on social media portrayals. This increasing trend necessitates that surgeons adopt a more rigorous evaluation framework to mitigate risks and eliminate candidates whose motivations may stem from superficial or transient influences. Furthermore, the ethical dimension of patient selection criteria cannot be overlooked, particularly when considering non-board-certified surgeons operating in spaces influenced by social media trends.

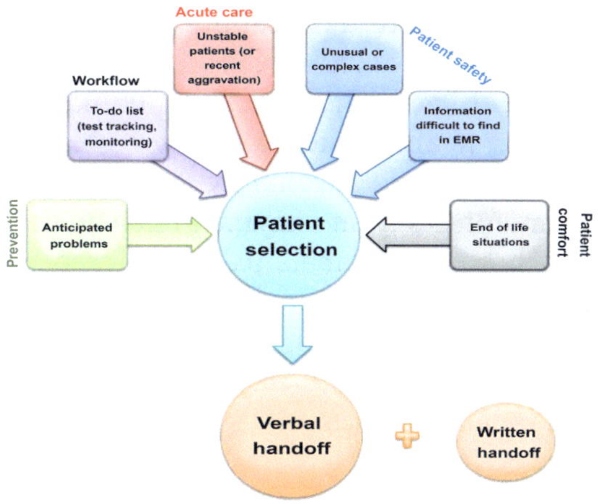

Figure 2.13. Patient selection criteria.

Source: https://www.researchgate.net/profile/Katherine-Blondon/publication/316492217/figure/fig2/AS:667844584935428@1536237965244/Criteria-for-patient-selection.png.

The prevalence of non-board-certified plastic surgeons offering services outside of their training raises significant concerns about patient safety and the quality of care delivered. Scarcella et al. (2022) note that many of these surgical practices exist without sufficient regulatory oversight, leading to a potential risk for patients who may not fully understand the implications of choosing such providers. Consequently, it is vital for both the surgical community and potential patients to critically evaluate the qualifications and motivations of medical professionals. Implementing strong patient selection protocols not only enhances surgical outcomes but also safeguards individuals from potential harm in an increasingly commercialized and sometimes misleading landscape of cosmetic surgery (Figure 2.13).

2.4.1. Assessing Medical History

Assessing medical history is a critical aspect of the principles underlying cosmetic and reconstructive surgery. A comprehensive medical history provides vital insights into a patient's overall health, previous surgical experiences, and potential complications. The importance of gathering accurate data cannot be overstated, as adverse outcomes in surgical procedures can be significantly influenced by undiagnosed underlying health issues. Moreover, conditions such as congenital adrenal hyperplasia (CAH), which manifests from enzyme deficiencies that lead to hormonal imbalances, underscore the necessity for thorough evaluations. In light of recent advancements in understanding these conditions, including improved diagnostic methods and treatment options, surgeons must remain vigilant in their assessments to tailor surgical interventions appropriately. Consequently, meticulous attention to a patient's medical history not only fosters a safer surgical environment but also enhances the prospects for successful outcomes (Claahsen-van der Grinten et al., 2021). In reconstructive surgery, the assessment of medical history extends beyond general health to include psychological factors, which are equally significant. Understanding a patient's mental fortitude and emotional readiness for surgery is paramount, as psychological well-being can influence both the decision to embark on surgical procedures and the recovery trajectory. For example, individuals with conditions like peripheral lymphedema may experience complexities that amalgamate physical deformities with psychological stressors. Current clinical guidelines emphasize the need to incorporate psychosocial assessments alongside physical health checks. By doing so, surgeons can ensure that patients are mentally equipped to handle the intricacies of surgery and subsequent recovery, thereby reducing the likelihood of complications associated with poor mental health. Thus, the nuanced exploration of a patient's psychological landscape is an integral component of a comprehensive medical history assessment (Consensus Document, 2020). Finally, a detailed assessment of medical history should address family medical history and genetic predispositions that can influence surgical outcomes. Being informed about hereditary conditions allows surgeons to devise more effective, personalized treatment plans that anticipate potential complications. For instance, conditions like CAH may not only affect hormonal profiles but can also predispose individuals to various health challenges that might complicate surgical procedures. Therefore, identifying these risk factors can be pivotal in ensuring optimal patient safety and care during surgery. Moreover, an understanding of familial health patterns can assist in educating patients regarding their own potential health risks, empowering them to take informed steps toward their surgical journey. As such, the evaluation of medical history serves as the bedrock upon which effective and tailored cosmetic and reconstructive surgical practices are built (Claahsen-van der Grinten et al., 2021).

2.4.2. Psychological Evaluation

Psychological evaluation serves as a critical component in the context of cosmetic and reconstructive surgery. Understanding a patient's mental health and emotional state is essential for determining their suitability for surgical intervention. Such evaluations traditionally assess various factors, including body image, self-esteem, and underlying psychological issues. This process is vital, as surgical procedures can not only alter physical appearance but also influence mental health outcomes. A thorough psychological evaluation can identify potential issues related to unrealistic expectations and the motivations behind seeking cosmetic enhancement. It ensures that patients are mentally prepared for the transformation and understand the implications it will have on their lives beyond the surgical procedure. Moreover, the psychological impacts of undergoing cosmetic surgery extend beyond mere satisfaction with the aesthetic result. Research indicates that individuals often seek these interventions as a means to address deeper psychological concerns, such as the aftermath of childhood trauma or experiences of bullying. The interplay between mental health and cosmetic surgery illustrates a complex relationship where improvements in body image can bolster self-esteem and mitigate psychological distress. For example, patients who have experienced trauma may find that cosmetic surgery provides a pathway to healing and empowerment, allowing them to reclaim their sense of agency and self-worth.

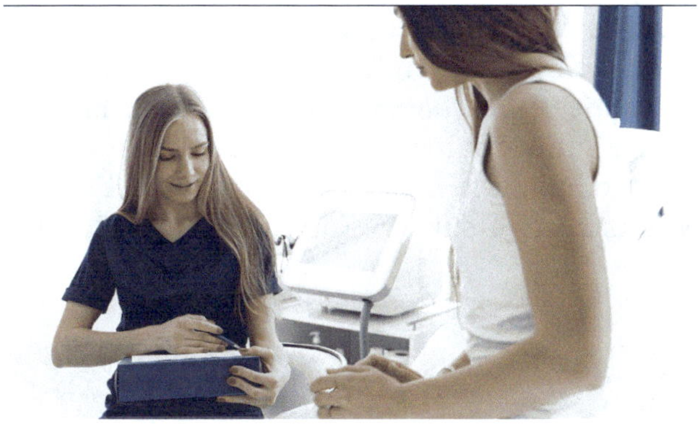

Figure 2.14. Psychological evaluation serves as a critical component in the context of cosmetic and reconstructive surgery.

Source: https://gfpsychology.com/wp-content/uploads/2020/05/Pre-surgical-psychological-evaluations-what-are-they.png.

However, it is equally important to consider the potential drawbacks, such as developing an obsessive desire for further procedures or distress stemming from the social stigma associated with cosmetic enhancements (Ip et al., 2019). Incorporating psychological evaluations into standard surgical practices not only aids in aligning patient expectations with outcomes but also fosters a holistic approach to treatment. The use of psychological assessments promotes a deeper understanding of each patient's unique experiences and emotional needs. Successfully navigating the complexities of body image and self-perception is central to optimizing surgical outcomes. Furthermore, when cosmetic surgery is performed without appropriate psychological support, it can lead to unwanted complications, both physically and mentally. Therefore, integrating psychological evaluations into the framework of cosmetic and reconstructive surgery is essential to ensure patients receive comprehensive care that addresses both their physical alterations and the psychological ramifications of those changes (Eom, 2020) (Figure 2.14).

2.4.3. Setting Realistic Expectations

Setting realistic expectations is critical in the field of cosmetic and reconstructive surgery, as patients often harbor preconceived notions about the outcomes of surgical interventions. Surgeons play a pivotal role in clarifying the potential benefits and limitations of procedures during preoperative consultations. A thorough understanding of individual patient needs, alongside a comprehensive assessment of their anatomical and psychological profiles, allows surgeons to tailor discussions focused on achievable results. Establishing these expectations not only cultivates patient satisfaction but also enhances the therapeutic alliance between provider and patient. This relationship is further underscored by the ethical principles governing aesthetic medicine, which necessitate that practitioners avoid exaggeration of outcomes that could lead to disappointment or dissatisfaction post-surgery. The ethical compass guiding surgical practice should prioritize patient well-being, fostering an environment where realistic goals are both communicated and understood (da Prato et al., 2024). Moreover, the advent of social media has intensified the challenges associated with setting realistic expectations. Patients frequently encounter idealized portrayals of surgical results that can warp their perceptions of what is attainable. The pervasive influence of digital imagery can prompt unrealistic aspirations that are largely unattainable within the context of individual anatomical variations and recovery processes. This discrepancy between social media representations and surgical realities necessitates an open dialogue about the importance of personalizing procedures to individual patient characteristics. Surgeons must engage in candid discussions regarding these images, contextualizing their implications to mitigate unrealistic expectations. Such conversations can empower patients to embrace individualized results while understanding that aesthetic enhancements improve their appearance rather than create a wholly new one. This proactive approach to patient education is essential in preserving ethical standards in cosmetic surgery (Puladi et al., 2023). Finally, fostering an environment that encourages open communication about expectations can significantly enhance surgical outcomes and patient satisfaction. By implementing a structured preoperative process that includes detailed consultations, visual aids, and possibly even simulations, surgeons can help patients visualize realistic outcomes more effectively. Emphasizing the importance of postoperative care and the natural progression of healing also contributes to sustained satisfaction. Patients should be made aware that the journey does not end with the surgical procedure; rather, it requires engagement in recovery protocols and periodic follow-ups to assess results. Ultimately, when patients comprehend the multifaceted nature of their surgical journey, they are less likely to harbor unrealistic beliefs about their results. This holistic approach underscores the essential principle of not only improving aesthetic appearances but prioritizing mental health and realistic self-perception, which is fundamental in the ethos of cosmetic and reconstructive surgery (da Prato et al., 2024).

Test Your Knowledge

1. What key medical conditions must be ruled out before planning a cosmetic or reconstructive procedure?
2. What psychological conditions should be screened for before approving a patient for cosmetic surgery?
3. How does discussing potential risks and outcomes improve satisfaction and informed consent?

2.5. Risks and Complications

Learning Outcome

1. Discuss the Common Risks Associated with Surgery
2. Explain the Long-term Complications
3. Focus on Managing Patient Safety

The field of cosmetic and reconstructive surgery, while offering transformative solutions for patients, is inherently fraught with various risks and complications. Each procedure, regardless of its perceived simplicity, carries the potential for adverse outcomes that may significantly impact patient health and satisfaction. Common risks include infection, poor wound healing, and complications associated with anesthesia. Such risks necessitate comprehensive preoperative assessments to ensure that patients are adequately informed and prepared for the potential consequences of surgery. Understanding these risks is crucial for fostering an open dialogue between surgeons and patients, enabling informed consent and aligned expectations regarding surgical outcomes as outlined in the principles of cosmetic and reconstructive surgery. Among the most concerning complications are those related to surgical techniques and individual patient responses to intervention. For instance, issues such as hematomas, seromas, or scarring can arise from surgical procedures, diminishing the aesthetic results that patients seek. Furthermore, the psychological impact of adverse outcomes cannot be overlooked; dissatisfaction with results can lead to long-term emotional distress and additional corrective surgeries. The joint consideration of these physical and mental health risks highlights the necessity for a multidisciplinary approach in managing patients pre- and post-operatively, ensuring that all aspects of a patient's well-being are taken into account in line with contemporary clinical practices that emphasize holistic care. Patients undergoing cosmetic and reconstructive procedures may also face unique challenges depending on their individual medical histories and the complexity of their conditions. For example, those with congenital disorders require tailored surgical approaches that consider the long-term implications of treatment on their health and quality of life. Such complexities are particularly pronounced in cases involving differences of sex development (DSDs), where surgical intervention must be approached with caution due to the profound implications on physical development and psychological well-being. The multidisciplinary team's role becomes critical in navigating these complexities, ensuring that not only are surgical risks effectively managed but also that patients' rights and experiences are prioritized throughout their treatment journey, as is stated in the evolving guidelines for DSD management, which emphasizes ongoing support and evidence-based care (Cools et al., 2018; Speiser et al., 2018) (Figure 2.15).

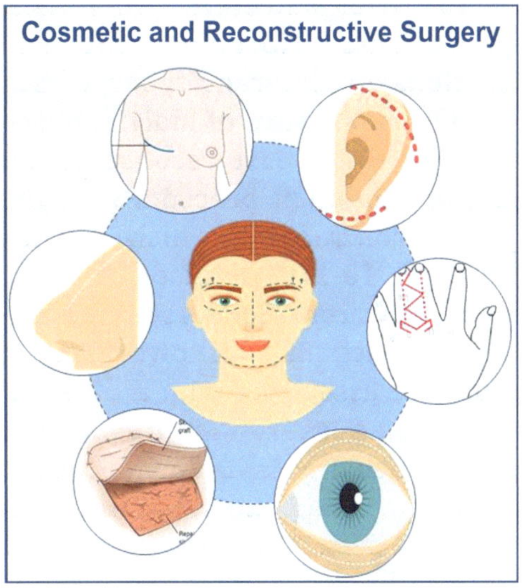

Figure 2.15. The field of cosmetic and reconstructive surgery.

Source: https://www.cosmeticandobesitysurgeryhospitalindia.com/blog/wp-content/uploads/2020/03/What-are-the-important-things-we-need-to-know-about-Reconstructive-and-Cosmetic-surgery-1.png.

2.5.1. Common Risks Associated with Surgery

In the context of cosmetic and reconstructive surgery, it is important for practitioners and patients alike to understand common risks to surgical procedures. The risks are highly dependent on the nature of the surgery undertaken. Examples of procedural complications, including infection, hematoma, and seroma, are common features of a variety of surgical methods. Especially in breast surgery, the risk for infection can range from 1% to as much as 10%, and is dependent on patient factors such as diabetes or obesity. Seroma development also occurs in 5% of patients and leads to complications following postoperative recovery. Early identification of these possible complications makes it easier for healthcare providers to optimize surgical planning and successful risk management, which equates to better outcomes and satisfaction among patients. Moreover, the specific complications of different types of surgery highlight the importance of individualized risk assessments. For breast reconstruction, for instance, implantation procedures have risks of capsular contracture, which develops in approximately 10-15% of cases, with a 1-5% chance of infection. Conversely, autologous tissue reconstructions have lower rates of flap failure but are associated with a different risk profile, including a very high frequency of fat necrosis, particularly in DIEP flap operations (10-15%). By taking the risks into account, physicians are better placed to inform patients about their choices so that they value both the benefits and potential drawbacks of each operation. This level of openness generates an environment of well-informed consent, part of ethical surgery practice. Lastly, the interaction between nutritional condition and operation outcome is another aspect often overlooked in cases of surgery. Poor nutritional condition can yield complications brought about by delayed wound healing, hypertrophic scars, and even infection, largely affecting the time of recovery and also the aesthetic results of interventions. As highlighted in the literature, the development of nutritional deficiencies prolongs postoperative complications, highlighting the importance of experts in the subject area conducting and acting on the nutritional needs of patients before being led into the operating room. By utilizing a proactive process that involves nutritional assessments, surgeons can optimize healing processes and enhance clinical outcomes, ultimately raising the quality of care in cosmetic and reconstructive surgery (Vitagliano et al., 2023; Ordóñez Guerrero, 2024).

2.5.2. Long-term Complications

The quest for aesthetic improvement through cosmetic and reconstructive surgery involves complex methods, but it is critical to note that long-term complications can occur, and they can significantly influence patient outcomes. These are complications that can arise in numerous forms, including pain that is long-lasting, discontent with the aesthetic outcome, and metabolic disorders. For example, in surgeries such as fat redistribution surgery, aimed at correcting deformities such as Barraquer-Simons Syndrome (BSS), long-term fat retention and metabolic stability are areas requiring closer examination. Although initial findings reflect gains in psychosocial health, the variability of fat graft retention necessitates ongoing follow-up and postoperative patient-specific care. Complications underscore the importance of prolonged preoperative evaluations to give proper expectations and prepare patients for upcoming challenges.

Addressing specific reconstructive procedures, the Keystone perforator island flap (KPIF) has demonstrated positive outcomes in vulvovaginal reconstruction patients. While initial functional and psychological results appear to be effective, long-term complications such as suture dehiscence and remote chronic pain or changed sensation are of concern. A case series of the KPIF technique ratified sufficient closure of large defects after surgery with minimal complications. However, it should be noted that a lack of immediate complication is no assurance of late result.

The implication for altered aesthetics and patient satisfaction can only fully emerge over the course of time, supporting the need for follow-up on the patient and lengthy evaluation of the surgical techniques used. Lastly, understanding these long-term implications is the foundation for good principles of reconstructive surgery. Satisfaction of the patient with cosmetic and reconstructive surgery transcends simply aesthetic outcome; it enters the realm of long-term health and general quality of life. Poor handling of post-operative complications can potentially lead to serious emotional trauma and disrupt the initial goals of surgery. When determining implications related to long-term complications, both flap procedures, like the KPIF and autologous fat grafting, involve a multidisciplinary approach in patient care.

The best example is postoperative metabolic effects in the case of patients with BSS, which require coordination of surgeons, endocrinologists, and mental health specialists to provide total care. The integration of these perspectives can enhance not only clinical outcomes but also patient happiness and welfare in the long term. These multi-dimensional strategies highlight the significance of awareness of long-term complications in ongoing refinement of the principles of cosmetic and reconstructive surgery (Figure 2.16).

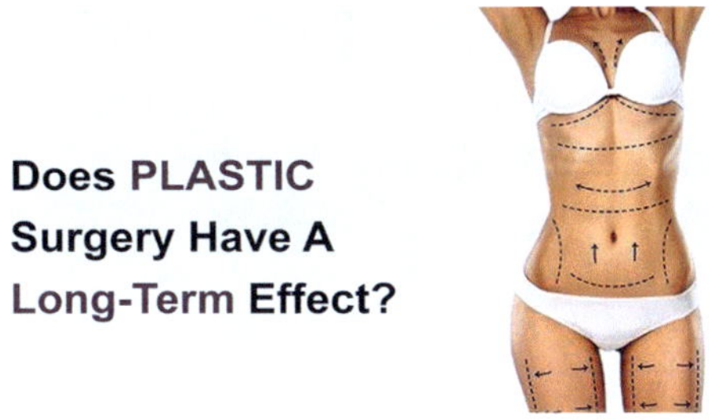

Figure 2.16. Long-term complications.

Source: https://www.divinecosmeticsurgery.com/wp-content/uploads/2024/01/Plastic-Surgery-Longevity.jpeg.

2.5.3. Managing Patient Safety

Patient safety management in cosmetic and reconstructive surgery is of extreme value, especially considering the increased popularity of new yet controversial procedures.

The increased access to elective procedures has necessitated the need for healthcare professionals to institutionalize patient safety protocols. Surgeons need to have thorough preoperative assessments that thoroughly review medical histories, psychosocial determinants, and realistic expectations of patients. These assessments are critical to minimizing complications and ensuring that patients correctly comprehend the risks of their procedure of preference. Furthermore, open communication between patients and healthcare workers preserves a climate of trust and openness such that there can be educated consent extending beyond paperwork to an actual discussion of potential outcomes and complications. The ethical component of managing clinical safety should also be taken into consideration, particularly in domains with controversy, such as female cosmetic genital surgery.

Doctors must critically assess the implications of their practices, particularly patient autonomy versus professional guidance. According to various analyses, the clinical and ethical rationale for new interventions like these tends to overlap with social trends and patient demand. Surgeons have to find their way through these complexities, adhering to professional standards which, at times, find disregard in the interest of entrepreneurial pursuits in the field of medicine.

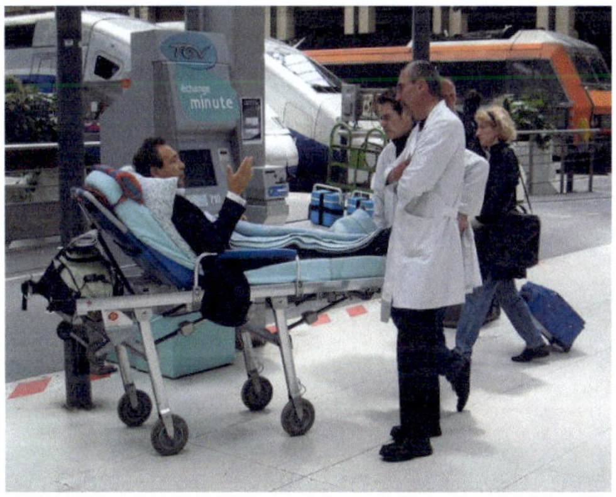

Figure 2.17. Managing patient safety in cosmetic and reconstructive surgery.

Source: https://endurid.com/wp-content/uploads/2013/01/patient-safety-manager-e1358541321945.jpg.

This highlights the role played by American Medical Association guidelines and recommendations of professional societies in defining best practices that not only ensure patient safety but also promote the ethical standards of the surgical profession (Clinch et al., 2011). Furthermore, the increase in prevalence of such procedures as female genital cosmetic surgery raises issues with the adequacy of available information on patient satisfaction and risks. There is a great deficit in strong evidence on efficacy and potential side effects since many of these procedures lack in-depth empirical studies that feed more conventional surgery practice. In order for this lacuna to be met, health practitioners and interested stakeholders must engage in continuous discourse and research that aims to pool comprehensive information towards the process of informing clinical practice. Through deliberation of individual and sociocultural determinants that inform the decision to undergo such procedures, clinicians become better equipped to address patient safety and set protocols that cater to medical as well as individual concerns in patients. This forward-thinking plan not only enhances patient safety but also contributes to an ethically stronger practice in the evolving realm of cosmetic and reconstructive surgery (Malone, 2025) (Figure 2.17).

Test Your Knowledge

1. What are the most frequently encountered intraoperative and postoperative risks in cosmetic surgery?
2. What long-term complications may arise after cosmetic procedures such as implants or facelifts?
3. How should surgeons respond when unexpected complications occur during or after surgery?

2.6. Postoperative Care

Learning Outcome

1. Focus on Importance of Follow-up Appointments
2. Know Recovery Process and Timeline
3. Discuss the Addressing Complications and Concerns

Effective postoperative care is critical in the practice of reconstructive and cosmetic surgery, and it determines the optimum outcome in patients. The patients undergoing surgery suffer some discomfort, bruising, and swelling that need to be controlled and monitored by practitioners. Postoperative care after the prescription made by Ambroise Paré and then later prescribed by Millard is crucial in making close follow-up care a priority. Patient comfort and strict compliance with rehabilitation regimens not only improve healing but also avoid complications like infection and wound failure. Patient communication at this phase is critical; professionals are to provide accurate instructions regarding drug consumption, activity restriction, and any sign of complication for immediate attention. Lastly, a general strategy towards postoperative treatment significantly enhances patient satisfaction and provides a good foundation for their subsequent recovery process (Rohrich et al., 2021). Patient education also significantly affects postoperative care in cosmetic and reconstructive surgery.

Patients should be educated about the expected recovery duration, possible side effects, and follow-ups. Through an open communication culture, surgeons encourage patients to be responsible for recovery processes. Active patient responsibility is also consistent with plastic surgery tenets that focus on preparation and compatibility of surgical intentions with patient desires. To this end, practitioners should engage patients in conversation regarding individual postoperative care plans. Showing patients how normal recovery is and when to report for follow-up decreases patient anxiety, enhances compliance with medical instructions, and thereby leads to better surgical outcomes. As patients know exactly what their recovery process is when they are told, they will be more likely to listen and obey, achieving greater safety and efficiency (Rohrich et al., 2021).

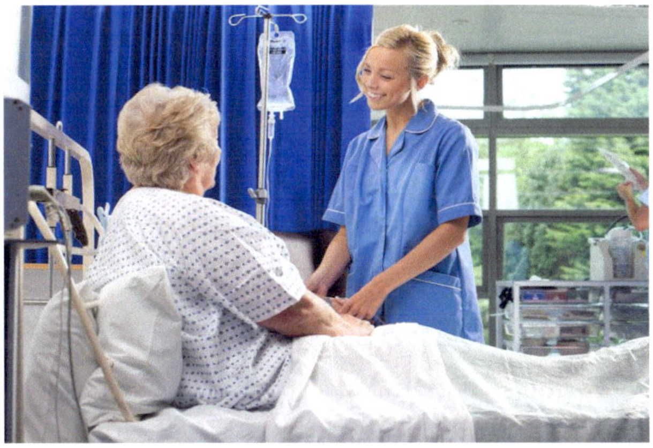

Figure 2.18. Effective postoperative care is critical in the realm of cosmetic and reconstructive surgery.

Source: https://media.post.rvohealth.io/wp-content/uploads/2020/08/postoperative-care_thumb.jpg.

Moreover, technology has transformed postoperative care, and new methods are employed in remote monitoring and patient involvement. Surgeons can perform postoperative follow-ups using telemedicine platforms, ensuring continuity of care and assessing patient complaints on time. The role of technology is not only to expand access but also to augment current surgical practice which is increasingly recognizing the utility of patient-centered care. Besides this, with wearable devices, patient parameters such as activity level and heart rate can be tracked, providing real-time data to aid in clinical decision-making. This technological advancement enables a more personalized postoperative care plan in accordance with the individual patient's needs. As plastic surgery keeps on evolving, these types of advancements will be vital in helping improve patient satisfaction and outcomes in the postoperative setting (Rohrich et al., 2021) (Figure 2.18).

2.6.1. Importance of Follow-up Appointments

The importance of follow-up visits to cosmetic and reconstructive surgery cannot be overemphasized because they are a critical part of the total patient care chain. The follow-up visits provide an invaluable chance for caregivers to monitor the results of the surgery and take care of any possible complications resulting from the initial operation. Through the follow-ups at regular intervals, surgeons can identify potential complications such as infection, scarring, or abnormal healing, which, if left untreated, can have a negative impact on visual results and patient satisfaction. Follow-up care also promotes feelings of safety and trust between the medical practitioners and the patient, which are very crucial to mental well-being as well as the general perception of success of the operations. Aside from physical outcome verification, follow-up visits offer the chance to discover the psychological impact of reconstructive and cosmetic surgery. The patients undergo dramatic emotional change following the surgery, and follow-up visits offer the appropriate atmosphere to discuss them. Through frank discussion of the patient's process, doctors can treat problems of self-esteem or fear that are triggered following the operation. Routine assessments in these visits allow practitioners to refer patients to relevant psychological care, thus ensuring a more holistic recovery process. Such integrated treatment also has the role of highlighting the importance of the patient-physician relationship by stressing the surgeon's commitment to the welfare of the patients in general. Ultimately, evidence supports the application of follow-up care as a way of enhancing surgical results as well as patient satisfaction. Research supports that consistent follow-up contributes to a positive change in long-term outcomes by ensuring correction and fine-tuning procedures are adequately and in a timely manner conducted when required.

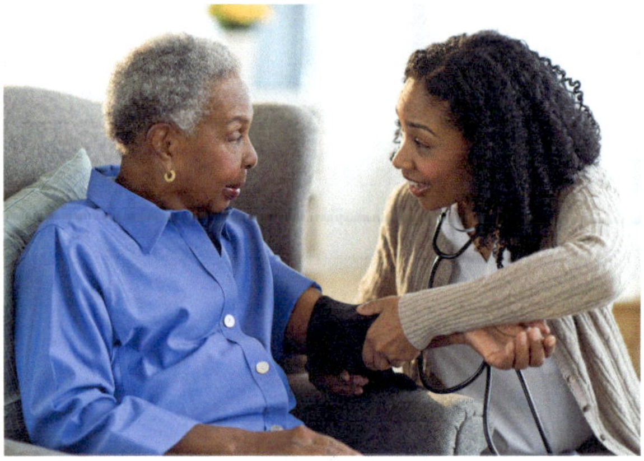

Figure 2.19. The role of follow-up appointments in the realm of cosmetic and reconstructive surgery.

Source: https://images.squarespace-cdn.com/content/v1/5d321403cc84dd0001efc483/1567092342174-ULQAUTD7C5XNX2VCBDKS/GettyImages-123317969.jpg.

For example, satisfaction with surgical outcomes is found to be greater in those patients who are advantaged with repeated follow-up consultations, as their schemes of treatment remain under continuous checking and corrective measures. Multidisciplinary practice is worth it; by combining the expertise of various health practitioners, like psychological and physical therapy, an adequate care plan can be made for each patient. This focus on continuous assessment and revision is in line with the guidance of experts in the discipline, who affirm that meticulous postoperative management is part of achieving the optimal results in cosmetic and reconstructive surgery (Kalaskar et al., 2016; Pandit et al., 2023) (Figure 2.19).

2.6.2. Recovery Process and Timeline

Healing subsequent to cosmetic and reconstructive surgery is a complex process essential to the success of the procedure overall. The healing process typically begins immediately after surgery, characterized by pain, bruising, and swelling. Patients are also usually advised to rest and avoid strenuous work throughout this phase, which varies from taking a few days' walk to a week, based on the type of surgery undergone. Coordination with health care providers is also important at this time since they can give first-hand guidance on pain management, wound dressing, and symptoms of complications needing emergency treatment.

Apart from that, compliance with postoperative instructions is highly likely to affect the healing process and, therefore, the role of active patient participation in its management right from the start. Upon completion of the initial healing process, patients usually shift to a more structured recovery program in the form of rehabilitation and follow-ups. This stage is dedicated to its return to regular activities and increasingly full mobility. Physical therapy can be initiated to aid healing, particularly with reconstructive surgery, when range of motion is a large factor to allow optimal function. Postoperative visits by the operating team are critically important since they allow for monitoring of healing, assessment of aesthetic outcome, and early intervention in the event of any issue. Additionally, the interaction of surgical outcome and psychological well-being can become more salient at this time, as individuals adjust to appearance and function following surgery. This underlines the requirement for a comprehensive recovery program that addresses both the physiological and psychosocial domains of care and makes an overall recovery program possible. The recovery process is very uncertain, depending on numerous variables like the type of surgery, the patient's age, and overall health. For instance, patients who undergo procedures like oncoplastic breast surgery may have different recovery patterns depending on the nature of the procedure and allied treatment modalities like radiotherapy, which needs to be considered within the recovery time (Wignarajah et al., 2023). On average, patients should expect to recover normal function within a few weeks, but months will pass before ultimate results are achieved, as the body recuperates and settles further. Indeed, the gradual process of healing from significant surgery can be daunting, demanding patience and understanding in the process. Lastly, building a conducive culture promoting recovery protocol follow-up and overall mental wellness will enhance the experience and outcomes of patients in cosmetic and reconstructive surgery (Toader et al., 2023).

2.6.3. Addressing Complications and Concerns

Meeting complications and issues in cosmetic and reconstructive surgery will guarantee maximum patient outcomes and satisfaction. More and more people are resorting to treatments like breast augmentation or liposuction, but they are ill-informed about the risks involved in such treatment. Complications like infection, scarring, and the psychologic effect of dissatisfaction especially do come with a prominent effect on a patients quality of life after surgery. As noted in literature, there is typically a discrepancy between strong evidence of the complications and outcomes of such operations, thus again reaffirming the necessity of close patient education and informed consent protocols. Increased incidences of female genital cosmetic operations are a perfect example where the patients and practitioners must sit down to discuss at length realistic expectations and risks of the operations (Malone, 2025).

Thus, actively resolving these issues can result in increased patient satisfaction and more effective surgeries. The evolutionary character of surgical methods also covers complications occurring during and following operations. New technologies in regenerative medicine, as well as new ideas in flap concepts, are promising in solving advanced reconstructive demands.

Literature indicates that techniques such as perforator flaps and bioengineered scaffolds radically improved functional return with lower rates of complications and better aesthetic outcomes (Bernal et al., 2024). For instance, regenerative techniques have been observed to witness remarkable improvement in wound healing and notable reduction in the rate of infections, which are crucial determinants of reconstructive cases. Yet, with these advancements, overall complication rates remain high, and the requirement for an accurate and effective comprehension by the operating personnel as well as the patients becomes critical.

Emphasis on ongoing research and the sharing of information about new surgical alternatives can assist in mitigating risks and establishing a strong groundwork for trust in the patient. Lastly, building an ethical and transparent culture between surgeons and patients is of utmost importance in terms of managing complications and issues in reconstructive and cosmetic surgery. Proper pre-operative evaluation cannot be overemphasized since pre-operative examinations usually detect underlying conditions that would otherwise raise the likelihood of complications during the process. No less important is the use of routine procedures of post-operative treatment to enable rapid recognition and handling of possible complications. As the popularity of cosmetic treatments becomes more widespread, medical practitioners must also increasingly function not merely to create aesthetic enhancements, but overall care embracing physical as well as psychic well-being. Through maintaining excellence in evidence-based practice, informed consent, and patient education, the specialty is well set to expand, ultimately lowering complications and increasing patient satisfaction with reconstructive and cosmetic surgery.

Test Your Knowledge

1. How do follow-up appointments help in identifying and managing delayed complications?
2. What factors influence the duration of recovery after common cosmetic procedures?
3. How should surgeons counsel patients experiencing anxiety or dissatisfaction during healing?

SUMMARY

The guidelines of cosmetic and reconstructive surgery are pivotal in enhancing patients quality of life and obtaining maximum surgical outcomes. The concordance of sound surgical methods is the top priority, as demonstrated by the success of intricate surgeries like augmentation ileocystoplasty and appendicocystostomy, whose meticulous planning and performance have been proven to improve children with severe bladder dysfunction significantly (Fofanov et al., 2021). This signifies the value of customized treatment plans that take each patient's unique needs and circumstances into account, ultimately leading to optimum outcomes. Second, optimizing the surgical process and adhering to established principles not only results in better physical recuperation but also psychological health since patients are given more confidence and improved socialization post-surgery. Additionally, the innovation trend within the specialty is such that growing emphasis on aesthetics, particularly for breast surgery, can be observed. The advancements in reduction, mastopexy, and augmentation of the breast reflect the surgeons' efforts to keep pace with changing techniques and new developing complications such as BIA-ALCL and BII (Roy et al., 2021). The more these types of complexities in aesthetic surgery become well understood, the more important it is to consider good principles of reconstructive surgery in addressing the difficulties presented by these complexities. Such ongoing advancement not merely facilitates patient safety but also breeds confidence in the surgical community, necessitating continued education and compliance with strict standards in cosmetic as well as reconstructive procedures. Last but not least, the necessity for enormous training and regulation in the field is impossible to overstate. With patients looking to achieve cosmetically perfect bodies, surgeons need to be trained in reconstructive surgery and aesthetic parameters. Crossovers between reconstructive and cosmetic surgery highlight the importance of an interdisciplinary model of education that is centered on patient care, psychological coping, and an appreciation for the possible risks (Roy et al., 2021). By deepening such values, the medical community can ensure quality practice that protects the welfare of patients but also supports the growth of the specialty. Finally, the intersection of aesthetic ideals and reconstructive imperatives leaves space for the future of innovation and patient-focused care.

Aesthetic and functional principles that guide cosmetic and reconstructive surgery are highly integrated, with special emphasis on the rehabilitation of form and function in the patients. The surgery is typically based on the understanding of the special needs of a case, which can include such factors as tissue viability, size of the defect, and severity of the specific condition of the patient. Taking a patient-focused philosophy, surgeons try to maximize the results for each patient by using methods specifically designed for the individual patient's needs. This basic principle is a guiding mandate for cosmetic reconstruction and repair of both the acquired and congenital defects alike, ultimately to enhance the general quality of life in such patients. The second significant aspect of modern surgical practice is the use of newer methods, such as flaps and vascular grafts, to optimize the viability of reconstructive endeavors. The use of vascular grafts has also arisen as a required alternative in situations requiring additional tissue support, particularly in the most severe cases of the lower extremity, as more recent evidence has testified. For instance, from 2010 to 2015, there was a clinical series with successful outcomes in patients who required microsurgical reconstruction, and with regard to this, arterial and venous grafts played a critical role in facilitating optimal repair. The ability to restore blood supply to areas of tissue is essential in reconstruction success, illustrating the importance of knowledge of vascular anatomy as being the foundation of the success of surgical procedures (Cordova et al., 2017). Selection of reconstructive procedures also can make or break not only the aesthetic outcome but also the recovery period and incidence of complications of surgical procedures. Retro comparison of the perforator propeller flaps (PPFs) and free flaps (FFs) indicated remarkable discrepancies in complication rates and healing times and guided the surgeon on the optimal procedure for every defect. Although PPFs were found effective in some conditions, FFs picked up pace with the decreased rates of complications and increased recovery time (Cajozzo et al., 2017). Therefore, appropriate comprehension of the principles of flap selection and application is necessary to attain maximum surgical efficacy, best care, and outcome in cosmetic and reconstructive surgery.

KEY TERMS FROM THIS CHAPTER

- Aesthetic Balance
- Proportion
- Tissue Viability
- Scar Formation
- Flap Reconstruction
- Functional Restoration
- Body Contouring
- Symmetry
- Reconstructive Ladder
- Wound Healing
- Tissue Expansion
- Graft Survival
- Facial Aesthetics
- Soft Tissue Management

CRITICAL THINKING QUESTIONS

1. **The main difference between cosmetic and reconstructive surgery is:**
   a. Cosmetic surgery improves function only
   b. Reconstructive surgery improves appearance only
   c. Cosmetic surgery enhances appearance; reconstructive restores form and function
   d. Both focus solely on aesthetics
2. **The reconstructive ladder represents:**
   a. Increasing levels of cosmetic difficulty
   b. A hierarchy of reconstructive options from simple to complex
   c. Facial nerve branches
   d. Types of scar patterns
3. **Which of the following is the simplest step on the reconstructive ladder?**
   a. Local flap
   b. Free flap
   c. Skin graft
   d. Primary closure
4. **The success of a flap largely depends on:**
   a. Skin color
   b. Vascular supply
   c. Patient age
   d. Muscle tone
5. **Which suture technique is best for reducing wound tension?**
   a. Simple interrupted
   b. Vertical mattress
   c. Subcuticular continuous
   d. Purse-string

Short Answer Questions

1. What is the fundamental difference between cosmetic surgery and reconstructive surgery?
2. Define the reconstructive ladder and list its main steps.
3. What are the key principles of tissue handling during surgery to minimize scarring?
4. Explain the concept of "aesthetic units" in facial reconstruction.
5. What factors determine the choice of flap versus graft in reconstructive surgery?
6. What is the importance of vascular supply in flap design?

Answers to Critical Thinking Questions

1. (c) 2. (b) 3. (d) 4. (b) 5. (b)

REFERENCES

1. Ávalos, N. J. A., Lupercio Romo, C. D., Cuadra Casillas, A., Ibarra Aguayo, D., Torres Somarriba, W. M., Flores Tavizón, E., Estrada, A. T., et al. (2025). Surgical management of lipodystrophy in Barraquer-Simons syndrome: Autologous fat redistribution and reconstructive strategies for acquired partial lipodystrophy. *International Journal of Medical Science and Clinical Research Studies*. https://www.semanticscholar.org/paper/5e3cac25999659170bb65e09ab0a4a4b8f8b9bfe (accessed on 14th July 2025).
2. Bellon, J. R., Burstein, H. J., Frank, E. S., Mittendorf, E. A., & King, T. A. (2020). Multidisciplinary considerations in the treatment of triple-negative breast cancer. *CA: A Cancer Journal for Clinicians, 70*, 432–442. https://doi.org/10.3322/caac.21643 (accessed on 14th July 2025).
3. Bernal, J. G. T., Galindo, A. S., García, M. F. R., Javier, L., et al. (2024). *Advances in flap surgical techniques and regenerative approaches for reconstruction of extensive defects in cutaneous squamous cell carcinoma: A systematic review of functional and aesthetic outcomes*. https://core.ac.uk/download/635338710.pdf (accessed on 14th July 2025).
4. Bora, P., & Sen Majumdar, A. (2017). Adipose tissue-derived stromal vascular fraction in regenerative medicine: A brief review on biology and translation. *Stem Cell Research & Therapy, 8*. https://doi.org/10.1186/s13287-017-0598-y (accessed on 14th July 2025).
5. Buttura da Prato, E., Cartier, H., Margara, A., Molina, B., Tateo, A., Grimolizzi, F., & Spagnolo, A. G. (2024). The ethical foundations of patient-centered care in aesthetic medicine. *Philosophy Ethics and Humanities in Medicine, 19*. https://doi.org/10.1186/s13010-024-00151-1 (accessed on 14th July 2025).
6. Cajozzo, M., Cordova, A., D'Arpa, S., Innocenti, M., et al. (2017). *Retrospective analysis in lower limb reconstruction: Propeller perforator flaps versus free flaps*. https://core.ac.uk/download/153398075.pdf (accessed on 14th July 2025).
7. Carmichael, K., & Mokbel, K. (2016). Evolving trends in breast surgery: Oncoplastic to onco-aesthetic surgery. *Archives of Plastic Surgery, 43*, 222–223. https://www.semanticscholar.org/paper/72ad7891d4acaa385335310d8d65d730a6d0b684 (accessed on 14th July 2025).
8. Citgez, B., Yigit, B., & Bas, S. (2022). Oncoplastic and Reconstructive Breast Surgery: A Comprehensive Review. *Cureus, 14*(1), e21763. https://doi.org/10.7759/cureus.21763(accessed on 14th July 2025).
9. Citgez, B., Yigit, B., & Bas, S. (2022). Oncoplastic and Reconstructive Breast Surgery: A Comprehensive Review. *Cureus, 14*(1), e21763. https://doi.org/10.7759/cureus.21763(accessed on 14th July 2025).
10. Claahsen-van der Grinten, H. L., Speiser, P., Ahmed, S. F., Arlt, W., Auchus, R. J., Falhammar, H., Flück, C. E., et al. (2021). Congenital adrenal hyperplasia—Current insights in pathophysiology, diagnostics, and management. *Endocrine Reviews, 43*, 91–159. https://doi.org/10.1210/endrev/bnab016 (accessed on 14th July 2025).
11. Clinch, N. C., Osland, A., & Wang, C. (2011). *Legitimizing Radical New Medical Services*. https://core.ac.uk/download/70426040.pdf (accessed on 14th July 2025).
12. Cools, M., Nordenström, A., Robeva, R., Hall, J. C., Westerveld, P., Flück, C. E., Köhler, B., et al. (2018). Caring for individuals with a difference of sex development (DSD): A consensus statement. *Nature Reviews Endocrinology, 14*, 415–429. https://doi.org/10.1038/s41574-018-0010-8 (accessed on 14th July 2025).

13. Cordova, A., D'Arpa, S., Pirrello, R., Roggio, A., et al. (2017). *Vascular grafts and flow-through flaps for microsurgical lower extremity reconstruction.* https://core.ac.uk/download/153398914.pdf (accessed on 14th July 2025).

14. Corvetto, E., Proto, A., Fais, M., Locati, V., Russo, M., Figus, A., Candotti, G., et al. (2019). EP1179 keystone flap application in vulvo-perineal reconstructive surgery: A case series of patients with vulvar cancer. *International Journal of Gynecological Cancer, 29*, A609–A609. https://www.semanticscholar.org/paper/0a603190ef3ae5d8e7ec3728aa03d65f7a855dc5 (accessed on 14th July 2025).

15. Cristel, R. T., Demesh, D., & Dayan, S. (2020). *Video conferencing impact on facial appearance: Looking beyond the COVID-19 pandemic. Facial Plastic Surgery & Aesthetic Medicine, 22*, 238–239. https://doi.org/10.1089/fpsam.2020.0279 (accessed on 14th July 2025).

16. Eom, K. S. (2020). Single-stage reconstruction with titanium mesh for compound comminuted depressed skull fracture. *Journal of Korean Neurosurgical Society, 63*, 631–639. https://doi.org/10.3340/jkns.2019.0181 (accessed on 14th July 2025).

17. Fofanov, O. D., Jurtseva, A. P., Zinyak, B. M., Dotsenko, Y. R., & Fofanov, V. O. (2021). The own experience of reconstructive-plastic operations on the bladder in children. *Pediatric Surgery Ukraine.* https://doi.org/10.15574/ps.2021.72.43 (accessed on 14th July 2025).

18. International Society of Lymphology. (2020). The diagnosis and treatment of peripheral lymphedema: 2020 consensus document of the International Society of Lymphology. *Lymphology, 53.* https://doi.org/10.2458/lymph.4649 (accessed on 14th July 2025).

19. Ip, K. T. V., & Ho, W. W. Y. (2019). Healing childhood psychological trauma and improving body image through cosmetic surgery. *Frontiers in Psychiatry, 10.* https://doi.org/10.3389/fpsyt.2019.00540 (accessed on 14th July 2025).

20. Karadžić, K. (2021). *Radiation Monitoring System. Book of Abstracts.* https://doi.org/10.21175/rad.abstr.book.2021.28.20 (accessed on 14th July 2025).

21. Kazimierczak, N., Kazimierczak, W., Serafin, Z., Nowicki, P., Nożewski, J., & Janiszewska-Olszowska, J. (2024). AI in orthodontics: Revolutionizing diagnostics and treatment planning—A comprehensive review. *Journal of Clinical Medicine, 13*, 344–344. https://doi.org/10.3390/jcm13020344 (accessed on 14th July 2025).

22. Lowe, B. (2017). *Slathered, zapped, nipped, and tucked: An ethical analysis of cosmetic dermatology.* https://core.ac.uk/download/129153456.pdf (accessed on 14th July 2025).

23. Malone, J. (2025). *Women and Genital Cosmetic Surgery.* https://core.ac.uk/download/pdf/30677491.pdf (accessed on 14th July 2025).

24. Masià, J. (2020). The largest multicenter data collection on prepectoral breast reconstruction: The iBAG study. *Journal of Surgical Oncology, 122*, 848–860. https://doi.org/10.1002/jso.26073 (accessed on 14th July 2025).

25. Meyer-Szary, J., Luis, M. S., Mikulski, S., Patel, A., Schulz, F., Tretiakow, D., Fercho, J., et al. (2022). The role of 3D printing in planning complex medical procedures and training of medical professionals—Cross-sectional multispecialty review. *International Journal of Environmental Research and Public Health, 19*, 3331–3331. https://doi.org/10.3390/ijerph19063331 (accessed on 14th July 2025).

26. Ordóñez Guerrero, A. L. (2024). Unveiling complexities: A comprehensive narrative review of complications in cosmetic and reconstructive breast surgery. *Global Journal for Research Analysis*. https://www.semanticscholar.org/paper/e9590c272baee4aa72aae69a4a6005d63ba1ddb1 (accessed on 14th July 2025).

27. Pandit, P., Murkey, S. P., Agarwal, A., Jaiswal, A., & Agrawal, S. (2023). Understanding fibroadenoma of the breast: A comprehensive review of pre-operative and post-operative clinicopathological correlations. *Cureus*. https://doi.org/10.7759/cureus.51329 (accessed on 14th July 2025).

28. Pressman, S. M., Borna, S., Gomez-Cabello, C. A., Haider, S. A., Haider, C. R., & Forte, A. J. (2024). AI and ethics: A systematic review of the ethical considerations of large language model use in surgery research. *Healthcare, 12*, 825–825. https://doi.org/10.3390/healthcare12080825 (accessed on 14th July 2025).

29. Puladi, B., Gsaxner, C., Kleesiek, J., Hölzle, F., Röhrig, R., & Egger, J. (2023). The impact and opportunities of large language models like ChatGPT in oral and maxillofacial surgery: A narrative review. *International Journal of Oral and Maxillofacial Surgery, 53*, 78–88. https://doi.org/10.1016/j.ijom.2023.09.005 (accessed on 14th July 2025).

30. Reddy, K., Gharde, P., Tayade, H., Patil, M., Reddy, L. S., & Surya, D. (2023). Advancements in robotic surgery: A comprehensive overview of current utilizations and upcoming frontiers. *Cureus*. https://doi.org/10.7759/cureus.50415 (accessed on 14th July 2025).

31. Rohrich, R. J., Dayan, E., & Xue, A. S. (2021). Social media in plastic surgery: The future is now? *Plastic & Reconstructive Surgery, 148*, 125S–126S. https://doi.org/10.1097/01.prs.0000794940.66507.3f (accessed on 14th July 2025).

32. Rohrich, R. J., Timberlake, A. T., & Afrooz, P. N. (2017). Revisiting the fundamental operative principles of plastic surgery. *Plastic & Reconstructive Surgery, 140*, 1315–1318. https://doi.org/10.1097/prs.0000000000003909 (accessed on 14th July 2025).

33. Rohrich, R. J., Timberlake, A. T., & Afrooz, P. N. (2021). Revisiting the fundamental operative principles of plastic surgery. *Plastic & Reconstructive Surgery, 148*, 117S–120S. https://doi.org/10.1097/01.prs.0000794928.23166.06 (accessed on 14th July 2025).

34. Rohrich, R. J., Weinstein, A., & Stuzin, J. M. (2020). Plastic and reconstructive surgery at 75: Stronger, better, and always changing. *Plastic & Reconstructive Surgery, 147*, 249–257. https://doi.org/10.1097/prs.0000000000007516 (accessed on 14th July 2025).

35. Roy, P. G., Yan, Z., Nigam, S., & Maheshwari, K. (2021). Aesthetic breast surgery: Putting in context—A narrative review. *Gland Surgery, 10*, 2832–2846. https://doi.org/10.21037/gs-20-892 (accessed on 14th July 2025).

36. Santoni, S., Gugliandolo, S. G., Sponchioni, M., Moscatelli, D., & Colosimo, B. M. (2021). 3D bioprinting: Current status and trends—A guide to the literature and industrial practice. *Bio-Design and Manufacturing, 5*, 14–42. https://doi.org/10.1007/s42242-021-00165-0 (accessed on 14th July 2025).

37. Scarcella, J., Guo, Y., & Yu, V. J. (2022). Shopping on social media for a cosmetic surgeon? The impact that truth in advertising laws have had on who is behind the most popular social media accounts that are advertising cosmetic surgery practices. *Plastic & Reconstructive Surgery Global Open, 10*, 35–35. https://doi.org/10.1097/01.gox.0000898488.05525.7b (accessed on 14th July 2025).

38. Sonnenfeld, D., Mogari, D., & Rothberg, A. D. (2016). *A review of selection criteria used by medical scheme advisers to approve or deny procedures with a cosmetic component.* https://core.ac.uk/download/478309425.pdf (accessed on 14th July 2025).

39. Speiser, P., Arlt, W., Auchus, R. J., Baskin, L. S., Conway, G. S., Merke, D. P., Meyer-Bahlburg, H. F. L., et al. (2018). Congenital adrenal hyperplasia due to steroid 21-hydroxylase deficiency: An Endocrine Society clinical practice guideline. *The Journal of Clinical Endocrinology & Metabolism, 103*, 4043–4088. https://doi.org/10.1210/jc.2018-01865 (accessed on 14th July 2025).

40. Sullivan, D. C., Chung, K. C., Eaves, F. F., & Rohrich, R. J. (2021). The level of evidence pyramid: Indicating levels of evidence in plastic and reconstructive surgery articles. *Plastic & Reconstructive Surgery, 148*, 68S–71S. https://doi.org/10.1097/01.prs.0000794868.07051.b4 (accessed on 14th July 2025).

41. Toader, C., Eva, L., Tătaru, C. I., Covache-Busuioc, R. A., Bratu, B. G., Dumitrascu, D. I., Costin, H. P., et al. (2023). Frontiers of cranial base surgery: Integrating technique, technology, and teamwork for the future of neurosurgery. *Brain Sciences, 13*, 1495–1495. https://doi.org/10.3390/brainsci13101495 (accessed on 14th July 2025).

42. Vitagliano, T., Garieri, P., Lascala, L., Ferro, Y., Doldo, P., Pujia, R., Pujia, A., et al. (2023). Preparing patients for cosmetic surgery and aesthetic procedures: Ensuring an optimal nutritional status for successful results. *Nutrients, 15*. https://www.semanticscholar.org/paper/b1f58b938270317122bdc9547797d4e6a0d6a592 (accessed on 14th July 2025).

43. Wignarajah, P., Malata, C. M., & Benson, J. R. (2023). Oncoplastic and reconstructive breast surgery. *Frontiers in Oncology, 13*. https://doi.org/10.3389/fonc.2023.1176915 (accessed on 14th July 2025).

44. Zargarbashi, R., Panjavi, B., & Bozorgmanesh, M. (2023). Congenital hypoplastic thumbs treated by staged nonvascularized MTP joint transfer for absent MCP joints and abductor digiti minimi tendon transfer for opposition: A case series study. *BMC Musculoskeletal Disorders, 24*. https://doi.org/10.1186/s12891-023-06165-8 (accessed on 14th July 2025).

PATIENT ASSESSMENT AND SURGICAL PLANNING IN COSMETIC FACIAL

3

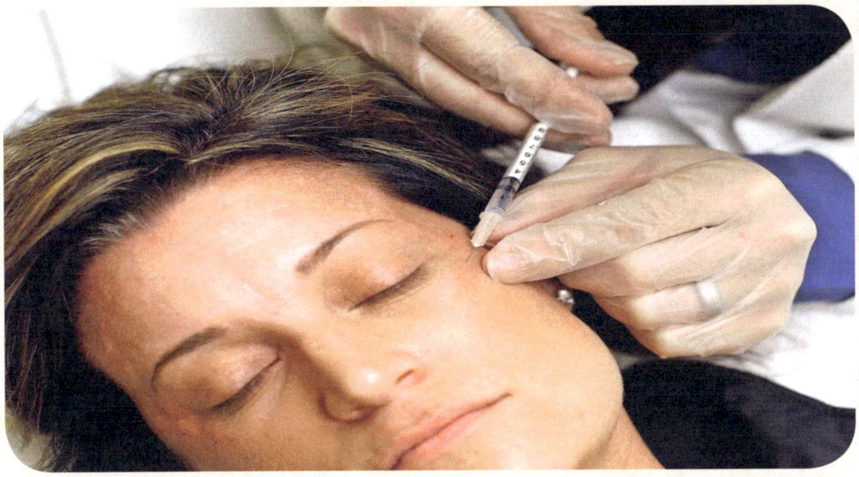

LEARNING OBJECTIVES

After studying this chapter, you will be able to:

1. Describe the patient history role;
2. Describe the physical examination methods;
3. Emphasize patient expectations and goals;
4. Discuss risk assessment and management;
5. Emphasize surgical planning strategies;
6. Understand ethical considerations in cosmetic surgery.

Introduction

The art of cosmetic facial surgery demands thorough knowledge of patient evaluation and surgical planning to gain the optimal results. The purpose of such an essay is to introduce the importance of systematic evaluation processes that dictate surgical decisions. Such an evaluation would typically involve not only a thorough medical history and physical examination but also evaluation of the patient's psychological readiness for surgery. It is only when those intricate variables are known that surgeons can responsibly weigh patient expectations against obtainable outcomes. Furthermore, an elementary knowledge of the most recent operative techniques and developments enhances the ability to tailor treatments in response to specific patient needs, thus improving overall levels of patient satisfaction and safety rates. Moreover, successful cosmetic facial surgery cannot be achieved without meticulous planning and preparation. Preoperative evaluations are extremely important in identifying any underlying medical conditions or contraindications that will complicate procedures or healing. Evidence-based guidelines, such as those distilled in a recent review of the literature that encompassed 293 relevant studies on patient evaluation and operative techniques, are key blueprints for practitioners. They reinforce the importance of collaboration among health care providers due to the fact that the collective input leads to diagnostic accuracy and treatment planning in the ever-evolving practice of cosmetic surgery. Adherence to these protocols not only reduces potential complications but also enhances overall patient care quality throughout the course of surgery. Finally, the application of revolutionary research and current evidence to surgical planning can significantly enhance patient outcomes. The constant updating of clinical guidelines, such as those organizations propose in times of crises such as the COVID-19 pandemic, reflects the demand that practitioners remain current. By the incorporation of evidence-based recommendations for preoperative care and surgical techniques, surgeons are enhanced in being competent to address the unique challenges presented in cosmetic facial surgery. This commitment to staying updated regarding new knowledge finally accrues to the advantage of surgical technique, enhanced patient assessment, and a more solid foundation for informed decision-making in cosmetic facial surgery (Aziz et al., 2020; Geiger et al., 2021).

Definition of Cosmetic Facial Surgery

Cosmetic facial surgery is a branch of medical science that deals with the improvement of facial aesthetic appearances through surgery. It is a wide field of surgery encompassing numerous procedures from small procedures like dermal fillers to complex procedures like facelift and rhinoplasty. The overall purpose is to make facial features more beautiful and to rectify asymmetry so that patients can equate their body with their self-perception. With the growing need for cosmetic treatments, experts in the specialty are faced with compromising the need for beauty versus safety, requiring extensive patient evaluation before any type of surgical planning can be done. These evaluations are critical as they assist in the determination of specialized needs, expectation management, and customized planning of surgical procedures. The importance of thorough patient assessment in cosmetic facial surgery cannot be overstated since it sets the stage for successful surgical outcomes. Effective assessment is a matter of understanding a patient's history, psychological readiness, and aesthetic needs. The assessment process also allows surgeons to detect any anatomical issues or causes of potential surgical complications. For example, a history of past medical illnesses can reveal contraindications that could complicate an advance-scheduled procedure. Accordingly, surgery planning needs to be directed by this multiaxial assessment to generate a customized approach that serves not merely the anatomical requirements but also the psychological demands of the patient's expectations. Such strict screening maximizes outcomes and satisfaction for the patient while minimizing complications through optimal surgery planning. As the art of cosmetic facial surgery is constantly changing, it is essential that all practitioners remain current with present practice and guidelines. Evidence-based guidance is essential for the aim of ensuring optimal practice is being adhered to in both patient assessment and surgical planning. For instance, the use of expert panel guidance on surgical diagnostic and therapeutic approaches can be a useful resource for handling challenging cases. Also, due to the recent global pandemics, including COVID-19, rapid literature reviews have underscored the need for flexible responses in clinical practice, including cosmetic facial surgery. Such developments highlight the necessity of surgeons being intelligent and adaptable, such that every facet of care for the patient, from assessment to postoperative care, is guided by recent research as well as professional consensus, as proposed by Aziz et al. (2020); Geiger et al. (2021) (Figure 3.1).

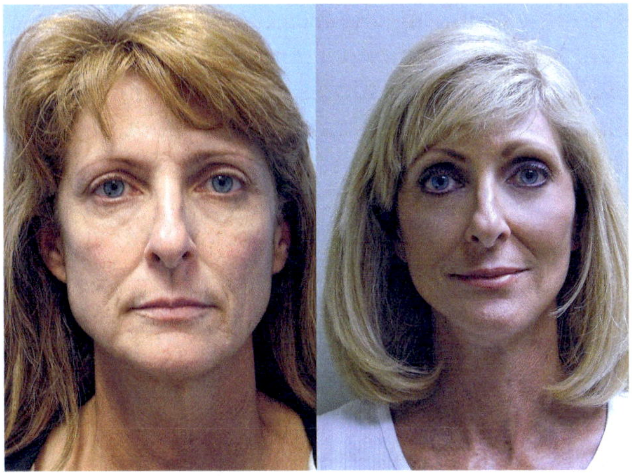

Figure 3.1. Cosmetic facial surgery.

Source: https://external-content.duckduckgo.com/iu/?u=https%3A%2F%2Fi.pinimg.com%2Foriginals%2Fa9%2F3c%2F32%2Fa93c32805ff62c82121cc79c8791717d.jpg&f=1&nofb=1&ipt=84ffb80ea365a38e73e709e6f19cafff40a368b3c01e5274494b01725faed32b.

Importance of Patient Assessment

Patient evaluation in cosmetic face surgery cannot be undervalued. Proper evaluation is the cornerstone of successful results as it helps surgeons acquire critical information about a patient's history, physical examination, and psychological status. This multi-faceted approach ensures that practitioners are in a position to individualize treatment on the basis of detailed needs, leading to enhanced levels of satisfaction. Research indicates that knowledge of a patient's motivations and expectations is an integral component of this, as unaligned goals are the cause of dissatisfaction, regardless of the technical success of the procedure. Therefore, preliminary assessment is not merely a formality of the process but an important interaction that determines the whole direction for cosmetic surgery, and the surgeon and patient become fully synchronized in their objectives for the procedure outcome. Moreover, patient assessment provides an environment in which preoperative consultation can be performed with sensitivity and prudence, and obtaining informed consent is of utmost importance. It allows the surgeon to inform the patient of the potential risks, benefits, and limitations associated with the procedure effectively. Open communication during this period not only brought about trust but also enabled patients to decide based on their course of treatment. With an era of information readily available from varied sources reaching out to patients and, more often than not, leading to misinterpretation or skewed perspectives about cosmetic procedures, thorough assessment is the priority. By engaging in a thorough clinical conversation founded on clinical experience, surgeons can realistically address unrealistic expectations, alleviate fears, and ultimately enhance general patient satisfaction. The conversation is also supplemented by evidence that highly individualized information delivery significantly contributes to patient confidence in surgical decision-making, emphasizing the need for extensive assessment procedures in improving surgical planning. Also, the evolving nature of artificial intelligence and technology brings implications for the future of cosmetic facial surgery patient assessment. While mechanisms such as AI platforms have proven viable when it comes to providing accurate information about operations, as has recently been emphasized through research, they cannot entirely replace human beings. For instance, ChatGPT's ability to provide critical information on procedures like rhinoplasty is promising but ultimately also points to the drawback of AI in delivering individualized advice (Xie et al., 2023). Human emotion, expectation, and apprehension are better understood through face-to-face assessments, allowing for individualized feedback that can't be offered by AI. Thus, the integration of traditional methods of evaluation with technology will boost the process of assessment to deliver extensive care to patients while maintaining the element of humanity in cosmetic surgical planning. In this the multifaceted interface between technology and customized care, patient assessment continues to be one of the cornerstones to enable the ultimate success of aesthetic surgery.

Overview of Surgical Planning Process

The preoperative planning for cosmetic facial surgery is a crucial process that begins with a thorough evaluation of the patient. This includes establishing patients' medical history, aesthetic intent, and psychological preparation for surgery. Based on physical examinations, digital photography, and discussions about expectations and potential risks of various procedures, an entire assessment is made. Further, this step is essential in establishing a relationship between the patient and the surgeon and developing a trusting atmosphere and open communication. Engaging patients extensively at this initial phase enhances their familiarity with the operation process, which plays a critical role in their satisfaction with the outcome. It is also necessary that surgeons analyze the psychological aspects that will influence the patient's perception of his or her body and the result, with the knowledge that unrealistic expectations are the cause of dissatisfaction post-surgery. Following the process of patient evaluation, surgical planning shifts to the technicalities of the procedure itself. This entails choice of the most appropriate surgical technique and technology suitable to the patient's particular anatomical and aesthetic demands. Up-to-date advancements, such as the utilization of ultrasonic osteotomes, have revolutionized surgical processes to enable higher accuracy in altering bones while preserving adjacent tissues. For instance, findings indicate that the application of tools like Piezosurgery results in better micromorphological outcomes and roughness values of osteotomized bone surfaces compared to traditional techniques (Anesi et al., 2014). A good surgical plan should also include anesthesia, postoperative management, and planning for potential complications. Such systemic planning ensures that all elements are addressed in a holistic fashion, allowing for the overall setup for a successful surgical outcome. Finally, the surgical planning process culminates in a detailed blueprint for the operation that guides the entire process. This plan is not just worried about the technical aspects of the surgery but also about the logistics, such as planning and resources. Effective communication between the surgical team, including the anesthesiologists and nurses, is essential to execute this plan effectively. A unified environment allows the sharing of ideas and changes as needed during the surgery, taking into consideration any unexpected complications that might arise. The use of research-supported methods and procedures, such as those discussed in studies on osteotomy methods, is essential to optimizing patient safety and maximizing healing outcomes (Kalaskar et al., 2016). Lastly, accurate surgical planning is imperative to the achievement of optimal aesthetic results, risk avoidance, and facilitation of a rewarding patient experience in cosmetic facial surgery (Figure 3.2).

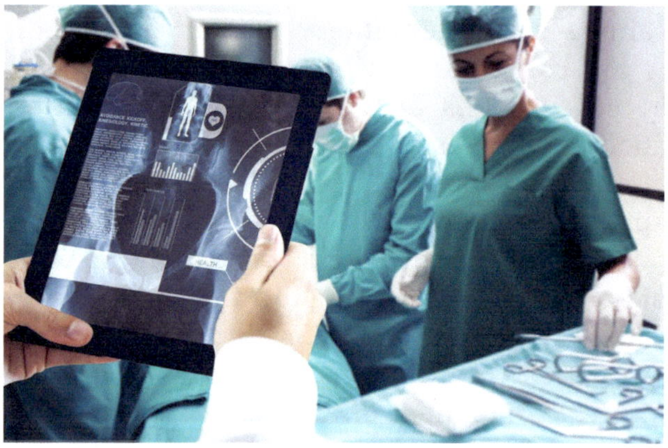

Figure 3.2. The surgical planning process in cosmetic facial surgery.

Source: https://cdn.prod.website-files.com/651c148151215 43d83a69af8/67994ad223af1a9d6bcd38ad_BLOG%202021-05-08%20Reimagining%20Surgical%20Planning.webp.

3.1. The Role of Patient History

Learning Outcome

1. Discuss the Gathering Comprehensive Medical History
2. nderstand Psychological Factors
3. Explain the Assessing Previous Surgical Experiences

Accurate patient history assessment is the building block of cosmetic facial surgery. Complete patient history enables surgeons to identify pre-existing medical conditions, past surgical histories, and potential hereditary factors that would affect the results of surgeries. All these precautions are considered necessary since factors like pre-existing illnesses or allergies have a significant effect on the choice of surgical techniques and equipment utilized in procedures. For instance, information about a patient's history of anesthesia can influence decisions regarding sedation techniques, minimizing complications during surgery. Further, this history facilitates the adjustment of postoperative care plans to offer patient safety and satisfaction as key priorities in surgical care. Through the meticulous history of the patient, surgeons are able to make a better grasp of each person's own situation, which is indispensable for effective surgical planning and better outcomes for patients. In addition to patient-specific surgical optimization, inquiry into a patient's psychosocial history is also part of the preoperative evaluation process. Cosmetic facial surgery patients typically possess specific aesthetic desires based on their personal experience, cultural background, and psychological state. Open communication of these factors can reveal deeper motives and expectations. Practitioners can more accurately determine realistic goals vs. dangerous ideals (Geiger et al., 2021). Mental health background, including conditions like body dysmorphic disorder, is of particular interest because it may necessitate special attention or other management plans prior to surgery. Placing this element of patient history at the beginning not only establishes the trust between the patient and surgeon but also ensures that any additional care or intervention that may be required is identified along the course of surgery. Further, the dynamic nature of evidence-based guidelines emphasizes the importance of gathering and assessing patient history. Preoperative evaluations according to the uncomplicated comprehension of every patient's medical history are recommended by the guidelines. For instance, patient history-based diagnosis of salivary gland malignancy can inform diagnostic workup and therapeutic intervention appropriately (Jörgen Slots, 2017). As clinical knowledge and facts change, so does the necessity to integrate older patient data with new emerging clinical facts. This integration informs best patient management strategies, the best surgical decision-making, and ultimately the best results. The ability to combine past information with current best practice not only confirms the importance of patient-centered care but also summarizes the evolving standards in cosmetic facial surgery, reflecting a significant shift towards more sophisticated, individualized treatment protocols (Figure 3.3).

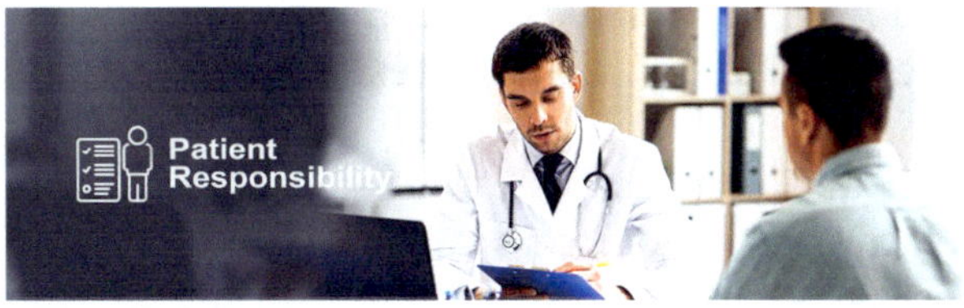

Figure 3.3. The accurate assessment of patient history.

Source: https://external-content.duckduckgo.com/iu/?u=https%3A%2F%2Fcleopatrahospitals.com%2Fmedia%2Ff1sh2jbk%2Fpatient-responsbi-ity-pic-2.jpg&f=1&nofb=1&ipt=8ad6d9fa21e47246a0136e175b17e672e5842cc681165bb0a9c06e9db2ccf294.

3.1.1. Gathering Comprehensive Medical History

Taking thorough medical history is an important aspect of patient assessment in the setting of cosmetic facial surgery. This is the pathway through which potential risks and contraindications can have an effect on surgical outcomes. For instance, a thorough examination of a patient's history, past surgical history, and medications must be undertaken in order to identify complications that could ensue, such as interactions with anesthetics or exacerbation of existing diseases. In addition, knowledge of the patient's psychosocial history, such as their expectations and emotional well-being, offers important insight into their motivations and fears about the procedure. This more complete consideration not only adds to the safety of the surgical treatment but also makes the results congruent with the patient's individual objectives, which in turn encourages satisfaction with the outcome. In addition to the usual components of medical history, questioning about some aspects, such as history of previous aesthetic treatments, family medical history, and chronic pain syndromes, is necessary for total evaluation of risk. For instance, careful attention must be given in cases like trigeminal neuralgia, which may influence the selection of surgery rationally and practically. By analyzing data from past medical histories and diagnostic tests, including imaging tests, surgeons can design a customized surgery plan in advance with anticipation of potential problems. The relationship between patients' histories and responses to treatments substantiates the necessity to individualize surgical methods. Deliberate planning significantly contributes to the success rates of procedural outcomes and minimizes post-operative complications, in line with proper practice in cosmetic surgery. Moreover, encouraging open discussion while taking the medical history can enable a better collaborative environment between the patient and surgical team. Permitting patients to express concerns, preferences, and past experiences empowers them to be more compliant with pre-operative orders and have greater satisfaction with the surgical procedure. The use of standardized measures can also help clinicians evaluate measures like the patient's level of anxiety and quality of life, thus creating a holistic picture of the patient's health status. It not only helps in better pre-operative planning but also aids in assuring follow-up after surgery, which addresses complications effectively. Lastly, this cross-disciplinary process reflects the contemporary movement in medicine, where patient-centered care is the most important aspect of cosmetic facial surgery in order to obtain optimal results and patient well-being in the surgery process (Figure 3.4).

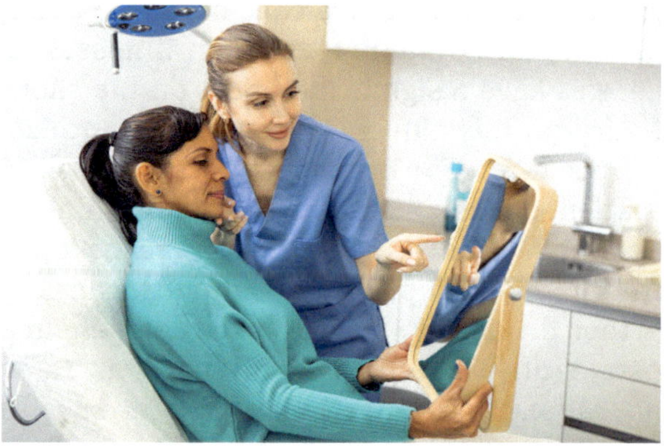

Figure 3.4. Gathering a comprehensive medical history.

Source: https://ambrdfcs.org/wp-content/uploads/2023/09/what-to-expect-at-a-facial-cosmetic-surgery-consultation.jpeg.

3.1.2. Understanding Psychological Factors

The psychological factors influencing patient assessment and surgical planning in cosmetic facial surgery are multifaceted and critical in achieving adequate results. It is essential to determine a patient's reasons for cosmetic surgery because such reasons are so embedded with personal self-image and self-worth. A comprehensive psychological evaluation can not only reveal the apparent desires for beauty alteration but also the underlying states of body dysmorphic disorder and anxiety. These disorders have the potential to distort patients' body image perceptions and affect satisfaction after surgery. Besides, clinicians must avoid having excessively positive expectations, which might lead to disappointment. Surgeons can adjust their technique to suit individual patients for treating these psychological factors and develop a goal-setting and therapy culture that is essential for cosmetic surgery success. Rapport building and communication in cosmetic facial surgery have fundamental roles in comprehending a patient's psychological situation. The initial consultation presents a good opportunity for surgeons to evaluate patients emotional readiness and expectations. Clinicians can elicit patients thoughts and feelings regarding the perceived flaws and desired improvements by active listening. Moreover, surgeons must make sure that their recommendations consider the psychological constitution of the patient in order to avoid the traps of dissatisfaction. Psychosocial assessment can guide surgeons in developing an integrated view of the patient such that they can individualize surgical plans that not only consider aesthetic goals but also prioritize emotional wellness. Such individualization is a component of having surgery perceived as life-enhancing rather than correctional. Post-operative psychological support is also important in maintaining patient satisfaction with cosmetic facial surgery. According to the procedure, patients can experience a range of emotions, from euphoria to regret. Surgeons should anticipate providing emotional support and full follow-up care to overcome potential psychological resistance to satisfaction. Follow-ups after surgery on a routine basis can also help determine any signs of depression or anxiety, allowing timely intervention if indicated. Research underscores that the best possible outcomes of cosmetic surgery are not simply a function of technical ability but also of understanding and dealing with the psychological aspects of recovery. With the addition of psychological support during preoperative assessments and follow-up after surgery, practitioners can have a deep impact on long-term patient satisfaction and overall success of cosmetic surgery procedures, ultimately leading to better correlation between patient outcomes and initial expectations and wishes (Figure 3.5).

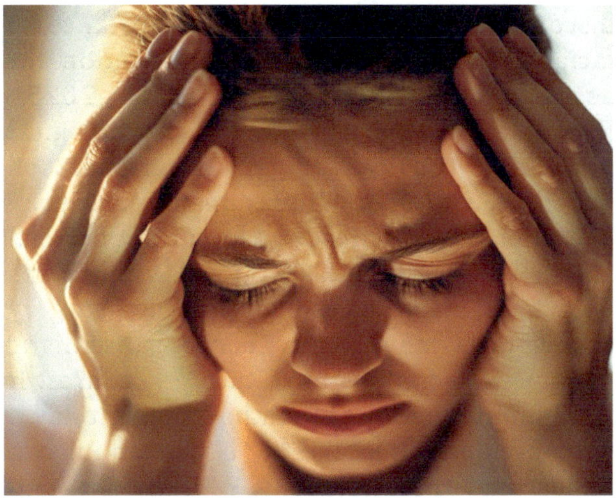

Figure 3.5. The psychological factors influencing patient assessment.

Source: https://external-content.duckduckgo.com/iu/?u=https%3A%2F%2Fimg.freepik.com%2Fpremium-photo%2Funderstanding-psychological-factors-influencing-chronic-pain-management_1247965-37725.jpg&f=1&nofb=1&ipt=8349ee4592e9110d201c90abee4c68214d6ced3709ea1f310836ecb869615e08.

3.1.3. Assessing Previous Surgical Experiences

The assessment of previous surgical experiences is an integral part of patient evaluation, in this case, cosmetic facial surgery. Knowledge of a patient's surgical history allows the firm assessment of his or her anatomical frame and affective responses to past surgeries. When evaluating prior surgeries, one should consider the outcomes, the complications that arose, and the patients' satisfaction. Such evaluations not just influence future procedure decisions but can also reveal underlying pathologies that require a tailored approach. For instance, patients with a history of facial surgeries are bound to present altered anatomical structures as a result of past interventions, which must be studied diligently to optimize surgical planning and patient satisfaction in future cosmetic procedures, as supported by recent scientific discoveries that highlight the importance of facial asymmetry patterns identification for aesthetic outcomes (Koppert et al., 2025). In addition to the physical, the psychological impacts of previous surgery experiences on patients can never be underestimated. A majority of patients who present for cosmetic facial surgery have complex emotional connections with their history of surgeries. Prior surgery experiences may create fear or unrealistic surgical expectations for future procedures. It is therefore vital that operating teams sit down with patients and candidly explain things to understand their concerns, expectations, and history of surgeries to their satisfaction. The assessment of these psychological elements is a part of creating an individualized surgical plan that aligns with the patient's aesthetic and emotional goals. Additionally, the patient-focused skill of the surgeon is reflected not only in trust establishment but also in greater overall satisfaction with outcomes, eventually creating a more agreeable setting for successful surgical encounters (Avetikov et al., 2024). Moreover, during the assessment process, the history of previous complications and how they were resolved can provide valuable information to plan for surgery. Accurate records should be maintained regarding any complications, healing issues, or dissatisfaction that accompanied previous surgeries. Such data can assist in planning the strategy by surgeons, whether to opt for less aggressive techniques or select a better postoperative care regimen, especially in complicated surgical histories of patients. Additionally, what the subtleties of previous surgery outcomes enable is improved patient education regarding expectations and risks from subsequent interventions. Informed discussion on the basis of the patient's history of procedures can lead to a patient-driven decision-making process, to a more comprehensive understanding of how previous experiences set the direction for future cosmetic intervention (Koppert et al., 2025).

Test Your Knowledge

1. Why is obtaining a comprehensive patient history essential for accurate diagnosis and treatment planning?
2. How can psychological factors such as anxiety, stress, or coping style influence a patient's medical or surgical outcomes?
3. What aspects of a patient's previous surgical experiences should clinicians assess to anticipate potential complications or patient concerns?

3.2. Physical Examination Techniques

Learning Outcome

1. Discus Visual Assessment of Facial Features
2. Explain the Palpation and Functional Assessment
3. Focus on Documentation of Findings

Physical examination techniques utilized in cosmetic facial surgery are integral components of patient assessment and operative planning. Thorough evaluation begins with a thorough patient history, including medical and cosmetic complaints. The patient's expectation, history of previous surgeries, and any medical conditions that can influence the result of surgery should be known by the surgeon. Assessment of facial morphology and facial symmetry is of utmost significance, as they influence the aesthetic results of surgeries tremendously. From visual inspection to palpation of discrete tissues, these types of examination techniques assist surgeons in creating customized surgery plans to accommodate the patient's desires and anatomical realities.

Apart from visual and tactile evaluation of soft tissues, functional assessments of the face also form a crucial component of preoperative workup. Surgeons need to evaluate facial nerve function and muscle tone to identify any asymmetry or restriction that will influence surgical decision-making. These measurements of function are the patient's skin quality, thickness, and elasticity, which are key determinants of which surgical approaches will best fit each patient. Understanding these variables enables clinicians to forecast potential complications and help facilitate optimal patient outcomes. Besides, the comprehensive approach facilitates an interactive consultation between patient and surgeon that lays the ground for multidisciplinary decision-making promoted by guidelines like the 2023 International Evidence-based Guideline (Teede et al., 2023). Finally, advanced imaging modalities may be used to supplement traditional examination habits, offering a detailed insight into facial anatomy. Imaging modalities like digital imaging or 3D photography allow surgeons to see the likely results of surgical procedures and convey these predicted results in an effective manner to patients. This type of technology facilitates the identification of particular areas that need intervention and improves the accuracy of surgical planning. Furthermore, marrying all this data with the findings of the physical exam results in an overall picture of what the patients require, finally leading to more tailored and effective treatment plans. As referenced in the recent patient management guidelines across various domains of medicine, evidence-based practice must be the driving force behind decision-making for surgery to minimize risk and maximize general patient satisfaction (Geiger et al., 2021) (Figure 3.6).

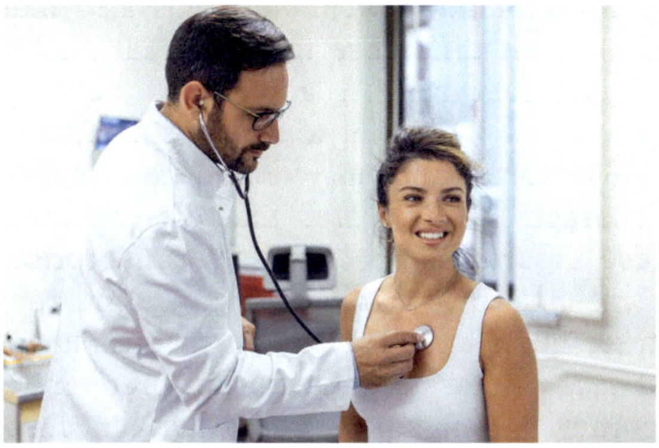

Figure 3.6. The physical examination techniques utilized in cosmetic facial surgery.

Source: https://external-content.duckduckgo.com/iu/?u=https%3A%2F%2Fmeridianhealthcare.net%2Fwp-content%2Fuploads%2F2022%2F03%2FPatient-receiving-a-physical-exam.jpg&f=1&nofb=1&ipt=8910389910f0bd8d8373480c6c5941dad259cb8fca8be7483d3ffda06cd4b713.

3.2.1. Visual Assessment of Facial Features

Visual evaluation of facial features is the bedrock within the field of cosmetic facial surgery and the initial step in patient evaluation and surgical planning. The ability to recognize subtle variations in facial features, from proportion and symmetry to overall appearance, is relied upon by surgeons for evaluation of an aesthetically good-looking face. A good visual inspection allows surgeons to create a longer profile of the patient's facial structure, drawing attention to aspects such as facial element congruence and overall harmony. This is not a subjective assessment; it relies on established aesthetic norms that are used to guide the surgery. Assisted by emerging technology, this visual assessment can then be supplemented by the use of imaging modalities and data analysis. Thus, the integration of newer technologies makes the diagnostic process easier, eventually enhancing decision-making and making the surgery plan compatible with the aspirations of patients and anatomical considerations. Progress made in artificial intelligence (AI) and 3D simulation technology has also made a significant difference in the visual analysis of facial features. AI algorithms have the capability of processing and analyzing intricate facial features, allowing for the identification of characteristic features that direct surgery. These algorithms, particularly convolutional neural networks, are most appropriate to extract important features from medical images and face photos to enhance the preoperative accuracy. Supplying surgeons with accurate information about facial structure, AI becomes a useful contribution in preoperative planning and outcome prediction. The combination of AI with traditional visual assessment methods results in a more advanced interpretation of patient anatomy, with space for tailor-made surgical techniques. As the discipline of cosmetic surgery embraces these advanced technologies, the boundaries between artistic intuition and algorithmic accuracy blur, enabling greater surgical outcomes that more closely approximate patient wishes (Rokhshad et al., 2023). Moreover, visual analysis of facial features not only serves as a vehicle of surgical planning but also as a critical component in patient and surgical team training. With the application of 3D printing and simulation techniques, surgeons can illustrate potential outcomes so that patients can better understand what realities are after surgery. This participatory approach facilitates improved patient consultations in which individuals can become active players in the decision-making process. By utilizing 3D models and simulation, there is open communication between patients and surgeons as treatment goals are explained, while expectations are managed. Notably, these techniques facilitate practicing complex procedures and refining surgical plans before stepping into the operating room. With ever-evolving aesthetic principles, the interactive process among visual assessment, technology, and patient education will not only dictate surgical outcomes but reshape the patient experience in cosmetic facial surgery (Meyer-Szary et al., 2022) (Figure 3.7).

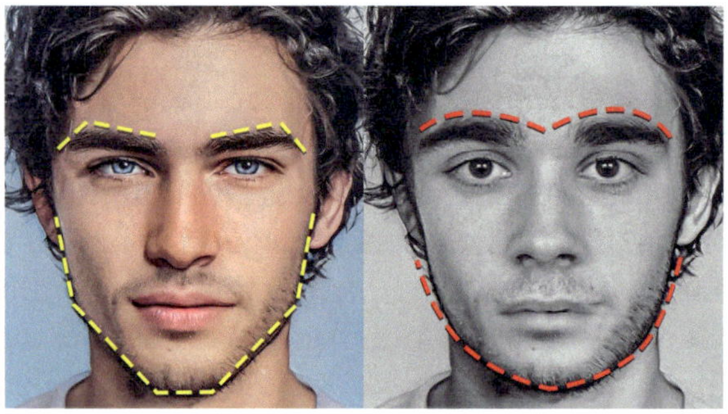

Figure 3.7. The visual assessment of facial features.

Source: https://external-content.duckduckgo.com/iu/?u=https%3A%2F%2Fi.ytimg.com%2Fvi%2FOxJ8K3T4Yl8%2Fmaxresdefault.jpg&f=1&nofb=1&ipt=c10a8ec968fd4010c6ad642c0e7be1d78f330a79fe2b74b7902ced5108119532.

3.2.2. Palpation and Functional Assessment

The functional assessment by palpation is a mainstay in the patient evaluation stage of cosmetic facial surgery. Palpation is this hands-on method that allows surgeons to systematically assess facial anatomy, not only assessing cosmetic but also functional aspects, such as muscle tension and tissue integrity. Careful palpation identifies concealed anatomical landmarks, providing information regarding individual variations that can influence surgical outcomes. Effective palpation enables the examiner to identify tension points or soft tissue pathology, which may reflect underlying conditions for consideration in planning surgery. The inclusion of functional assessment in the form of facial expression measurement and muscle activity allows procedure appropriateness to be determined. This technique ensures that surgical interventions are as per the patient's own facial anatomy and function-based profile, ultimately resulting in the best aesthetic results and preservation of facial dynamics. In facial cosmetic surgery, the accuracy of palpation and functional assessment is a significant factor in deciding the success of surgery. Literature reveals that patients who have severe gender dysphoria are more likely to have a higher demand for facial feminization procedures, such as rhinoplasty and mandible reduction, in which precise anatomical information must be considered during pre-surgical planning (Yu et al., 2022). By utilizing a lot of palpation, surgeons can estimate the degree of malleability of the tissue as well as assess any potential complications due to underlying factors. This assessment not only guides the selection of the surgical techniques but also allows practitioners to anticipate the extent of possible modification required to achieve the desired aesthetic results. Further, incorporation of functional assessments within the assessment process allows for ease of determining risks inherent in functional impairment, thereby allowing for a comprehensive understanding that directly impacts the surgical approach used. The long-term rewards of successful palpation and functional evaluation extend beyond the first surgery itself and into the larger postoperative process. Successful initial examinations can lead to increased patient satisfaction and a greater quality of aesthetic outcomes. For instance, in the management of conditions such as fibrous dysplasia, meticulous evaluation of the affected anatomy through palpation will guide the surgeons' decision towards wholesale excision and not conservative recontouring (Gbujie et al., 2021). Such a decision is critical, as improper assessment of the extent of anatomical deformities will compromise functional and aesthetic results. Overall, the integration of palpation and functional assessment encourages a patient-centered process of cosmetic facial surgery to ensure every surgical plan is individually tailored to not only meet aesthetic objectives but also optimize the patients' functional well-being.

3.2.3. Documentation of Findings

Recording of findings in cosmetic facial surgery is the foundation of effective patient assessment and surgical planning. Clinicians must document in-depth details of facial asymmetry, which, in the majority of instances, is pivotal in establishing aesthetic outcomes. Studies show that high facial asymmetries can greatly influence patients' perceptions of their appearance and emotional expressions. Thus, meticulous documentation of such asymmetries, especially those with specific rotation patterns along the xyz axes, enhances surgical planning and ensures that patients' expectations are conscientiously synchronized with potential outcomes (Koppert et al., 2025). By incorporating sound documentation procedures, surgeons can establish a tailored strategy for each case, thereby optimizing surgical methods and patient satisfaction in general. Documentation also extends beyond observation; it involves assessments based on state-of-the-art imaging studies and feedback from patients. The use of high-resolution digital photography and controlled lighting enables specialists to obtain accurate renderings of facial forms, as this provides consistent and reliable analyses of rotation and symmetry. As mentioned in current literature, rightward and leftward rotation is prevalent among various populations, which underscores the need for inclusive measures that consider both individual differences in anatomy as well as overall patterns. Standardized documentation procedures, combined with group evaluation by independent examiners, ensure that variation in original reports is captured, improving validity in the assessment process (Koppert et al., 2025). This deliberative process not only assists in laying out the prime surgical targets but also establishes a partnership of trust between the patient and the operating team. The incorporation of patient satisfaction forms into the documentation process also enriches planning in cosmetic facial surgery. Employment of standardized questionnaires and panel ratings can offer valuable input regarding patients' satisfaction with outcomes following blepharoplasty. Research indicates that proper pre- and post-surgical documentation enhances understanding of intervention impact on facial topography and overall aesthetics. This feedback process enhances continuous improvement in surgical technique and enhances sensitivity to patients' wishes and needs. Hence, thorough reporting of outcomes is part of the definition of success in cosmetic surgery, which not only affects clinical practice but also further assists patient education and ultimately leads to more accurate and satisfactory surgical treatments.

Test Your Knowledge

1. What key facial characteristics should be evaluated during the visual assessment portion of a physical examination?
2. How does palpation contribute to understanding functional issues or abnormalities in the facial structures?
3. Why is accurate and detailed documentation important after completing the physical examination?

3.3. Patient Expectations and Goals

Learning Outcome

1. Discussing Desired Outcomes
2. Focus on Managing Unrealistic Expectations
3. Explain Importance of Clear Communication

Goals and expectations of the patient in cosmetic facial surgery are a critical foundation for successful surgical planning and outcome. Recognition of these assumptions enables surgeons to tailor their approaches to align with what patients are thinking for themselves. This begins via consultations, where the professionals must have serious conversations to discuss the motivations behind a patient seeking specific procedures. By actively listening and encouraging open communication, surgeons can separate more realistically possible wishes from less realistically possible ones. Such transparency not only supports the creation of mutual understanding but also enhances patient satisfaction following surgery. In addition, as patient-centered care becomes increasingly a priority within cosmetic clinics, the capacity to accurately assess and respond to such expectations has a far-reaching impact on quality control in ensuring a pleasant experience and achieving aesthetic objectives in line with patient intent. With the constant stream of evolving technological developments, they are increasingly being drawn into shaping patient expectations and surgical planning in cosmetic facial surgery. Mobile apps and artificial intelligence (AI) are now essential in informing patient decisions. Patients can utilize these systems to view outcomes, providing more informed discussion between patient and surgeon on what can be done and what should be done. For instance, mobile applications that simulate cosmetic alterations permit patients to experiment with alternate appearances, thereby demystifying their expectations prior to formal surgical consultation. This integration of high-tech technology helps fill the gap between patient expectation and operating room reality and eventually constitutes a more interactive relationship in the therapeutic process. The patients can now enter their operations with clearer, more precise expectations, which has a direct relation to higher satisfaction rates at procedure end, further enhancing the value of such advanced techniques towards improved patient care (Vargas et al., 2025). Moreover, the construction of algorithms in clinical practice serves to underline the importance of individualized care plans with unique patient information. As identified in recent literature, algorithms allow systematic assessment of patient needs and guide surgeons to individualized surgical approaches appropriate to particular goals. Systematic application of algorithms optimizes the likelihood of successful surgical outcomes because it allows surgeons to foresee and optimize intervention outcomes. By doing so, surgeons can provide realistic timelines and recovery expectations as well as opportunities for long-term satisfaction with results. This not only improves the surgical experience but also gives rise to improved all-around quality of life after intervention, a measure of commitment to providing optimal aesthetic outcomes with fewer complications and risks. Leveraging such advancements, healthcare providers can make sure that patients' expectations are met with more efficiency and compassion in cosmetic facial surgery (Tukeshov et al., 2024) (Figure 3.8).

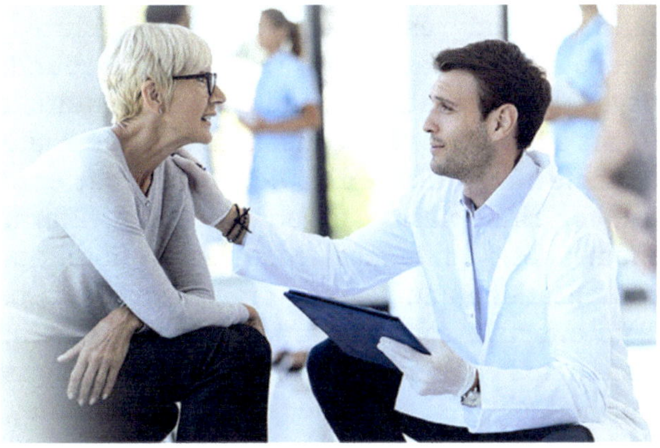

Figure 3.8. Patient expectations and goals.

Source: https://external-content.duckduckgo.com/iu/?u=https%3A%2F%2Fadit.com%2Fstorage%2Ffiles%2Fnavigating-patient-expectations-setting-realistic-goals-for-treatment.jpg&f=1&nofb-1&ipt=d1849957a3c0cf8fba2ef22102d54bf939592825b0f6d8dcad307253dd7901a4.

3.3.1. Discussing Desired Outcomes

In cosmetic facial surgery, describing desired results to patients is a critical component of the patient assessment process. The articulation of patients' aesthetic ideals allows surgeons to create individualized surgical plans according to their specific needs. During initial consultations, clinicians must engage in adequate discussions to discover the patients' expectations, fears, and self-assessed physical features. This understanding is supported when patients verbally communicate explicit desires regarding augmentation or alterations, e.g., alteration of the nose shape or jawline definition. Moreover, studies have found that surgeries, especially to address gender dysphoria, can lead to improved psychological well-being and patient satisfaction when these desires are clearly articulated and realized (Yu et al., 2022). Thus, collaboration not only facilitates a trusting relationship between the patient and the surgeon but also enhances chances for positive surgery results. Application of preoperative assessment to match surgery with desired results cannot be overstated. Thorough evaluation of medical background, psychological readiness, and physical condition forms a basis for valid consent and appropriate expectations. For example, when patients ask for rhinoplasty, surgeons need to inform them about anatomical constraints, potential complications, and the recovery period required. This effective communication at this point in time helps establish a basis on which patients can actually visualize the potential outcomes, which minimizes postoperative dissatisfaction. These assessments also allow surgeons to identify any issues of the mind that could influence outcomes, particularly in procedures aimed at correcting big flaws of self-image (Rohrich et al., 2000). Through meticulous planning and evaluation, the operating team is able to best advise patients regarding how their personal desires match with functional and aesthetic potential. Lastly, negotiation of desired outcomes is not merely a procedural step but an integral component of patient-centered care in cosmetic facial surgery. The individualized approach requires practitioners to employ both subjective and objective measures in terms of evaluation of improvements and satisfaction levels following the surgery. Surgeons have to utilize methods such as imaging technology and measurement analysis to give patients realistic expectations, while the final results harmonize with their natural facial structure. The integration of surgeons' suggestions and patients' comments not only enhances surgery precision but also assists in establishing a mutual understanding of results. Such a cooperative endeavor reaffirms the problem of patient autonomy and satisfaction, as evidenced by findings that present higher levels of satisfaction if patients feel that their personal preferences have been respected in the course of surgery (Yu et al., 2022). Active exploration of hoped-for expectations is thus critical to effective patient assessment and surgical planning.

3.3.2. Managing Unrealistic Expectations

Management of unrealistic expectations in cosmetic facial surgery is a critical component of patient care with a direct impact on surgical results. The patients arrive with idealized ideals regarding beauty because of social media, celebrity status, and personal aspiration. This means the mismatches between what the patients desire and what can potentially be achieved by surgery. A thorough initial patient assessment, therefore, should include an open discussion of likely outcomes, limitations, and the realistic potential of cosmetic surgery.

These discussions assist in gaining a better understanding of patients' motivations and having a clearer idea of setting realistic goals, ultimately guiding the planning process of surgery to a better and more satisfactory patient outcome. Additionally, the use of advanced technologies like artificial intelligence may enhance the preoperative consultation process by assisting in communicating potential outcomes in visual terms. Using Generative Adversarial Networks (GANs) to produce realistic images that are associated with the anticipated changes in a patient's appearance will assist in demonstrating multiple outcomes while making things clearer about what is achievable. As mentioned, the created images have reflected biases, mostly featuring lighter-skinned women, thus requiring caution and ethical considerations in representation in educational materials in cosmetic surgery (Lim et al., 2023). Through the responsible use of such tools, surgeons can avoid risks of misaligned expectations, with the end result being higher patient satisfaction rates. Finally, the importance of addressing defensive practices in the clinical scenario of cosmetic surgery cannot be overstated. Defensive medicine presents itself as a response to complaints from patients, where doctors may be extra careful so they will not get complaints, leading to excessive procedures or tests (Eftekhari et al., 2023).

This not only complicates the patient's process but can also bring about increasing healthcare costs and loss of trust in the patient-provider relationship. Through the promotion of simple communication and ethics in expectation management, cosmetic surgeons can build a more empathetic environment with more focus on patient care and trust. Enhanced patient assessment procedures, driven by innovative technological options, will lead the way in maximizing surgical planning and maintaining the integrity of cosmetic surgery practice (Figure 3.9).

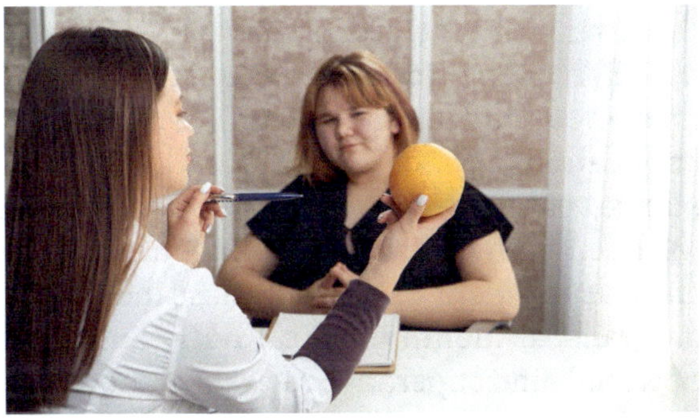

Figure 3.9. Managing unrealistic expectations.

Source: https://external-content.duckduckgo.com/iu/?u=https%3A%2F%2Fcosmeticfact.com.au%2Fwp-content%2Fuploads%2F2023%2F06%2F4R-53.webp&f=1&nofb=1&ipt=eec488de7db2c731d6a77fcd0ca432ce39bce4f8d42c6ef74a460f6fbea64526.

3.3.3. Importance of Clear Communication

Effective communication is a cornerstone in the context of cosmetic facial surgery, particularly at patient assessment and surgical planning. When surgeons thoroughly inform patients of procedures, risks, and outcomes, the patients are in a position to make informed decisions regarding their treatment. This openness will facilitate a trusting relationship between practitioner and patient that is essential in overcoming any complications and ensuring expectations are aligned with realities.

Additionally, a well-formulated conversation can result in a shared understanding of what aesthetic results are expected, thereby minimizing the chances of postoperative dissatisfaction.

When patients understand and are heard, they can more effectively comply with preoperative and postoperative directives, enhancing overall surgery results. Secondarily, it facilitates diagnosing any underlying psychological pathology concomitant with cosmetic procedures. The vast majority of patients undergo surgery due to personal or societal pressure, most commonly issues of self-esteem and body image. These need to be addressed openly so surgeons can adjust their treatment accordingly.

For instance, the psychological impact of conditions like strabismus has a significant influence on the quality of life of a patient, as seen through research that indicates how such conditions affect self-esteem as well as social relationships (Astle et al., 2016). Through an understanding and consideration of such aspects in open conversation, doctors are capable of making sounder decisions for the psychological preparation of patients for surgical procedures. Also, applying advanced technologies such as Piezosurgery® involves effective communication in a way that provides the patient with an understanding of the novel techniques used. Surgeons must describe the advantages and limitations of various osteotomy methods, like those described in comparative studies of conventional and ultrasonic osteotomes (Anesi et al., 2014). This level of openness enables patients to possess a full awareness of their surgical options and a feeling of empowerment in medical decision-making. Finally, good communication not only enhances patient satisfaction but also makes an enormous difference in the result of surgery, as well-informed patients are likely to have realistic expectations and be actively involved in their postoperative care.

Test Your Knowledge

1. Why is it important for clinicians to identify and address unrealistic patient expectations early in the consultation?
2. What strategies can clinicians use to ensure patients fully understand the limitations and potential results of a procedure?

3.4. Risk Assessment and Management

Learning Outcome

1. Identifying Potential Surgical Risks
2. Evaluating Patient Health Status
3. Developing a Risk Mitigation Plan

Effective risk assessment and management are crucial components in cosmetic facial surgery because of the multifaceted interplay between a patient's physiological status and operative outcomes. Comprehensive patient evaluation before any operation involves examination of both physiological and psychological parameters that may affect healing, as well as satisfaction with outcome. An in-depth understanding of the patient's medical background, including present diseases, allows for early detection of potential complications during the planning stage of surgery. By the inclusion of findings from various sources of diagnosis, professionals are able to anticipate complications and implement risk management strategies most ideal for the particular patient's requirement, ultimately enhancing the surgical process and result. Furthermore, surgical complications can be minimized significantly through the utilization of a formalized nutritional evaluation, particularly in high-risk patient groups. Surgery recipients who have cosmetic facial reconstruction can experience nutritional insufficiency-related complications, which can impair healing. For instance, patients with head and neck cancers have been shown to develop malnutrition, yet clinical assessment using body mass index (BMI) alone fails to identify critical nutritional risks that would affect operative recovery (Chowdhury et al., 2025). Thus, utilization of such measures as Nutrition Risk Screening (NRS) is required in an effort to better identify individuals at risk so that proper dietetic interventions can be instituted in a timely fashion. By taking into account nutritional needs before the fact, operating rooms can provide an environment for support conducive to optimal recovery and reduce postoperative complications. Further, the interrelationship between psychological health and physical health also supports the value of a comprehensive risk management approach to cosmetic facial surgery. Incorporating psychological assessments in patient screening will reveal problems like body dysmorphic disorder or unrealistic expectations for desired outcomes. Identification of such risks enables surgeons to initiate crucial preoperative discussions and, when necessary, refer patients to mental health professionals for help. In identification not just of the physical aspect of surgical risk but also the psychological aspect, practitioners can position themselves better to handle patient expectations and satisfaction after surgery. Thus, this comprehensive approach to risk estimation, with both psychological and physiological elements, can potentially enhance overall success in surgery and the safety of patients in cosmetic facial surgery.

3.4.1. Identifying Potential Surgical Risks

Estimation of probable surgical risks is an important element in the patient assessment process of cosmetic facial surgery. Thorough evaluation begins with a thorough history of the patient that encompasses medical diseases, prior surgical history, and any family predisposition to healing and recovery. Underlying states of disease, such as diabetes, cardiovascular disease, or autoimmunity, significantly augment perioperative risks. Substances such as cigarette smoking and alcohol also discourage healing and increase complication rates. Through careful risk assessment, surgeons can tailor surgical plans that are sensitive to each patient's unique profile, optimizing both outcomes and safety. Proper identification and management of these risks are critical in informing patients completely and, eventually, in making them satisfied with their surgery. Surgical risk assessment extends beyond personal health histories; it entails thoughtful evaluation of the surgery itself. Each cosmetic facial surgery modality carries inherent risks, from infection and scarring through to complications of nerve injury or hematoma development. Surgeons must also consider the complexity of the operation and the anticipated recovery time. For instance, more complex operations will carry a larger potential risk than minimally invasive procedures and therefore necessitate a more advanced preoperative strategy. In addition, understanding the patient's expectations and psychological readiness is necessary to avoid discontent after the operation.

Addressing these procedural hazards in an integrated fashion allows the surgical staff to create a better and more individualized surgical plan, thereby enhancing the outcome and satisfaction of the patient and decreasing the possibility of postoperative complications. Continuing the discussion of surgical hazards implies recognition of how these assessments influence postoperative treatment. Risk identification before treatment allows effective management methods, including tailored postoperative care and vigilant monitoring measures. For instance, those undergoing surgery that significantly alters facial contours can be assisted by further follow-up care to closely monitor for swelling or infection. Similarly, those with higher risks can be compelled to go through more intensive preoperative education and psychiatric evaluation to prepare them for the reality of surgery. The nuances of patient care that arise from thorough risk identification have the potential to significantly enhance patient experience and surgical outcomes. To this end, a sound understanding of what can potentially be risky in surgery, guided by ongoing research and clinical advancements, is essential to furthering the overall image of cosmetic facial surgery (Jörgen Slots, 2017; Topalian et al., 2020) (Figure 3.10).

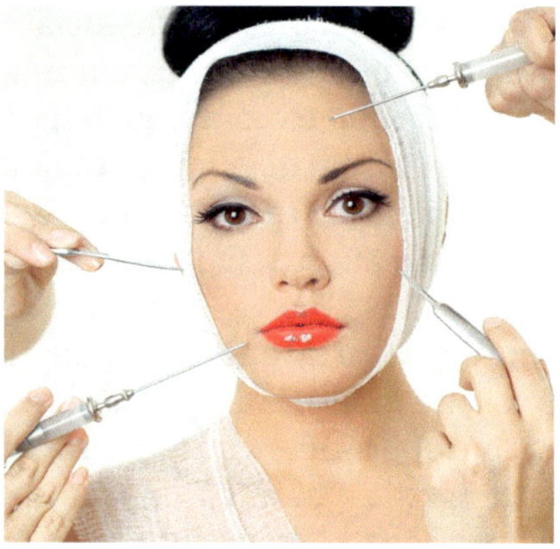

Figure 3.10. The identification of potential surgical risks.

Source: https://external-content.duckduckgo.com/iu/?u=https%3A%2F%2Fsurgeryvip.com%2Fwp-content%2Fuploads%2F2014%2F07%2Fplastic-surgery-scars.jpg&f=1&nofb=1&ipt=03dfc939328b3c98f54df92b25887f4de914075d47339b0f6d66ef61ea0adff7.

3.4.2. Evaluating Patient Health Status

Evaluation of patient health status plays an essential role in the practice of cosmetic facial surgery, as it has a direct bearing on planning and results of surgery. An accurate evaluation involves close examination of medical history, health status at the time, and mental condition. For instance, preoperative examinations may identify such variables as comorbidities influencing the surgery or the recovery process. As proposed in current research, higher preoperative SF-12 scores are significantly correlated with improved postoperative outcomes of facial reconstruction surgery (Wu et al., 2024). Medical screening that addresses both physical and emotional needs is thus a key to effective patient evaluation, enabling surgeons to tailor their surgical intervention accordingly. Besides medical history, patient medical screening should further include psychological testing. Identification of the mental health status of the patient is most important, particularly when it comes to cosmetic surgery, whose success hinges on self-esteem and body image. Gender dysphoria, for instance, may be a factor for a patient seeking a specific surgery, as demonstrated in research among transgender and nonbinary individuals with high gender dysphoria (Yu et al., 2022). These evaluations will permit patient requirements to be anticipated and expectations managed, which will increase satisfaction levels. By the inclusion of a holistic overview of patient health, surgeons are not just able to treat physical change but also foster an environment conducive to psychological well-being. Furthermore, the inclusion of health screenings within surgical planning permits the selection of effective methods and recovery processes postoperatively. Evaluation of age, body mass index (BMI), and fitness allows decisions on surgical approaches in a manner that minimizes complications. For example, evidence suggests that underweight patients will have higher rates of postoperative infections, which emphasizes the importance of tailored preoperative measures (Yu et al., 2022). Furthermore, information on sociodemographic factors, such as insurance status and geography, allows for more equitable care and resource distribution. Therefore, meticulous patient health status evaluation not only optimizes the success of surgery but also ensures each patient is given individualized care he or she needs for a successful encounter with cosmetic facial surgery.

3.4.3. Developing a Risk Mitigation Plan

Due to the complicated nature of cosmetic facial surgery, developing a plan of risk reduction is essential, particularly in light of the multicultural patient populations and various levels of ethics-based standards governing the provision of care. An efficient risk mitigation process begins with a complete patient evaluation, such as identification of present medical conditions, lifestyle choices, and mental readiness for surgery. Surgeons must engage the patient in conversations to reach a definitive understanding of their medical history, goals, and potential psychological impacts of cosmetic change. This initial contact is paramount in determining patient expectations while, at the same time, addressing potential complications experienced in surgical procedures. By increasing transparency and awareness, professionals can prepare better for the inherent risks of surgical procedures, thereby leading to improved patient outcomes and satisfaction rates in cosmetic surgery. In addition to patient assessment, risk mitigation in cosmetic facial surgery must incorporate effective surgical planning. This phase involves a thorough consideration of the surgical technique and technology involved, and a detailed understanding of the individualized anatomical variables encountered by each patient. Surgeons are supported to adopt evidence-based practice supported by current research and clinical guidelines, which can minimize recovery complications. For instance, the application of sophisticated imaging and 3D modeling technology can provide surgeons with enhanced visualizations of the operating site, thereby enabling more precise and individualized surgical procedures. Furthermore, integrating collaborative practice can enhance the surgical team's ability to cope with unanticipated problems that can occur during the operation and consequently result in improved patient care and safety. Lastly, there is a need to establish a balanced risk reduction plan through continuous evaluation and refinement of the plan with emerging new information and technology within the industry. Continuous professional education through learning and training can make surgical teams remain vigilant on the latest advancements in patient safety and surgery techniques. Furthermore, adherence to systems of post-operative monitoring and follow-up will aid in early detection and management of potential complications. Data from historical cases, such as those identified in relevant studies, can inform adjustments of surgical techniques and risk mitigation strategies. Emphasizing flexibility as a point of emphasis encourages ongoing practice and future practice in cosmetic facial surgery to be prioritized through paying ongoing focus on patient safety and satisfaction, which is paramount to upholding discipline, credibility and integrity (Cajiao, 2023; Yu et al., 2022) (Figure 3.11).

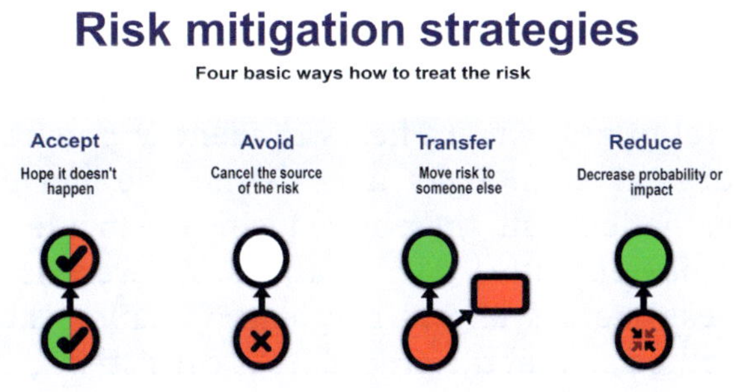

Figure 3.11. Developing a risk mitigation plan.

Source: https://external-content.duckduckgo.com/iu/?u=https%3A%2F%2Faptien.com%2Fuploads%2Fkb_block_image%2Fwhat-are-risk-treatment-strategies%2Fmedium_four-basic-risk-mitigation-strategies.png&f=1&nofb=1&ipt=b97f7e321fafc236b709712e6be4c1bfebc83c9bd8ce40de51a51eb8ef691c3d.

Test Your Knowledge

1. What common surgical risks should be discussed with patients during the risk assessment process?
2. How does a patient's overall health status influence their suitability for surgery and potential postoperative outcomes?
3. What key components should be included in an effective risk-mitigation plan prior to surgery?

3.5. Surgical Planning Strategies

Learning Outcome

1. Discus the Creating a Tailored Surgical Plan
2. Focus on Selecting Appropriate Surgical Techniques
3. Explain Considering Postoperative Care

It is crucial in cosmetic facial surgery to develop successful outcomes for patients through careful surgical planning. One of the building blocks of such planning is a general assessment of the patient's anatomical structure and aesthetic desires. The use of advanced imaging techniques, such as three-dimensional facial scans, allows surgeons to well visualize underlying bone anatomy and soft tissue dynamics, making way for personalized treatment strategies. This level of assessment helps to identify potential surgical challenges and define the perfect aesthetic result, thereby reducing the incidence of postoperative complications. Awareness of these factors allows surgeons to tailor their method so that the procedure is consistent with the patient's expectations and preserves facial functional and aesthetic integrity. Additionally, the selection of appropriate surgical procedures and instruments is important during the surgical planning process. New technology has ensured the availability of such tools as ultrasonic osteotomes, which offer significant advancements over the traditional method. According to studies, these ultrasonic devices, such as Piezosurgery®, enhance the precision of osteotomies without unnecessary soft tissue damage, which is paramount in cosmetic surgery where subtlety is essential (Anesi et al., 2014). Secondly, incorporating an awareness of micro-morphologies and roughness values into bone manipulation within the sphere helps to optimize the healing processes after surgery. Lastly, the integration of the most recent technologies into surgical strategies not only optimizes patient safety but also facilitates successful recovery as well as aesthetic satisfaction. Lastly, collaboration between the patient and the surgical team contributes significantly to successful surgical planning. Engaging patients in their own surgical experience ensures that expectations are appropriately understood and managed. Information regarding the surgical process, outcomes to be expected, and recovery is central to facilitating well-informed choice-making. Application of pedicled perforator flaps for partial breast reconstruction demonstrates how surgical planning can be individualized to address individual patient needs while designing aesthetically pleasing outcomes (Cillino et al., 2010). By encouraging open communication and realistic expectations, the operating team is able to develop a partnership that ultimately gains the patient's overall experience and satisfaction with his or her cosmetic surgery process (Figure 3.12).

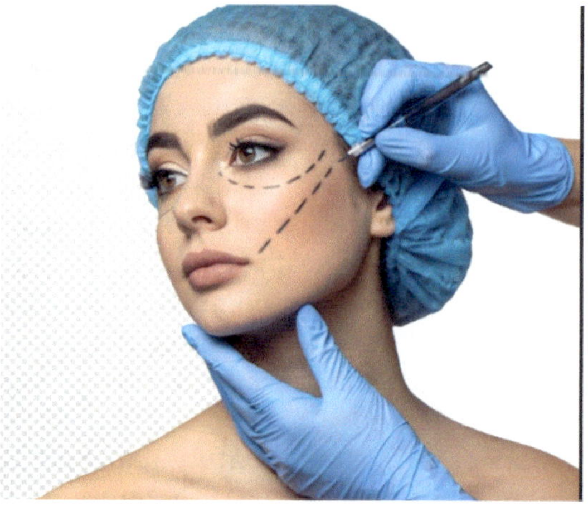

Figure 3.12. In cosmetic facial surgery, meticulous surgical planning.

Source: https://external-content.duckduckgo.com/iu/?u=https%3A%2F%2Fimg.freepik.com%2Fpremium-psd%2Ffacial-surgery-planning-doctor-marking-face_1086464-821.jpg&f=1&nofb=1&ipt=58979a7267a99c429f70ec7d8c0b0df20f87d5a6b1d4f17bf415069006115368.

3.5.1. Creating a Tailored Surgical Plan

The process of developing an individualized surgical plan in cosmetic facial surgery begins with a detailed patient evaluation that is extremely important in order to achieve individualized treatment results. This evaluation includes assessment of the patient's facial appearance, history and factors, and psychological suitability for surgery. Careful facial examination involves the examination of symmetry and proportions because disordered facial asymmetry can heavily affect perceived beauty as well as emotional facial expression. According to recent observations, asymmetries of the face must be accurately treated to match the patient's cosmetic desires, with a focus on a meticulously thought-out surgical approach considering elements such as facial rotation due to age and inherent asymmetries of the patient (Koppert et al., 2025).

By applying standardized evaluation techniques, surgeons can distinguish between different types of asymmetries and design strategies to address them in an effective manner, ultimately enhancing aesthetic and functional outcomes for the patient. A personalized surgical plan must also consider the specific characteristics of the patient overall, including gender, ethnicity, and idiosyncratic facial attributes. For example, for gender-affirming procedures, such as male-to-female surgeries, clinicians must navigate numerous masculine features—wide chins and high hairlines—whom they must dramatically reconstruct with surgery. Facial feminization surgery, as revealed in recent work, addresses performing an adequate clinical assessment and subsequently adopting a customized approach to each patient's requirements, with surgical modifications being in harmony with the ideal result desired (Shams et al., 2009). This meticulous planning allows surgeons to formulate a sequence of phased procedures to treat hard and soft tissue alterations. The level of customization provides for more natural-appearing results in the postoperative period, which is important in cosmetic surgery, where patient satisfaction is highly reliant on perceived improvement. Moreover, the success of an individualized surgical plan does not lie solely on surgical skills but on the team player bonding between patient and surgeon. Communication is the key to understanding the patient's expectations and delivering these appropriately into real intraoperative results. Surgeons must enlighten patients regarding the potential risks, benefits, and limitations of their surgeries and facilitate an active decision-making approach that upholds the patient's desires and anxieties (Koppert et al., 2025). Through an open discussion, professionals can achieve enhanced patient confidence and engagement, ultimately leading to greater satisfaction with surgical encounters. This combined environment has the consequence of putting patients at ease, knowing that their unique facial characteristics will be considered, thereby advancing the art of aesthetic facial surgery in the form of personalized planning.

3.5.2. Selecting Appropriate Surgical Techniques

The selection of appropriate surgical techniques in cosmetic facial surgery is essential to the achievement of optimal patient results. Surgeons are responsible for performing a comprehensive assessment involving not just the anatomical problem but also the patient's specific aesthetic goals and medical history.

Technique selection is strongly related to factors like the extent of the procedure, the outcomes to be obtained, and the specific anatomical structures being targeted. According to the American Society of Clinical Oncology's definition, practitioners should use evidence-based guidelines in scheduling operations. Such guidelines also entail preoperative evaluations, which are most relevant to guide the surgical approaches adopted so as to ensure optimal safety as well as outcomes (Geiger et al., 2021). Furthermore, each surgical approach should take into consideration multidisciplinary advice, combining the views of a number of experts so as to achieve the best available option for the patients specific needs.

This common platform allows for prolonged study of the patient's state in relation to parameters like skin quality, tissue laxity, and structural anatomy that is more profound. For example, procedures like rhytidectomy may be perfectly suited for facial rejuvenation in high-skin-laxity patients, while non-surgical procedures like injectables may be perfect for minimal enhancements.

Comprehensive training in these various techniques is required for surgeons to conduct tailored interventions that adapt to patients' cosmetic requests (Niemiec et al., 2020). Postoperative considerations also play an important role in selecting surgical techniques. Surgeons must anticipate the process of recovery, probable complications, and the overall pattern of recovery in relation to different approaches. Techniques minimizing scarring and speeding up recovery, such as endoscopic methods, are increasingly encouraged to dispel concerns over obvious postoperative changes. In addition, maintaining an open dialogue with patients throughout the operating process greatly influences levels of satisfaction, making them feel included in making the decision. Lastly, better insight into surgical technique, patient-centered planning, and evidence-based guidelines underpins the selection of techniques that produce good cosmetic outcomes and the health of the patient (Niemiec et al., 2020).

3.5.3. Considering Postoperative Care

Postoperative care for cosmetic facial surgery is an aspect that is instrumental in impacting patient outcomes and satisfaction. Following surgical intervention, recovery of the operation requires specially tailored management techniques to achieve optimal healing and esthetic results. It is crucial for health care professionals to implement complex postoperative programs comprising pain relief, infection prevention, and wound care. The early postoperative period is often accompanied by patient education about awareness of complications, such as overswelling or infection, hence empowering the patients with information that fosters active participation in their recovery (Geiger et al., 2021). Consequently, formal follow-up visits are essential in monitoring progress towards healing, in addressing concerns, and in incorporating necessary adjustments to care plans to ultimately optimize the overall surgical outcome.

Additionally, those patients who are post-cosmetic facial surgery may have varying degrees of physical and emotional response in the postoperative period, which requires vigilant response. Psychological impacts following surgery can range from depression after the surgery to unrealistic expectations regarding outcomes. Thus, inclusion of psychological care services in the postoperative treatment is vital in the context of handling such emotional aspects (Geiger et al., 2021).

Besides, health care providers can implement evidence-based interventions that are both patient-centered and responsive to the feedback of the patients. For instance, practices that offer personalized pain management choices or use minimally invasive techniques can facilitate quicker recovery and better patient satisfaction. Accordingly, collaborative learning, where a culture of shared decision-making is fostered, can significantly enhance postoperative care experiences with a focus on addressing the physical as well as psychological needs. Finally, the integration of innovations in surgical techniques and therapeutic adjuvants will also facilitate postoperative care for cosmetic facial surgery. The use of immune checkpoint blockade therapies, as shown in current literature, is a revolutionary approach that would enhance recovery results through optimized healing and reduced inflammatory responses. Pursuing these new lines of treatment calls for intense collaboration among surgical teams, oncology professionals, and caregiver patients to help address the complexities of treatment. The multi-disciplinary treatment not only boosts the postoperative model of care but also follows best practices as outlined in prevailing clinical guidelines (Geiger et al., 2021). By careful assessment and planning, patients can achieve the desired cosmetic results, reduce complications, and enhance their postoperative experience (Figure 3.13).

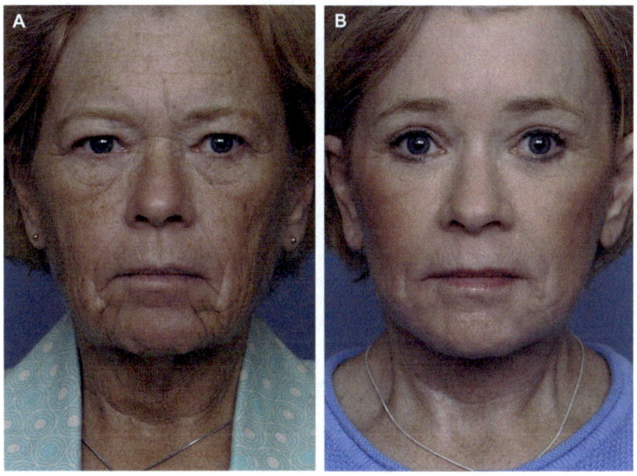

Figure 3.13. Considering postoperative care.

Source: https://external-content.duckduckgo.com/iu/?u=https%3A%2F%2Fwww.facialplastic.theclinics.com%2Fcms%2F10.1016%2Fj.fsc.2019.09.010%2Fasset%2Fe53971e5-96ce-4718-85c0-1e5ad3a85508%2Fmain.assets%2Fgr3_lrg.jpg&f=1&nofb=1&ipt=e7258b59149c3d83c2b450c9229cf66369c6ba0c11216b9eb8956d4482894099.

Test Your Knowledge

1. What factors should be evaluated when creating a tailored surgical plan for an individual patient?
2. How do surgeons determine which surgical techniques are most appropriate for achieving the desired outcome?
3. Why is it essential to consider postoperative care during the preoperative planning phase?

3.6. Ethical Considerations in Cosmetic Surgery

Learning Outcome

1. Discuss the Informed Consent Process
2. Focus on Addressing Ethical Dilemmas
3. Explain Importance of Patient Autonomy

Ethical considerations are paramount in cosmetic surgery, as they directly impact outcomes and satisfaction among patients. The decision to undergo procedures such as Facial Feminization Surgery (FFS) is driven by more than a desire for beauty, but also by psychological and social drivers. Physicians must walk the tight rope of complex motivations and ensure patients are making decisions based on complete information. As noted in the current debate, virtual planning and morphing using artificial intelligence can deliver accurate surgical results, but they also raise ethical concerns in terms of patient autonomy. Providers need to hold the interests of patients in balancing the need to fulfill expectations with the interest in advancing realistic outcomes and dealing with implied psychological implications at the preoperative assessment phase. This emphasizes the necessity of conducting proper consultations that are not merely focused on cosmetic aims but also patients' psychological health and well-being. Professionalists have an ethical obligation to defend vulnerable individuals who undergo cosmetic surgery, for example, those who are transgender, who are usually under greater scrutiny and subjected to immense social pressures. Informed consent is more challenging in such cases, since surgeons need to ensure prospective patients are adequately informed regarding the risk, benefit, and limitation of surgery. The significance of making intensive patient evaluation cannot be overstated, particularly concerning emotional readiness and alleviation of gender dysphoria potential. Ethical practice obliges surgeons to have candid discussions with patients regarding their expectations and the reality of surgical outcomes, encouraging a supportive and respectful attitude. Such responsibility is needed to steer clear of regret or dissatisfaction with the outcome of surgery and to uphold the integrity of the profession. Furthermore, cosmetic surgery involving machine learning introduces new ethical considerations that need to be addressed by practitioners.

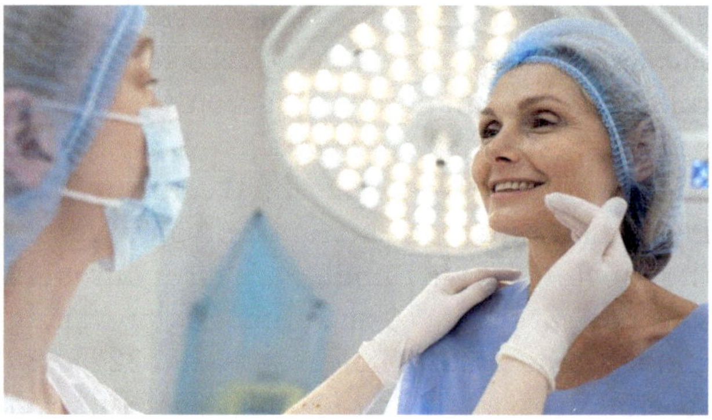

Figure 3.14. Ethical considerations in cosmetic surgery.

Source: https://external-content.duckduckgo.com/iu/?u=https%3A%2F%2Ffitcoding.com%2Fwp-content%2Fuploads%2F2024%2F09%2FUntitled-design-2024-09-04T233034.240.jpg&f=1&nofb=1&ipt=77bd1f0c51ba24fdcd4790aa2ebad89e3fd850ab2266b60fffbbcfb62d30e7d3.

As recognized in current literature, machine learning algorithms provide more precise preoperative assessments by analyzing varied patient data and surgical outcomes. While these technologies have the potential to significantly improve surgical planning and predict outcomes, problems of data privacy, algorithmic bias, and technology over-reliance must be considered. Surgeons and practices must instill robust data protection measures and ensure that algorithms are trained on diverse datasets to avoid exacerbating existing inequalities in treatment for patients. Cosmetic surgery should not replace but augment the human element of care, so it is a requirement that ethical considerations in patient assessment and planning for surgery be placed front and center in practice (Figure 3.14).

3.6.1. Informed Consent Process

The informed consent process is central to ethical medical care, particularly in cosmetic facial surgery. It is the method by which patients gain a complete understanding of the treatments that they are considering, including the potential benefits, risks, and alternatives. Through developing a collective decision-making culture, surgeons facilitate patients to make an educated choice that is commensurate with their respective needs and expectations. The process is not ritual in its nature but involves open communication and active involvement to enable patients to possess a realistic perception of surgical outcomes. This openness is critical in that it paves the way for a trusting patient-surgeon relationship and ultimately yields patient satisfaction and adherence to post-operative instructions. For the management of the process of details in informed consent, there has to be comprehension of the imperative of individualized communication. The surgeon must be ready to tailor explanations to various levels of comprehension by patients, particularly for complex procedures such as rhinoplasty. This is underscored by evidence that patient-friendly language can improve understanding and eventually render the decision-making process more effective. Furthermore, the deployment of visual aids and electronic media can help demystify complicated surgical information, thereby enabling patients to envision hypothetical outcomes. Coupled with an analysis of patient attitudes and expectations towards cosmetic outcomes, these steps consolidate the informed consent process. Most significantly, ongoing testing of patient understanding throughout the preoperative phase can also further develop the consent process to ensure that it is responsive to patients' needs but is still ethical (Xie et al., 2023). Lastly, informed consent for cosmetic facial surgery also needs to deal with the evolving world of medical technology and innovation. The introduction of new materials and techniques, such as polycaprolactone fillers, necessitates reevaluation of what constitutes adequate information for patients. As demonstrated by recent research, novel treatments have the potential to yield meaningful cosmetic benefits but also create concerns regarding safety and effectiveness. Plastic surgeons must stay current with research and clinical recommendations to advise patients on pertinent information on emerging alternatives and how they may influence surgery plans. Through the use of informed consent discussions grounded in contemporary evidence, such as safety protocols and adverse event management strategies, surgeons are able to educate patients to make informed, educated decisions regarding their cosmetic procedure (Marie-Christen et al., 2020). This progresses the commitment to patient care and ethical practice within the intricate realm of cosmetic surgery.

3.6.2. Addressing Ethical Dilemmas

Ethical decision-making in cosmetic facial surgery is critical to patient health and professional integrity. Because surgery is incorporated into self-concept, practitioners must cope with unique issues related to patient motivation and expectations. Surgeons must ensure that they conduct thorough patient evaluations to distinguish attainable goals from unrealistic ideals. A clear understanding of a patient's emotional and psychological state can prevent postoperative disappointments. Ethics also encompasses informed consent, where patients have to be fully informed about the risks and implications of their intended procedures. Through effective open communication and honesty, surgeons can establish a feeling of trust, thus allowing patients to make appropriate decisions about their surgical procedures. Artificial intelligence, particularly in cosmetic facial surgery, makes ethical decision-making even more complex. As technological advancement has brought with it enhanced preoperative assessment and intraoperative planning ability, it does come with potential ethical concerns, such as the potential for over-reliance on algorithmic recommendations. Surgeons must carefully examine the implications of incorporating tools like large language models into practice. As suggested by recent literature, the implementation of such models, as promising as they potentially are for patient communication and education, raises gigantic ethical concerns to be considered carefully before they are implemented in clinical settings (Puladi et al., 2023). It is then important that professionals balance technological advantages with necessary human reasoning so that ethical requirements are not undermined. Italicized version. Moreover, the impact of cultural norms on patients' internal concept of beauty and the demand for surgically induced enhancement provides another ethical challenge in cosmetic facial surgery. Numerous patients will likely be driven by external forces rather than internal motivations, resulting in concerns about cultural pressures, self-concept and decision-making. Surgeons need to consider such cultural pressures and establish a culture encouraging genuine patient autonomy. Therefore, the inclusion of individualized care considering individual psychosocial factors is needed in addressing such concerns. Additionally, it is important to anticipate how changing patterns of body image perception can affect patient outcomes and satisfaction levels. Formulation of this field must include ongoing argumentation on ethics in practice so that patient well-being remains the focal point in cosmetic surgery interventions (Lei-Cao et al., 2023).

3.6.3. Importance of Patient Autonomy

The patients' autonomy value in cosmetic facial surgery cannot be overstressed. While people undergo the surgical procedure to enhance their appearance, they ought to have the necessary information to make independent decisions regarding their treatment. Patient autonomy in this sense entails a right over one's medical choice, as per one's values, desires, and ambitions. This principle is particularly paramount in cosmetic surgery, where operations like blepharoplasty not only place a premium on physical outcomes but also on the fulfillment of personal expectations. A significant role here for surgeons is to ensure that patients are well informed and are in a position to make effective decisions about their operating plans. Failing to respect patient autonomy can lead to discontent with outcomes and undermine the surgeon-patient therapeutic alliance, illustrating the necessity of shared decision-making in the field. Inclusion of patient autonomy fundamentally alters the character of the process of surgical planning, most significantly during the assessment stage.

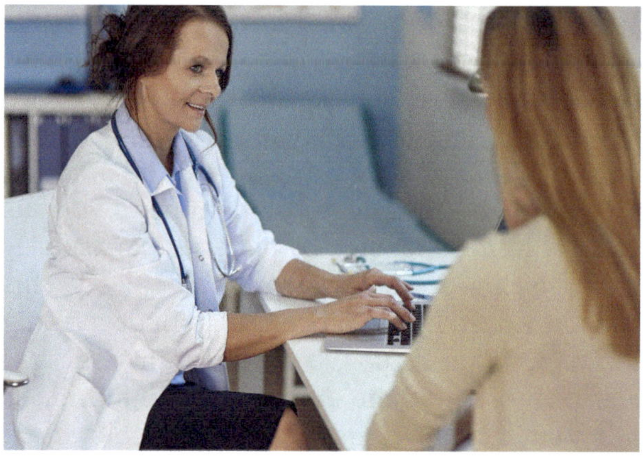

Figure 3.15. The importance of patient autonomy in cosmetic facial surgery cannot be overstated.

Source: https://external-content.duckduckgo.com/iu/?u=https%3A%2F%2Fdomf5oio6qrcr.cloudfront.net%2Fmedialibrary%2F9451%2FiStock_78445461_MEDIUM.jpg&f=1&nofb=1&ipt=29e4ba73880faa9a999579b8745fcb0b78b61b2911af826d13c6fcb006619eb9.

Surgeons are compelled to hear out individual conceptions of their patients, acknowledging their reasons and concerns for various procedures. For example, in assessing facial asymmetry, as highlighted in the case of facial rotation and its aesthetic implication, patient engagement comes into the picture when individualizing surgical intervention to suit specific needs (Koppert et al., 2025). This assists in harmonizing the patient's expectations with the provided treatment plan, which can then enhance satisfaction with the outcome. Moreover, patient engagement in their treatment reinforces patient agency to experience an even more positive general surgery experience. Practitioners honor patient autonomy by stressing open communication and shared decision-making, which enhances a culture of interdependence that is best suited for successful surgical experience. Moreover, the issue of patient autonomy is also rooted in ethical issues in the practice of cosmetic face surgery. Surgeons play a twofold role of articulating their patients' best interests while remaining respectful of their autonomy and personal choice. As covered in assessing blepharoplasty outcome, patient satisfaction is linked with the comprehensiveness of preoperative assessment and shrewd surgical planning (Zhang et al., 2024). This two-way role is a delicate balancing act; surgeons must ensure patients are not only choosing procedures to meet their goals of beauty but also that they make safe and appropriate choices based on their medical history and physical exams. Therefore, establishing an environment of trust through respectful dialogue and comprehensive education ultimately empowers patients. The resulting collaboration enhances satisfaction and qualitative outcomes in cosmetic surgery, verifying the central importance of patient autonomy in modern surgical practice (Figure 3.15).

Test Your Knowledge

1. What key elements must be included in a thorough informed consent process for cosmetic surgery?
2. How should clinicians approach ethical dilemmas that arise when a patient's desired procedure may not be in their best interest?
3. Why is respecting patient autonomy essential in cosmetic surgery decision-making?

SUMMARY

The intricacy of patient assessment and surgical planning in cosmetic facial surgery verifies the overriding importance of an integrative approach. Effective results of surgery are dependent on thorough evaluations, considering not just the physical factors but also the psychological and emotional needs of the patients. With the improvement in life expectancy and consequent increase in patients seeking cosmetic enhancements, professionals are finding themselves more often needing to address conditions that can arise, like those related to gingival and cosmetic factors, that may be particularly relevant in facial work. Moreover, expansion of knowledge regarding mucogingival deformities puts significant emphasis on the need for practitioners to remain updated with anatomical determinants of surgical success and patient satisfaction overall (Cortellini et al., 2018). Multidisciplinary care, with integration of knowledge from all aspects of health care, will be essential in preserving positive outcomes. Furthermore, surgical planning entails appreciating a person's unique anatomical and physiological characteristics. The evaluation stage has to take into account not only the aesthetic goals of the patient but also the potential impact of surgical interventions on short-term and long-term oral health. As evidenced by studies, conditions like mucogingival defects significantly undermine aesthetic outcomes, leading to patient dissatisfaction unless adequately assessed preoperatively (Cortellini et al., 2018). Likewise, periodontal health complications also require conservative management methods as a first line of treatment, only opting for surgical procedures where they are specifically indicated. A balance, therefore, of aesthetic desires with strict health evaluation will have the implication of optimizing patient results along with reducing risk factors associated with surgical procedures. Lastly, the evolution of cosmetic facial surgery necessitates practitioners to adhere to a promise of continuous education and optimization of best practice to meet the evolving needs of patients. As the materials used in surgery change and techniques advance, so too should understanding of associated ailments such as periodontitis and how these impact aesthetic treatments. Prioritizing patient education and patient self-care will similarly be crucial in guaranteeing successful long-term results. Specifically, the health of the periodontal tissue also has a striking impact on influencing the outcome of cosmetic surgery, and this highlights the importance of interdisciplinary consultation in formulating and applying surgical management. Through recognition of the relationship between patient health, desired look, and potential for surgery, practitioners are able to better control the complexities of cosmetic facial surgery, ultimately to the advantage of enhanced patient satisfaction and general well-being.

The correct surgical planning is a general process that is included in successful cosmetic facial surgery. It begins with meticulous patient evaluation that examines the person's specific anatomical features, medical background, and psychological readiness for surgery. Understanding the patient's goals and expectations is critical; discrepancies between patient desires and surgical outcomes will lead to discontent. The assessment includes physical exams and may employ imaging modalities to aid in the visualization of hidden structures. Also, tissue elasticity, quality of skin, and bone structure underneath are evaluated to provide valuable information for individualizing procedures. Through proper evaluation, surgeons can develop a tailored plan for surgery that takes into consideration the aesthetic issues and functional needs, as well as ensuring that the interventions chosen are suitable for the individualized patient parameters. One of the most important aspects of surgical planning is choosing surgical methods that minimize complications while maximizing outcomes. Advances in technology, including bone ultrasonic osteotomes, have made it possible to evolve beyond traditional methods of bone surgery in the aesthetic field. Studies have indicated that ultrasonic-assisted devices possess advantages over traditional techniques in providing smoother surfaces of bone and reducing damage to the surrounding soft tissues, which promotes quicker healing and better aesthetic results (Anesi et al., 2014). A surgeon's experience with the equipment and techniques directly influences the preparation of the operating environment and the recovery process anticipated. Furthermore, surgical planning must take into account individual variation, such as ethnic facial anatomical variations, which play significant roles in the final aesthetic results. Understanding these variations allows for more tailored treatment, maximizing the success of the operation. Finally, the inclusion of preoperative simulations and postoperative protocols is a critical aspect of the surgical planning process. Preoperative simulation may enable the surgeon and patient to visualize the likely outcome, which promotes more harmonious expectation agreement. Communication for postoperative care is also important to facilitate optimal recovery and prevent complications. Individualized care plans are also emphasized by evidence that reports anthropometric variation among different populations and how they may influence surgical technique (Durairajanayagam, 2011). Inclusive models of management encompassing both the surgical procedures and the postoperative care not only ensure patient satisfaction but also ensure optimal healing processes. Combining these elements in the planning model for surgery ensures an integrative approach to patient treatment in cosmetic facial surgery, leading to more predictable and satisfying results.

KEY TERMS FROM THIS CHAPTER

- Facial Proportions
- Symmetry Evaluation
- Facial Landmarks
- Skeletal Framework Analysis
- Medical History
- Patient Expectations
- Risk Assessment
- Aesthetic Analysis
- Skin Quality Assessment
- Soft Tissue Assessment
- Photographic Documentation
- Psychological Evaluation
- Candidacy Criteria
- Facial Aging Patterns

CRITICAL THINKING QUESTIONS

1. **The first step in cosmetic facial surgical planning is:**
   a. Choosing the surgical technique
   b. Preoperative imaging
   c. Patient consultation and history-taking
   d. Selecting anesthesia type
2. **Which factor is MOST important when evaluating a patient's suitability for cosmetic facial surgery?**
   a. Age
   b. Psychological stability and expectations
   c. Occupation
   d. Hair color
3. **In aesthetic facial analysis, symmetry is evaluated mainly through:**
   a. Vertical and horizontal reference lines
   b. Skin color
   c. Ear size
   d. Dental alignment
4. **A patient with body dysmorphic disorder (BDD) is generally considered:**
   a. A good candidate for cosmetic surgery
   b. A high-risk candidate requiring psychiatric referral
   c. Suitable only for injectables
   d. Eligible for surgery after consent
5. **Which preoperative assessment is essential for rhinoplasty planning?**
   a. Visual acuity test
   b. Airway assessment and nasal breathing evaluation
   c. Hearing test
   d. Neck flexibility test

Short Answer Questions

1. What role does facial symmetry play in preoperative facial aesthetic evaluation?
2. Explain the significance of preoperative photography in cosmetic facial surgery.
3. What clinical features should be assessed during nasal evaluation for rhinoplasty planning?
4. What are the main facial proportions used to guide cosmetic surgical planning?
5. How does skin quality influence the choice of surgical technique in facial aesthetic procedures?

Answers to Critical Thinking Questions

1. (c) 2. (b) 3. (a) 4. (b) 5. (b)

REFERENCES

1. Anesi, A., Cavani, F., Chiarini, L., Ferretti, L., et al. (2014). Preliminary findings of a potentiated piezosurgical device at the rabbit skull. https://core.ac.uk/download/80171725.pdf (accessed on 14th July 2025).
2. Astle, A. T., Foulsham, T., & McGraw, P. V. (2016). The consequences of strabismus and the benefits of adult strabismus surgery. https://core.ac.uk/download/76972262.pdf (accessed on 14th July 2025).
3. Avetikov, D., Havryliev, V., Ivanytska, O., Ivanytskyi, I. O., Yatsenko, P., & Lokes, K. P. (2024). Peculiarities of clinical presentation, diagnosis, and treatment for injuries of the large salivary glands. Ukrainian Dental Almanac. https://www.semanticscholar.org/paper/2794e9390b2f6da5ba29152cfb731ab69309f586 (accessed on 14th July 2025).
4. Aziz, S., Arabi, Y. M., Alhazzani, W., Evans, L., Citerio, G., Fischkoff, K., Salluh, J. I., et al. (2020). Managing ICU surge during the COVID-19 crisis: Rapid guidelines. Intensive Care Medicine, 46, 1303–1325. https://doi.org/10.1007/s00134-020-06092-5 (accessed on 14th July 2025).
5. Barnett, S. L., Choe, J., Aiello, C., & Bradley, J. P. (2023). Facial feminization surgery: Anatomical differences, preoperative planning, techniques, and ethical considerations. Medicina, 59. https://www.semanticscholar.org/paper/a11049586e66b659fae40171ec9e7127f8b85d7f (accessed on 14th July 2025).
6. Cajiao, X. (2023). Colombia and medical tourism. Voices in Bioethics. https://www.semanticscholar.org/paper/7d33445bf62fbe0067e7cdeda2cf8301f14ad6fe (accessed on 14th July 2025).
7. Cao, L. M., Zhong, N. N., Li, Z. Z., Huo, F. Y., Xiao, Y., Liu, B., & Bu, L. L. (2023). Lymph node metastasis in oral squamous cell carcinoma: Where we are and where we are going. Clinical and Translational Discovery, 3. https://doi.org/10.1002/ctd2.227 (accessed on 14th July 2025).
8. Christen, M. O., & Vercesi, F. (2020). Polycaprolactone: How a well-known and futuristic polymer has become an innovative collagen-stimulator in esthetics. Clinical Cosmetic and Investigational Dermatology, 13, 31–48. https://doi.org/10.2147/ccid.s229054 (accessed on 14th July 2025).
9. Cillino, M., Cordova, A., D'Arpa, S., Liuzza, M., et al. (2010). Algorithm of partial breast reconstruction with pedicled perforator flaps. https://core.ac.uk/download/53293997.pdf (accessed on 14th July 2025).
10. Claahsen-van der Grinten, H. L., Speiser, P., Ahmed, S. F., Arlt, W., Auchus, R. J., Falhammar, H., Flück, C. E., et al. (2021). Congenital adrenal hyperplasia—Current insights in pathophysiology, diagnostics, and management. Endocrine Reviews, 43, 91–159. https://doi.org/10.1210/endrev/bnab016 (accessed on 14th July 2025).
11. Cortellini, P., & Bissada, N. F. (2018). Mucogingival conditions in the natural dentition: Narrative review, case definitions, and diagnostic considerations. Journal of Periodontology, 89. https://doi.org/10.1002/jper.16-0671 (accessed on 14th July 2025).
12. Durairajanayagam, S. (2011). Anthropometric measurement of the lip-nose complex among young adults in Kuala Lumpur, Malaysia. https://core.ac.uk/download/143644123.pdf (accessed on 14th July 2025).

13. Eftekhari, M. H., Parsapoor, A., Ahmadi, A., Yavari, N., Larijani, B., & Shamsi Gooshki, E. (2023). Exploring defensive medicine: Examples, underlying and contextual factors, and potential strategies – A qualitative study. BMC Medical Ethics, 24. https://doi.org/10.1186/s12910-023-00949-2 (accessed on 14th July 2025).

14. Gbujie, E. A., Dahillo, D. F., Fulorunso, B. E., Nwankwo, O., Quadri, B., Egbe, B., Bello, B., et al. (2021). Surgical treatment of monostotic cranio-facial fibrous dysplasia: Changing the narratives. International Journal of Otolaryngology and Head & Neck Surgery, 10, 49–59. https://www.semanticscholar.org/paper/786a89ac90674dacc5e9d62395b40dd5899b90b4 (accessed on 14th July 2025).

15. Gehl, J., Serša, G., Matthiessen, L. W., Muir, T., Soden, D. M., Occhini, A., Quaglino, P., et al. (2018). Updated standard operating procedures for electrochemotherapy of cutaneous tumors and skin metastases. Acta Oncologica, 57, 874–882. https://doi.org/10.1080/0284186x.2018.1454602 (accessed on 14th July 2025).

16. Geiger, J. L., Ismaila, N., Beadle, B. M., Caudell, J. J., Chau, N. G., Deschler, D. G., Glastonbury, C. M., et al. (2021). Management of salivary gland malignancy: ASCO guideline. Journal of Clinical Oncology, 39, 1909–1941. https://doi.org/10.1200/jco.21.00449 (accessed on 14th July 2025).

17. González-González, A. M., Soto-Goñi, X. A., Hallal-Peche, F., & Sánchez-Romero, E. A. (2025). Interdisciplinary approach in ophthalmic trigeminal neuralgia: A case report. Electronic Journal of General Medicine. https://www.semanticscholar.org/paper/d63f16b4d65d93910200924fe0510d1f930025e3 (accessed on 14th July 2025).

18. Koppert, E., & Yi, K. (2025). Observational study of facial rotation patterns. The Journal of Craniofacial Surgery. https://www.semanticscholar.org/paper/ee4ee7c035c5c3adaf31a5df50d70511561394e1 (accessed on 14th July 2025).

19. Lim, B., Seth, I., Kah, S., Sofiadellis, F., Ross, R. J., Rozen, W. M., & Cuomo, R. (2023). Using generative artificial intelligence tools in cosmetic surgery: A study on rhinoplasty, facelifts, and blepharoplasty procedures. Journal of Clinical Medicine, 12, 6524–6524. https://doi.org/10.3390/jcm12206524 (accessed on 14th July 2025).

20. Meyer-Szary, J., Luis, M. S., Mikulski, S., Patel, A., Schulz, F., Tretiakow, D., Fercho, J., et al. (2022). The role of 3D printing in planning complex medical procedures and training of medical professionals—Cross-sectional multispecialty review. International Journal of Environmental Research and Public Health, 19, 3331–3331. https://doi.org/10.3390/ijerph19063331 (accessed on 14th July 2025).

21. Mir, M., & Maurya, R. (2023). Precision and progress: Machine learning advancements in plastic surgery. Cureus, 15. https://www.semanticscholar.org/paper/5664bda3626dc002698aeb24bd72d365bff7dcbb (accessed on 14th July 2025).

22. Deepak M. Kalaskar, Peter E. Butler, Shadi Ghali. (2016). Textbook of Plastic and Reconstructive Surgery. ISBN: 978-1-910634-37-0 (Hbk.) https://core.ac.uk/download/79526588.pdf

23. (accessed on 14th July 2025).

24. Niemiec, B. A., Gawor, J., Nemec, A., Clarke, E., McLeod, K. C., Tutt, C., Gioso, M. A., et al. (2020). World Small Animal Veterinary Association global dental guidelines. Journal of Small Animal Practice, 61, 395–403. https://doi.org/10.1111/jsap.13113 (accessed on 14th July 2025).

25. Pal Chowdhury, K., Barman, D., & Sengupta, A. (2025). A retrospective study on nutrition risk assessment and nutritional management of head and neck cancer patients undergoing surgery in a tertiary care teaching hospital. Annals of Medical Science & Research. https://www.semanticscholar.org/paper/1ed12b95bdadaad80e72422ff400b5ed2cff4a30 (accessed on 14th July 2025).

26. Puladi, B., Gsaxner, C., Kleesiek, J., Hölzle, F., Röhrig, R., & Egger, J. (2023). The impact and opportunities of large language models like ChatGPT in oral and maxillofacial surgery: A narrative review. International Journal of Oral and Maxillofacial Surgery, 53, 78–88. https://doi.org/10.1016/j.ijom.2023.09.005 (accessed on 14th July 2025).

27. Rohrich, D., & Muzaffar, A. (2000). In search of the ideal nose. Plastic and Reconstructive Surgery, 105(7), 2568–2569. https://www.semanticscholar.org/paper/b5c804682a00b0d2e85b7de325b9eb2adfa70ca8 (accessed on 14th July 2025).

28. Rokhshad, R., Keyhan, S. O., & Yousefi, P. (2023). Artificial intelligence applications and ethical challenges in oral and maxillo-facial cosmetic surgery: A narrative review. Maxillofacial Plastic and Reconstructive Surgery, 45. https://doi.org/10.1186/s40902-023-00382-w (accessed on 14th July 2025).

29. Shalini, G., Parameswaran, R., Parameswaran, A., & Vijayalakshmi, D. (2025). Ortho-surgical management of a patient with short face syndrome. Oral Health Research and Clinical Evidence. https://www.semanticscholar.org/paper/64595502de9b778fa60f23ab0d5060c0ed2c4188 (accessed on 14th July 2025).

30. Shams, M. G., & Motamedi, M. (2009). Case report: Feminizing the male face. Eplasty, 9. https://www.semanticscholar.org/paper/ed9307c50ef1ca81c4c2628cc996caa6823a8d62 (accessed on 14th July 2025).

31. Slots, J. (2017). Periodontitis: Facts, fallacies and the future. Periodontology 2000, 75, 7–23. https://doi.org/10.1111/prd.12221 (accessed on 14th July 2025).

32. Teede, H., Tay, C. T., Laven, J. J. E., Dokras, A., Moran, L., Piltonen, T., Costello, M., et al. (2023). Recommendations from the 2023 international evidence-based guideline for the assessment and management of polycystic ovary syndrome. The Journal of Clinical Endocrinology & Metabolism, 108, 2447–2469. https://doi.org/10.1210/clinem/dgad463 (accessed on 14th July 2025).

33. Topalian, S. L., Taube, J. M., & Pardoll, D. M. (2020). Neoadjuvant checkpoint blockade for cancer immunotherapy. Science, 367. https://doi.org/10.1126/science.aax0182 (accessed on 14th July 2025).

34. Tukeshov, S., Nurdinov, B., Mamatov, U., Alybaev, U., & Kadyraliev, U. (2024). Employing algorithms in cosmetic facial surgery. Bulletin of Science and Practice. https://www.semanticscholar.org/paper/3cdbed971990c813540e649b6fb1f77632b470a9 (accessed on 14th July 2025).

35. Vargas, N., Hamrah, D., & Serra, M. M. (2025). Artificial intelligence technologies and mobile applications in cosmetic surgery: Trends and recommendations. The American Journal of Cosmetic Surgery. https://www.semanticscholar.org/paper/ea17007c0be0c709b415d0ecfa57c92d79ff5764 (accessed on 14th July 2025).

36. Wu, L., Tang, S., Jiang, J., & Li, K. (2024). Construction of a predictive model for the effectiveness of plastic surgery and repair in patients with facial basal cell carcinoma. American Journal

of Cancer Research, 14(12), 5798–5811. https://www.semanticscholar.org/paper/42454037831911ae880424ea3c190b139f050b58 (accessed on 14th July 2025).

37. Xie, Y., Seth, I., Hunter-Smith, D. J., Rozen, W. M., Ross, R., & Lee, M. (2023). Aesthetic surgery advice and counseling from artificial intelligence: A rhinoplasty consultation with ChatGPT. Aesthetic Plastic Surgery, 47, 1985–1993. https://doi.org/10.1007/s00266-023-03338-7 (accessed on 14th July 2025).
38. Yu, A., Ference, E., Ge, M., Su, P., Smith, S., Moayer, R., Levin, K. M., et al. (2022). Facial plastic and reconstructive surgery poster presentations. Otolaryngology–Head and Neck Surgery, 167, P182–P192. https://www.semanticscholar.org/paper/e467d5d0d3f13c11f7cf2c4402802ca47316c419 (accessed on 14th July 2025).
39. Yurtkal, M. C. (2024). Optimizing hysterectomy: A prospective comparative analysis of surgical techniques and their impact on women's lives. Journal of Personalized Medicine, 14. https://www.semanticscholar.org/paper/5e7631760e0e90e09b3a66084e5dfdebfd105d9f (accessed on 14th July 2025).
40. Zhang, Q., Wang, F., Hu, Q., & Ma, X. (2024). Assessment of the cosmetic effect of eye bag surgery on facial morphology changes. Academic Journal of Medicine & Health Sciences. https://www.semanticscholar.org/paper/1f2b0d41f797628a2f2b9f8306df44af682bd3ac (accessed on 14th July 2025).

4

BLEPHAROPLASTY (EYELID SURGERY) IN FACIAL COSMETIC

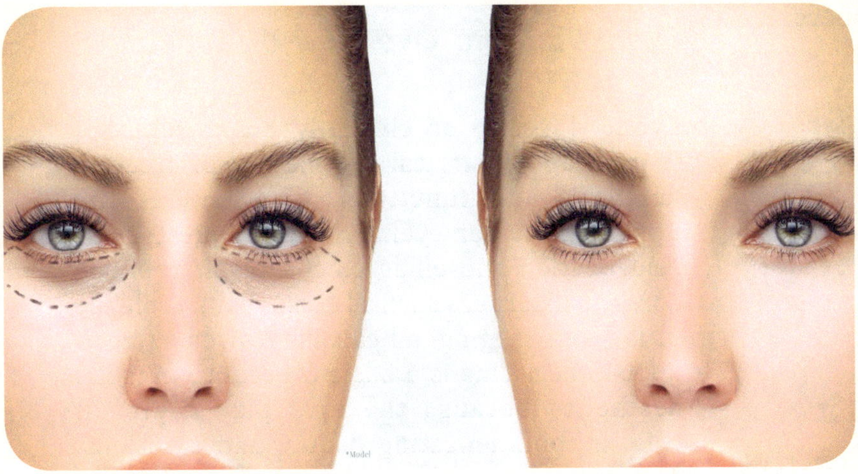

LEARNING OBJECTIVES

After studying this chapter, you will be able to:

1. Discuss the blepharoplasty types;
2. Explain indications for blepharoplasty;
3. Understand the procedure;
4. Highlight risks and complications;
5. Learn about the recovery process;
6. Assess psychological and social impacts.

Introduction

Blepharoplasty or eyelid surgery is a surgical procedure essentially intended to enhance the aesthetic look and functional capacity of the eyelids. As part of facial aesthetics, this procedure corrects typical issues related to aging, such as sagging eyelids, redundant skin, and bulging fat deposits under the eyes. Through eliminating or repositioning these tissues, blepharoplasty is capable of greatly transforming the facial look for a brighter and younger appearance. The popularity of the procedure is a result of its relatively uncomplicated nature and the notable impact it may have on one's overall appearance, usually augmenting other facial aesthetic treatments. Moreover, advancements in surgical techniques have rendered it even more accessible to a broader population, including those in search of treatment for both aesthetic and functional disability due to drooping eyelids. The significance of thorough preoperative consultation cannot be exaggerated in the case of blepharoplasty. The proper assessment should involve establishing patient history, possible complications, and establishing expectations, particularly in patients with medical conditions such as hypertension or diabetes. Anticoagulant medication users or those who have just undergone refractive surgery represent a high-risk factor during convalescence. Also, nutritional status will perform the wound healing function, so pre-operative screening shall extend beyond physical examination to include lifestyle. Besides improving the success of surgery, this holistic treatment provides a prevention of complications such as swelling or infection, and the overall procedure becomes more effective (Portilla et al., 2024).

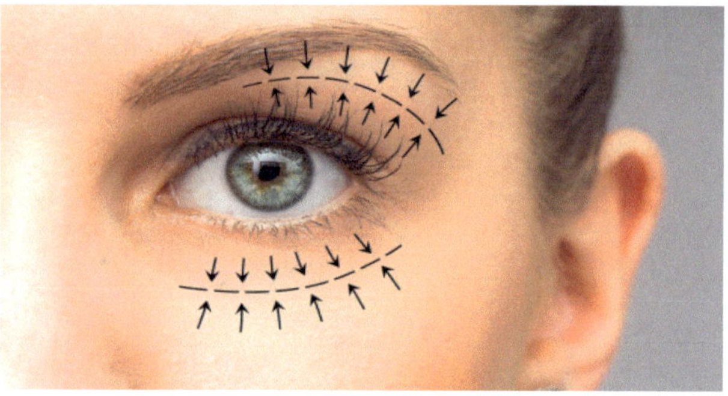

Figure 4.1. Blepharoplasty, commonly referred to as eyelid surgery.

Source: https://external-content.duckduckgo.com/iu/?u=https%3A%2F%2Ffacialsurgerycenter.com%2Fwp-content%2Fuploads%2Felementor%2Fthumbs%2FBlepharoplasty-qbannlvyu1qkx02x4gjsowhy3xqg6wdaw35z4awtqc.png&f=1&nofb=1&ipt=8cb86f2446290849075cc3cf0b114e059d3b76a6b3a6da426dc35cf9b948f41c.

The postoperative care is another imperative element that will affect the success of blepharoplasty. Patients, after undergoing surgery, must adhere to strict wound care instructions in such a way as to enable proper healing. While techniques such as continuous suturing and tissue glue can offer equal results in terms of time of healing, patient education is also vital for the correct care. Postoperative instructions not being followed strictly can lead to complications of eyelid malposition, dry eye syndrome, and wound dehiscence. Modern developments also consider the inclusion of minimally invasive procedures, such as laser treatment, into the recovery process to yield better outcomes. As facial beauty continues to advance, an understanding of postoperative complications will play a key role in minimizing complications and attaining patient satisfaction from blepharoplasty (Portilla et al., 2024) (Figure 4.1).

Definition and Overview of Eyelid Surgery

Eyelid surgery, or clinically blepharoplasty, is a group of surgical techniques for treating aesthetic and functional disorders of the upper and lower eyelids. Often requested for rejuvenation and enlargement, blepharoplasty corrects disorders such as excess skin, prolapse of fat, and sagging, all causing a tired or aged appearance. This is a basic procedure in facial aesthetics because the eyes play a pivotal role in communicating beauty and emotions. The prominence of eyelid surgery in cosmetic practice is not only due to its effectiveness but also due to the evolving desires of people who want to improve their facial features. As one of the most common aesthetic surgical procedures, blepharoplasty requires thorough knowledge of the anatomy of the eyelid to provide desirable results and results that seem natural, which adds further to the need for skilled professionals in this field (Filippo et al., 2024). Surgical techniques for blepharoplasty vary according to the patient's targeted need and the targeted area. For upper eyelid surgery, treatments commonly involve the removal of the excess fat and skin to redrape a more youthful look. In contrast, lower eyelid surgery may aim at decreasing bulging fatty pads and dark circles or puffiness under the eyes. A major trend in this field has been the shift towards conservative techniques, where the use of techniques that not just remove tissue but also help restore volume to enhance the natural contour of the eyelids is made. This conservativeness is consistent with contemporary beauty ideals favoring a fuller and restored appearance over a blunt or over-worked appearance. Understanding these nuances is the secret to surgeons modifying their approach to accommodate the specific patient requirements and preferences (Chuang et al., 2016). The practice of eyelid surgery cannot be emphasized enough with regard to the involvement of a multidisciplinary team. Blepharoplasty represents an area of overlap between aesthetic and functional surgery, and thus practitioners borrow from other specialties in medicine, like plastic surgery and ophthalmology.

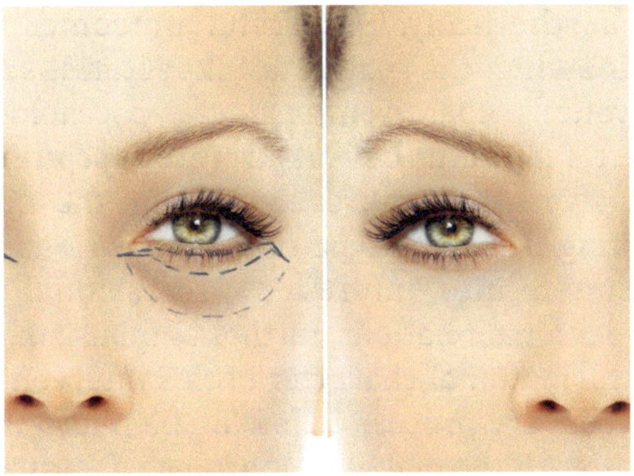

Figure 4.2. An overview of eyelid surgery.

Source: https://external-content.duckduckgo.com/iu/?u=https%3A%2F%2Fpereaclinic.com%2Fwp-content%2Fuploads%2F2022%2F04%2FEYELID-SURGERY-scaled.jpg&f=1&nofb=1&ipt=e6810ab6a28506b1495d69d1485e81f747119ad25ea328e6b414550531dc5bb1.

This overall training enables the surgeons not just to enhance the aesthetic beauty but also to achieve proper function and health of the eyelids. With technological advancement in surgery, procedures such as minimally invasive surgery and the use of adjunctive technologies like lasers have become the order of the day. This necessitates ongoing research and professional development in this ever-evolving field as a prerequisite for practitioners. These advances have opened new windows of opportunity for improved healing and patient satisfaction, and eyelid surgery is therefore an ever-changing branch of facial aesthetics in contemporary medical practice (Chuang et al., 2016; Filippo et al., 2024) (Figure 4.2).

Historical Context and Evolution of the Procedure

The blepharoplasty, or eyelid surgery procedure, has come a long way over the centuries from primitive methods to highly sophisticated surgical procedures. Historical evidence reveals that in ancient Egypt, too, healers performed simple surgical procedures to correct eyelid deformities and trauma for the twin reasons of health and beauty. The focus on duality remained right through ancient Roman years when physicians documented eyelid surgeries in medical texts. The contemporary concept of blepharoplasty, however, came into existence in the middle of the 20th century when technological developments in anesthetic and surgical methods provided for more precise techniques. Physicians started to embrace principles centered on restoring not just the functional aspect of vision but also beautifying appearance, as societal values regarding beauty and youthfulness broadened. During the late 20th century, blepharoplasty saw a resurgence in popularity as part of a growing social interest in cosmetic improvement and anti-aging procedures. The time saw a turning point as practitioners increasingly began to use eyelid surgery as a standard cosmetic procedure for rejuvenating facial appearance. Innovative events and congresses, such as the annual congress of the Italian Association of Plastic Aesthetic Surgery (AICPE), highlighted these innovations and provided a platform for specialists to exchange innovative methods (Riggio, 2024). Consequently, directly due to this, a variety of approaches evolved, with varying techniques that were precisely designed to address individual patients' needs. This period of emphasis on personal aesthetic goals only further cemented blepharoplasty in the cultural awareness, coupling the procedure with notions of freedom and beauty in contemporary society. Evolving medical rhetoric regarding blepharoplasty has only further associated the procedure with ethical and social concerns surrounding aging and femininity. Research in the realm of beauty standards in contemporary times points out how medicalization has led to specific women's appearance expectations as they grow older. Herein, practitioners opt to market blepharoplasty not only as corrective surgery but as a corrective technique against the perceived deterioration of health with increasing age (Pussetti, 2021). This convergence of ethics and aesthetics entwines the history of blepharoplasty, under which patients must struggle with cultural demands alongside making personal choices regarding their bodies. The development of this procedure thus reflects broader cultural values and the complicated politics of gender performance in beauty, highlighting how personal decision-making is greatly reliant on prevailing aesthetic norms and societal values.

Importance of Blepharoplasty in Facial Aesthetics

Blepharoplasty, or eyelid surgery, is an important aspect of facial beauty enhancement since it addresses the signs of aging that appear on the eyelids, typically one of the initial areas to be affected. In addition to removing drooping skin and fat, the surgery also brings an overall lift to the face, significantly improving a youthful and bright appearance. With evolving values of aesthetics towards a more holistic definition of beauty, blepharoplasty becomes an integral part of the overall scenario of dermatological and surgical corrections. Portilla et al. (2024) explain that developments in oncologic treatment of aging increasingly focus on minimizing invasive procedures, making blepharoplasty a better option for enhancing facial appearance with quicker recovery. The interplay between new surgical methods and technological innovation continues to enhance the safety and effectiveness of this procedure, further solidifying its position as an aesthetic mainstay. The psychological effects of blepharoplasty also render it essential in facial aesthetics. Low self-esteem is a universal response from most individuals caused by perceived imperfections around their eyes, including bulging skin and puffiness. Through such corrections, blepharoplasty has the potential to significantly enhance the self-view and self-confidence of an individual. One such study presented in Nieć et al. (2024) illustrates the extent to which patient readiness and preoperative consultation can influence the outcome, both functionally and aesthetically. Successful outcomes rely on knowing the patients' expectations and motivations. Apart from aesthetics, psychological benefits should be taken into account as well, given that improvements for the better resulting from this type of surgery are usually translated into improved professional and interpersonal relations, further emphasizing the transformational character of this intervention. The recovery process following blepharoplasty is an area of the highest importance that directly affects patient satisfaction and the ultimate result. It must be properly prepared for and cared for postoperatively to have an uneventful healing course, as outlined in Nieć et al. (2024). Swelling and bruising are a couple of potential recovery complications, thus necessitating careful patient selection and appropriate preoperative assessment. Significance of lifestyle factors—diet and medications—on recovery enhances the need for an integrative treatment plan. With the increased popularity of blepharoplasty among cosmetic surgeons, innovation in standardized protocols regarding patient preparation and post-treatment will be critical. To ensure patients are given the best possible care throughout, practitioners are able to optimize the efficacy of blepharoplasty and further cement its status as a leading facial aesthetic procedure.

4.1. Types of Blepharoplasty

Learning Outcome

1. Discuss Upper Eyelid Blepharoplasty
2. Explain Lower Eyelid Blepharoplasty
3. Focus on Transconjunctival Blepharoplasty

Blepharoplasty in facial aesthetics serves many cosmetic and functional purposes with respect to the eyelids. Blepharoplasty can be classified as upper and lower blepharoplasty, both differing in approach and outcome. Upper blepharoplasty is meant to erase surplus skin and fat above the eyes to offset sagging that affects vision and creates a tired appearance. This is particularly beneficial in elderly patients whose eyelids have dropped with age. In contrast, lower blepharoplasty addresses the underside of the eyes, removing or redraping fat deposits responsible for puffiness, along with further correction of looseness of skin. These techniques are not only limited to aesthetic purposes but also to improved eye function, which further underscores the multi-faceted benefit of these surgical procedures. Ethnic considerations are also important in determining the type of blepharoplasty performed as anatomical variation significantly affects outcomes. An example is that, in certain ethnic populations like the Hazara, unique genetic features render combined eyebrow lifting and upper blepharoplasty necessary for optimal outcomes. The combined treatment allows for the genetic correction of low eyebrows, which may create a perception of drooping eyelids. In 163 patients, Hazara women were observed to yield notable improvement under the overall method, highlighting the importance of customized surgical planning to accommodate individual anatomical needs (Azimi, 2024). Non-Hazara individuals, by contrast, should be able to obtain acceptable results utilizing isolated blepharoplasty, which highlights the importance of tailoring surgical procedures to accommodate diverse population groups. Beyond traditional surgical techniques, blepharoplasty's evolution has seen the incorporation of advanced non-surgical and minimally invasive treatments that are attractive to individuals unwilling to submit to more invasive facial renewal processes. Injectables, such as fillers and thread lifts, offer alternatives for patients afraid of the risk associated with surgery, allowing for discreet rejuvenation without the long recovery of traditional blepharoplasty (Portilla et al., 2024). Furthermore, the technological progress, including laser therapy, has allowed for easier postoperative healing and less scarring, enhancing patient satisfaction. Hence, the procedure of blepharoplasty is continuously adapting to accommodate patient interests at the cost of compromising aesthetic goals with safety and efficacy, making its use relevant in contemporary facial aesthetics (Figure 4.3).

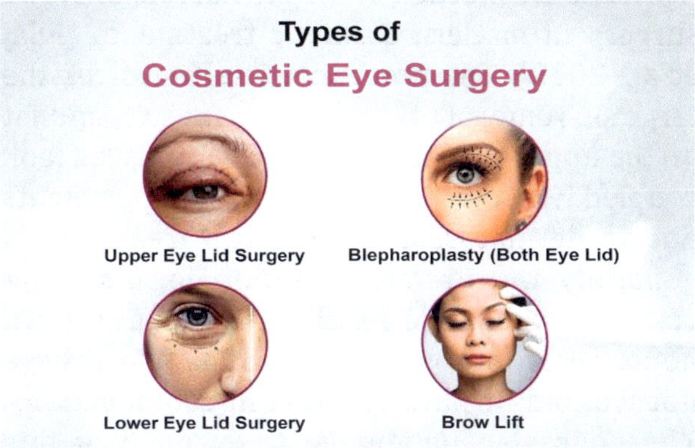

Figure 4.3. The blepharoplasty serves multiple purposes.

Source: https://www.google.com/url?sa=i&url=https%3A%2F%2Fwww.mmjoshieyeinstitute.com%2Fblog%2Fdifferent-types-of-cosmetic-eye-surgeries%2F&psig=AOvVaw1mPonEUMJnwleUJXI8z1HZ&ust=1751986820874000&source=images&cd=vfe&opi=89978449&ved=0CBQQjRxqFwoTCMij9tKBq44DFQAAAAAdAAAAABAE.

4.1.1. Upper Eyelid Blepharoplasty

Upper eyelid blepharoplasty, or the surgical procedure designed to revive the eyelids, is an essential procedure employed to enhance facial looks. As age catches up with people, they start losing their youthful appearance and acquire dermatochalasis, an overabundance of skin and fat in the area of the eyelids, leading to a tired appearance. Not only does the condition lead to an ugly appearance, but it also cause vision loss in severe cases. Most noticeably, though, are the hoods over the eyelids that bother patients seeking this operation because they can give the face a more serious, deeper look. Blepharoplasty only succeeds if there is a meticulous evaluation of the facial structure so that the operative design satisfies the wishes of the patient as well as the international facial balance. The rejuvenative effect of the procedure is not only about restoring youth but also about enhancing the patient's self-esteem and confidence about her looks, a reflection of the pivotal role of eyelid surgery in modern cosmetic treatments (Filaj et al., 2023). The procedure itself involves the targeted removal of excess skin, muscle, and fat on the upper eyelids, resulting in a renewed look coupled with correcting functional impairments due to dermatochalasis. Surgical treatment is generally the preferred option for its long-standing and stable results, particularly when nonsurgical interventions, such as fillers, have not worked or have resulted in complications. The Caucasian patient is an example of this kind of case because frequent injections with hyaluronic acid resulted in side effects, such as eyelid heaviness. By undergoing upper eyelid blepharoplasty, the medical team solved both the functional and aesthetic problems by carefully excising the surplus tissue and rebuilding the original shape of the eyelids. Postoperative evaluation revealed a satisfaction score that was very high among patients, affirming the success of blepharoplasty in reversing the signs of aging as well as enhancing visual fields (Maione et al., 2021). Lastly, upper blepharoplasty is the summation of cosmetic and functional surgery and how cosmetic issues are predominantly used to decide on surgery. Not only does the surgery redefine the upper lid but also collectively refines the overall facial appearance, contributing to a more youthful and lively look.

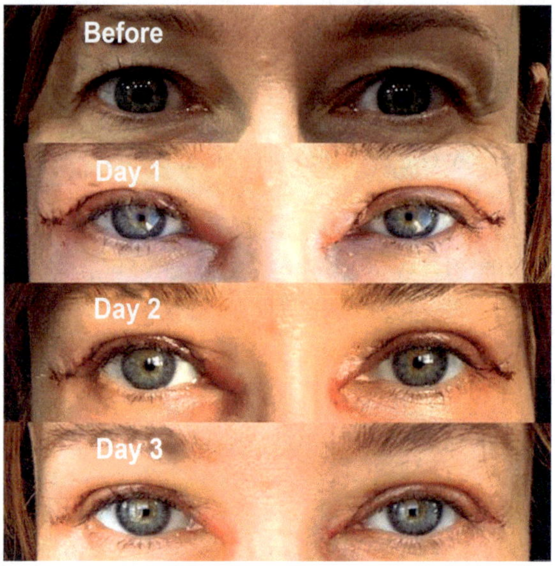

Figure 4.4. Upper eyelid blepharoplasty, a surgical procedure designed to rejuvenate the eyelids.

Source: https://tabanmd.com/wp-content/uploads/2021/03/Slide-2A-upper-blepharoplasty-healing.jpg.

The addition of ancillary procedures such as brow lifting or facial rejuvenation techniques, can complement overall results and patient satisfaction. With each continued advance in surgical technique and postoperative care, the potential for optimization of the best aesthetic result increases, further establishing upper eyelid blepharoplasty in the grand canvas of facial aesthetics. The importance of a sound surgical plan and meticulous technique cannot be underestimated, as both have a part to play in the success and naturalness of the aesthetic outcome (Filaj et al., 2023) (Figure 4.4).

4.1.2. Lower Eyelid Blepharoplasty

As a core procedure in facial aesthetics, lower eyelid blepharoplasty addresses cosmetic and functional concerns related to the lower eyelids. The surgical process is primarily designed to eliminate excess skin as well as fat deposits, thereby reducing the appearance of bags and wrinkles that have the tendency to make the person look tired or aged. The patient typically goes in for the procedure not only for cosmetic reasons but also to enhance peripheral vision disabled by sagging eyelids. With the different methods, including transconjunctival and external approaches, the operation can be tailored to each individual's aesthetic and anatomical needs. Studies have indicated patient satisfaction levels after the surgery to be incredibly high, which indicates the success of the surgery in restoring the area of the lower eyelid. Finally, lower eyelid blepharoplasty is an integral component of cosmetic surgery, not just changing looks but also self-esteem and confidence in patients. The postoperative recovery period following lower eyelid blepharoplasty is crucial to ensuring optimal outcomes. Patients' health as well as compliance with postoperative orders are key in this process. Appreciation for the value of preoperative consultations, which assess potential complications and patients' expectations, is essential. Research has established that patients with comorbidities, such as diabetes and hypertension, are capable of longer healing and increased complications, which makes patient selection very important when planning for surgery (Nieć et al., 2024). Appropriate wound care and dealing with potential complications, such as dry eye syndrome and edema, also enhances rapid healing. The role of nutrition also cannot be overstated, because it directly influences the healing of wounds and repair of tissues. Therefore, an excellent recovery experience can be perceived by effective communication between patients and surgeons regarding expectations and procedures for care. In all, facial aesthetic fields, lower eyelid blepharoplasty is the best example of the synergy between surgical approaches and complete treatment of patients. The technique has evolved over the past several years, such as noninvasive adjuncts that are secondary to surgical outcomes, as outlined in recent reviews (Portilla et al., 2024). Fillers and skin-tightening modalities are significant aspects in enhancing aesthetic outcomes with low recovery. The evolution of technology and materials, such as continuous sutures and applications of lasers, has also advanced the process of surgery. These developments not only improve procedural efficiency but also contribute to finding aesthetic satisfaction that patients pursue. Lower eyelid blepharoplasty, being popular and effective, still remains a core issue in the debate on facial rejuvenation within aesthetic medicine, citing the synergy between surgical intervention and comprehensive patient care (Figure 4.5).

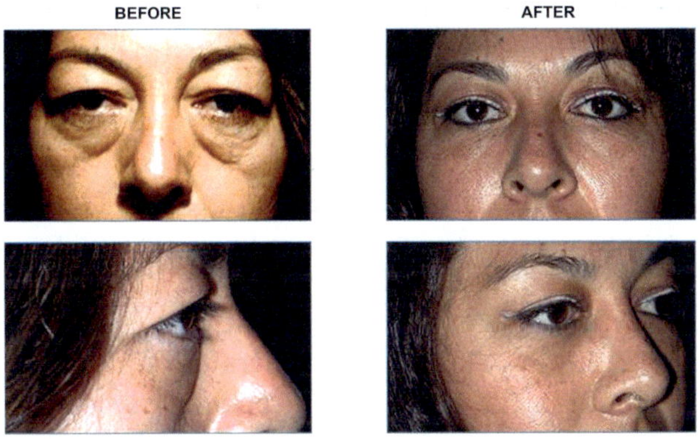

Figure 4.5. As a pivotal procedure in facial aesthetics, lower eyelid blepharoplasty addresses aesthetic and functional concerns related to the lower eyelids.

Source: https://www.google.com/url?sa=i&url=https%3A%2F%2Fwww.mdeyecare.org%2Fservices%2Ffacial-cosmetic-surgery%2Flower-eyelid-surgery%2F&psig=AOvVaw0dCBMYtnA1JpzOlPCFy8Dr&ust=1751986721342000&source=images&cd=vfe&opi=89978449&ved=0CBQQjRxqFwoTCNjX2aeBq44DFQAAAAAdAAAAABAM.

4.1.3. Transconjunctival Blepharoplasty

Transconjunctival blepharoplasty is a favorite blepharoplasty procedure because of its minimally invasive method of rejuvenating the lower eyelids. This surgical treatment is achieved through a cut within the conjunctival lining, thereby eliminating visible scars on the surface of the skin. As a result, the patient ends up with a more attractive outcome with less downtime. The focus on precise fat removal and the preservation of the overlying tissues decreases the risk of complications, a consideration that is especially critical in cosmetic surgery, where both form and function are important. In addition, the transconjunctival approach is a more targeted intervention, addressing problems of fat protrusion without running into pitfalls of more traditional techniques, like overresection of the skin and subsequent eyelid laxity degrading facial beauty (Zhang et al., 2025). Assessing the success of transconjunctival blepharoplasty, findings indicate that incorporation of fat repositioning techniques further enhances aesthetic results. As the aging process causes the lower eyelid to change, including the development of clearly defined tear troughs and eye bags, procedures must be compatible with these problems. Science has proven that the combination of orbital septal fat repositioning and transconjunctival procedures can work very effectively to correct both tear trough deformities as well as overall eyelid skin quality. A recent study of patients undergoing transconjunctival blepharoplasty reasserted that combined surgical technique in such a procedure had good patient satisfaction rates, with a considerable number reporting better appearance of the lower eyelid and lower postoperative complications (Yordanov, 2025). This indicates that transconjunctival blepharoplasty is not only effective but also an innovative strategy for personal aesthetic treatments in facial rejuvenation. Moreover, the rapid healing that comes after transconjunctival blepharoplasty is another important feature behind its high popularity. The patients experience less postoperative discomfort and less swelling compared to standard lower eyelid surgeries. This rapid recovery makes it particularly well-suited for individuals with active lifestyles, who desire to eliminate their downtime as much as possible while still achieving their desired cosmetic outcome. The accomplishment of such a surgical intervention, combined with adjunctive techniques such as fat grafting or SVF-gel injection, remains evidence of its versatility and lasting impact on facial aesthetics. By providing the capability to perform tough yet refined treatment of lower eyelid rejuvenation, transconjunctival blepharoplasty not only enhances beauty but also enhances the quality of life of the patient, positioning it as one of the leading candidates in cosmetic surgery (Zhang et al., 2025).

Test Your Knowledge

1. What anatomical concerns are typically addressed with upper versus lower eyelid blepharoplasty?
2. What are the primary differences in incision placement and tissue handling between upper eyelid, lower eyelid, and transconjunctival blepharoplasty?

4.2. Indications for Blepharoplasty

Learning Outcome

1. Discuss the Cosmetic Reasons for Eyelid Surgery
2. Explain Functional Implications of Eyelid Conditions
3. Focus on Age-Related Changes and Their Impact

Blepharoplasty, or surgery of the eyes, is predominantly indicated for aesthetic and functional purposes. The operation is typically sought by the patient to resuscitate apparent signs of aging, like sagging skin, puffiness, and bulbous eye bags, that can mar an otherwise youthful appearance. Since the eyelid skin is very thin and delicate, it tends to age faster than other facial skin. This surgical intervention not just freshens up the eyes but also plays an important role in completing the facial loveliness as a whole. Moreover, patients with sagging eyelid skin also possess possible visual field obstruction, thus functional outcomes become an important aspect in preoperative assessment as well as in preserving patient satisfaction following surgery. Besides aesthetic reasons, another significant indication for blepharoplasty is enhancing the quality of life of the patient. Functional disabilities, like impaired vision from sagging eyelids, can lead to handicaps in daily functioning in specific situations and cause psychological distress. Studies have shown impressive quality of life enhancements, such as reduction of headache frequency and enhancement of vision-based quality parameters post-upper blepharoplasty. The combined effect of aesthetic advantage and functional gain demonstrates the importance of addressing both these aspects simultaneously. This combined approach explains the high patient satisfaction rates quoted by patients, which is a reflection of the benefits overall that blepharoplasty provides beyond attractiveness (Costa et al., 2023). In addition, advances in surgical techniques have expanded the indications for blepharoplasty so that more patients can benefit from this procedure. Non-surgical treatments, like plasma sublimation, are designed to advance traditional techniques, with encouraging outcomes and less recuperation time. The application of coenzyme Q10 postoperatively has also proved beneficial in skin improvement and healing, further increasing the efficacy of the surgery. These advances highlight the dynamic nature of blepharoplasty and prove its adaptability according to the distinct requirements of every patient. With ongoing development of technology and our understanding of the outcomes, blepharoplasty indications will continue to rise, as more patients will demand it as a solution to both cosmetic and functional eyelid concerns (Costa et al., 2023).

4.2.1. Cosmetic Reasons for Eyelid Surgery

Cosmetic indication is the prime reason for performing blepharoplasty, or eyelid surgery, most of the time, particularly due to age. When the skin loses its elasticity and the supporting tissues undergo physiological change, drooping eyelids may create a fatigued and aged look. Not only does it influence the beauty quotient, but it also influences self-esteem and social life. The majority of patients who come for this procedure are dissatisfied with their appearance, and it influences their self-esteem and social relationships. By rejuvenating the eyelids to a youthful shape, blepharoplasty is not only a renewing operation that increases facial attractiveness but also emotional well-being, aligning with contemporary beauty and youth ideals of society. Besides, the cosmetic aspect of blepharoplasty extends beyond aesthetics; the operation can also remove functional obstacles caused by surplus skin or fat around the eyelids. In certain cases, such structural alterations disrupt vision, and normal functioning becomes difficult. Esthetic rejuvenation through eyelid surgery thus has twofold benefits—improving both the manner in which an individual looks and the manner in which he or she can see. Blending of surgical techniques with non-surgical methods in facial aesthetic surgery serves to reflect the evolving nature of cosmetic therapies aimed not just at maximizing external beauty but also at improving ocular function. As research continues to uncover more advanced options for rejuvenation, the fusion of function and form in eyelid surgery gains increasing significance (Portilla et al., 2024).

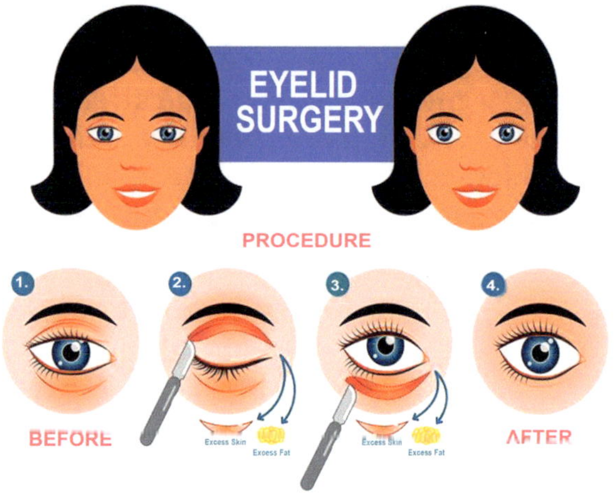

Figure 4.6. Cosmetic reasons for eyelid surgery.

Source: https://www.kelsey-seybold.com/-/media/Project/KelseySeybold/KelseySeyboldClinic/Images/Blog-Images/Plastic-Surgery-Body-Images/eyelid-surgery-graphic.jpg?w=70%25&hash=B83A1A8F2ED6D63AD41C130A035A73C0.

In addition, preoperative interviews have a considerable role in assessing the suitability of candidates for blepharoplasty, especially their expectations and medical history. Familiarity with the anticipated results, potential complications, and recuperation processes allows patients to make educated decisions. Moreover, collaboration with problems like general well-being and lifestyle factors significantly influences the surgical process and result. As stated in the majority of studies, well-informed and clearly defined expectations among patients are those who achieve higher satisfaction scores following the surgery. Common understanding among surgeons and patients protects against misaligned expectations and results in improved aesthetic outcomes and reduced recovery time. Thus, the ophthalmic universe of eyelid surgery isn't just cosmetic repairs; it's about a whole-dimensional comprehension of the patient's needs and condition to be able to provide the best outcome (Nieć et al., 2024) (Figure 4.6).

4.2.2. Functional Implications of Eyelid Conditions

The functional implications of eyelid disorders are more than cosmetic and profoundly impact people's daily lives and psychological well-being. Ptosis or loose skin, for example, can hinder vision and result in severe visual impairment. Patients will struggle with restricted peripheral vision, which will complicate activities like reading, driving, or even watching television. Further, the discomfort caused by eyelid conditions, ranging from irritation to chronic fatigue, is itself capable of producing a low quality of life. Through blepharoplasty, not only can physical symptoms be alleviated, but facial appearance as a whole is rejuvenated by surgery, so functional and aesthetic problems are addressed simultaneously. With the ongoing improvement in surgical technology, so too does understanding of the various functional consequences that can follow eyelid conditions. Patients may have an inability to fully close the eyelids, leading to exposure keratitis, with the cornea becoming compromised due to uncontrolled exposure. The functional limitation necessitates a surgical intervention that is not only cosmetically corrective but also aimed at restoring ocular well-being. Progress in recent procedure techniques and anesthesia has enhanced surgeries like blepharoplasty, which are currently safer and more effective, allowing for tailored interventions for the correction of chosen functional impairment. According to recent studies, high evidence is present of increased quality of life and satisfaction rates in relation to better visual function after surgery, indicating the double benefit of such procedures (Nieuwenhuis et al., 2023). There is also a psychosocial factor present in the functional impacts of eyelid disorders because the visibility of the condition leads to social apprehension and lower self-esteem. Those patients suffering from drooping eyelids or other cosmetic issues will be made to feel self-conscious, and this impacts their social interactions and working lives. In addition, blepharoplasty is reported by many people to make them look younger and more confident, further indicating the role of aesthetics in contributing to functional well-being. In treating eyelid conditions, it is important to consider this psychological factor since improving the appearance of a patient can improve their feelings and become more interactive and mentally healthy socially. Thus, filling the gap between both cosmetic and functional purposes to undergo blepharoplasty makes an integrated strategy that considers physical and emotional factors, showing modified paradigms in facial esthetics (Portilla et al., 2024).

4.2.3. Age-Related Changes and Their Impact

Aging impacts the face with an array of modifications that may have a significant impact on facial appearance, particularly in the eyes. During aging, there are various factors responsible for a decrease in the elasticity of skin and loss of subcutaneous fat, which are finally held responsible for the facial appearance normally seen with increasing age. For instance, the skin on the eyelids becomes loose and thin, adding not only to a worn-out or tired appearance but also to peripheral vision blockade. Further, muscles used for eye-positioning assistance may weaken, which again adds to such problems. The concurrent action of such changes may result in loss of beauty perception according to society, which impacts self-esteem as well as social relationships. Correcting these age changes with surgical procedures, such as blepharoplasty, can restore youthful vitality and address cosmetic concerns, positively affecting the well-being of an individual. The applicability of surgical methods such as blepharoplasty is supported by the need patients have for a better aesthetic outcome. Age-associated periorbital alterations pose the void to be filled with procedures that not only seek to enhance superficial appearance but also address the underlying anatomical structure. As per research, procedures like deep rhytidectomy have their best results by addressing both the skin and deeper planes of tissues, enhancing the general facial harmony, as evidenced in the seen visual enhancement in studies focused on the long-term results of plastic surgeries conducted on the face (Бондарєв et al., 2024). Rejuvenation of youthful contours and drooping eyelid reduction through blepharoplasty can restore an individual's facial outline, instilling a feeling of contentment that aligns with postoperative healing expectations.

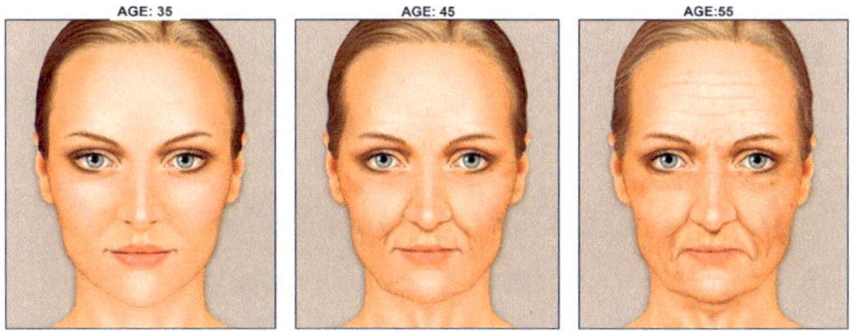

Figure 4.7. The aging process brings about a myriad of changes that significantly impact facial aesthetics.

Source: https://external-content.duckduckgo.com/iu/?u=https%3A%2F%2Fpreventouscosmetic.com%2Fmedia%2F220bac7a-3803-462f-9e73-effe22b5220c.jpeg&f=1&nofb=1&ipt=ea9c1f6edb8767704088cd7757f5fccb9e81b6bfff3bc8ba006b1ff1d8a8d22d.

Also, the aesthetic plastic surgery specialty is constantly evolving by implementing new research discoveries and technical improvements to improve surgical technique. Conferences such as the Italian Association of Plastic Aesthetic Surgery's (AICPE) annual congress promote new methods and offer useful information about the evolving face of facial aesthetic treatments (Riggio, 2024). While the professionals convene to discuss alterations with age and consequences, a collaborative effort towards enriching the blepharoplasty technique has been observed. This collaboration of established techniques and novel developments supports the clinician in a greater appreciation of the patient's desires and in maximizing surgical outcomes. With meticulous preoperative planning and delivery, blepharoplasty evolves from a procedure of rejuvenation to a holistic method respecting the nuances of aging, eventually reasserting the importance of aesthetic integrity in facial surgery (Figure 4.7).

Test Your Knowledge

1. What cosmetic concerns commonly lead patients to seek eyelid surgery (blepharoplasty)?
2. How can certain eyelid conditions create functional problems that make blepharoplasty medically necessary?
3. In what ways do age-related changes to the eyelids affect vision, appearance, or eyelid function?

4.3. The Surgical Procedure

Learning Outcome

1. Discuss the Preoperative Consultation and Assessment
2. Explain Surgical Techniques and Approaches
3. Focus on Anesthesia Options and Patient Comfort

Blepharoplasty, or eyelid surgery, is an extremely intricate surgical procedure correcting eyelid defects like loose muscles, fat, and skin. The operation is commonly requested for cosmetic reconstruction as well as for the restoration of functional issues, for instance, reduced peripheral vision caused by sagging eyelids. The surgery involves opening along natural folds of the eyelids to reduce the visibility of scarring, thereby retaining the looks. Fat and excess skin can be removed or redistributed, depending on skillful technique, to restore symmetry and a rejuvenated appearance post-surgery. Such precision not only creates improved cosmetic appearances but can contribute significantly to patients' self-esteem and satisfaction levels, and is thus a significant component of facial beauty. The choice of surgery typically depends on the individual requirements of patients and anatomical considerations. Traditional blepharoplasty is primarily focused on excision or distortion of tissue, but new technology has introduced advanced techniques such as transconjunctival blepharoplasty, which does not even involve exterior incisions and is less invasive. Improvements, such as the application of laser technology, have offered more accurate tissue removal with less swelling and recovery. With developments in surgery, the application of noninvasive adjuncts like dermal fillers or procedures like plasma sublimation is also being utilized as complementary therapy to enhance the end result as much as possible. Most importantly, these techniques are also being blended together to produce a natural, youthful look without compromising the stability of the eyelid's architecture, thereby optimizing the longevity of the surgical outcome while ensuring patient satisfaction. The effects of blepharoplasty extend beyond aesthetics; there is also a crossover with overall health results. There has been research to show that this procedure can lead to improved psychological states and social confidence, especially in individuals whose self-image is based on how their eyes appear. Besides, as put forward in recent research, dietary habits and nutrition are vital for healthy skin, focusing on a general strategy for pre- and postoperative care (Costa et al., 2023). The supplementation with some nutrients may enhance healing, increase skin elasticity, and maximize surgery outcomes. With new developments in ocular aesthetics, more and more it is clear that combining surgical techniques with total lifestyle modifications like nutritional supplementation can offer optimal outcomes, not only for aesthetics, but also for quality of life.

4.3.1. Preoperative Consultation and Assessment

Proper preoperative consultation and evaluation are integral to the planning of surgery and the success of blepharoplasty. The initial phase facilitates the clinician to evaluate the patient's medical history, such as any of the chronic illnesses like hypertension or diabetes, which are vital during the anticipation of postoperative recovery and complications. For instance, patients with these basic conditions experience longer recovery times as well as insufficient scar formation, hence the significance of tailored preoperative interventions (Nieuwenhuis et al., 2023). Moreover, this assessment promotes open communication about the patient's expectations in an effort to determine that surgical goals are consistent with desired aesthetic outcomes. Enjoying such aspects not only reduces the risk of dissatisfaction post-surgery but also enhances informed consent, improving the quality of care provided. Other than medical history evaluation, aesthetic assessment during preoperative consultation is a significant determinant of blepharoplasty success. Clinicians use a variety of measurement methods, including standard scales, to measure factors such as eyelid position, lid crease shape, and facial harmony overall to take accurate measurements. Recent research shows that post-surgery patient satisfaction may be directly related to preoperative measurement and aesthetic correlation with patient expectations (Nieuwenhuis et al., 2023). The measurement ensures that any deviations from the look that the patient wants and the potential outcome are thoroughly dealt with. By establishing realistic aesthetic goals and informing patients of the limitations of surgery, health care professionals can decrease unrealistic expectations and enhance satisfaction with final outcomes. This discussion also serves to strengthen the therapeutic relationship between clinician and patient. Preoperative visits are more than medical assessments; they involve conversations regarding lifestyle behaviors that affect surgical outcomes. For example, the nutrition of patients and habits such as smoking have a significant effect on wound healing, underlining the importance of holistic assessments before surgery (Nieć et al., 2024). The implementation of a preoperative optimization policy, for example, dietary recommendations and cessation of deleterious behaviors, can improve recovery and decrease complication rates. In addition, treatment of these issues consolidates the shared duty of clinician and patient toward surgical success. As surgical methods in blepharoplasty develop, standardization of preoperative procedures and accessibility to everyone become imperative to improve patient safety and ensure the optimal result in aesthetic procedures (Figure 4.8).

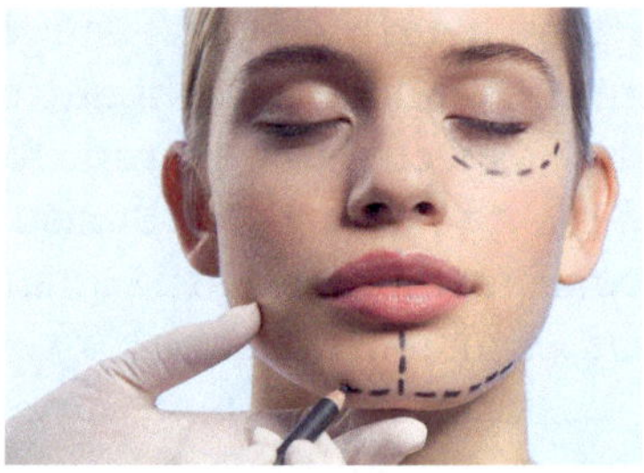

Figure 4.8. A comprehensive preoperative consultation and assessment.

Source: https://www.artefacial.com/wp-content/uploads/2017/10/valoracion-preoperatoria-1.jpg.

4.3.2. Surgical Techniques and Approaches

Evolution of the surgical techniques in blepharoplasty mirrors the increased demand for aesthetic eyelid surgery, resolving a vast array of patient problems. Traditional surgical procedures involve incisions along the creases of the natural folds of the eyelid to remove excess skin, fat, and muscle in trying to recreate the look of a younger eyelid. Based on upper versus lower eyelid surgery, the methods may vary considerably, with upper blepharoplasty usually doing no more than correct loose skin and excess fat and lower blepharoplasty to correct puffiness and dark circles caused by herniated fat pads. The use of accurate measurements in conjunction with dissection methods allows optimal preservation of periorbital anatomy, yielding natural results and minimizing complications. With the refinement of the techniques, aesthetic outcomes meeting patient expectations are sought, and such requires an understanding of anatomical features and potential surgical modifications comprising optimal eyelid beauty. Apart from conventional surgical techniques, the incorporation of minimally invasive techniques in blepharoplasty has also revolutionized the landscape of facial aesthetic surgery. Fat grafting and the use of thread lifts exemplify the dichotomy of surgical and non-surgical modalities to achieve optimal rejuvenation of the eyelids. Such as fat grafting, which has been praised for its ability to restore volume in the periorbital region, not just enhance facial attractiveness, but also establish a smoother and more youthful contour. Similarly, thread lifting with threads like polydioxanone (PDO) and polylactic acid (PLA) threads is employed as an adjunct procedure to enhance skin laxity, providing patients with a less invasive option that generally bears less downtime and recuperation. As highlighted by the most recent trends in aesthetic medicine, the evolution of these techniques is a manifestation of a broader direction towards both effective and less invasive anti-aging solutions (Portilla et al., 2024). Moreover, the introduction of laser treatments is revolutionizing recovery and aesthetic outcomes of blepharoplasty procedures by offering patients a diversified array of therapeutic options. As in surgical application, carbon dioxide lasers proved themselves to be excellent at treating various dermatoses of aging skin condition-related fine wrinkles and lines that are so typical for the eyelids (Penev, 2022). The ablative controlled component of CO_2 lasers provides for easy targeting of skin remodeling with a lot of constructive damage and minimal destructive damage, thus ensuring maximum patient recovery and satisfaction. With traditional surgery, laser therapy can effectively enhance the integrity of eyelid skin to make the skin more cosmetically attractive, smoother, and tighter. This two-dimensional approach, which combines surgical expertise with technology in the guise of laser therapy, characterizes the current trend in facial aesthetic surgery, particularly in blepharoplasty.

4.3.3. Anesthesia Options and Patient Comfort

The selection of appropriate anesthesia methods is most critical in achieving patient comfort during blepharoplasty, a procedure aimed at enhancing the facial appearance of the eyelids.

The most traditional and widely employed has been local anesthesia supplemented with sedation to facilitate cooperation and minimize pain in the patient. This procedure is improved by the possibility of targeting particular areas that require surgical intervention, with the patient still fairly awake and able to converse as a means of communication with the surgical team. The success of local anesthesia in managing pain in blepharoplasty highlights the importance of understanding patient fears and wishes for their operating room procedure. Letting patients know what anesthetics will be used may greatly enhance their comfort levels and reduce anxiety, which can lead to improved surgical outcomes. Local anesthesia is not the only avenue for blepharoplasty; general anesthesia also has the potential, particularly for patients who may have extreme anxiety or require a more extensive surgery.

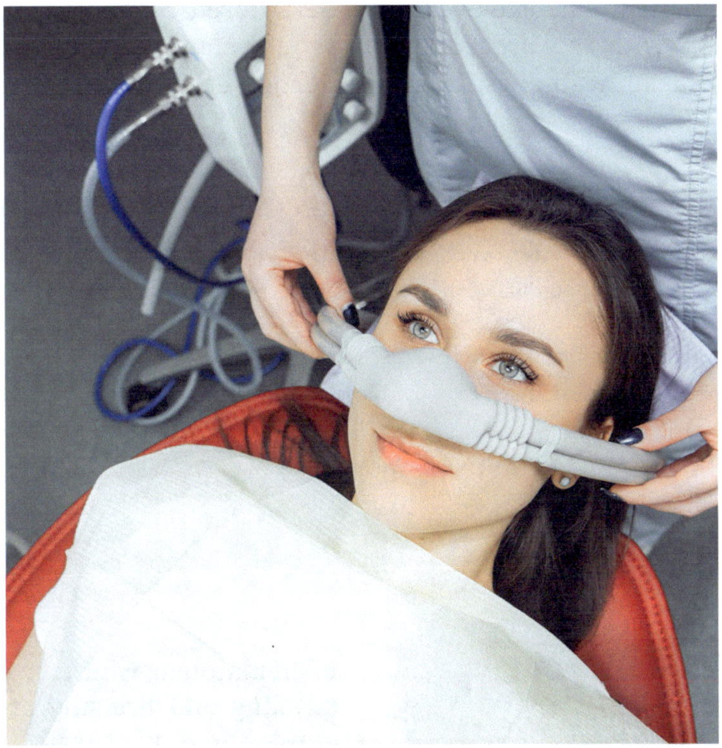

Figure 4.9. The selection of appropriate anesthesia options is critical in achieving patient comfort during blepharoplasty.

Source: https://external-content.duckduckgo.com/iu/?u=https%3A%2F%2Fcms.bayareaimplantperio.com%2Fwp-content%2Fuploads%2F2023%2F10%2Fmobile-hero-sedation-.jpg&f=1&nofb=1&ipt=8124b2231891095bc0a200f5b263a610296f10b3131ad59604c943b27bdc0ad4.

Though deeper in the level of sedation, this type of anesthesia requires careful consideration due to its potential dangers and monitoring requirements during surgery. Ensuring the optimum safety and comfort of the patient comes first, and anesthesiologists are particularly engaged in this through evaluation of individual health records and surgery requirements. As pointed out in the literature, advancements in anesthesia techniques and equipment are continually refining safety profiles to the extent that even more anxious patients can now enjoy a more comfortable ride. Such adaptability in the use of anesthesia is a significant contributing factor to patient satisfaction in the context of facial aesthetic surgery, such as blepharoplasty. Consequently, additional advancements in minimally invasive techniques and other modalities, such as laser therapy, have become increasingly prevalent compared to the application of eyelid surgery for both cosmetic enhancement and comfort. Integration of such technology provides the potential to achieve incorporation of the various modalities with specific regimens of anesthesia, thereby providing an improved patient outcome overall and patient satisfaction with the procedure. With the evolution of facial aesthetics, there has been a focus on creating less traumatic therapies that do not compromise outcome. Progressions such as CO_2 laser therapy for rejuvenation and resurfacing offer additive options to traditional surgical treatments, not just enhancing the safety and comfort of the patient but also the efficacy of the aesthetic outcome. With our continuing assessment and integration of these developments, surgical techniques and anesthetic care protocols can be tailored by clinicians to fulfill the specific requirements of their patients (Penev, 2022; Portilla et al., 2024) (Figure 4.9).

Test Your Knowledge

1. What key evaluations are performed during the preoperative consultation to determine a patient's suitability for blepharoplasty?
2. How do different surgical techniques and approaches vary in addressing upper versus lower eyelid concerns?
3. What factors influence the choice of anesthesia for blepharoplasty, and how does each option affect patient comfort?

4.4. Risks and Complications

Learning Outcome

1. Discuss the Common Risks Associated with Blepharoplasty
2. Focus on Potential Complications and Their Management
3. Explain Importance of Choosing a Qualified Surgeon

Risks and complications of blepharoplasty are of highest priority in treating its safety and efficacy in facial beauty. One such common postoperative complication is the formation of hematoma, where it can lead to apparent swelling and bruising of the eyes, potentially concealing aesthetic results. Immediate postoperative management is sometimes recommended by surgeons to be vigilant against such an occurrence. Furthermore, dryness and irritation can result from altering the function of the eyelid, and lubricating eye drops need to be applied during the period of recuperation. Furthermore, infection, while rare, needs to be guarded against tightly because it can severely delay recovery as well as produce unacceptable cosmetic outcomes. Stringent compliance with proper surgical principles and postoperative routines can prevent most of these complications, emphasizing the importance of selecting an experienced surgeon highly proficient in eyelid surgery techniques. Another equally significant issue raised through blepharoplasty is that of asymmetry or displeasing aesthetic results. Due to how sensitive eyelid anatomy is, slight variations in technique will produce asymmetrical eyelid heights or contouring. It is particularly pertinent in pre-existing anatomical variation cases, where such parameters can make surgery difficult to pursue. Studies suggest that patient dissatisfaction can be associated with such aesthetic results and, in most cases, leads to the need for revision surgery. To avoid such complications as much as possible, meticulous preoperative assessment and realistic counseling about expected outcomes are necessary. The introduction of adjunctive treatments like PDO thread lifts, as delineated in the present literature, has proved to contribute to aesthetic outcomes while also providing an integrative approach to the rejuvenation of the face, proposing a possible way of improving patient satisfaction scores among patients undergoing blepharoplasty (Park et al., 2024). Secondly, the patients need to be aware of the long-term implications of blepharoplasty, such as the need for subsequent surgical interventions in the future. As time goes on in the aging process, the results of the original surgery may fade and leave patients desiring further improvement to maintain their intended appearance. The interaction between the initial surgery and future cosmetic needs underscores the imperative of full patient education before performing the procedure. Complications such as residual scarring or eyelid positional asymmetry could also necessitate revisional surgery, further mentally and financially stressing the patient. Therefore, adequate preoperative counseling, including potential long-term consequences, is required in shielding the patient from the realities of eyelid surgery, especially given that the cosmetic advantages of blepharoplasty may perpetuate a cycle of continuous seeking of facial feature enhancement (James et al., 2024).

4.4.1. Common Risks Associated with Blepharoplasty

Blepharoplasty, despite being commonly performed for its cosmetic benefits, entails a host of risks that potential patients must consider. One of the high risks is the development of postoperative complications such as infection, bleeding, or hematomas. These complications may result from the procedure itself or from inappropriate care following the procedure. Infections, in particular, are at high risk because they can lead to additional complications such as scarring or further surgical procedures. In addition, the risk of uncontrolled bleeding can threaten the healing process; hence, careful patient choice and proper surgical technique are critical to avoid such risks. Keeping these points in mind is crucial for patients who are going to undergo blepharoplasty, as knowledge of the potential risks can enhance more educated decision-making on the patient's side regarding surgery and recuperation. The second common danger of blepharoplasty is its aesthetic outcome, which can be less than what the patient anticipates. Eyelid asymmetry of shape or suboptimal eyelid contouring could result, in most instances, from surgical technique, pre-existing anatomical status, or individual healing response. Unrealistic expectations on some occasions could result in a state of dissatisfaction, and, therefore, strict preoperative evaluation is recommended. Surgeons should carefully counsel patients in formulating realistic expectations based on individual assessment and photographic examination. Significantly, the emotional reaction to such outcomes should also be considered, as they can include emotional distress and disappointment. So, communication during the preoperative period is most essential in keeping potential dissatisfaction with aesthetic outcomes at bay. Moreover, ongoing side effects such as dry eye syndrome or ptosis (droopy eyelids) are major risks following blepharoplasty. Dry eyes may be encountered in patients due to disrupted tear film or eyelid function changes after surgery, and such effects result in irritation and chronic visual disturbances. Ptosis may also develop as a consequence of skin and muscle detachment or over-resection and may need to be corrected with surgery. The late effects of such side effects contribute much to changing daily activities and the general quality of life. Therefore, careful surgical planning and postoperative management are essential to prevent these risks. Accordingly, potential patients must consider these, having comprehensive discussions with their surgeons on not only the cosmetic benefits but also the long-term consequences of blepharoplasty on their eye health and functional outcomes (Costa et al., 2021; Lim et al., 2023) (Figure 4.10).

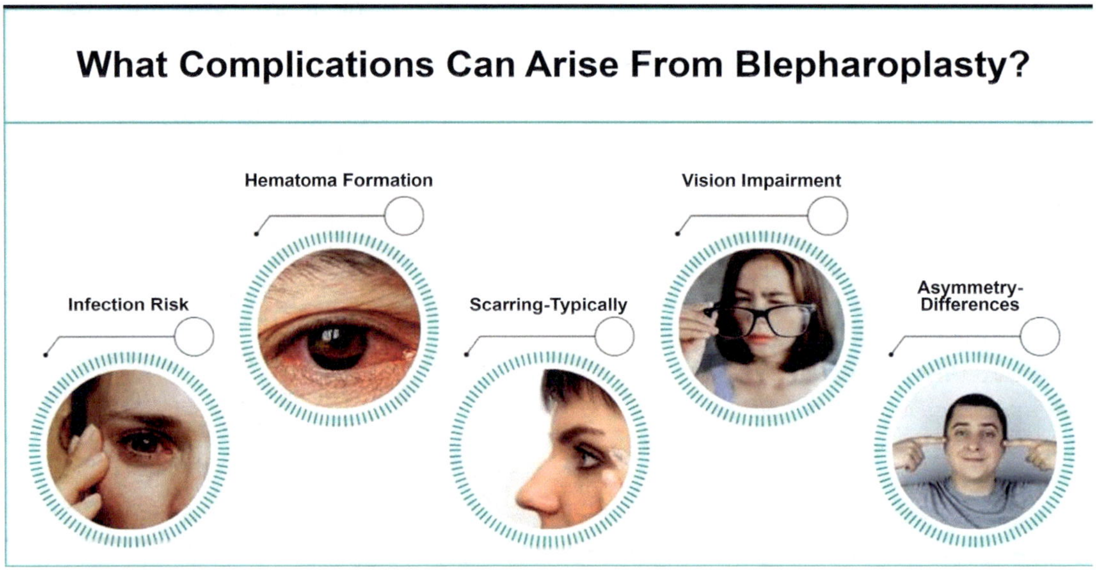

Figure 4.10. Common risks associated with blepharoplasty.

Source: https://www.drtarekaesthetics.com/wp-content/uploads/2023/11/What-Complications-Can-Arise-From-Blepharoplasty-1024x538.jpg

4.4.2. Potential Complications and Their Management

Blepharoplasty, though an extremely popular and generally safe operation to enhance facial appearance, comes with possible complications that must be carefully considered and managed. Swelling and bruising post-surgery are to be expected and will usually resolve themselves in a few weeks' time. The practitioner must, however, pay attention to infection or bleeding tendency, which can be symptoms of deeper issues. Underlying medical conditions, such as diabetes or hypertension, result in extended recovery periods and impaired scarring. By doing thorough preoperative testing to identify these risks, surgeons can adapt their technique to minimize the complications and optimize the healing outcome. Besides, good postoperative care is crucial; direct teaching on wound care can significantly influence the recovery time, and thus patient education is an integral component of the total management plan for blepharoplasty complications (Portilla et al., 2024). Another complication could be eyelid malposition, where the eyelids fail to close after the surgery, presenting functional as well as cosmetic problems. To manage this risk, preoperative evaluation must incorporate the assessment of eyelid anatomy and function so that precise planning for surgery can be undertaken. If there is malposition, it may be corrected by realignment surgery or by the use of corrective appliances to aid in maintaining eyelid position during healing. Dry eye syndrome is another common complication of blepharoplasty, perhaps secondary to altered eyelid function or reduced tear production. Its treatment involves adaptive therapies through artificial tears or punctal plugs, depending on the severity. Regular follow-up postoperative visits are required to observe these conditions so that early intervention is possible once complications arise (Portilla et al., 2024). Finally, wound dehiscence may occur if the incision fails to heal properly, a complication that is generally dependent on the nutrition of the patients and adherence to postoperative care principles. Balanced diet is an important aspect in wound healing, and patients need to be advised to have a good diet before and after surgery to maximize recovery. Between sutures and tissue glue, healing time will either be affected or not be affected, but both are approximately equal in eradication of postoperative pain. Surgeons must make patients aware of the importance of care during the initial weeks following surgery since proper postoperative care can avoid the majority of complications of blepharoplasty, hence enhancing general patient satisfaction with the result (Nieć et al., 2024).

4.4.3. Importance of Choosing a Qualified Surgeon

The decision to undergo blepharoplasty, or eyelid surgery, is not one to be made lightly; it dramatically alters both shape and function. Therefore, the importance of selecting an expert and competent surgeon cannot be emphasized enough. A good surgeon possesses the technical expertise and knowledge required to deliver visually pleasing results while mitigating surgical-related risks. Such expertise allows them to avoid possible complications, such as uneven eyelid placement or scarring, that can adversely affect the patient's overall appearance and satisfaction. Moreover, a qualified surgeon's competence to analyze individual facial structures makes it possible to have a custom surgical intervention according to each patient's own requirement, facilitating the optimal outcome in both function and esthetics. Thus, possessing the right choice in a surgeon is the cornerstone for an effective blepharoplasty experience, not just treating the physical demand but also enhancing the psychological well-being of patients needing rejuvenation. Choosing an experienced surgeon is also crucial to ensuring patient safety during the procedure. Prospective patients should realize that surgical procedures, even blepharoplasty, come with inherent risks like infection, complications from anesthesia, and disappointing outcomes. An experienced surgeon practices under the most stringent safety precautions and practices good pre-operative screening to ensure that patients are good prospects for the procedure.

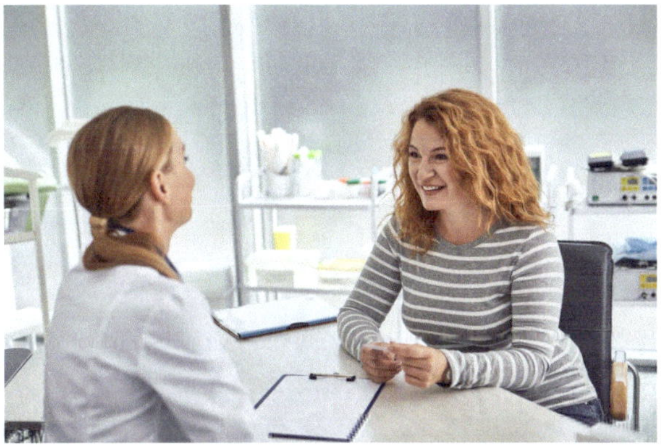

Figure 4.11. Importance of choosing a qualified surgeon.

*Source:*https://external-content.duckduckgo.com/iu/?u=https%3A%2F%2Fwww.columbusplasticsurgery.com%2Fimg%2Fasset%2FYXNzZXRzL2hlcm9zL2lzdG9jay0xMTI1NjYyOTY1Lmp wZw%3D%3D%3Fw%3D1024%26fm%3Dwebp&f=1&nofb=1&ipt=d87f0c2235e8b42d58023e1127b5e3f95c8e2930ca53f26a07400fba68d98c5c.

They provide thorough pre-operative visits that evaluate medical history, current health status, and potential risk factors, which result in informed decisions (Bosniak, 1990). And a skilled surgeon will likely perform the procedure in accredited facilities with advanced technology and attendant personnel, further enhancing patient safety. Ultimately, the use of a well-trained surgeon reduces to a large extent the risks of blepharoplasty and makes patients more confident in undergoing the surgery. Beyond safety and aesthetic outcomes, patient satisfaction and after-care are influenced by choosing to employ a well-trained surgeon. A successful surgeon not only performs the surgery but also places a lot of importance on proper aftercare, necessary for achieving desirable results. It includes providing instructions for post-operative care, managing pain or discomfort, and scheduling follow-up visits to monitor recovery. An effective surgeon also has good communication with patients, paying attention to manage inquiries and expectations throughout the treatment (Bosniak, 1990). This rapport is a central element of the overall surgical experience since patients who are heard and cared for will have better chances of favorable outcomes and reduced anxiety. Therefore, selecting an effective surgeon ultimately benefits as part of a holistic blepharoplasty approach, advocating for the merit of informed choices toward aesthetic enhancement (Figure 4.11).

Test Your Knowledge

1. What common risks are associated with blepharoplasty, and how frequently do they occur?
2. How should potential complications—such as infection, asymmetry, or dry eyes—be identified and managed?
3. Why is selecting a qualified and experienced surgeon critical for reducing the likelihood of complications in blepharoplasty?

4.5. Recovery Process

Learning Outcome

1. Focus on Immediate Postoperative Care
2. Know Timeline for Healing and Activity Resumption
3. Discuss Long-Term Care and Follow-Up

The postblepharoplasty healing process is the most critical factor that can profoundly influence the patient's satisfaction and success of the surgical procedure. Postoperative management knowledge is indispensable in the optimization of healing and prevention of complications. Preoperative condition, nutritional status, and adherence to postoperative instructions are key factors in determining the duration and quality of recovery. Comorbid patients, such as those with diabetes or hypertension, may recover for a longer time and have more complications, for which individual postoperative care plans are needed. Effective education on potential complications, such as swelling, dry eye syndrome, and wound dehiscence, is necessary in educating the patient and reducing his/her expectations (Portilla et al., 2024). Lastly, active recovery that addresses the needs of the patient optimizes superior aesthetic results and maximizes patient satisfaction throughout healing. Management of the postoperative course is equally important since this time can be filled with pain and emotional stress for patients. After eyelid surgery, puffiness and swelling are common, which take some time to settle. The use of appropriate wound care techniques, including the placement of cool compresses and medications as needed, may minimize pain and aid in healing. The recovery process involves adherence to personal guidelines regarding physical activity, cleanliness, and follow-up visits, all of which are important to the prevention of complications. Furthermore, evaluation of the effectiveness of different closure techniques—i.e., running sutures vs. glue—is instrumental in affecting recovery. Research has indicated that both methods yield similar healing times but that practice preference may be influenced by information regarding postoperative pain (Portilla et al., 2024). Clinicians can enhance recovery results and reinforce the aesthetic success of blepharoplasty operations by applying best practices in postoperative care. In addition to accurate care and control, emotional and psychological support during the recovery period is required. Aside from altering physical appearances, blepharoplasty also has a tendency to influence patients' self-perception and confidence. As such, the psychological aspect of recovery cannot be taken lightly. Support structures, including family support and professional guidance, can go a long way in addressing patients' emotional condition at this juncture. Establishing elaborate preoperative consultations also allows one to identify patients' psychological readiness, which is crucial in preparing for postoperative emotions. Multidisciplinary treatment involving physical recovery and emotional counseling is essential for an all-inclusive recovery process. With facial aesthetics evolving, maintaining a focus on improving recovery methods will be key to optimizing patient outcomes and satisfaction for blepharoplasty procedures (Nieć et al., 2024) (Figure 4.12).

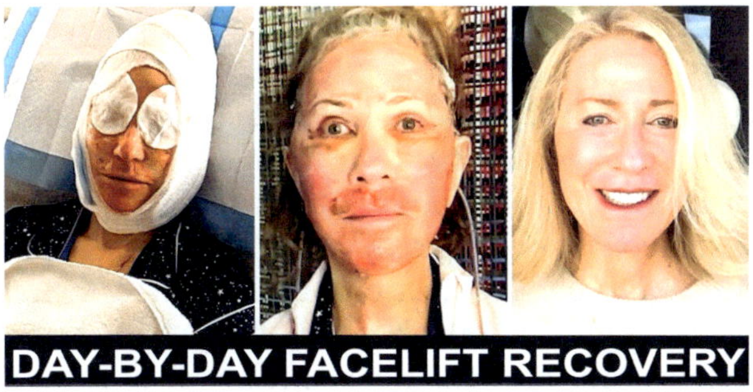

Figure 4.12. The recovery process following blepharoplasty.

Source: https://external-content.duckduckgo.com/iu/?u=https%3A%2F%2Fi.ytimg.com%2Fvi%2FZ7CWld6HLHs%2Fmaxresdefault.jpg&f=1&nofb=1&ipt=cdbee7900e63672a262ebdf6b7e0c0e01ca2d0e11a6c23c924678597ef6e8b1a.

4.5.1. Immediate Postoperative Care

Postoperative care immediately following blepharoplasty is crucial in ensuring optimal recovery and minimizing complications. For the initial hours after surgery, patients are often monitored under close watch in a controlled setting to determine stability and address any ensuing problems that may develop, i.e., excessive bleeding or heightened pain. The eyelids are extremely sensitive and typically become bruised and swollen after the procedure, which involves the application of cold compresses to alleviate edema and discomfort. Also, adherence to prescribed medications like analgesics and antibiotics in a strict manner is required to prevent infection and pain relief. Observation of the individual over this phase of time allows the care practitioners to review the patient's response to the intervention and make adjustments to care plans accordingly to provide interventions in a timely manner whenever needed. In conclusion, an effective immediate postoperative care plan can enhance patient satisfaction and result in successful surgery. As the recovery from the blepharoplasty proceeds, attention now shifts to instructing the patient in proper self-care measures that are essential to allow an uneventful recovery. It is at this time of particular importance to emphasize the importance of keeping the skin around the surgery clean and dry so as not to develop infections. Patients are typically instructed how to gently clean the eyelids and apply topical medications as indicated when necessary. Also, they must be taught not to do heavy exercise, bending, or lifting for at least a few weeks following surgery to prevent stressing the extremely delicate tissues.

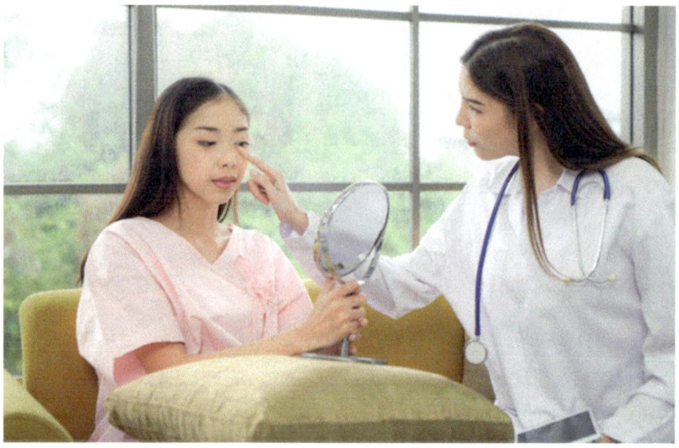

Figure 4.13. The immediate postoperative care following blepharoplasty.

Source: https://external-content.duckduckgo.com/iu/?u=https%3A%2F%2Fimg.freepik.com%2Fpremium-photo%2Fbeauty-doctor-explains-cosmetic-surgery-postoperative-care_159755-10797.jpg&f=1&nofb=1&ipt=109d2161bd5a737f898b5458aed5ae5ab40ae9a42e231087fa750b709d6729d3.

Good communication about anticipated changes, such as transient fluctuating bruising and swelling, helps manage patient expectations and reduces anxiety. Adequate patient education, along with judicious postoperative monitoring, is essential to keep the healing process within normal limits. Lastly, follow-up visits are a part of the continuum of postoperative care shortly after surgery, so the care team can evaluate the healing and to react to any problems. Visual examination on follow-up visits examines eyelid position, symmetry, and overall cosmetic outcome. Selective use of other imaging technologies is employed to estimate internal structures altered by the surgery. It is also a time for clinicians to prioritize patient-reported outcomes (PROs), which, as discovered in the instance of gender-affirming procedures, highlight the importance of patient satisfaction with postoperative results (Gursky et al., 2024). Moreover, professional congresses, such as the annual congress of the Italian Association of Plastic Aesthetic Surgery (AICPE), are essential places for sharing information on global care approaches and postoperative management innovations, further counseling best practices within the field (Riggio, 2024). Regular follow-up appointments enhance the support system for patients, enhancing their recovery process (Figure 4.13).

4.5.2. Timeline for Healing and Activity Resumption

The healing time course following blepharoplasty, or eyelid surgery, is a critical component of the process with a profound impact on patient satisfaction. In the majority of instances, patients can expect to have early bruising and swelling dissipate in the first week following surgery. During this time, patients are typically told to maintain a low level of activity to aid recovery. They aim to reduce the risk of complications. It is important that candidates for surgery understand that the recovery period may vary based on the individual's own healing response, which also depends on factors like age, health, and adherence to post-surgical instructions. Moreover, resumption of normal activities gradually is advised so that patients might return to light activities within 10 days, but not to rigorous exercises for some weeks afterward. This programmed healing is essential in obtaining the optimal aesthetic and functional results following eyelid surgery. As their body heals, patients typically experience relief from post-operative symptoms like discomfort, dryness, and sensitivity. Most individuals can resume moderate physical activity and a relatively normal way of life within two to four weeks following surgery. Interestingly, adherence to prescribed medication and follow-up appointment compliance are significant contributing factors to this healing timeline. Patients are typically asked to avoid the sun and strenuous activity until fully cleared by their surgeon, as these activities will have a significant impact on swelling and scarring outcomes.

When patients reach the one-month mark, they become generally more satisfied with their visual results, reporting a sense of increased confidence, a key to determining the success of blepharoplasty for cosmetic reasons. Gradual adaptation to activity and social involvement is a manifestation of the equilibrium between healing and normalcy restoration. Ultimately, knowledge of healing and return of activity timelines can enable patients to expect reasonably well following blepharoplasty. For further recovery support, various surgeons also recommend some post-surgery practices, like cold compresses to manage swelling and drugs as prescribed to manage pain. The patients must also remain vigilant for potential signs of complications, which will help in timely intervention in case of any issues. As reinforcement of this emphasis on patient education, recent literature highlights the advantages of minimally invasive techniques that enable quicker recovery in cases that are relevant to eyelid surgery. All such advancements, for example, as in parallel lines of the like of oral and maxillofacial surgery, attest to the ongoing advancement in surgical principles for the sake of optimal healing and esthetic results to enhance the patient's overall experience in facial aesthetics (Costan, 2020; Araujo, 2025).

4.5.3. Long-Term Care and Follow-Up

Long-term care and follow-up after blepharoplasty are an essential part of the delivery of optimal results for the patients. The cosmetic procedure, intended to raise eyelids and bring back facial beauty, needs close observation and follow-up postoperative care. Regular follow-up visits allow surgeons to watch for healing, spot complications such as hematoma or infection, and see the aesthetic result. The visits also provide an open communication between the patient and surgeon, allowing them to share concerns or unexpected appearance alterations. It is such active involvement that generates confidence and ensures that any challenge that will arise is addressed in good time, which is very important for achieving the desired results of improved eyelid function and shape. Long-term care challenges extend beyond the acute postoperative period, usually necessitating a more substantial intervention. Several patients are likely to acquire structural changes of the eyelid with the passage of time due to normal aging processes, potentially influencing surgical results.

Consequently, follow-up entails regular checking to evaluate not just the area of the wound but also the facial dynamics surrounding it, which is crucial for maintenance of desired cosmetic outcomes. The evidence suggests that other treatments, such as non-invasive skin procedures or other operations, can be required to counteract changes as a result of aging, rendering patients appear to be in their younger years. By establishing an intensive follow-up program, medical practitioners can navigate patients through the fluctuating angles of their facial appearances. Complications can arise following surgery, so professionals should already have methods for managing such complications effectively. For instance, with the practice of intricate surgical procedures, such as postseptal upper eyelid weight implantation, such complications as extrusion and asymmetry have been reduced to a minimal level. Studies indicate fewer complications with this approach than with traditional methods, which is of more significance in patient care (Rail et al., 2024). Follow-up on a regular basis will enable us to identify any complications jeopardizing the outcomes of the first surgery. Further, since aesthetic improvements are inextricably connected to psychological well-being, patient compliance through ongoing care can lead to a high level of patient satisfaction and overall health. This multi-faceted long-term care approach fosters improved aesthetic results and healthy patient-physician relationships. The evolving nature of aesthetic needs throughout the aging process even further supports the use of adaptive follow-up strategies (Alhashem et al., 2024).

Test Your Knowledge

1. What are the key steps in immediate postoperative care following blepharoplasty to ensure proper healing?
2. How does the typical timeline for healing influence when patients can safely resume normal activities?
3. Why is long-term follow-up important, and what aspects of eyelid health are monitored during this period?

4.6. Psychological and Social Impacts

Learning Outcome

1. Discuss Effects on Self-Image and Confidence
2. Explain the Social Perceptions of Aesthetic Surgery
3. Focus on Patient Satisfaction and Quality of Life

The psychological consequences of blepharoplasty, or eyelid surgery, extend beyond mere physical enhancement and into the very essence of self-concept and self-esteem. Patients typically report dramatic changes in their perceptions of self after surgery, with the majority reporting a rejuvenated and increased confidence. The modification is particularly powerful in social interactions, where reversibility of appearance can lead to modifications in social activity. The procedure has also been linked to reduced anxiety regarding social judgment, as individuals feel better integrated in the cultural perception of beauty. These psychological advantages underscore the importance of aesthetic surgery as a tool of self-improvement to facilitate greater participation in a society that is more attuned to visual looks as an indication of worth and professional capability. This component emphasizes how surgical interventions can impact mental well-being directly by enhancing a feeling of personal self. At the societal level, blepharoplasty also has an impact on individuals' behavior towards their roles and relationships in society. In cultures in which physical appearance is closely linked to social value, such as in Chinese urban society, the decision to undergo eyelid surgery can be motivated by the need to pursue traditional views of beauty that symbolize success and modernity. "Weizheng," or micro cosmetic surgery, is an emerging trend in which women, particularly the post-1980 generation, undergo these beautification procedures to negotiate their position within society. The testified benefits of achieving a desired appearance—larger double-lidded eyes and a youthful appearance—can foster increased social mobility and acceptance. This not only testifies to individual reasons but to the underlying social pressures that construct beauty standards, revealing the advanced connection between individual preference and cultural context within cosmetic surgery (Lotti et al., 2022).

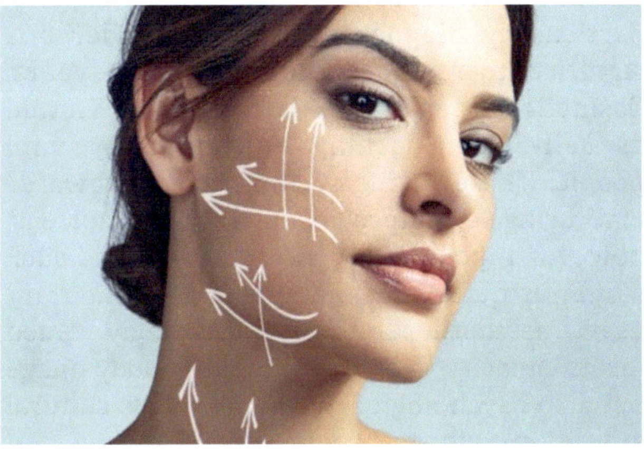

Figure 4.14. Psychological and social impacts.

Source: https://external-content.duckduckgo.com/iu/?u=https%3A%2F%2Fmegaglobalnews.com%2Fwp-content%2Fuploads%2F2023%2F11%2Fsdfdfsdg 2023-11-06T140551.060.jpg&f=1&nofb=1&ipt=eadf1c88cdaacee36ace14fba82b2b189eecd2a1d8ab84846c7e30823ab18143.

Also, the psychological effect of blepharoplasty is found to overlap with social dynamics, ultimately influencing how people see the world around them after the procedure. The surgery can be a form of empowerment for people who feel marginalized due to appearance, as they are now in charge of their bodies as well as the perception of society towards them. This empowerment has a tendency to result in more professional opportunities since individuals have a better attitude, and this can subsequently promote better job opportunities and social networking achievements. This connection between self-perception and career development makes apparent the social implications of aesthetic interventions. Moreover, emotional recovery from surgery generally comprises a regained sense of self, where the patient feels that his or her outer form finally coincides with his or her inner self, which ensures greater levels of relation with others and positive feedback cycle in enriching one's social life and mentality (Penev, 2022) (Figure 4.14).

4.6.1. Effects on Self-Image and Confidence

The effect of blepharoplasty on self-confidence is considerable because this form of cosmetic surgery brings major changes to one's appearance, especially around the eyes. To most individuals, the eyes are a significant communication and expression hub. As time goes by and aging finally reaches them, sagging eyelids and puffiness can project tiredness or even negativity at the expense of the person's confidence. Patients tend to notice renewed vigor and confidence following surgery since they have a younger and more vibrant image. The response to heightened aesthetics is usually immediate, altering the manner in which one views oneself. As confidence improves due to improved image, the ripple effect can have far-reaching influences on social life and interpersonal relationships, illustrating the delicate balance between appearance and perception of oneself. Furthermore, the psychological impacts of blepharoplasty are not only superficial but also impact emotional status and social functioning. The findings in upper eyelid blepharoplasty indicate substantial improvements in a variety of patient reports on psychological and social functioning. After surgery, patients have higher self-esteem and favorable attitudes toward their lives, which ultimately lead to more social interaction and improved relations with other people. The advantages of such alterations suggest that the cosmetic improvements achieved through surgery make a significant contribution to overall quality of life. Strict research, such as that utilizing FACE-Q questionnaires, enables an in-depth understanding of these findings, underscoring the role of patient-centered care in cosmetic surgery. The positive impact of blepharoplasty on self-esteem and confidence highlights the necessity of continued research and standardized assessment in cosmetic surgery.

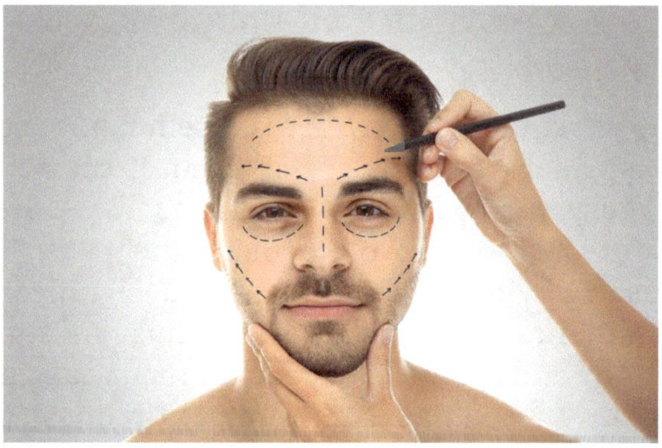

Figure 4.15. The effects of blepharoplasty on self-image are profound.

Source: https://external-content.duckduckgo.com/iu/?u=https%3A%2F%2Fdelrayplasticsurgery.com%2Fwp-content%2Fuploads%2F2020%2F08%2Fman-cosmetic-surgery.jpg&f=1&nofb=1&ipt=4825a41fd482fc15cdebc3ca8e3c815f43d5b1b41501d627276867bd78682a90.

Conferences such as those held by societies like the Italian Association of Plastic Aesthetic Surgery (AICPE) are essential to the exchange of information and best practice in aesthetic surgery. By bringing together acknowledged experts and caretakers, such encounters generate dialogue regarding patient results and improving techniques, eventually giving way to improved aesthetic results and patients' self-image. Improved understanding and application of findings from robust studies, such as the one assessing complete effects of upper eyelid surgery, can result in more informed decision-making by prospective patients, including both functional and aesthetic results. Thus, the promise of change presented by blepharoplasty to optimize self-image and confidence is an important area to continue exploring in facial aesthetics (Figure 4.15).

4.6.2. Social Perceptions of Aesthetic Surgery

The social attitudes towards aesthetic surgery, particularly blepharoplasty, have undergone significant transformation in recent years. Cosmetic surgeries have hitherto been viewed as self-esteem-lacking endeavors by vain people. The evolving societal culture towards embracing self-improvement and self-choice is, however, repositioning the debate around such surgeries quite substantially. In contemporary usage, aesthetic surgery is increasingly valued for its capacity to enhance not only body image but also psychological well-being. This cultural alteration reflects broader social trends that prioritize independence and self-determination, allowing patients to pursue treatments like blepharoplasty as a means of living a better life, thereby displacing traditional notions of beauty and self-esteem that had the effect of dichotomizing cosmetic treatment attitudes. In particular, empirical evidence highlights the beneficial impacts of blepharoplasty on social relationships and self-esteem of the patients. In a study, patients who were operated on the upper eyelid experience significant quality of life gains oriented to psychological and social functioning, as evidenced by findings of studies implementing standardized measuring tools like the FACE-Q questionnaire (Vasović et al., 2024). These studies recognize that beauty satisfaction most often results in greater social confidence, reducing insecurity and improving interpersonal relations. Therefore, these pleasant patient-reported results reflect the notion that aesthetic surgeries are not merely cosmetic but also contribute greatly to individuals' well-being, enabling them to blend into society seamlessly and enhancing their self-perception within societal beauty ideals. By contrast, even with the rising popularity of aesthetic surgery, there still remains today a complicated social landscape tainted by ambivalence. Some people may perceive the likes of blepharoplasty as frivolous or as an exhibition of vanity, reinforcing stigma that will keep individuals away from intervention. Ambivalence towards surgical enhancement also often intersects with common narratives about age, beauty, and gender, which create sophisticated attitudes based on individual values and social norms.

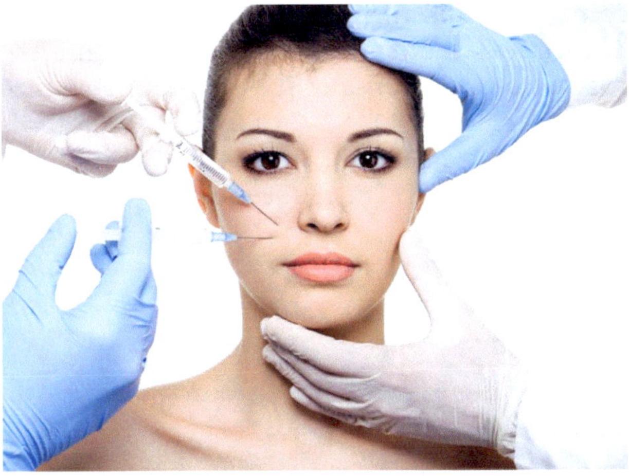

Figure 4.16. The social perceptions surrounding aesthetic surgery.

Source: https://external-content.duckduckgo.com/iu/?u=https%3A%2F%2Fcdndailyexcelsior.b-cdn.net%2Fwp-content%2Fuploads%2F2020%2F07%2Ftop-plastic-surgery-countries.jpg&f=1&nofb=1&ipt=500bf344588d60f17a3c80c5d6744b5bc7d86f0b7eecbda1eea38e6ffa3b9b8c.

Particularly, gender roles also play a critical role to the extent that women may be socialized to adhere to certain standards of beauty and thereby drive the number of cosmetic surgeries upward among them. Addressing these conflicting social attitudes is crucial to the development of a culture where individuals are free to make well-informed choices about their aesthetic looks without fear of stigma or censure, again highlighting the need for yet more discussion and information about the psychosocial benefits of such treatments (Figure 4.16).

4.6.3. Patient Satisfaction and Quality of Life

Patient satisfaction with blepharoplasty is, of course, associated with several determinants affecting the aesthetic outcomes experienced by the subjects post-surgery. In one study involving 583 patients, it was observed that a substantial majority, 63%, of treatment outcome satisfaction variability could be accounted for by a combination of patient factors, clinician ratings, and postoperative outcomes (Nieuwenhuis et al., 2023).

Of these, the most significant contributory factor came from patient-reported outcomes gathered following the surgery, highlighting the importance of patients' perception of their cosmetic change and resulting quality of life. This puts a spotlight on an approach to methodology within cosmetic surgery that is patient-orientated, whereby understanding individual patients' expectations can impact surgical intervention and postoperative management, further elevating overall satisfaction levels. Secondarily, postoperative time is also very important when planning patient satisfaction, particularly improvement in perceived quality of life following blepharoplasty.

Findings of the study highlight that satisfaction is highly related to improvements in facial looks as measured in FACE-Q scales, which assess several quality of life and aesthetic areas (Nieuwenhuis et al., 2023). The patients also gain not only a new appearance but also a new level of confidence and self-esteem, which has a significant bearing on their overall way of life.

This transformation increases the significance of aesthetic procedures in attaining psychological well-being, thus proving that successful surgery results transcend change in body to affect patients' mental states and social interactions. The marriage of both surgical and non-surgical methods, as mentioned in the dynamic future of facial aesthetics, is key to the attainment of patient satisfaction. The evolution of minimally invasive procedures and dermatological adjuncts enhances traditional methods like blepharoplasty, giving patients a greater number of options best applicable to their requirements. This diversified approach enables practitioners to counter the complicated nature of aging and aesthetic demands, subsequently elevating patient levels of satisfaction. As the field evolves, maintaining attention on individualized treatment plans for consideration of both surgical outcomes and personal quality of life measurements will be paramount in maximizing patient contentment and satisfaction with eyelid surgery (Figure 4.17).

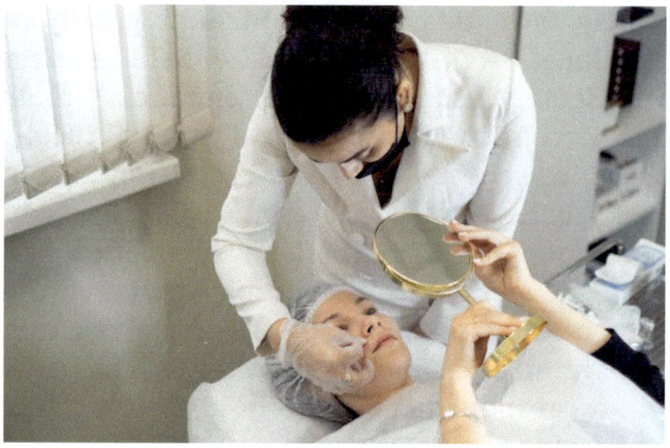

Figure 4.17. Patient satisfaction and quality of life.

Source: https://external-content.duckduckgo.com/iu/?u=https%3A%2F%2Fimg.freepik.com%2Fpremium-photo%2Fpatient-views-her-facial-treatment-results-testament-cosmetic-precision-quality-care-leads-client-empowerment_941451-7403.jpg&f=1&nofb=1&ipt=2e734acfae625d74e5d344f758c6560dfffd2f58346137fdd92ec1803c968a67.

Test Your Knowledge

1. How can blepharoplasty affect a patient's self-image and overall confidence?
2. Why is patient satisfaction an important measure, and how does it relate to quality of life after surgery?

SUMMARY

The summary of an essay on blepharoplasty includes not just the aesthetic and functional benefits of eyelid surgery but also emphasizes the overriding significance of an adequate preoperative assessment and patient selection. The success of the result is based on possessing true knowledge about the personal condition of every patient, comorbidities such as hypertension and diabetes, which can actually impact postoperative recovery and complications, as has already been stated in the study. Proper preparation of patients is not ancillary but instead affects the entire surgical process and, ultimately, wound healing and aesthetic satisfaction. This indicates it is important that practitioners adopt evidence-based practices and carry out comprehensive consultations that consider patient expectations as well as make clear possible risks and benefits of the procedure (Nieć et al., 2024). Furthermore, the innovation of surgical techniques, including the exploration of fibrin tissue adhesives, represents a significant step towards minimizing complications resulting from traditional suture closure. Suture techniques, while efficacious, are shown to cause scarring and pain that will decrease patient satisfaction. The advent of biomaterials like fibrin tissue adhesives offers potential alternatives through the enhancement of healing and a decline in surgical morbidity, but with flaws. A balanced overview of these techniques is warranted, since the demand for innovation in eyelid surgery should not be greater than the value of established techniques (Silva et al., 2011). Both conventional and new techniques reflect a more complete consideration of treatment possibilities for patients. Blepharoplasty ultimately pursues more than mere cosmetic improvement; it pursues the return of natural beauty and enhancement of functional abilities. The assessment of outcomes in eyelid surgery need not be limited to redo rates and complications but can include patient satisfaction, healing, and scar formation, all of which are significant determinants of the success of the surgery overall. Subsequent research should attempt to design holistic outcome measures that encapsulate these diverse factors and, in doing so, enable a richer understanding of recovery and satisfaction after surgery. With blepharoplasty, one of the most sought-after cosmetic treatments, patient education, refinement of techniques, and outcome measures are still progressing the field of facial aesthetics immensely (Silva et al., 2011; Nieć et al., 2024).

In the field of facial aesthetics, blepharoplasty, which is otherwise known as eyelid surgery, is increasingly recognized for its capability to restore youthful eyes. This procedure not only rectifies functional disabilities, such as defective vision resulting from droopy eyelids—but also enhances the beauty of the face as a whole. As people endeavor to present themselves with a youthful and energetic image, blepharoplasty is a key component of this pursuit of beauty. By removing the excess muscle, skin, and fat around the eyelids, the surgery has the capability of radically altering both looks and confidence, thus underlining the surgery's dual aesthetic and functional worth. On the whole, this redemptive process hints at the intricate role that surgical procedures play in the overall climate of the standards of beauty in our contemporary era. Moreover, blepharoplasty's stakes are greater than its surface-level, immediate attraction since patient motivations and expectations depend on social conceptions of beauty. Cultural norms of society often dictate why people get cosmetic surgery, particularly in societies where youthfulness is equal to success and good health. The interaction suggests that blepharoplasty is no longer merely a cosmetic surgery; it also reflects societal norms and values concerning beauty. In interpreting these implications, health professionals must approach the consultation room with an awareness of the psychosocial issues at play, including self-image anxiety and social pressure. The procedure of blepharoplasty is therefore complicit with a wider debate about identity and authenticity, echoing assumptions drawn from broader debates in aesthetic surgery and media representation. Finally, ongoing study and professional discussion within the field also reinforce the evolving applicability of blepharoplasty within cosmetic practice. Conventions such as the Italian Association of Plastic Aesthetic Surgery (AICPE) annual congress are instrumental in the sharing of knowledge and advancements in procedures, patient treatment, and ethics. The emphasis on evidence-based care and patient-driven approaches determines the future of aesthetic surgery in that it enables practitioners to refine their skill level and stay up to date with the latest trends. By enhancing a culture of continuous learning and collaboration, such professional gatherings maximize the efficacy and safety of blepharoplasty so that it can remain a valid option for facial rejuvenation. This style permits the advancement of blepharoplasty to reflect not only individual wants but also the general evolution of aesthetic medicine as a respected field.

KEY TERMS FROM THIS CHAPTER

- Upper Eyelid Blepharoplasty
- Transconjunctival Approach
- Eyelid Crease
- Orbital Septum
- Skin Redundancy
- Lateral Canthopexy
- Eyelid Ptosis
- Lower Eyelid Blepharoplasty
- Subciliary Incision
- Fat Prolapse
- Pretarsal Muscle
- Lid Laxity
- Medial Canthal Tendon
- Dermatochalasis

CRITICAL THINKING QUESTIONS

1. **The primary goal of upper eyelid blepharoplasty is to:**
   a. Correct nasal deviation
   b. Remove excess skin and fat from the upper eyelid
   c. Lift the brows
   d. Correct refractive errors
2. **Which structure forms the main barrier between eyelid fat and the skin-muscle layer?**
   a. Orbicularis oculi
   b. Orbital septum
   c. Levator aponeurosis
   d. Tarsal plate
3. **A common functional indication for upper eyelid blepharoplasty is:**
   a. Cosmetic enhancement alone
   b. Obstruction of visual fields
   c. Changing eye color
   d. Increasing eyelid pigmentation
4. **Lower eyelid "bags" are primarily caused by:**
   a. Overactive orbicularis
   b. Prolapse of orbital fat
   c. Increased tear production
   d. Excessive blinking
5. **The transconjunctival approach in lower blepharoplasty is preferred when the patient has:**
   a. Significant extra skin
   b. Fat herniation without skin excess
   c. Brow ptosis
   d. Deep crow's feet

Short Answer Questions

1. What are the main aesthetic indications for upper eyelid blepharoplasty?
2. What are common functional indications for blepharoplasty?
3. What is the role of the orbital septum in eyelid aging and surgical planning?
4. How is lower eyelid laxity assessed preoperatively?
5. What are the major risks and complications associated with blepharoplasty?
6. What is the purpose of the pinch test during lower eyelid evaluation?
7. How does skin quality affect the choice between transcutaneous and transconjunctival approaches?

Answers to Critical Thinking Questions

1. (b) 2. (b) 3. (b) 4. (b) 5. (b)

REFERENCES

1. Isabela Rombaldi Costa1*, João Pedro Rombaldi Costa2, Melina da Silva Costa1, Alyne Macedo1, Gabriela Batauz Lisboa3, Maria Fernanda Farah Fadel3, Natalia Hirt Viana e Silva1, Ana Luisa Nogueira Abumussi1 (2023). *Major considerations of clinical findings of eye aesthetic and skin treatment with the use of dietary therapy, plasma, and coenzyme Q10: A systematic review.* International Journal of Nutrology.Vol 16 Iss 2. https://core.ac.uk/download/622812164.pdf (accessed on 14th July 2025).

2. Alhashem, M., Alsuwaida, M., Algamdi, M. A., Alhaddad, A. A., Khairi, A. R., & Bajawi, A. M. (2024). Effect of maxillofacial surgery on facial growth and development. *Journal of Healthcare Sciences.* https://www.semanticscholar.org/paper/9b4fe584448b7a68fe06fd2b5ac9239e0dcce3f9 (accessed on 14th July 2025).

3. Araujo, M. J. (2025). *New minimally invasive technique for the treatment of labia minora hypertrophy: Vulvar endolifting.* https://www.amwc-conference.com/content/dam/markets/aest/amwc-conference/2025/pdf/AMWC2025-Abstratcs.pdf (accessed on 14th July 2025).

4. Azimi, H. (2024). Assessing the efficacy of blepharoplasty in Afghan people residing in Kabul. *Afghanistan Journal of Basic Medical Science, 2*, 21–27. https://doi.org/10.62134/ajbms/v2.i2.khatamuni.3 (accessed on 14th July 2025).

5. Chuang, J., Barnes, C., & Wong, B. J. F. (2016). Overview of Facial Plastic Surgery and Current Developments. *Surgery journal (New York, N.Y.), 2*(1), e17–e28. https://doi.org/10.1055/s-0036-1572360(accessed on 14th July 2025).

6. Bondariev, R. V., & Logvinov, Y. O. (2024). Visual comparative analysis of the effectiveness of SMAS and deep rhytidectomy. *The Ukrainian Journal of Clinical Surgery, 91*, 38–42. https://doi.org/10.26779/2786-832x.2024.6.38 (accessed on 14th July 2025).

7. Bosniak, S. L. (1990). *Cosmetic Blepharoplasty.* Lippincott Williams & Wilkins. http://books.google.com/books?id=6pNsAAAAMAAJ&dq=Importance+of+choosing+a+qualified+surgeon+for+blepharoplasty+in+facial+aesthetics&hl=&source=gbs_api (accessed on 14th July 2025).

8. Portilla, A. S. P., Portilla, C. S. P., Palacios, G. S. G., Rodríguez, B. S. P., Castillo, S. G. A., Espin, N. E. P., & Pita, G. P. M. (2024). The integration of surgical and dermatological techniques in the treatment of cutaneous aging: multidisciplinary approaches and clinical outcomes - a comprehensive systematic review of current literature. *International Journal of Research in Medical Sciences, 12*(5), 1659–1667. https://doi.org/10.18203/2320-6012.ijrms20240943(accessed on 14th July 2025).

9. Costa, J., Steinmetz, A., & Delgado, E. (2021). Clinical signs of brachycephalic ocular syndrome in 93 dogs. *Irish Veterinary Journal, 74.* https://doi.org/10.1186/s13620-021-00183-5 (accessed on 14th July 2025).

10. Costan, V. V. (2020). *Insights into oral and maxillofacial surgery: From practice to research.* https://www.umfiasi.ro/ro/academic/programe-de-studii/doctorat/Documents/Abilitare/2020/Domeniul%20Medicina%20dentara/Conf.%20univ.%20dr.%20COSTAN%20Victor-Vlad/02_Tez%C4%83_abilitare.pdf (accessed on 14th July 2025).

11. De Silva, J. (2011). *The evaluation of fibrin tissue adhesive for skin closure following eyelid surgery.* https://core.ac.uk/download/19085637.pdf (accessed on 14th July 2025).

12. Di Filippo, J., Gagliano, C., Grando, M., Miotti, A., et al. (2024). *Fat management in upper*

blepharoplasty: Addition or subtraction blepharoplasties, how and when. https://core.ac.uk/download/614033783.pdf (accessed on 14th July 2025).

13. Nieć, M., Olejarz, Z., Nowak, K., Drygała, Z., Wyrwał, J., Zielińska, Z., ... Krasuska, M. (2024). Factors influencing the length of the recovery period after blepharoplasty: a review of the latest data. *Journal of Education, Health and Sport, 59*, 183–208. https://doi.org/10.12775/JEHS.2024.59.012(accessed on 14th July 2025).
14. Filaj, V., Fida, M., Kola, E., & Kola, I. (2023). The importance of counseling, planning and choosing the proper surgical technique for optimal results in the upper face. *Albanian Journal of Trauma and Emergency Surgery*. https://www.semanticscholar.org/paper/279dd8383b350cf27eafc7af6746525e38a6d250 (accessed on 14th July 2025).
15. Gursky, A. K., Chinta, S. R., Wyatt, H., Belisario, M. N., Shah, A., Kantar, R. S., & Rodriguez, E. D. (2024). A comprehensive analysis of genioplasty in facial feminization surgery: A systematic review and institutional cohort study. *Journal of Clinical Medicine, 14*, 182–182. https://doi.org/10.3390/jcm14010182 (accessed on 14th July 2025).
16. Hollander, M. (2022). *Upper Blepharoplasty: Aesthetic and Functional Aspects*. https://core.ac.uk/download/518788184.pdf (accessed on 14th July 2025).
17. James, A. J., Assi, P. E., Torres-Guzman, R. A., Nemani, S. V., Saad, M., Kalmar, C., Perdikis, G., et al. (2024). Optimizing safety and aesthetics in facial feminization: Laryngoscopic-assisted chondrolaryngoplasty (2019–2023). *The Journal of Craniofacial Surgery, 36*, 750–753. https://www.semanticscholar.org/paper/aab90af66a829606ef6a01299f727fbaacf8bd37 (accessed on 14th July 2025).
18. Lim, B., Seth, I., Kah, S., Sofiadellis, F., Ross, R. J., Rozen, W. M., & Cuomo, R. (2023). Using generative artificial intelligence tools in cosmetic surgery: A study on rhinoplasty, facelifts, and blepharoplasty procedures. *Journal of Clinical Medicine, 12*, 6524–6524. https://doi.org/10.3390/jcm12206524 (accessed on 14th July 2025).
19. Lotti, V. (2022). *What women want: An analysis of cosmetic surgery and social achievements in contemporary urban China*. https://core.ac.uk/download/614350451.pdf (accessed on 14th July 2025).
20. Maione, L., Vinci, V., Costanzo, D., Battistini, A., Lisa, A., & Di Maria, A. (2021). Upper eyelid blepharoplasty following hyaluronic acid injection with improved facial aesthetics and eye symptoms: A case report. *Journal of Medical Case Reports, 15*. https://www.semanticscholar.org/paper/9a97df247f412d658ed49a15edfb6fa9d1fbc2b5 (accessed on 14th July 2025).
21. Ng Man Chuen, C. (2024). *Interrogating authenticity: Understanding East Asian female pop music in the Western cultural sphere*. https://doi.org/10.32920/26046658.v1 (accessed on 14th July 2025).
22. Nieuwenhuis, D., Hazenkamp, L. S., Hummelink, S., Luong, M., et al. (2023). *Factors associated with treatment outcome satisfaction six months after upper blepharoplasty: A large cohort study*. https://core.ac.uk/download/588748279.pdf (accessed on 14th July 2025).
23. Park, J. H., Jeong, J. W., & Park, J. U. (2024). Advanced facial rejuvenation: Synergistic effects of lower blepharoplasty and ultrasound guided mid-face lift using polydioxanone (PDO) threads. *Aesthetic Plastic Surgery, 48*, 1706–1714. https://www.semanticscholar.org/paper/dc27fd3cad06e8e682135475775d19dabf848f82 (accessed on 14th July 2025).

24. Penev, Y. (2022). *Laser resources for facial rejuvenation and aestheticisation // Възможности за лазерно подмладяване и естетизиране на кожата на лицето.* https://core.ac.uk/download/578416857.pdf (accessed on 14th July 2025).

25. Portilla, A. S. P., Portilla, C. S. P., Palacios, G., Rodríguez, B. S. P., Castillo, S., Espin, N. E. P., & Pita, G. P. M. (2024). The integration of surgical and dermatological techniques in the treatment of cutaneous aging: Multidisciplinary approaches and clinical outcomes – A comprehensive systematic review of current literature. *International Journal of Research in Medical Sciences, 12*, 1659–1667. https://doi.org/10.18203/2320-6012.ijrms20240943 (accessed on 14th July 2025).

26. Pussetti, C. (2021). Because you're worth it! The medicalization and moralization of aesthetics in aging women. *Societies, 11*, 97–97. https://doi.org/10.3390/soc11030097 (accessed on 14th July 2025).

27. Rail, B., Bhatia, S. S., & Rozen, S. (2024). Upper eyelid postseptal weight placement for treatment of paralytic lagophthalmos: Long-term outcomes. *Journal of Reconstructive Microsurgery*. https://www.semanticscholar.org/paper/ce47b01f15ebf1c0c9057712b8ac1fb5fcabf673 (accessed on 14th July 2025).

28. Riggio, E. (2024). Report on the 11th National Congress AICPE (Associazione Italiana di Chirurgia Plastica Estetica) held in Rimini, Italy, 12–14 April 2024. *Surgical Techniques Development, 13*, 122–161. https://doi.org/10.3390/std13020009 (accessed on 14th July 2025).

29. Vasović, D. D., Karamarković, M., Jovanović, M., Stojičić, M., Rašić, D., Marjanović, I., Kalezić, T., et al. (2024). Comprehensive evaluation of quality of life following upper eyelid blepharoplasty: A prospective analysis. *Medicina, 60*, 500–500. https://doi.org/10.3390/medicina60030500 (accessed on 14th July 2025).

30. Yordanov, Y. P. (2025). Combined surgical approach for safe and effective rejuvenation of the lower eyelids. *Acta Medica Bulgarica, 52*, 14–20. https://doi.org/10.2478/amb-2025-0003 (accessed on 14th July 2025).

31. Zhang, H., Zhang, Y., Lu, Z., Qian, J., Ye, Z., & Xiaohui, L. (2025). Application of orbital septal fat repositioning combined with SVF-gel fillers in lower blepharoplasty. *Journal of Craniofacial Surgery*. https://doi.org/10.1097/scs.0000000000011289 (accessed on 14th July 2025).

RHYTIDECTOMY (FACELIFT) AND NECK LIFT

5

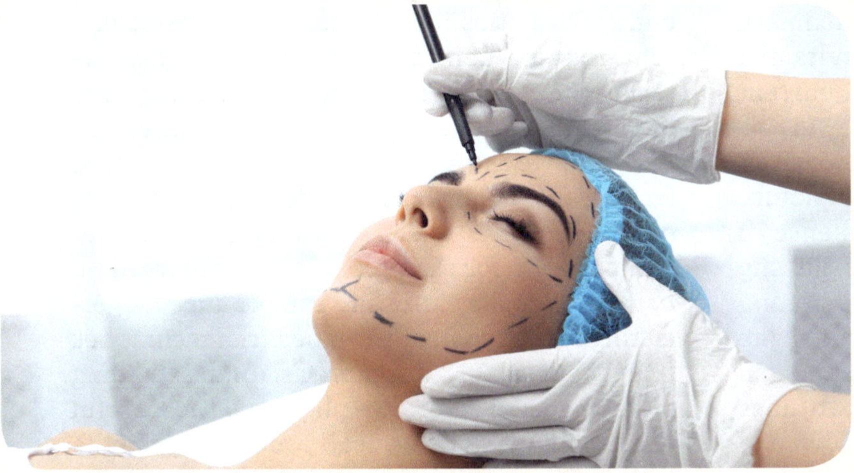

LEARNING OBJECTIVES

After studying this chapter, you will be able to:

1. Discuss the historical background;
2. Describe the types of facelift procedures;
3. Consider neck lift procedures;
4. Understand indications for surgery;
5. Evaluate risks and complications in rhytidectomy;
6. Learn about recovery and aftercare.

Introduction

Cosmetic facial surgery has evolved enormously in recent years, and perhaps no field has benefited more than rhytidectomy, the widely used slang term for facelift. As people more and more look to improve their appearance, knowing the functional ramifications and results of such treatments becomes increasingly important. The increasing demand for facelifts and neck lifts is an expression of larger societal trends in aesthetics, aging, and self-image. In addition, the ease of access to information via the internet places information at patients' fingertips to use in making their decisions. In this regard, Google Trends analysis has assessed the relationship between internet search trends and volumes of cosmetic surgery procedures and revealed nuanced correlations capturing patient preference for such interventions (McGuigan & Trinh, 2022). For this reason, practitioners and patients alike must gather comprehensive information about rhytidectomy and neck lifts to navigate this complex environment. Improvements in surgery have transformed the way rhytidectomy and neck lifts are carried out, with an added focus on minimizing risks and enhancing recuperation periods. Aggressive traditional techniques have been replaced by more sophisticated methods, which focus on safety and patient satisfaction. The advent of the S-Plus lift, a new technique that blends other surgical aspects together, is a good example. By employing long flap superficial musculo-aponeurotic system (SMAS) methods, the S-Plus lift minimizes complications and also optimizes results in rejuvenation (Hopping et al., 2010). The method has set the benchmark for less invasive but longer-lasting results and greater patient comfort and addresses current expectations about cosmetic surgery. As the demand for rhytidectomy and neck lifts increases, it is more crucial to look at the larger picture behind these cosmetic procedures. A sense of the demographics of the individuals getting the procedures done and why they are getting them helps shape the argument regarding the aesthetic treatments. This greater demand can also be attributed to social shifts in attitudes to aging and looks, as well as to the power of the media image. Secondly, the low complication rates of technologies like the S-Plus lift indicate a fruitful path towards minimizing risks of cosmetic procedures that could promote greater acceptance and active engagement by potential candidates (Hopping et al., 2010). Thus, a thorough review of rhytidectomy and neck lifts offers not only insight into medical innovation but also into evolving patient mindsets within a rapidly changing social context.

Definition of Rhytidectomy

The word rhytidectomy gets its etymology from the Greek words rhytis for wrinkle and ektomē for cutting away or excision. In contemporary medical terminology, rhytidectomy specifically refers to the surgical procedure commonly called a facelift, which is performed to reduce the noticeable marks of aging, particularly of the face and neck. This procedure corrects sagging skin, jowls, and folds of the face by tightening and lifting up the underlying soft tissue, potentially restoring a more youthful facial contour. Technological advancements in surgical techniques over the years have given rise to more natural-looking aesthetic outcomes, given that surgeons are better at sculpting facial structures to achieve the desired outcomes with minimal complications (Azizzadeh & Lu, 2024). This evolution follows the enhanced understanding of the complex interplay between the skin, underlying muscles, and supporting connective tissues necessary for optimal rejuvenation. Central to rhytidectomy lies the technique used in achieving optimal aesthetic outcomes. The surgery generally involves multiple techniques, including traditional facelifts and deep plane facelifts, that emphasize different aspects of facial rejuvenation. A deeper plane facelift, for example, allows more freedom to maneuver the SMAS and can produce longer-lasting results than more superficial techniques (Talei et al., 2024). It is a precise understanding of the facial vectors at play and the careful execution of the surgical procedure that is necessary to determine whether or not the procedure is a success. Through rigid surgical methods, including SMAS suspension and careful tissue dissection, facial surgeons aim not just for a restored appearance but also for patient safety and satisfaction. Of paramount concern in rhytidectomy is the vector of lift, meaning the precise direction tissues are lifted during the procedure. A facelift success also heavily depends on aligning the lifting vectors in the direction of the natural vectors of descent of aging, thereby enhancing the final aesthetic result (Talei et al., 2024). Research shows that primary and revision facelifts are associated with typical vectors specific to each patient's anatomy, which demands an individualized approach to surgical correction. The proper identification and control of such vectors can be the deciding factor when it comes to achieving a natural and harmonious appearance post-surgery. The art of rhytidectomy thus puts as much emphasis on surgical skill as on a deep understanding of facial dynamics, ultimately leading surgeons to the goal of delivering exceptional aesthetic results while maintaining the integrity of facial expression (Figure 5.1).

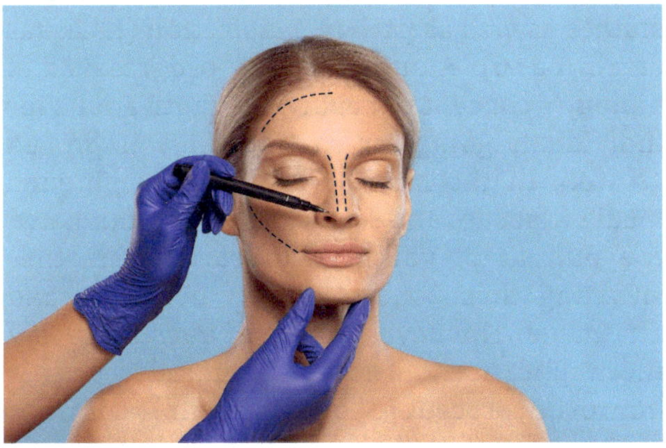

Figure 5.1. The term rhytidectomy.

Source: https://external-content.duckduckgo.com/iu/?u=https%3A%2F%2F149727273.v2.pressablecdn.com%2Fwp-content%2Fuploads%2F2024%2F01%2FLS7cUEXjDQ3biM8YLBiz9L44VAw1sbAhK8Lai6WZ6SV8HFt7RgQr9YvgydeiaollaQuMwCsZJ3s5nP5YjY_vnA_Bw3DYuLRoEPxL2u49v4VFkKk1_Bh_oqGB0rVp-1.png&f=1&nofb=1&ipt=6d7b02a76e40a596ccc1729d481110ad7e7e8855e7ef92e864236cc922cc3aa4.

Importance of Facial Aesthetics

Facial attractiveness is an important aspect of human interaction, which affects perceptions of attractiveness, professionalism, and confidence. The face is an important mechanism for the transmission of emotions and social cues, which underscores the importance of possessing a pleasing face. Youthfulness is equated with attractiveness in most cultures, and hence individuals seek all forms of treatments as reactions to signs of aging. Aging can be caused by internal factors like genetics and external factors like environmental stressors and result in loss of skin elasticity, texture, and facial contours. The desire to become more beautiful through methods like rhytidectomy (facelift) and neck lift reflects society's emphasis on maintaining youthful and handsome appearances, which can greatly affect career and social prospects, self-esteem, and psychological well-being. Recent developments in surgical and non-surgical facial rejuvenation treatments mirror the evolving standards of facial beauty. Recent approaches include a range of procedures, far beyond traditional surgical methods, to include less invasive measures like fillers and injectables that correct a range of patient desires and aesthetic needs. The synergy of dermatologic techniques and surgical operations allows for more extensive treatment of the aesthetics of the face, where patients can achieve tremendous rejuvenation with minimal risk and downtime. Portilla et al. (2024) underline the need for the application of a combination of surgical and non-surgical techniques in achieving optimal outcomes in facial aesthetics. By realizing the plurality of the treatments available, patients are able to make informed decisions based on their aesthetic preferences in a manner that avoids risks associated with more invasive treatments. Additionally, the applicability of facial aesthetics can also be viewed according to age-related changes and how these impact the modes of treatment. Different ranges of ages bring different features of aging and different ideals of beauty, and thus, a tailored approach to the treatment is necessary. For instance, individuals in their 20s may receive preventive procedures to maintain youthful features, while those between the ages of 50 and 60 may require more aggressive measures to address the specific signs of aging. Cohen et al. (2023) also observe that with growing understanding of facial changes by decade, doctors can treat individuals better based on individual need and expectation. This personalized treatment program not only enhances the overall effectiveness of aesthetic treatments but also provides a genuine and accommodating environment for patients to optimize facial beauty, thereby positively affecting their quality of life (Figure 5.2).

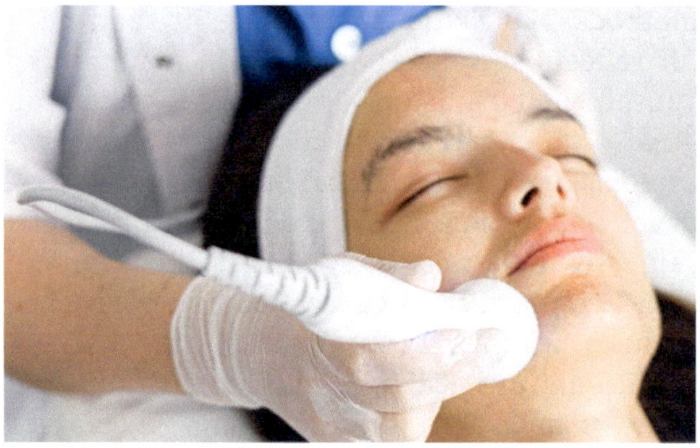

Figure 5.2. Facial aesthetics play a critical role in human interactions.

Source: https://external-content.duckduckgo.com/iu/?u=https%3A%2F%2Fwomenfitnessmag.com%2Fwp-content%2Fuploads%2F2023%2F04%2FBenefits-Of-Facial-Aestheti.jpg&f=1&nofb=1&ipt=275b68b098b8e735eb7cb8138792dd1f726e117cbf352812aa323384db8a142a.

5.1. Historical Background

Learning Outcome

1. Evolution of Facelift Techniques
2. Discuss the Key Figures in Cosmetic Surgery
3. Focus on Milestones in Rhytidectomy Development

Historically, rhytidectomy, also popularly known as facelift surgery, began in the early 20th century and marks a significant milestone in the history of cosmetic surgery. In the early years, the procedures were rudimentary and were aimed at tightening the skin alone with no anatomical knowledge of the face. Early plastic surgery innovators, such as Dr. Erich Lexer, experimented with numerous trial methods that led to modern aesthetic surgery. Lexer's contribution was instrumental, as it highlighted not only the necessity to raise the skin but also to move deeper tissue in order to achieve a more natural and permanent outcome. With progression in the field of surgery and technology over the decades, facial rejuvenation options have been expanded, which has led a primitive procedure to its current advanced level during contemporary times, evidence of a continuous process that is driven by scientific studies as well as patient satisfaction (Kalaskar et al., 2016). Along with the progression of biology's concept of beauty, the motivations for individuals going for rhytidectomy improved as well. In the mid-20th century, heightened media exposure and celebrity society stimulated the pursuit of youthful appearance, further situating these operations as desirable and attainable. The development of anesthesia and the application of aseptic techniques greatly improved procedure safety, making cosmetic surgery more attractive to an ever-broadening population. Concurrently, cultural narratives surrounding aging evolved; vanity and self-indulgence came to be seen increasingly not only as self-indulgent but as empowerment. Concurrently with this cultural shift, rhytidectomy became associated with imagery of renewal and youth, reinforcing a paradigm in which individuals actively sought to express their inner energy with external appearances, uncovering deeply ingrained societal values about youth and beauty (Camm et al., 2025). Methods of rhytidectomy continued to evolve with advancements in medical technology and greater understanding of aesthetics. Minimally invasive techniques introduced during the latter part of the 20th century, such as endoscopic methods, brought additional possibilities for candidates for surgery who might otherwise have avoided intrusive surgery due to fears regarding extended periods of recovery and notable scarring. These developments not only improved patient outcomes but also encouraged further research into other technologies such as neck lifts, which were increasingly popular as standalone procedures or in combination with facelifts. These advances signify more than mere technical improvement; they represent a growing acknowledgment of the psychosocial character of cosmetic surgery, where individual beauty ideals, self-image, and mental well-being converge to redefine the field of individual health and identity in contemporary popular culture (Kalaskar et al., 2016).

5.1.1. Evolution of Facelift Techniques

The development of techniques for the facelift has mirrored a wider change in cosmetic surgery towards techniques that are less invasive and more effective at rejuvenating the face. Traditionally, methods used for the facelift centered around tightening the facial skin to reverse the effects of aging. Yet, within the last few decades, the specialty has branched out to encompass a range of techniques that take into account the anatomical structures underlying the face. Techniques such as the Superficial Musculoaponeurotic System (SMAS) facelift surgery have gained popularity. The technique enhances repositioning of not just the skin but also the deeper tissues, yielding more natural and long-lasting results. Correspondingly, facial anatomy and how changes in aging take place in this anatomy are vital in guiding surgical correction to allow for personalized treatment plans that target individual patient needs. In addition to surgical procedure advancements, the incorporation of non-invasive technology has revolutionized facial aesthetic surgery. Patients are now more focused on seeking less invasive options to traditional surgery that are quicker and involve less risk. Non-surgical procedures such as filler injections and thread lifts have become popular choices that facilitate dramatic facial rejuvenation without requiring extensive recovery. Techniques such as the Minimal Access Cranial Suspension Lift (MACS) and volumetric methods using hyaluronic acid (HA) fillers are typical of this trend. In minimizing the invasiveness of surgery without sacrificing efficacy, these treatments both appeal to a broader population as well as encourage discussion regarding the optimal balance of efficacy and patient safety in cosmetic procedures (Portilla et al., 2024). In addition, the evolution of face-lift surgeries emphasizes a three-dimensional method for rejuvenation of the face using both surgical and dermatological therapy. The progress has brought forth greater insight into balancing surgical facelifts with such adjunctive therapies as fat grafting and laser skin resurfacing. Addition therapies optimize aesthetic outcomes, not just tightening and eliminating redundant skin, but also revolumizing deflated tissue and smoothing skin texture. The coming together of these diverse techniques represents a paradigm in the aesthetic surgical process from strictly surgical to a general definition of facial rejuvenation. This evolution encompasses the ongoing drive to refine techniques, ensure patient satisfaction, and adapt to patients' desires for having a youthful appearance (Portilla et al., 2024) (Figure 5.3).

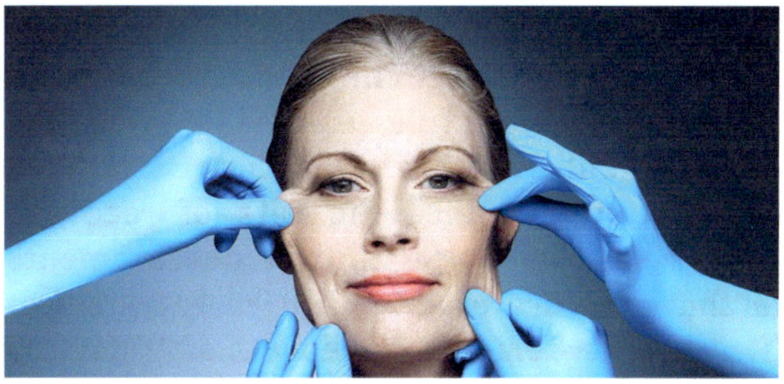

Figure 5.3. The evolution of facelift techniques reflects a broader shift.

Source: https://external-content.duckduckgo.com/iu/?u=https%3A%2F%2Fprimehairtransplant.com%2Fwp-content%2Fuploads%2F2025%2F01%2Ffacelift-technique-1.jpg&f=1&nofb=1&ipt=6365fc0bc39f835f6eaf131b24fff84b061cdf03a9040e9c3db0b51e9f4a59c4.

5.1.2. Key Figures in Cosmetic Surgery

Cosmetic surgery has been shaped to a great degree by leading individuals whose contributions have set benchmark methods for procedures such as rhytidectomy and neck lifts. Such trailblazers as Dr. Thomas Rees and Dr. Ivo Pitanguy have worked significantly to bring aesthetic surgery to the status of a respected medical specialist. Dr. Rees, often called the father of facelift surgery, introduced new methods that focused on maintaining natural contours of the face and the removal of excess skin. His work paved the way to breaking away from older practices towards approaches that were based on patient safety and satisfaction after the procedure. Dr. Pitanguy also emphasized psychological health in patients, as he understood that cosmetic surgery goes beyond external appearance and affects self-esteem and identity. This integrated perception of surgery renders the need to study major players in this field in an attempt to comprehend current practice apparent. The evolution of cosmetic surgery, particularly of facelifts and neck lifts, has been influenced by a series of innovative procedures that have been led by major players. Advances in technology have also played a significant role, as is evident from the development of minimally invasive methods designed to enhance the rate of recovery and overall safety. Significant developments in this area are examined in recent medical literature to demonstrate how energy devices and liposuction have refined the face and neck. For instance, developments in rhytidectomy procedures were pioneered to provide the optimal outcomes with minimal scarring and recovery. Having experienced surgeons who continue to push the boundaries of aesthetic treatments emphasizes the necessity for rigorous training and expertise in the field. These advancements allow for informed treatment decisions, positioning practitioners to deliver more for their patients in ways they want and achieving desired aesthetic outcomes (Kalaskar et al., 2016). The sociocultural dimension of cosmetic surgery cannot be denied, particularly regarding how opinion makers shape public perception and patient choice. Research suggests a correlation with enhanced positive body image and more social acceptance, locating cosmetic surgery in the broader context of identity and self-expression (Castro et al., 1996). An understanding of the intricacies of personal motivation toward aesthetic procedures is important for practitioners. For example, an understanding of the psychological undertones of surgery enables surgeons not only to address physical problems but also emotional and social stress that patients experience. Hence, the contributions of prime stakeholders in cosmetic surgery go beyond technical prowess; they entail an ongoing understanding of how aesthetic procedures relate to cultural expectations and personal identity. Such considerations emphasize the need for a biopsychosocial approach in this rapidly expanding field (Figure 5.4).

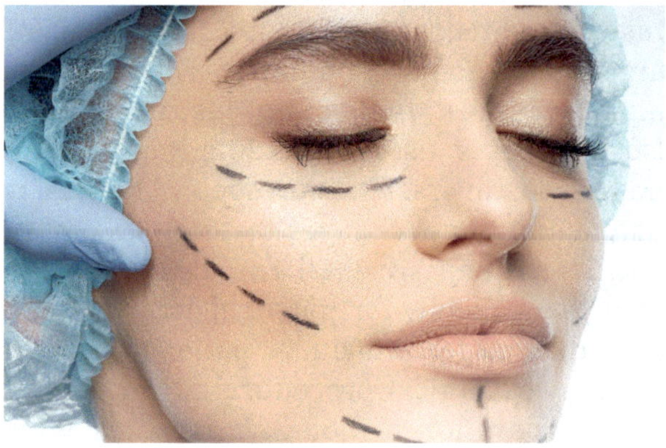

Figure 5.4. Key figures in cosmetic surgery.

Source: https://external-content.duckduckgo.com/iu/?u=https%3A%2F%2Fwww.phoenixmag.com%2Fwp-content%2Fuploads%2F2023%2F05%2FPHM0623SASCosmetic-Surgery01-scaled.jpg&f=1&nofb=1&ipt=10fbe57c9195cf8b03e93f2a9ba8ff2e2fc5a04534396e683b71924b655ebf4f.

5.1.3. Milestones in Rhytidectomy Development

The evolution of rhytidectomy development has been characterized by milestone breakthroughs that reflect a continually refined understanding of facial anatomy and surgical techniques. Early facelifts focused primarily on the superficial skin layers, with a tendency to create a pulled-back and unnatural appearance. While surgeons gained knowledge about the deeper layers, methods developed to incorporate the extensive manipulation of soft tissue. The development of the superficial musculoaponeurotic system (SMAS) during the latter half of the 20th century was a turning point; it permitted smoother lifting and shifting of facial structures with better results. The procedure then became linked with not just aesthetic enhancement but also increased patient safety and reduced recovery time. By considering these previous milestones, it is clear that it is simpler to realize the complexity and efficacy of present techniques used in present rhytidectomy operations (Azizzadeh & Lu, 2024). In still more recent history, the advent of minimal invasive techniques is another significant milestone in rhytidectomy development. The introduction of the Rhytidoplasty Through Minimal Incisions (Rhythmic) offers an attractive alternative that precludes the shortcomings of traditional facelift operations, providing scarring and prolonged healing. Physicians employ the technique with minimal incisions, reducing scarring by wide margins while achieving aesthetic improvement comparable to traditional methods. The new procedure offers vast facial rejuvenation with minimal disruption to underlying structures. Interestingly, patients have shown increased cervicofacial angles and treated vertical frown lines with minimal surgery. These changes highlight a new era of procedural finesse with safety and natural outcomes being paramount, marking a departure from the past in facial surgery (Castillo-Campos et al., 2022). Further milestones in the growth of rhytidectomy are also contributed to by continuous innovation in surgical techniques and the introduction of technologies. Increasingly sophisticated surgical devices and imaging equipment have produced increasingly precise and safer procedure options. Above all, advances in knowledge regarding facial nerve anatomy have been crucial in minimizing such complications as facial palsy. As surgeons strive to maintain essential anatomical structures during facelifts, the development of nerve integrity-sparing techniques has become more predictable and has resulted in more gratifying results. Such attention to detail not only complements the aesthetic outcomes but also highlights the significance of one-stop patient treatment in rhytidectomy surgeries. With the evolving discipline, such milestones instill hope for continual advancements in rhytidectomy and neck lift operations (Azizzadeh & Lu, 2024).

Test Your Knowledge

1. Understand and use of the SMAS (superficial musculoaponeurotic system) in facelift surgery.
2. Which major milestones—such as the advent of deep-plane facelift techniques or the incorporation of endoscopic methods—marked shifts toward more natural outcomes and longer-lasting results in the evolution of facelift surgery?

5.2. Types of Facelift Procedures

Learning Outcome

1. Discuss about Traditional Facelift
2. Understand the Mini Facelift
3. Know Non-Surgical Facelift Options

The history of facelift surgery has come a long way, from the older surgical techniques to newer, more minimally invasive procedures. Classic rhytidectomy encompasses the total facelift, which addresses the whole face, lifting sagging skin and restoring contours. This procedure, though, tends to leave such facial scars and can disrupt the natural facial anatomy with a less pleasing result for certain patients. On the other hand, modern techniques prefer subtlety and renewal, combining surgical procedures with dermatology technology in order to meet specific needs and aesthetic desires. Minimally invasive treatments have facilitated rejuvenation with less danger and reduced downtime, acceptable to a larger clientele. Of the various types of facelift surgery, the mini facelift has gained popularity due to its targeted approach and less intrusive procedure. This procedure often targets the jawline and lower face, giving a younger look without the long recovery that usually comes with a full facelift. Smaller incisions and a smaller surgical footprint characterize the mini facelift compared to its conventional alternative, reducing scarring (Portilla et al., 2024). Those patients who want to obtain a mid-lifting effect without undergoing a more intricate procedure will often find the mini facelift to be an acceptable alternative. Perhaps more significantly, however, this treatment can be easily combined with other non-surgical treatments, such as dermal fillers or Botox, to aggregate overall results in an effort to meet individual standards of beauty and need. Another new treatment that is gaining widespread popularity in facial rejuvenation is the thread lift. This technique employs certain threads made from materials such as polydioxanone (PDO) to tighten skin non-surgically, providing a quick result with minimal downtime (Portilla et al., 2024). The threads are inserted strategically below the skin in such a way that loose tissue can be lifted without a lengthy series of surgical procedures. Thread lifts appeal to patients who desire an instant, effective solution to facial aging without the irreversibility of traditional facelifts. Secondly, the benefits extend beyond mere lifting, since the threads stimulate the production of collagen, which also leads to long-term rejuvenating effects on the skin. With the inclusion of such minimal invasive methods, patients enjoy a broader array of treatments suited to their personal concerns of aging, thus improving the world of facial rejuvenation surgery (Figure 5.5).

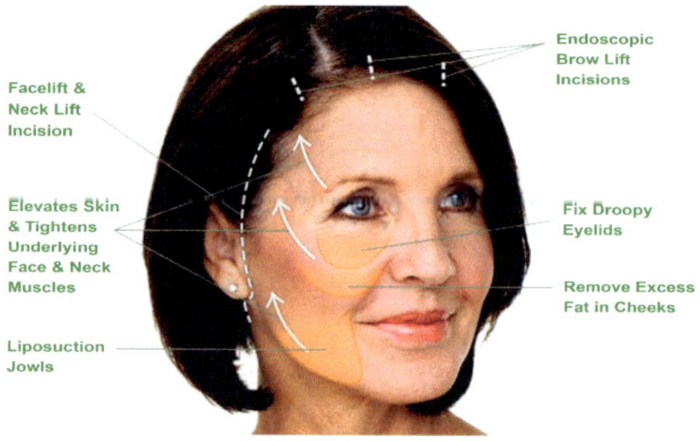

Figure 5.5. The landscape of facelift procedures has evolved significantly over the years.

Source: https://external-content.duckduckgo.com/iu/?u=https%3A%2F%2Farticles.mymeditravel.com%2Fwp-content%2Fuploads%2F2019%2F06%2Ffacelift-graphic-1050x600.jpg&f=1&nofb=1&ipt=aec0e6ac5b323174b9d80087ddb59a659955be14167c70c52712cdafe5369dbd.

5.2.1. Traditional Facelift

The traditional facelift, also known scientifically as rhytidectomy, is a surgical intervention utilized to revive the youthful appearance of the face by addressing sagging skin, wrinkles, and facial volume loss. The procedure often involves incisions that are mapped out along the hairline, traced around the ears, and, in some cases, to the region behind the ears. With these cuts, the loose skin is excised and muscles and connective tissue underneath are tightened to create a smoother and more chiseled facial contour. How successful a facelift is primarily a matter of the surgeon's ability at proportionate beauty balance and preservation of the natural look because an unnatural or even theatrically augmented result can ruin the overall intention of the surgery. Achievement of aesthetic harmony is most critical for patient satisfaction, particularly because an ideal chin and jawline greatly increase facial beauty, as the facial aesthetic literature highlights (Newberry & Mobley, 2019). Postoperative complications have the capability of enormously impacting the recovery and outcome that accompany traditional facelift procedures. Hematomas, or the localized collections of blood outside vessels, are one of the most common complications of aesthetic surgery. These may cause pain, swelling, and in some cases, the necessity for additional surgery to repair. Identification of the risk factors for the development of hematoma and deployment of prevention measures in the perioperative setting is crucial for the best management of patients. Reduction of trauma to the vascular facial tissues is done through maneuvers employed by surgeons, while preoperative assessment determines those patients who are at higher risk. By putting hematoma prevention and treatment first, caregivers may optimize overall patient satisfaction and reduce the occurrence of postoperative complications (Hood et al., 2018). The traditional facelift has also been adapted to incorporate multiple adjunctive procedures that can further optimize the overall result and address several issues simultaneously. For instance, a combination with other procedures like eyelid surgery or brow lifting can provide overall face rejuvenation. Secondly, with the worth of a balanced face shape becoming increasingly familiar, chin augmentation has emerged as a complementary procedure to create a better-defined lower third face. With implants or fillers, surgeons can achieve a more balanced and beauty-enhanced jawline, and chin augmentations are thus an important factor in facelift planning (Newberry & Mobley, 2019). As surgical methods and instruments advance, the traditional facelift continues to be a significant option for clients who wish to undo the aging process, with both functional and aesthetic enhancement when undertaken with meticulous planning and seasoned execution (Figure 5.6).

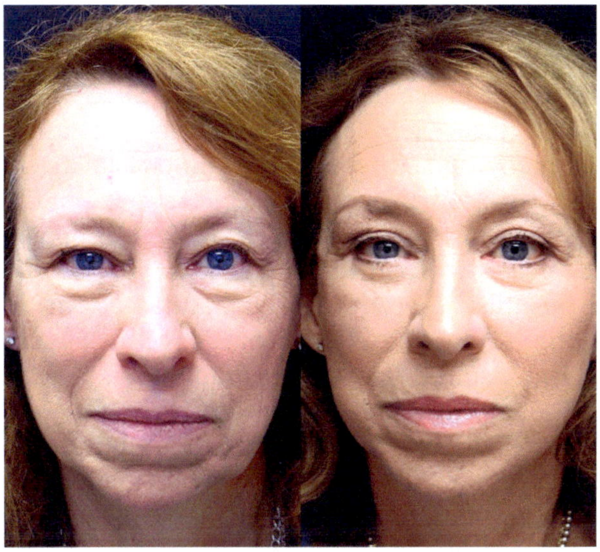

Figure 5.6. The traditional facelift.

Source: https://external-content.duckduckgo.com/iu/?u=https%3A%2F%2Ffacelift-rhytidectomy.com%2Fwp-content%2Fuploads%2F2017%2F05%2FTraditional-Facelift-Before-And-After.jpg&f=1&nofb=1&ipt=d7fea7b3cf20f90001db3b4708f8daf980d37d70e229574399a3ed771dc336a6.

5.2.2. Mini Facelift

The process of aging greatly impacts facial and neck appearance, such that the decline in facial volume and formation of skin laxity leads to undesirable aesthetic alterations. Traditional facelift techniques produce conspicuous structural alterations and potential complications and thus may not be offered to many candidates. Conversely, the mini facelift has been a more attractive choice for individuals seeking to correct mild to moderate aging signs with less invasiveness. Notably, this procedure maximally tightens the skin without compromising the natural appearance and hence preserves the underlying anatomical structure of the face. By specifically targeting the lower face and neck, a mini facelift can rejuvenate the appearance without the extensive recovery period associated with more conservative rhytidectomies, treating issues effectively without the negative effects of scarring and facial anatomy distortion typical of larger procedures (Kao et al., 2023). The latest research upholds the mini facelifts as an excellent modality for treating mild facial aging. Short-scar rhytidectomies, which are one of the minimal incision methods, have been reported to provide significant benefits, especially for candidates with early manifestations of aging. Review of 1,000 consecutive short-scar rhytidectomies showed favorable results with few complications; suture extrusion was the most frequent complication, found in only 14.8% of the patients, and severe complications such as nerve damage or skin necrosis were significantly absent (Tanna et al., 2008). The infrequent development of complications speaks to the efficacy and safety of treatments. The outcomes encourage practitioners and potential candidates to consider mini facelifts a viable option against traditional methods, particularly given that techniques evolve and better patient outcomes follow. Mini facelifts' appeal transcends their technical benefits; they also respond to patients' increasing requests for personalized aesthetic treatments. The majority of individuals today choose procedures that yield rejuvenating results with minimal downtime in returning to normal life. The shorter recovery time in the mini facelift not only addresses patients' cosmetic requirements but also aligns with the demands of modern lifestyle, with work and other obligations being significant discouragers to staying off work for long periods. Furthermore, by maintaining natural facial contours, the procedure balances safety and aesthetic wishes. Since the evidence grows for the effectiveness and legitimacy of mini facelifts, it is increasingly obvious that such innovative techniques appeal especially well to a clientele with an active desire for subtle and effective rejuvenation strategies (Tanna et al., 2008) (Figure 5.7).

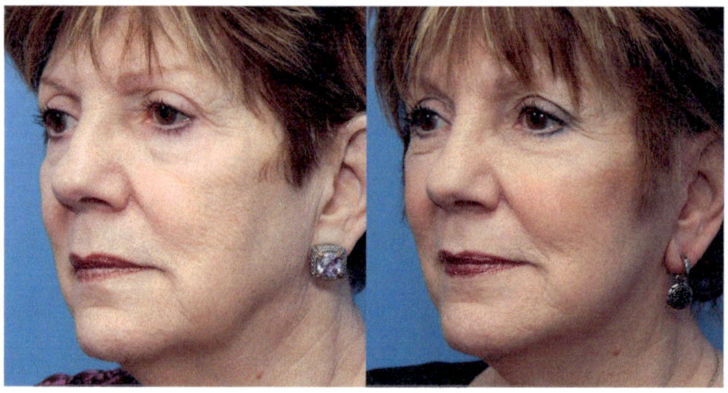

Figure 5.7. Mini facelift.

Source: https://external-content.duckduckgo.com/iu/?u=https%3A%2F%2Fwww.datocms-assets.com%2F54152%2F1632332827-05949040-2644-4b1a-be24-de0bec199f18.jpg&f=1&nofb=1&ipt=51d4d891032a2ff878effdc3cad05b10cfb375cfdd3ffb6e4055dfa755b9ac9c.

5.2.3. Non-Surgical Facelift Options

In aesthetic medicine, non-surgical facelifts have become increasingly popularly accepted as they can shorten recovery time and avoid the risks that come with invasive procedures. Techniques such as Ultherapy and fat grafting are particularly popular for their efficiency in tightening skin and volumizing. Ultherapy, utilizing ultrasound technology, stimulates collagen production in the deeper layers of the skin and results in a natural lifting effect over time. Fat grafting is more about harvesting fat from areas of the patient's body and transferring it to the face to restore volume and outline contours without the need for invasive surgery. These methods are characteristic of the shift from surgical rhytidectomy to a less invasive, more comprehensive method of facial rejuvenation, one that is appropriate for an emerging population desiring less rather than encumbrancing effects of surgery (Portilla et al., 2024). A second evolving frontier in non-surgical facelift is the use of energy-based devices, permitting tissue contraction and skin tightening. Techniques involving lasers, radiofrequency, and ultrasound have emerged as welcome alternatives for patients who want cosmetic improvements with minimal lost time. Renuvion™, for instance, utilizes helium gas-created plasma energy and radiofrequency to facilitate the controlled heating of tissue that will contract the skin without inordinate thermal destruction. The ability to deliver successful results in a less invasive technique is attractive, as it reduces the risks typically associated with surgical facelifts, such as prolonged recovery and potential complications. This technology can also be used in various applications, such as subdermal techniques or as an adjunct to traditional rhytidectomies, demonstrating its value in the broader context of facial rejuvenation (Leake et al., 2021). Secondly, advancements in thread-lifting treatments provide another convincing non-surgical option for appearing youthful. Using threads such as polydioxanone (PDO) threads, the treatment entails threading away dissolvable sutures underneath the skin, which lift and hold it up and concurrently stimulate collagen creation. The surgery is quite minor and can be performed with the use of local anesthesia, with patients recovering rapidly to return to normal activity within hours. Results can be dramatic, with improvement in skin laxity and facial shape as a whole. As the popularity of non-surgical rejuvenation continues to grow, it is crucial for clinicians to remain abreast of new technology and techniques. Identifying these non-surgical alternatives not only enhances the satisfaction of patients but also corroborates the notion that the pursuit of youthful beauty can be maximized by means of complex and less provocative procedures, expanding the horizon of options beyond traditional surgery (Portilla et al., 2024) (Figure 5.8).

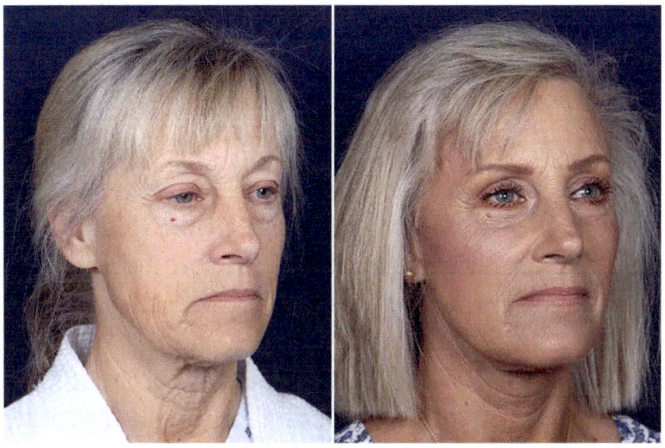

Figure 5.8. Non-surgical facelift options.

Source: https://external-content.duckduckgo.com/iu/?u=https%3A%2F%2Fwww.beckerplastics.com%2Fwp-content%2Fuploads%2F2022%2F12%2Fpatient-4063-facelift-before-after-1.jpg&f=1&nofb=1&ipt=c9ccd82fb73f566949e81f1bcb425b65cdc8def64832f57f55ac36cfa70259ec.

Test Your Knowledge

1. What areas of the face and neck does a traditional facelift typically target, and how does it differ in invasiveness compared to other facelift techniques?
2. Why is a mini facelift often recommended for patients with mild to moderate sagging, and what is its main advantage regarding recovery time?
3. What are two common non-surgical facelift treatments, and how do they improve facial appearance without incisions?

5.3. Neck Lift Procedures

Learning Outcome

1. Definition and Purpose of Neck Lift
2. Explain the Techniques Used in Neck Lifts
3. Differences Between Neck Lift and Facelift

Neck lift surgery, in some cases a standout component of facial rejuvenation, is meant to correct age-related alterations in the neck, such as sagging skin, fat accumulation, and muscle banding. As one ages, the loss of collagen and subcutaneous fat changes result in the development of jowls and a less distinct jawline. The neck lift is used to redefine this region by eliminating loose skin and facial muscle tightening underneath it, and the result is a more youthful, smoother profile. Neck lift can be done in combination with rhytidectomy (facelift) for facial rejuvenation. Minimally invasive techniques have also become the focus, which have shorter recovery time and higher patient satisfaction. As per a report on the advancements in facial rejuvenation, various modalities, including injectable fillers and thread lifts, can be used in conjunction with surgical interventions, which can ultimately enhance the general outcome of neck lift surgery (Li et al., 2022). The psychological impact of a neck lift cannot be ignored and may be significant. Patients undergo this surgery not only for aesthetics but also for better self-esteem and social quality of life. Social preoccupation with appearing young will encourage individuals to undergo surgery that will yield a younger profile of the neck. Plastic surgeons must be aware of the emotional motivations behind such choices. Complete preoperative assessments should consider patients' expectations to obtain realistic outcomes. In addition, detailing the possible benefits as well as possible issues, such as hematoma formation, a commonly faced postoperative issue, can equip patients with the necessary information to make informed decisions about their treatment (Hood et al., 2018). A well-informed patient is also more likely to achieve a satisfactory result, again underlining the importance of full consultations before going in for surgery. Postoperative care is also essential for the success of neck lift surgery. After surgery, patients are made to adhere to some rules to achieve optimal healing and prevent complications. These include not overexerting the body, not taking some medications that can predispose to hematoma, and following up with the surgical team from time to time. Non-adherence to follow-up with postoperative protocols can result in complications, and hematomas rank among the most prevalent complications encountered. They can cause delayed healing, increased pain, and in some cases, revision surgery. Therefore, it is crucial that both practitioners and patients remain vigilant during the postoperative period. Overall, the success of neck lifting surgery is supported by an overall approach based on patient education, proper management of realistic expectations, and prudent postoperative monitoring to an optimum aesthetic result (Figure 5.9)

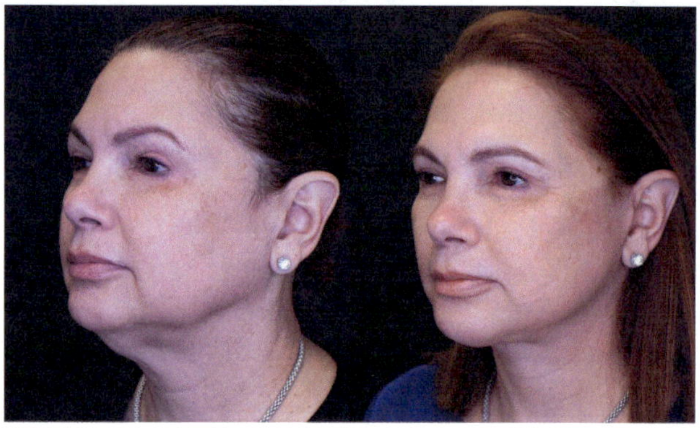

Figure 5.9. Neck lift procedures.

Source: https://external-content.duckduckgo.com/iu/?u=https%3A%2F%2Frodriguezfelizmd.com%2Fgallery%2Fface-neck%2Fneck-lift%2F11%2F02.jpg&f=1&nofb=1&ipt=2a9b88dbf7fbe066fd2d797600ee4fa840377ebf7ed3a14a15c2d7a1730417e2.

5.3.1. Definition and Purpose of Neck Lift

The neck lift, also clinically known as cervicoplasty, is a refined surgical process meant to strengthen the cosmetic appearance of the neck. The procedure targets essentially the redundant skin, looseness of the muscles, and unwanted fat that causes a creased or sagging appearance. These problems typically arise due to natural processes of aging, sun exposure, and inherited characteristics, and result in platysmal banding or a double chin. By addressing these, a neck lift effectively rejuvenates the neck region so that it aligns with the facial contour. The objective is to reclaim a more youthful and refined appearance, and this makes the individuals gain confidence in their beauty profile. Barring cosmetic appearance, the role of a neck lift also extends to psychological and social spheres. For most, an aged neck makes them appear less attractive as a whole, leading to lower self-esteem. With this procedure, they generally observe significant improvements in mental well-being and interpersonal relationships. Besides, as a part of a general aesthetic process, a neck lift can be coupled with a facelift to create an overall rejuvenation effect. Individuals who go through both processes and merge them are usually capable of achieving a balanced natural appearance, regaining a new concept of self that is advantageous to their general well-being. These results exemplify the multifaceted benefits related to aesthetic processes like the neck lift. The surgical process of a neck lift has also been enhanced to ensure that the procedure is safer and more effective. Recent techniques prefer to use minimally invasive surgeries, such as endoscopy, which reduces healing time and scarring and adds to the patients' comfort during surgery. Advances in surgical procedures have also led to more tailored procedures, which allow for customized treatment protocols based on specific patient anatomy and preferences. Neck lift potential is also supported by recent evidence indicating factors such as vitamin D levels could have some bearing on the healing process of the surgery and end result (Trifan et al., 2023). This provides an opportunity for surgeons to incorporate holistic methods into pre- and post-surgery care. Lastly, the purpose of a neck lift not only enhances physical appearance but also contributes to a broader appreciation of aesthetic surgery as a convergence between health and cosmetic care (Walker et al., 2018).

5.3.2. Techniques Used in Neck Lifts

Neck lift techniques differ, with each being unique in addressing particular patient concerns with signs of aging and sagging tissues in the cervical region. A fundamental basis of any neck lift procedure is the clear understanding of the underlying anatomy. Knowledge of the platysma muscle, cervical fat pads, and planes of connective tissues guides ideal surgical outcomes. The classic neck lift, limited incision neck lift, and endoscopic methods give surgeons the choice of offering customized procedures based on patient requirements. This customization allows for minimal scarring and customized adjustments in skin tightening and reduction of fat, a consideration of particular relevance in achieving maximum patient satisfaction and natural-appearing results as surgical rejuvenation becomes a consideration of increasing relevance among populations pursuing cosmetic enhancement (Lin et al., 2022). Among the commonly applied methods, the submental approach and deep plane neck lift are gaining prominence due to their effectiveness in addressing moderate to severe laxity of the neck. The submental approach is where a small incision is made under the chin, giving better access to deeper tissues with reduced visibility of scarring. It is an effective technique that redrapes skin and muscle, hence favored by clients with moderate laxity of the skin. In contrast, the deep plane neck lift is characterized by its thorough approach to elevating not just the skin but also deeper tissues, with a resultant more long-lasting restoration of neck contour. It is particularly suitable for individuals with advanced neck aging and offers a more complete rejuvenation by also addressing the remodeling of the subcutaneous volumetric changes apart from skin laxity, as described in recent reviews on surgical techniques of facial rejuvenation (Quatela et al., 2021). Augment adjunctive treatments following surgery to further enhance the outcomes of neck lift surgeries. Patients can also enjoy the synergy of both neck elevation methods along with non-surgical procedures such as injectables, chemical peels, or dermabrasions in treating finer wrinkles and textural inconsistencies. The synergy among the surgical and non-surgical methods not only rejuvenates the neck region but also contributes to a general harmonious appearance of the face and neck regions. Furthermore, understanding the dynamic process of facial aging necessitates an integrated approach that respects both gravity and volumetric alteration in the aging process. By employing mixed techniques, surgeons are in a position to considerably amplify the pleasing results of neck lifts, thus meeting the increasing demands for efficient and long-term facial rejuvenation procedures (Lin et al., 2022) (Figure 5.10).

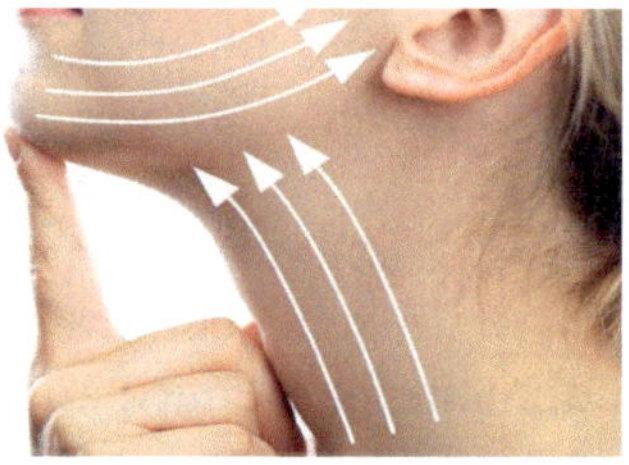

Figure 5.10. The techniques employed in neck lifts.

Source: https://external-content.duckduckgo.com/iu/?u=https%3A%2F%2Fcitizensjournals.com%2Fwp-content%2Fuploads%2F2023%2F06%2FHow-Neck-Lifts-Can-Turn-Back-the-Clock-680x350.jpg&f=1&nofb=1&ipt=ebc235312f591a70353c885194544782b5267e28149bf9f81914ff48741cc9f9.

5.3.3. Differences Between Neck Lift and Facelift

The distinction between a neck lift and a facelift lies in the specific regions of anatomy that they treat, as well as the type of aging signs that they correct. A facelift, or rhytidectomy, addresses the mid to lower face, addressing such issues as sagging, deep nasolabial folds, and jowls that are often secondary to the loss of elasticity and facial volume loss. On the other hand, a neck lift addresses the space on the neck, reviving sagging skin, excess fat, and banding of the muscles, which may lead to an older-looking aspect.

Even if both procedures can contribute to a more youthful general appearance, they address different targets that encourage patients to choose one or another based on their aesthetic issues and desired outcomes. Another significant distinction lies in the surgical technique utilized in these procedures.

A facelift most commonly involves ear incisions to enable lifting and tightening of the underlying facial muscles, as well as removal of excess skin. The procedure can vary, with some surgeons employing minimally invasive techniques that can potentially shorten recovery periods. On the contrary, a neck lift typically is accompanied by incisions in the back of the ears and beneath the chin, designed to eliminate unwanted skin and fat while repositioning muscles of the neck for a more symmetrical silhouette.

The nature of the technique utilized may significantly influence the experience of recovery, possible complications, and final results, thus influencing patients' choices regarding the treatments. Furthermore, the recovery periods and accompanying risks of each treatment are also different. Facelifts come with swelling and bruising that can persist for several weeks, since the face must heal from underlying tissues being manipulated. Aftercare can involve compression garments and limited activities in the recovery phase. Patients who receive neck lifts may experience the same swelling and pain, yet since the area of incisions is less conspicuous, they may feel more comfortable in social situations sooner. It is also worthwhile to mention the potential complications of both procedures, for instance, hematoma formation, which may be encountered after both a facelift and a neck lift. Research shows that proper treatment, for instance, the administration of atenolol and tranexamic acid, can significantly minimize such complications and increase patient satisfaction (Fagundes et al., 2014; Chávez Díaz et al., 2024).

Test Your Knowledge

1. What is the primary purpose of a neck lift, and which common aesthetic concerns does it address?
2. What are two techniques commonly used in neck lift procedures, and how does each improve the appearance of the neck?
3. How does a neck lift differ from a facelift in terms of the areas treated and the goals of each procedure?

5.4. Indications for Surgery

Learning Outcome

1. Discuss the Age-Related Changes in the Face and Neck
2. Explain the Genetic Factors Influencing Skin Elasticity
3. Focus on Psychological Motivations for Undergoing Surgery

The decision to perform rhytidectomy, or facelift, is supported by several clinical and cosmetic indications. The procedure is commonly performed in patients as a means of addressing severe facial aging features, such as sagging skin, deep nasolabial folds, and neck bands. These facial alterations are due to natural processes of aging, inheritance, and environmental factors. A thorough examination of a patient's facial structure, tissue laxity, and overall dermal quality is critical to establishing candidacy for surgery. Beyond cosmetic concerns, there are also psychological motivations that encourage individuals to go through the transformation process, and thus, patient expectations and mental preparedness need to be addressed. This thorough evaluation guarantees that surgery is in accordance with the patient's wishes and yields satisfactory results, ultimately contributing to both physical form and self-esteem. In addition, certain medical conditions have a profound impact on whether to suggest rhytidectomy and neck lift procedures. For instance, patients suffering from severe skin laxity as a result of weight fluctuations or menopause will derive substantial benefit from surgery. In some cases, facial injuries or congenital deformities in the past may cause unevenness of facial features, and the patients will need correction surgically. In those patients with too much sun damage or skin textural aberrations, combined procedures can correct these conditions and thereby make the facelift effective. The surgeons have to make a calculation of the overall health of the patient, considering skin elasticity and potential to heal, to get the optimum during surgery. These overall evaluations ensure that not just are applicants physically fit to undergo surgery, but that they are also emotionally prepared to accept the needs of postoperative care and recovery. Extension of indications for surgery occurs when adjunctive procedures are used as an addition to rhytidectomy. Among such adjuncts, removal of the buccal fat pad has gained attention for its cosmetic significance in facial contour. By removing this localized fat area, surgeons can enhance the prominence of the zygoma, creating a more youthful and harmonious facial outline, which is in perfect concordance with the inverted triangle of beauty principle (Moura et al., 2018).

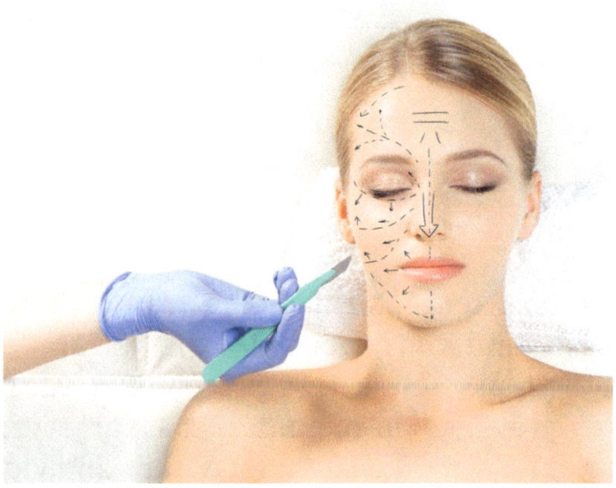

Figure 5.11. The decision to pursue rhytidectomy, commonly referred to as a facelift, hinges on several clinical and aesthetic indications.

Source: https://external-content.duckduckgo.com/iu/?u=https%3A%2F%2Fdrsidle.com%2Fwp-content%2Fuploads%2F2021%2F01%2Ffacial-plastic-surgery-scaled.jpg&f=1&nofb=1&ipt=3f8a4659c263f67788af879efc1f04ca072a1718f2c33b9e0eb31b7202d3b3c0.

While the overall goal remains rejuvenation of the integrity of faces, there is a need to consider approaches that simultaneously uplift and sculpt, thus addressing multiple aesthetic concerns in a single surgery session. Also, the technique of thread-lift sutures, as advanced as it is becoming, is noteworthy for its lesser but reasserting efficacy in non-surgical uplift. Awareness of these adjunct solutions bolsters surgical thinking, as it maintains the surgical strategy in synchrony with the patient's aesthetic goals for optimal outcomes (Gülbitti et al., 2018) (Figure 5.11).

5.4.1. Age-Related Changes in the Face and Neck

With advancing age, the face and neck also undergo profound physiological changes that have a dramatic impact on appearance. The skin undergoes a progressive thinning process, which decreases elasticity and moisture content, leading to the development of wrinkles, sagging, and a generally tired look. Age-related alterations of the supporting musculature may add to these influences. Loss of muscle tone brings about what is commonly referred to as jowls, with the sagging, redundant skin under the jawline. These effects not only affect beauty but also personal self-esteem and social life, prompting many to consider surgical interventions like rhytidectomy (facelift) and neck lift as methods of rejuvenation and personal empowerment (Pourdanesh et al., 2016). The aging effects also extend to the subcutaneous tissues of the neck and face, where thinning in the fat results in gauntness or emptiness, notably in the cheeks and temples. The thinning of the subcutaneous fat, combined with gravitational forces, induces an exaggerated loss of definition of the contours of the face, tending to enhance sagging skin. These transformations are external signs of aging, often striking a dramatic contrast between one's still youthful internal state and others' perception of an aging face. To this end, therefore, rejuvenating a younger-looking face becomes most important to many, with surgical procedures offering targeted corrections to these very familiar signs of aging (Badin et al., 2011). Apart from surgical interventions, non-surgical techniques have gained wide popularity as adjunctive treatment to correct facial and neck alterations resulting from aging.

Therapies such as aesthetic massage were found to stimulate physiological responses of the skin that could support the results of surgical treatments. Aesthetic massage would improve blood circulation, initiate collagen synthesis, and increase water levels in the skin, all contributing to a brighter and more youthful-looking face. However, while the non-surgical treatments work, they can require a specialized technique in order to treat the individual's specific needs, especially where there is extensive sagging of the skin or excessive fat deposit (Badin et al., 2011). Hence, the integration of both surgical and non-surgical procedures will prove to yield the best results for individuals contemplating the rejuvenation of the face and neck regions.

5.4.2. Genetic Factors Influencing Skin Elasticity

Genetic influences on skin elasticity are a vital consideration in planning surgeries such as rhytidectomy (facelift) and neck lift. As one ages, skin elasticity function diminishes as a result of diminished collagen and elastin production, the proteins required to keep the skin firm and flexible. Genetic predisposition is an important factor in protein synthesis and degradation. For example, those with a family history of extreme skin aging or specific dermatoses may present with more severe and earlier manifestations of diminished skin elasticity. The genetic factor, especially genes controlling the synthesis of collagen, emphasizes the importance of personal considerations in surgery. Genetic influences, as the role to be performed accentuates the importance of preoperative assessment, where persons with good genetic backgrounds may enjoy more favorable surgical outcomes as well as longer-lasting results following surgery, while less desirable genetic backgrounds might require additional technologies or supportive interventions to achieve satisfactory aesthetic goals. Environmental factors also play a role in genetic predisposition to determine skin elasticity, particularly in cosmetic procedures like rhytidectomy. Whereas genetic predisposition lays the groundwork for healthy skin, extrinsic factors, like sun exposure, air pollution, and lifestyle factors, can accelerate the loss of skin elasticity. For instance, ultraviolet (UV) radiation can degrade collagen and elastin fibers, which enhance the hereditary tendency towards skin aging. Therefore, it is essential to know a patient's environmental exposure, which is inherited to some extent by patterns of behavior within their family, when planning for surgery. Cosmetic treatment breakthroughs, coupled with technological advances, allow surgeons to tailor treatments based on each patient's genetic and environmental profiles. This awareness not only enhances postoperative satisfaction but also enables clinicians to recommend additional preventive treatments to reverse the effect of aging on skin elasticity in their patients in the long term. Lastly, the convergence of genetic information and technology in cosmetic procedures has transformed the field of aesthetic surgery, specifically for rhytidectomy and neck lifts. As demand continues to increase, driven by cultural changes towards self-improvement and social media, cosmetic procedures are growing more sophisticated. Fedorchenko (2024) also identifies the role of technology innovation in enhancing procedural outcomes via customization of treatment based on the unique genetic profile of a patient. Through enhanced technology in such procedures, minimally invasive treatment is becoming increasingly popular due to its offering less damage to the skin without reducing effectiveness. Kalaskar et al., 2016 also explain how varying the range of treatments can lead to compounded effects, even for people with genetic issues that make it hard to handle them using conventional approaches. By understanding how genetic and environmental forces interact, cosmetic surgeons can develop integrated treatment plans that honor the individual complexities of each patient's skin elasticity, ensuring more successful and more satisfying outcomes (Figure 5.12).

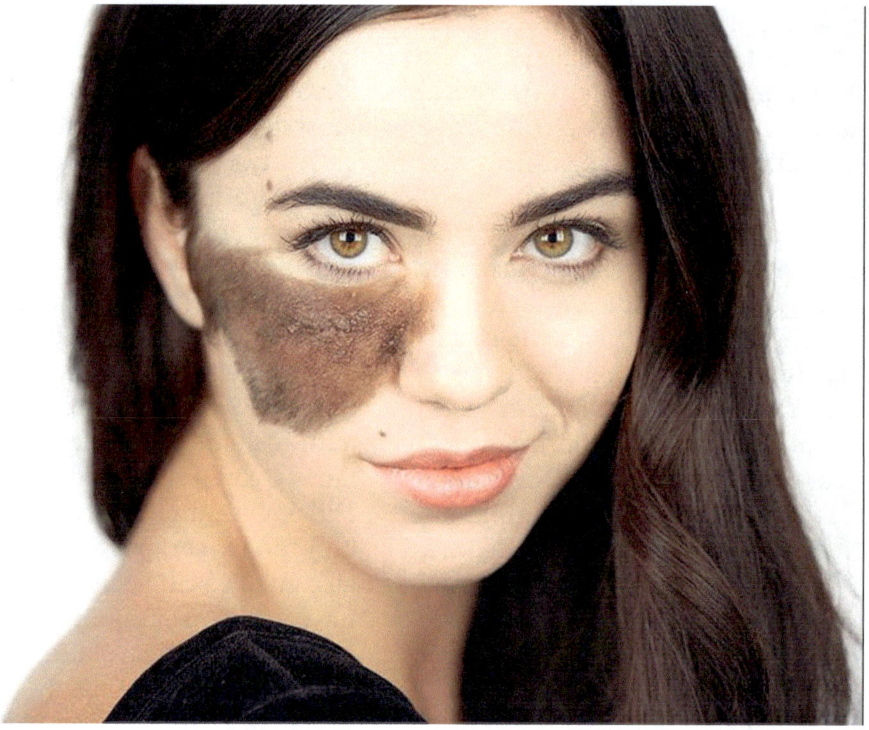

Figure 5.12. The genetic factors influencing skin elasticity.

Source: https://colecosmeticskincare.com/wp-content/uploads/2025/01/cassandra-naud-800-2126a3dacc4740a48ca66a9058a181dd.jpg.

5.4.3. Psychological Motivations for Undergoing Surgery

The need to look younger tends to motivate people to seek surgical procedures such as rhytidectomy, commonly known as a facelift, and neck lift surgery. These surgeries hold the potential for restabilizing a younger appearance, and this has extensive psychological consequences. During a period when the pursuit of a younger face is prevalent, patients tend to attend these cosmetic surgeries in an effort to boost their self-confidence and increase their acceptability. Literature establishes that increasing numbers of individuals have turned to aesthetic improvements not only for vanity but even as a form of therapy to combat the psychological pain that accompanies aging. Thus, such motivations can be intricately embedded within the fabric of an individual's concept of self and overall well-being, mandating the motivation for surgical interventions as a way of restoring self-esteem and public acceptance, an observation included in more recent studies (Castle et al., 2006). With shifting societal norms and increased exposure to cosmetic treatments, psychology is also a factor involved in whether a person decides to undergo procedures like facelifts. The modern environment, where social media permeates everything, provides for constant comparison and serves to create a want of physical perfection that was not so easily available in previous generations. The individual may perceive a younger appearance as being attractive and versatile in their social or professional sphere, thus prompting them to consider surgery. Moreover, the psychological impacts of aging, coupled with the demands of society, may instigate feelings of inadequacy, prompting individuals to seek cosmetic alterations. This social process is facilitated by the growing demand for aesthetic treatments, as a sign of transformation in the public's attitudes towards cosmetic surgery as more than just cosmetic alterations; instead, they are viewed as means to enhanced psychological welfare (Fedorchenko, 2024). Motives to undergo surgical treatments, particularly for the elderly, illustrate complex interplays among social pressure and desires. For others, going for rhytidectomy or a neck lift is the outcome of desiring greater control over their aging process and visual narrative of their lives. This desire is usually fueled by deeper psychological desires, such as the desire to avoid the emotional effects of aging, such as decreased self-esteem and social standing. As theories of psychological identity and self-concept suggest, facial appearance has a great social impact and influences interpersonal relationships. Thus, the decision to undergo surgery is most often brought into relief by a need to be accepted and validated, a drive that restively restores one's sense of authority and selfhood. As techniques advance and become safer and more effective, the psychological motivations behind such choices will necessarily shift as well, further solidifying society's significance placed on youth and beauty (Castle et al., 2006).

Test Your Knowledge

1. What age-related changes in the face and neck most commonly indicate the need for cosmetic surgery?
2. How can genetic factors influence a patient's skin elasticity and their suitability for facial or neck procedures?
3. What psychological motivations might lead someone to pursue cosmetic surgery, and why is evaluating these motivations important?

5.5. Risks and Complications

Learning Outcome

1. Discuss the Common Surgical Risks
2. Explain the Potential Complications Specific to Rhytidectomy
3. Focus on Importance of Choosing a Qualified Surgeon

Complications and risks of rhytidectomy and neck lift operations are matters of utmost concern for the patient as well as the surgeon. Surgical risks such as infection, hematoma, and anesthesia complications are always present in each invasive procedure. Hematomas, or blood accumulation outside blood vessels, can occur during the postoperative period and may necessitate additional surgery to prevent undesirable outcomes. Infection, although uncommon, can affect healing times as well as result in complications such as scarring or necrosis of tissues. The intricate surgical anatomy of facial layers delineated by Locketz et al. (2020) indicates how crucial it is to traverse these structures properly in a bid to avoid such hazards during surgery. Understanding the subtleties of these potential complications assists surgeons in preparing and preventing complications that may arise during or after the procedure. Surgical edema and ecchymosis are also major risks that may profoundly affect patient satisfaction. Swelling is unavoidable, yet excessive edema can form lengthy recovery time and an unsatisfying cosmetic result. Recent evidence, as examined by Locketz et al. (2020), shows that the use of tranexamic acid (TXA) has the possible effect of reversing these conditions through the reduction of post-operative bruising and swelling. However, evidence regarding the efficacy of TXA is still scarce and drastically variant among studies. Patient anatomical nuances, along with individual healing patterns, contribute to such outcome uncertainty. Therefore, the practitioners should ensure proper preoperative counseling in which realistic expectations regarding swelling and its impact on the overall process of recovery are given. The second significant complication involves nerve injury, which may occur during rhytidectomy due to the intricate network of facial nerves. Damage to these nerves can lead to temporary or, in a few cases, permanent changes in facial sensation and motor function, which have a significant impact on a patient's satisfaction with the outcome of surgery and quality of life. Surgeons must therefore exercise extreme caution to identify and preserve these critical structures during surgery. How to understand the anatomy used in facial rejuvenation surgery, as stipulated in Hashem et al. (2019), cannot be overstated. With facial surgery techniques improving by the day, obtaining optimal patient safety while pursuing aesthetic enhancement is a key dilemma in cosmetic surgery.

5.5.1. Common Surgical Risks

The incidence of complications of surgery with rhytidectomy, or facelift surgery, is a serious issue that cannot be overlooked. Facial anatomy cannot be dissected with such complexity and therefore requires utmost care, and dissections can lead to numerous complications. Hematomas, which are confined collections of blood outside the blood vessels due to damage to the vessels during the procedure, are frequent among patients. Facelift surgeries are particularly risky in this case, where there is excessive manipulation of connective tissues. Apart from that, infection is a serious complication that can lead to prolonged recovery and disfiguring results. Awareness of these common risks of surgery is significant to both surgeons and patients as it determines the decision-making process and emphasizes selecting competent surgeons who will be in a position to avoid these risks effectively (Pourdanesh et al., 2016). Another major complication that arises when undergoing facelift and neck lift surgeries is nerve damage, which takes the form of facial paralysis or dysesthesia. These are caused by the intricate interaction of the nerves with anatomical structures that are being moved during a procedure. The marginal mandibular nerve, for instance, may be inadvertently injured and lead to asymmetry of expressions and loss of muscle function in parts of the face. While the majority of the damage to the nerves is reversible, some nerve injuries are permanently devastating, fundamentally altering the quality of a patient's life. Extensive preoperative assessments and meticulous surgical techniques must be employed in order to minimize such risks and ensure maximum functioning of the facial tissues post-surgery (Carneiro et al., 2022). Apart from the immediate risks of surgery, patients must prepare for the long-term consequences of a facelift or neck lift. Scarring is common, with others experiencing hypertrophic scars or keloids that could be unsightly and worrisome. For example, postoperative adjustments such as methods of suturing can influence the formation of scars, and therefore, it is necessary that surgeons apply methods that promote optimal healing. Also, patients may have issues of sensitivity or pigmentation change of the skin that could be triggered by the surgical procedures. Awareness of such potential complications not only helps patients in terms of having realistic expectations but also brings to light the significance of thorough discussions with their surgeons prior to and subsequent to surgery. Hence, being well-educated about common surgical risks results in improved surgical outcomes and better-informed patients in decision-making (Pourdanesh et al., 2016) (Figure 5.13).

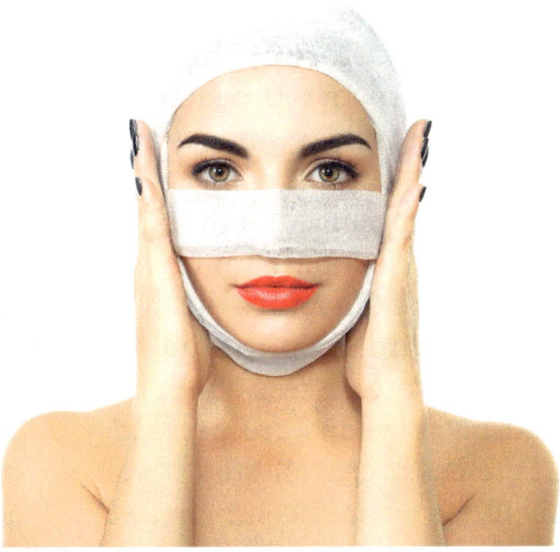

Figure 5.13. The incidence of surgical risks during rhytidectomy.

Source: https://drtorgerson.com/wp-content/uploads/2018/12/Plastic-Surgery-Risks-1.jpg.

5.5.2. Potential Complications Specific to Rhytidectomy

The practice of rhytidectomy, more commonly known as a facelift, is fraught with numerous potential complications for providers to navigate to achieve patient outcomes. One actual complication is the development of hematomas, which happen in 1% and 15% of cases. Hematomas result from the accumulation of blood between the skin flap and the underlying tissues as a result of inadequate vascular control during surgery or postoperative hemodynamic changes. Hematoma can impair healing and, in severe cases, lead to skin necrosis, necessitating relief of the complication by subsequent surgery. Thus, knowledge of the risk factors and application of preventive measures, such as meticulous surgical technique and postoperative regimens, is mandatory for reducing the risk of hematoma formation. In addition to hematomas, infection is also a frequent post-rhytidectomy complication. Surgical wounds are inherently susceptible to bacterial colonization, particularly in poor-risk patients who may harbor underlying diseases such as diabetes or immunosuppression. Infections can manifest as redness, increased drainage, and systemic signs such as fever, possibly requiring antibiotic therapy or surgical drainage. Proper preoperative evaluation of patients and scrupulous postoperative care are key features in the prevention of infection complications. The majority of surgeons emphasize ensuring sterile procedures throughout surgery and educating patients on signs of infection so that they can be identified and treated immediately (Kalaskar et al., 2016). Moreover, nerve injury, particularly of the facial nerve, poses a serious risk in rhytidectomy. Because of the intricate anatomy of the facial nerve, which innervates the facial musculature used for expression, careful dissection and identification of the nerve should be undertaken intraoperatively. Nerve injury can lead to facial asymmetry, weakness, or even paralysis of the affected side. Along with better techniques and equipment, these complications remain to be presented, which stresses the need for surgeons to employ their technical knowledge of anatomy and experience in order to minimize risks. Recent studies have demonstrated that the application of methods such as tranexamic acid (TXA) can assist in the minimization of intraoperative bleeding and theoretically reduce surgical dissection complications (Kalaskar et al., 2016).

5.5.3. Importance of Choosing a Qualified Surgeon

The choice of a skilled surgeon is extremely crucial while deciding between rhytidectomy (facelift) and neck lift surgery since it significantly determines the success, safety, and patient satisfaction. Specialist surgeons who are skilled in cosmetic surgery, particularly those who possess certified education in plastic and reconstructive surgery, possess the valuable experience that can enable them to overcome the complexities associated with these procedures. Their knowledge of facial anatomy and aesthetics is not only theoretical but also has a direct impact on their ability to deliver results that are both natural and harmonious. The aesthetic technique that is needed for cosmetic surgery cannot be overstated since it entails not only technical skill but also appreciation of the psychological load which patients must be allowed to carry. As the case in the Ouroboros metaphor, the repeated cycle of self-discovery and then the need for personal improvement underscores the importance of the physical makeover being left to a trained professional (Camm et al., 2025). Secondly, the technical nature of neck lift and face lift procedures requires that patients do their research extensively when selecting a trained surgeon. This is normally done through patient testimonials, before-and-after photo albums, and professional qualifications. Most professionals highlight the importance of board certification and membership in reputable surgical societies, ensuring these are indicators of a surgeon's commitment to maintaining high surgical standards. It is essential that prospective patients book consultations to gauge the surgeon's style, philosophy, and willingness to address every aspect of the procedure, including the risks and rehabilitation. The significance of open communication cannot be overstated, as it builds trust and allows the development of a stable surgeon-patient relationship. Ultimately, education allows patients to take charge of their surgery and minimize potential complications, thus enhancing their overall satisfaction (Kalaskar et al., 2016). Furthermore, complications resulting from poorly performed cosmetic procedures can have physical and psychological effects in the long run. Surgically inexperienced practitioners may result in unsatisfactory cosmetic outcomes, and subsequent corrective procedures at a cost to the patient in terms of finances and emotional distress. The patient may end up feeling regretful, losing self-esteem, or even develop chronic dissatisfaction with the way they look, illustrating the absolute need to select an appropriately trained practitioner. To that end, education and awareness about the credentials of would-be surgeons are necessary; diligence is nonetheless a crucial step in navigating the complexity of cosmetic surgery. Surgeons who are trained in sophisticated techniques and technologies and possess an understanding of facial aging considerations will be well poised to provide tailored treatment plans that are commensurate with individual patient goals. Ultimately, a skilled surgeon not only gives a more beautiful outcome but also safeguards the patient's mental and emotional well-being during the procedure (Camm et al., 2025) (Figure 5.14).

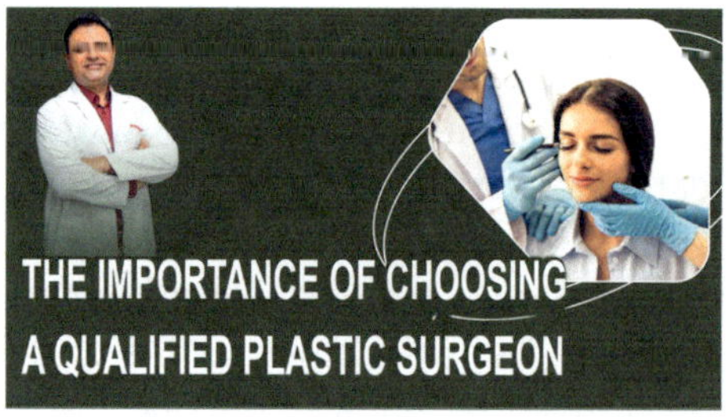

Figure 5.14. Importance of choosing a qualified surgeon.

Source: https://galwacarehospital.com/wp-content/uploads/2024/10/image-15.png.

Test Your Knowledge

1. What general surgical risks should patients be aware of before undergoing any cosmetic procedure?
2. What are two potential complications specific to rhytidectomy (facelift) surgery?
3. Why is selecting a qualified and experienced surgeon essential for minimizing risks and achieving optimal outcomes?

5.6. Recovery and Aftercare

Learning Outcome

1. Explain the typical recovery timeline
2. Discuss the post-operative care instructions
3. Focus on long-term maintenance of results

The process of recovery after a rhytidectomy or neck lift is crucial for achieving the best surgical outcomes. Postoperative management in the early stages typically consists of a brief stay in the hospital, where the patients are monitored for vital signs and complications. The first few days after surgery are typically characterized by swelling, bruising, and a sense of tightness throughout the face and neck area. The patients are instructed to maintain a head elevation and refrain from any strenuous effort during this time to minimize swelling and promote healing. Adequate hydration, optimal nutrition, and adherence to pain management protocols as ordered are essential to enable recovery. Also required are routine follow-up visits to the surgical staff to assure healing progress and address any patient anxiety regarding the condition of their postoperative status. These pre-emptive evaluations can have a substantive impact upon the general recovery process and mitigate risk for negative effects during the process of healing. Proper aftercare is critical to long-term results following rhytidectomy procedures, where education in self-care is required. The patient is typically advised to avoid direct sunlight and strenuous exercise for several weeks post-surgery since these can compromise healing. Topical agents and employing the same preoperative skincare routine can also avoid discomfort as well as scarring. Communication with medical professionals regarding potential questions or issues that arise during the recovery process is also highly recommended. Careful adherence to aftercare instructions not only promotes faster recovery but also better overall appearance of the surgery. Making sure patients read and comply with these aftercare protocols eventually becomes the key to maximizing the efficacy of the rhytidectomy or neck lift surgery. From a surgical precision as well as from the patient's recovery point of view, the procedures employed in performing rhytidectomy or neck lift directly affect the patterns of recovery.

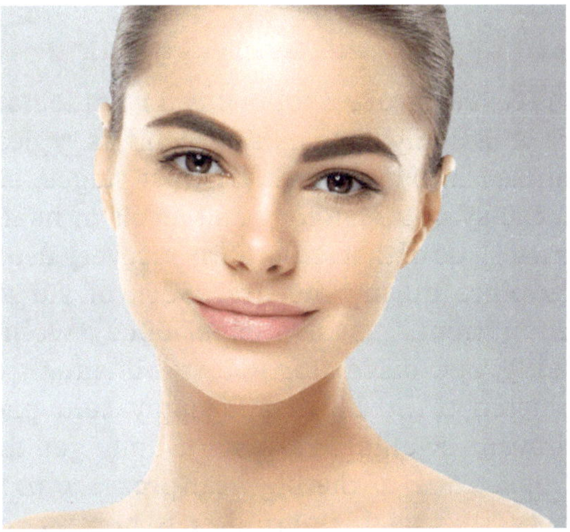

Figure 5.15. The recovery phase following a rhytidectomy.

Source: https://evexiamedspa.com/wp-content/uploads/2024/11/PRP-Recovery-and-Aftercare-What-to-Expect-After-PRP-Injections-Evexia-Medspa-McLean-VA.png.

Newer techniques, like minimally invasive techniques, have been developed that reduce postoperative complications and increase patient comfort. For instance, Piezosurgery Medical® has proven to be effective in maintaining bone through selective cutting of mineralized tissues, which would be beneficial when facial bone structures are utilized for lifting procedures. It is defined by association with more effective healing due to conserved surrounding soft tissues, which is particularly relevant upon recovery. Furthermore, the use of contemporary machinery and methods supports a smoother postoperative result through alleviation of pain and swift recovery, such that enhanced aftercare practices become imperative to satisfaction of the patient and achieving the coveted cosmetic aesthetic as emphasized in writings like the comprehensive manual Textbook of Plastic and Reconstructive Surgery (Kalaskar et al., 2016) and study of surgical tools and techniques (Anesi et al., 2014) (Figure 5.15).

5.6.1. Typical Recovery Timeline

The recovery process following a rhytidectomy, more commonly known as a facelift, is typically organized into a series of distinct stages, each with the symptomatology and levels of healing characteristic of that stage. Early recovery usually takes place during the first week of surgery, when patients usually experience swelling, bruising, and discomfort. Most individuals are instructed to lie down and apply cold packs to prevent swelling. Patients usually get tired and upset due to the physical pressure of the surgery. During this period, it is necessary to follow post-operative instructions meticulously since they guide the healing process and prevent complications. Moreover, support from caregivers or family members is often beneficial so that the patient can focus on healing without having to worry about medication routines or follow-up procedures. As the healing process extends to the second week, improvements are typically visible. Patients tend to complain less about swelling and bruising, leading to a more pleasing appearance that gradually works toward achieving the anticipated outcomes from the surgery. It is here that the majority of individuals will be prepared to resume light exercises and possibly even return to work, but heavy exercises should be avoided. Keeping a clean surgical area and clinic visits for follow-up cannot be overstated as these are critical in monitoring healing as well as any issues that may arise. Furthermore, with this stage, statistics from recent studies on facelift procedures, such as the modifications preferred for surgeries such as the R lift, indicate the advancements in minimizing downtime while still achieving esthetic outcomes (Saleh et al., 2021). By the end of six weeks, most of the patients resume their usual activities without any inherent restraint. Yet, complete recovery may take a few months, more specifically in residual swelling or numbness, which may persist. Patients are typically instructed to maintain a normal skin care routine and keep the surgical area out of the sun to prevent complications such as hyperpigmentation or suboptimal scarring. Notably, the advent of techniques that prioritize less downtime, like the altered en bloc facelift, has emerged as a feasible option for patients who desire to circumvent the recuperation challenges that typically characterize traditional methods (Meretsky et al., 2024). Lastly, knowing the normal recovery time enables people to have appropriate expectations and makes informed choices about their surgical encounter.

5.6.2. Post-Operative Care Instructions

Extensive post-operative care directions are essential in patients undergoing rhytidectomy (facelift) and neck lifts. Such directions usually comprise wound care, medication regimen, and activity restriction for optimal recovery outcomes. Patients are advised to have their surgical sites clean and dry, with the application of any prescribed ointments overseen by the physician. In addition, infection prevention and pain control are crucial; hence, patients should adhere to medication regimens, including antibiotics and pain medication. The clarity and comprehensiveness of such instructions can significantly influence compliance among patients, reducing the likelihood of problems like infection or dehiscence of the wound. A planned communication can be useful in making sure that every detail of post-operative care is communicated to the patient, thereby enhancing the overall experience and satisfaction rates from the surgery. The addition of educational tools such as patient information leaflets (PILs) can also improve the delivery of post-operative advice. A study indicates that the application of PILs has a direct positive effect on patient satisfaction and concordance for preoperative and postoperative care. For example, before the advent of PILs, there was a high rate of rescheduling due to miscommunication, which reduced once they were employed. The ability to have something tangible to refer to enables patients to read important instructions in their own time, decreasing misconceptions and fear of recovery. As far as rhytidectomy and neck lifts are concerned, a well-designed PIL can include particular instructions on how to recognize signs of complications, circulating exercises, and post-operative activity guidelines for a return to normal activity following surgery for easier recovery.

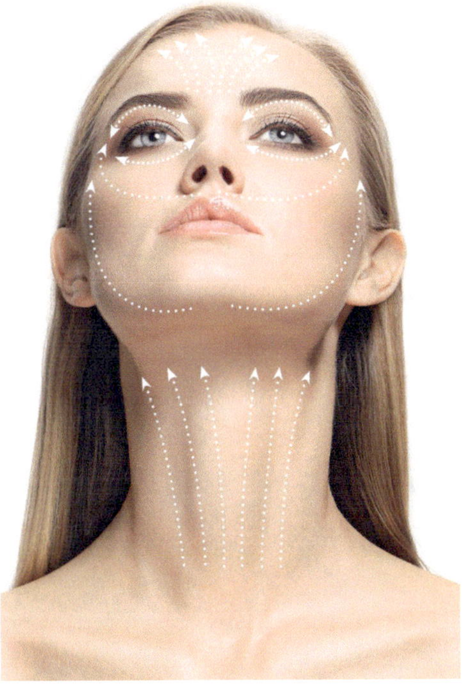

Figure 5.16. The post-operative care instructions are essential for patients undergoing rhytidectomy (facelift) and neck lift procedures.

Source: https://www.phuketpsi.com/wp-content/uploads/2022/07/1657166161031.jpg.

Moreover, the inclusion of emergency cognition aids, including using the THYRAID tool for post-thyroidectomy care, can be an indispensable resource for emergency presentations following facelift or neck lift surgery. While frequencies of serious complications may be small, anticipation of potential emergencies, such as profuse bleeding and airway obstruction, is essential. A structured system of early warning signs detection and immediate intervention can minimize adverse outcomes significantly. Systematic training of the healthcare team in the application of such mental aids can improve team communication, allowing for quick response when a complication arises. As can be seen in environments where organized emergency procedures are established, early intervention can promote patient safety and reassurance, which highlights the significance of thorough post-operative guidelines given to patients who have undergone aesthetic surgery (Bakshi et al., 2021; Phillips et al., 2022) (Figure 5.16).

5.6.3. Long-Term Maintenance of Results

Long-term preservation of outcome after rhytidectomy and neck lift surgery is an important issue to consider for both the patient and the surgeon. Creating long-lasting aesthetic enhancement entails more than what happens in the operating room initially; it means having a thorough appreciation for the process of aging and how aging influences facial contours throughout life. Techniques such as deep rhytidectomy, involving the treatment of deeper tissue planes, have been shown to provide superior and longer-lasting results compared to the more superficial techniques. Specifically, studies have identified that patients who received deep rhytidectomy have improved aesthetic outcomes and maintain these in the long term, as rated on the Merz scale and Global Aesthetic Improvement Scale (GAIS) (Bondariev

& Logvinov, 2025). The long-term permanence of these outcomes emphasizes the importance of surgical technique in the planning of operations for effective long-term rejuvenation. Issues of the patient, such as lifestyle, age, and skin quality, also bear great significance in maintaining facelift outcomes in the long term, in addition to surgical technique. Younger patients are more likely to have more long-term satisfaction with their outcome, partly due to having better skin elasticity and resiliency. Conversely, older patients may have difficulty obtaining results due to reduced muscle tone and elasticity of the skin. Furthermore, lifestyle choices such as sunlight exposure, smoking, and skin care affect the prolongation of the aging process and influence the longevity of surgical results. For instance, patients who get into the habit of sun protection and adopt healthy lifestyles are more likely to be long-term retainers of their youthful appearance than those who do not (Tao et al., 2025). This calls for emphasizing engaging patients in well-balanced lifestyle discussions during preoperative consultations. Finally, postoperative management and follow-up cannot be overemphasized in the longevity of surgical results. Regular follow-up appointments permit observation of the healing process and the solving of any ensuing problems, thereby ensuring maintenance of optimum results. Secondly, incorporation of non-surgical adjuncts, such as fillers or neuromodulators, can enhance and prolong the cosmetic improvements provided by a facelift or neck lift. These treatments, administered wisely, can treat the progressive reversal of the aging changes, giving patients a complete solution to sustaining their rejuvenated appearance. By monitoring and participating in their aesthetic process, patients can significantly prolong the life of their facelift and neck lift results, establishing a foundation for long-term satisfaction after surgery.

Test Your Knowledge

1. What is the typical recovery timeline following a facial cosmetic procedure, and which stages are most important for healing?
2. What key post-operative care instructions should patients follow to minimize complications and support proper recovery?
3. What long-term habits or maintenance strategies help preserve the results of facial or neck surgery?

SUMMARY

The Overview of a study into rhytidectomy and neck lift surgery emphasizes the dramatic impact these facial rejuvenation surgical treatments can have on patients requiring restoration of the facial appearance. In addition to addressing outward signs of aging, such as sagging skin and loss of definition in the face, these surgeries assist in enhancing self-esteem and overall health. As has been shown by progress in surgical techniques, e.g., deep plane facelifts, professionals have not ceased enhancing patient outcomes while restricting complications. As such, it is extremely important that those considering the procedure be subjected to extensive examinations to ensure optimal results and satisfaction. Since the psychological element of aesthetic transformation exists, patients must engage in realistic discussions regarding expectations and potential outcomes in relation to rhytidectomy and neck lift surgeries. Further, customized surgical planning is of the utmost significance. Success in a rhytidectomy or neck lift requires attention to each patient's specific anatomical features as well as to their goals for looks. Not only must surgeons be skilled, but they must also possess an artistic appreciation of facial movements so that they can create aesthetically pleasing results. Preoperative assessment, such as close regard for flexibility of the skin and face volume, are pillars of effective surgical intervention. Evidence confirms that a tailored method has enhanced satisfaction postoperatively, minimized complications, and maximized the duration. The use of modern techniques and technologies to perform a facelift continuously advances, establishing new standards for aesthetic surgery that significantly improve patient experience and results. Finally, ongoing improvement in rhytidectomy and neck lifts emphasizes the need for ongoing research and education in aesthetic medicine. By analyzing outcomes and building up optimized surgical procedures, surgeons can contribute to a repository of knowledge that drives best practice. Surgeons, scientists, and patients are working together, which gives rise to knowledge about the impact of these cosmetic procedures. Furthermore, through the incorporation of patient-provided outcomes and feedback as part of surgery procedures, patient care and treatment for potential future surgical subjects can be enhanced. As incorporated into the broader narrative of cosmetic surgery, what neck lifts and rhytidectomies illustrate is the intersection of medical competence and that basic human desire for self-perfection and rebirth and, therefore, the relevance of these procedures in modern surgical practice.

With advancing rhytidectomy, or colloquially known as facelift surgery, the incorporation of varied aesthetic techniques has been the hallmark issue in optimizing surgical outcomes. The procedure corrects facial sagging, wrinkles, and skin laxity, which significantly impact the patient's psychological status and self-perception. Advances in surgical techniques now permit a more individualized approach, catering to the individual patient's anatomy and desired aesthetic outcome. Further, improved pre-operative consultation and post-operative care have improved recovery times and patient satisfaction rates. Overall, it provides useful insight into the effectiveness of traditional facelift surgery while opening the door to new alternative therapies for facial renewal. Supplementing surgical procedures, non-surgical and minimally invasive interventions have gained popularity as effective alternatives for traditional rhytidectomy. Such technologies as Ultherapy and fat grafting also now overwhelm dermatology, offering rejuvenating effects without serious recovery in the guise of surgery. These treatments not only address epidermal signs of aging, but also support integrity of deeper structures, thereby helping to favor a more youthful appearance. Furthermore, treatments such as thread lifts, which involve materials such as polydioxanone (PDO), provide reliable alternatives to give lift and volume with no need for general anesthesia. The growing menu of treatment modalities supports the validity of an integrated approach in assessing anti-aging strategies, the synergistic benefit of multi-modal applications for optimal effects. As practitioners increasingly advocate a holistic solution to facial rejuvenation, the role of aesthetic massage procedures emerges as a significant contribution to surgical and dermatologic therapy. These treatments are designed to stimulate the physiological processes of skin and underlying tissues, enhance water potential, and restructure facial contours, potentially optimizing the effects of surgical treatments. Incorporation of aesthetic massage into anti-aging treatments can significantly improve patient outcomes by actively promoting tissue regeneration and optimizing metabolic processes. This non-surgical treatment also allows for customization in treatment protocols, attending to the needs and expectations of individual patients. Emphasizing the balance of patient education and realistic expectations, clinicians can take people through their aesthetic outcomes with minimal potential drawbacks associated with radical surgical decisions, improving satisfaction and safety in facial rejuvenation treatments.

KEY TERMS FROM THIS CHAPTER

- Superficial Musculoaponeurotic System (SMAS)
- Platysmaplasty
- Jowl Correction
- Skin Redraping
- Submental Liposuction
- Platysmal Bands
- Retroauricular Incision
- Platysma Muscle
- Neck Contouring
- Cervicofacial Rhytidectomy
- Facial Ligaments
- Subplatysmal Fat
- Periauricular Incision
- Hairline Incision

CRITICAL THINKING QUESTIONS

1. **The primary goal of a facelift (rhytidectomy) is to:**
   a. Remove facial fat completely
   b. Reposition sagging facial tissues and tighten the SMAS
   c. Improve skin pigmentation
   d. Enlarge facial muscles
2. **The SMAS layer is important in facelift surgery because it:**
   a. Contains all sensory nerves
   b. Provides structural support for soft tissues
   c. Houses salivary glands
   d. Is responsible for skin elasticity
3. **Injury to which nerve can cause lower lip asymmetry during facelift surgery?**
   a. Temporal branch of facial nerve
   b. Marginal mandibular nerve
   c. Oculomotor nerve
   d. Glossopharyngeal nerve
4. **The most effective technique for improving a sagging neck and platysmal banding is:**
   a. Chemical peel
   b. Botox alone
   c. Platysmaplasty
   d. Dermal fillers
5. **A key sign of facial nerve injury after facelift surgery is:**
   a. Blurred vision
   b. Difficulty closing the eye
   c. Loss of eyebrow shape
   d. Ear numbness

Short Answer Questions

1. What are the main aesthetic indications for performing a rhytidectomy (facelift)?
2. Why is the SMAS layer important in facelift surgery?
3. What anatomical structures must be carefully protected during a neck lift procedure?
4. What are the common complications associated with facelift surgery?
5. How does platysmaplasty improve the contour of the neck in neck lift procedures?

Answers to Critical Thinking Questions

1. (b) 2. (b) 3. (b) 4. (c) 5. (b)

REFERENCES

1. Allahyari Fard, S. (2018). *Kirurške i nekirurške metode pomlađivanja lica.* https://core.ac.uk/download/197825730.pdf (accessed on 14th July 2025).
2. Anesi, A., Cavani, F., Chiarini, L., Ferretti, et al. (2014). *Preliminary findings of a potenziated piezosurgical device at the rabbit skull.* https://core.ac.uk/download/80171725.pdf (accessed on 14th July 2025).
3. Azizzadeh, B., & Lu, R. J. (2024). Facial nerve considerations for the deep plane facelift and neck lift. *Facial Plastic Surgery, 40*, 687–693. https://doi.org/10.1055/s-0043-1777801 (accessed on 14th July 2025).
4. Badin, I., Gozhenko, O., & Zukow, W. (2011). *Face-lift with the use of an aesthetic massage technology: Strategy and tactics.* https://core.ac.uk/download/587245563.pdf (accessed on 14th July 2025).
5. Bakshi, S., Tambule, A., Panigrahi, A. R., & Pai, P. (2021). *Effect of patient information leaflet on working pattern and patient satisfaction level in a busy Indian day care operative theater complex. Journal of Anesthesiology, Clinical Pharmacology, 37*, 347–353. https://www.semanticscholar.org/paper/d32bc59703469cae3e2bd971eabaf5285e77e788 (accessed on 14th July 2025).
6. Bondariev, R. V., & Logvinov, O. Y. (2025). *Evaluation of immediate and long-term results of surgical correction of involutional changes of the face and neck. Kharkiv Surgical School.* https://www.semanticscholar.org/paper/0bee0575e9127859ebe459ac8ae0b877c5bcaf37 (accessed on 14th July 2025).
7. Butz, D. R., & Geldner, P. (2016). *The use of tranexamic acid in rhytidectomy patients. Plastic and Reconstructive Surgery Global Open, 4.* https://www.semanticscholar.org/paper/cfe838ee91146e7fd67c88fdfe10f41699bb28b8 (accessed on 14th July 2025).
8. Camm, E. M. (2025). *Narcissistic vulnerabilities experienced within the processes of change and development.* https://core.ac.uk/download/82963780.pdf (accessed on 14th July 2025).
9. Carneiro, S. C. D. A. S., Vasconcelos, B. C. E., Martins, E. S. A., Diniz, et al. (2022). *Complications associated with submental liposuction: A scoping review.* https://core.ac.uk/download/570980520.pdf (accessed on 14th July 2025).
10. Portilla, A. S. P., Portilla, C. S. P., Palacios, G. S. G., Rodríguez, B. S. P., Castillo, S. G. A., Espin, N. E. P., & Pita, G. P. M. (2024). The integration of surgical and dermatological techniques in the treatment of cutaneous aging: multidisciplinary approaches and clinical outcomes - a comprehensive systematic review of current literature. *International Journal of Research in Medical Sciences, 12*(5), 1659–1667. https://doi.org/10.18203/2320-6012.ijrms20240943 (accessed on 14th July 2025).
11. Castillo-Campos, P. (2022). *Rhytidoplasty through minimal incisions (Rhythmic). Aesthetic Surgery Journal Open Forum.* https://doi.org/10.1093/asjof/ojac059 (accessed on 14th July 2025).
12. Castle, D. J., & Honigman, R. (2006). *Aging and Cosmetic Enhancement.* https://core.ac.uk/download/pdf/8296058.pdf (accessed on 14th July 2025).
13. Chávez Díaz, M., De la Cruz Ku, G., Ziegler Gutiérrez, O. E., & Ziegler Rodríguez, et al. (2024). *Safety and outcomes in multiplane facial rejuvenation with tranexamic acid: A cohort study.* https://core.ac.uk/download/609795360.pdf (accessed on 14th July 2025).

14. Cohen, J. L., Goodman, G., Trindade de Almeida, A., Jones, D., Carruthers, J., Grimes, P. E., de Maio, M., et al. (2023). *Decades of beauty: Achieving aesthetic goals throughout the lifespan. Journal of Cosmetic Dermatology, 22*, 2889–2901. https://doi.org/10.1111/jocd.15968 (accessed on 14th July 2025).

15. Pourdanesh, F., Esmaeelinejad, M., Jafari, S. M., & Nematollahi, Z. (2016). Facelift: Current Concepts, Techniques, and Principles. InTech. doi: 10.5772/63150(accessed on 14th July 2025).

16. Fagundes, D. J., Gurgel, S. J. T., Hartmann, R. C. B., & Martins, et al. (2014). *O atenolol previne a formação de hematoma expansivo após ritidoplastia*. https://core.ac.uk/download/37711982.pdf (accessed on 14th July 2025).

17. Fedorchenko, Y. (2024). ANTI-AGING COSMETIC PROCEDURES: BENEFITS AND RISKS. *Anti-Aging Eastern Europe*, *3*(3), 135-140. https://doi.org/10.56543/aaeeu.2024.3.3.04(accessed on 14th July 2025).

18. Gülbitti, H. A., Colebunders, B., Pirayesh, A., Bertossi, D., & van der Lei, B. (2018). *Thread-lift sutures: Still in the lift? A systematic review of the literature. Plastic & Reconstructive Surgery, 141*, 341e–347e. https://doi.org/10.1097/prs.0000000000004101 (accessed on 14th July 2025).

19. Hashem, A. M., Couto, R. A., Duraes, E. F. R., Çakmakoğlu, C., Swanson, M., Surek, C., & Zins, J. E. (2019). *Fa*celift part I: History, anatomy, and clinical assessment. *Aesthetic Surgery Journal, 40*, 1–18. https://doi.org/10.1093/asj/sjy326 (accessed on 14th July 2025).

20. Hood, K., Kumar, N. G., Kaoutzanis, C., & Higdon, K. K. (2018). *Hematomas in aesthetic surgery. Aesthetic Surgery Journal, 38*, 1013–1025. https://doi.org/10.1093/asj/sjx236 (accessed on 14th July 2025).

21. Hopping, S. B., Janjanin, S., Tanna, N., & Joshi, A. (2010). *The S-Plus lift: A short-scar, long-flap rhytidectomy. Annals of the Royal College of Surgeons of England, 92*(7), 577–582. https://www.semanticscholar.org/paper/d4b5d2f4f679b377251541c10c48d0bc14291b0b (accessed on 14th July 2025).

22. Kao, C. C., & Duscher, D. (2023). The ponytail lift: 22 years of experience in 600 cases of endoscopic deep plane facial rejuvenation. *Aesthetic Surgery Journal, 44*, 671–692. https://doi.org/10.1093/asj/sjad382 (accessed on 14th July 2025).

23. Leake, D., & Lee, J. (2021). *Applications of Helium Plasma in Rejuvenation of the Face and Neck*. https://core.ac.uk/download/479935723.pdf (accessed on 14th July 2025).

24. Li, K., Meng, F., Li, Y. R., Tian, Y., Chen, H., Jia, Q., Cai, H., et al. (2022). *Application of nonsurgical modalities in improving facial aging. International Journal of Dentistry, 2022*, 1–18. https://doi.org/10.1155/2022/8332631 (accessed on 14th July 2025).

25. Lin, S. J., Veeramani, A., & Ebersole, T. G. (2022). *Face and neck lift. DeckerMed Plastic Surgery.* https://www.semanticscholar.org/paper/b884060bddd8efc6bfa578cf97d63772f7918fea (accessed on 14th July 2025).

26. Lo Castro, A. M. (1996). *Aspects of Physical Appearance and Clothing Behavior*. https://core.ac.uk/download/655000294.pdf (accessed on 14th July 2025).

27. Locketz, G. D., Lozada, K. N., & Bloom, J. D. (2020). *Tranexamic acid in aesthetic facial plastic surgery: A systematic review of evidence, applications, and outcomes. Aesthetic Surgery Journal Open Forum, 2*. https://doi.org/10.1093/asjof/ojaa029 (accessed on 14th July 2025).

28. McGuigan, K. C., & Trinh, L. (2022). *Do Google Trends correlate with the number of facial plastic surgery procedures performed in the United States? Facial Plastic Surgery, 39*, 160–163. https://www.semanticscholar.org/paper/cae3c1a946a347ec87d227f40f2f148f496217e0 (accessed on 14th July 2025).

29. Meretsky, C. R., Hausner, P., Flynn, B. P., & Schiuma, A. T. (2024). *A systematic review and comparative analysis of reconstructive rhytidectomy: Advantages, disadvantages, and patient outcomes. Cureus, 16*(10), e71006. https://www.cureus.com/articles/296838-a-systematic-review-and-comparative-analysis-of-reconstructive-rhytidectomy-advantages-disadvantages-and-patient-outcomes.pdf (accessed on 14th July 2025).

30. Moura, L. B., Spin, J. R., Spin-Neto, R., & Pereira-Filho, V. A. (2018). *Buccal fat pad removal to improve facial aesthetics: An established technique? Medicina Oral, Patología Oral y Cirugía Bucal.* https://doi.org/10.4317/medoral.22449 (accessed on 14th July 2025).

31. Deepak M. Kalaskar, Peter E. Butler, Shadi Ghali. (2016). *Textbook of Plastic and Reconstructive Surgery*. ISBN: 978-1-910634-37-0 (Hbk.) https://core.ac.uk/download/79526588.pdf (accessed on 14th July 2025).

32. Newberry, C. I., & Mobley, S. R. (2019). Chin augmentation using silastic implants. *Facial Plastic Surgery, 35*, 149–157. https://doi.org/10.1055/s-0039-1683867 (accessed on 14th July 2025).

33. Phillips, J. G., Eyeington, C., Mercer, I., Taylor, C., & Farrell, S. (2022). *THYRAID: A cognitive aid for the management of neck hematoma following thyroid surgery. ANZ Journal of Surgery, 92.* https://www.semanticscholar.org/paper/14a4214688cb80c32163286f031bb81933ee9e5c (accessed on 14th July 2025).

34. Ponce Vera, M. S., Criollo Jimenez, M. E., Idalgo, F. A., Pereira, S. S., Nunes, A. G., Kassis, E., Cicareli, Á. J. (2023*). Major evidence and guidelines for antibiotic therapy in implant dentistry: A systematic review. MedNEXT Journal of Medical and Health Sciences.* https://www.semanticscholar.org/paper/9499eb25c13ae04a87e716eb7e324e3fca2e1b51 (accessed on 14th July 2025).

35. Portilla, A. S. P., Portilla, C. S. P., Palacios, G., Rodríguez, B. S. P., Castillo, S., Espin, N. E. P., & Pita, G. P. M. (2024). The integration of surgical and dermatological techniques in the treatment of cutaneous aging: Multidisciplinary approaches and clinical outcomes – A comprehensive systematic review of current literature. *International Journal of Research in Medical Sciences, 12*, 1659–1667. https://doi.org/10.18203/2320-6012.ijrms20240943 (accessed on 14th July 2025).

36. Quatela, V., & Ahmedli, N. (2021). *The selection of facelift approach on the basis of midfacial ptosis. Facial Plastic Surgery, 37*, 149–159. https://www.semanticscholar.org/paper/a9e2580847d5d8705f3771e2e1dc3f1f00f7b2a7 (accessed on 14th July 2025).

37. Saleh, D. B., Brierley, N., & Riaz, M. (2021). *"R" face and neck lift: A modified technique for en-bloc facial rejuvenation. Plastic and Aesthetic Research, 8*(10). https://www.mrmriaz.com/s/3889.pdf (accessed on 14th July 2025).

38. Talei, B., Gould, D., & Ziai, H. (2024). Vectorial analysis of deep plane face and neck lift. *Aesthetic Surgery Journal.* https://www.semanticscholar.org/paper/d5cb6cd181b368ec115ea1e2e6cb07e3dc8a1b3c (accessed on 14th July 2025).

39. Tanna, N., & Lindsey, W. H. (2008). *Review of 1,000 consecutive short-scar rhytidectomies. Dermatologic Surgery, 34*, 196–203. https://doi.org/10.1097/00042728-200802000-00008 (accessed on 14th July 2025).

40. Tao, Y., Siu, L. L., Licitra, L., Burtness, B., Tahara, M., Rischin, D., Alves, G., et al. (2025). *Long-term results of the randomized, phase 3 KEYNOTE-412 trial of pembrolizumab (pembro) or placebo (pbo) plus concurrent chemoradiotherapy (CRT) for unresected, locally advanced head and neck squamous cell carcinoma (LA HNSCC). Journal of Clinical Oncology*. https://www.semanticscholar.org/paper/40117cfafb273accffca2d79d630e75f44a1cfae (accessed on 14th July 2025).

41. Trifan, D. F., Tirla, A., Moldovan, A. F., Moş, C., Bodog, F., Maghiar, T., Manole, F., et al. (2023). *Can vitamin D levels alter the effectiveness of short-term facelift interventions? Healthcare, 11*, 1490–1490. https://doi.org/10.3390/healthcare11101490 (accessed on 14th July 2025).

42. Walker, N. J., Crantford, J. C., Rudolph, M., & David, L. R. (2018). *Outcomes analysis of chief cosmetic clinic over 13 years. Annals of Plastic Surgery, 80*, 600–606. https://doi.org/10.1097/sap.0000000000001443 (accessed on 14th July 2025).

RHINOPLASTY (NOSE SURGERY)

6

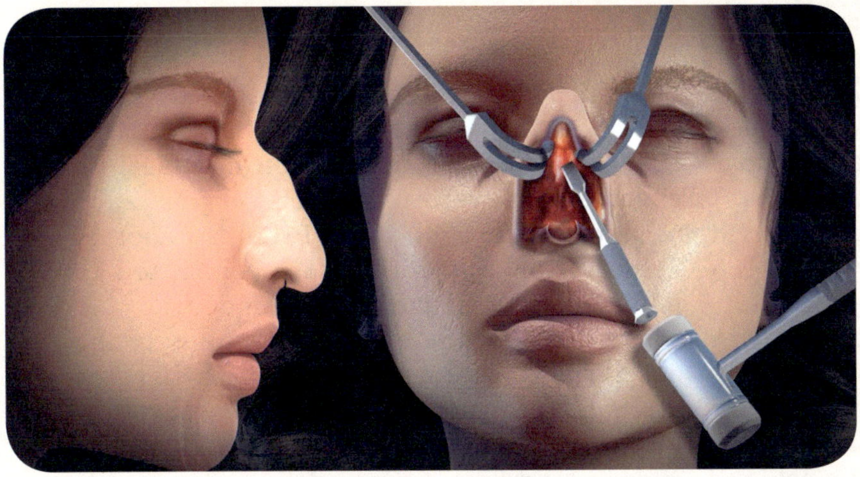

LEARNING OBJECTIVES

After studying this chapter, you will be able to:

1. Describe categories of rhinoplasty;
2. Describe indications of rhinoplasty;
3. Emphasize the process of rhinoplasty;
4. Understand risks and complications in rhinoplasty (nose surgery);
5. Evaluate the psychological effect of rhinoplasty;
6. Study cultural attitudes towards rhinoplasty.

Introduction

Rhinoplasty, also known as nose surgery, has emerged as one of the most sought-after cosmetic surgeries of contemporary medicine. This three-dimensional process is not merely aesthetic; it is a functional correction that can significantly improve the life of a patient. Individuals visit for rhinoplasty to correct birth defects, trauma, or to reverse aging effects, and this shows the universal appeal of the process. Besides its popularity, rhinoplasty has numerous intricacies that baffle even seasoned surgeons. The subtleties of nasal anatomy and individual notions of beauty demand both form and function acumen in the planning of surgery. Since the demand for rhinoplasty will continue to increase, it is increasingly significant that practitioners remain current with the numerous variables involved in achieving favorable outcomes. In rhinoplasty, both surgical and nonsurgical techniques may be distinguished, each of which is tailored to treat distinct patient needs. Nonsurgical rhinoplasty, or the liquid nose job, is a newer innovation consisting of injectable fillers to temporarily increase nasal contours. It is appropriate for individuals with very slight flaw who may not be ready to undergo invasive surgery. But the key point to bear in mind is that even nonsurgical procedures are not without risks. As the literature reports, the practitioner must possess an extensive knowledge of facial anatomy so as not to endanger the patient with future complications, varying from bruising to major vascular obstruction and skin necrosis (Czach et al., 2024). Thus, both techniques' efficacy and safety depend on the experience of the clinician and the selection of the patient. Also, intrinsic rhinoplasty difficulties present significant challenges to even skilled surgeons. Anatomical variations, aesthetic goals, and pre-existing medical conditions can affect surgical outcomes and risk (Torres & Marianetti, 2016). The danger of possible complications, both minor and significant, increases the burden of the decision for surgery, and therefore informed consent, as well as patient education, becomes most important (Torres & Marianetti, 2016). Improved surgeon-patient communication regarding anticipated outcomes and possible risks can make a more rewarding surgical experience. Ultimately, understanding the nuances of rhinoplasty and varying methodologies provided is essential in ensuring that patients are making entirely informed choices towards receiving surgery. By breaking down these important considerations, this essay hopes to enlighten the reader on the complexity of rhinoplasty and guide prospective patients through their decision.

Definition of Rhinoplasty

The word rhinoplasty, or nose surgery, refers to a variety of surgical procedures intended to enhance the nasal structure's aesthetic and functional characteristics. Typically categorized into two broad types, cosmetic rhinoplasty and reconstructive rhinoplasty, such surgical intervention rectifies not only the way one's nose appears but also its ability to perform its necessary functions, e.g., breathing. Cosmetic rhinoplasty seeks to improve facial harmony, most often by altering or reshaping the shape or size of the nose to address one's aesthetic requirements. Reconstructive rhinoplasty is applied, on the other hand, to repair anatomic deformities resulting from birth defects, injury, or disease and restore function and form. This polarity indicates the multifaceted character of rhinoplasty, which simultaneously accounts for patients' desires for beauty and addresses severe health concerns intrinsic to nasal integrity. In acknowledgment of growing refinement, methods in rhinoplasty have come to reflect a more precise understanding of nasal anatomy and the sophistication necessary to ensure optimal results. Technologies, such as the concept of New Extended Dorsal Preservation Rhinoplasty, are committed to minimal invasion methods intended for the conservation of the original structures of the nose. The new method employs partial and incomplete osteotomies, which allow surgeons to preserve the nasal pyramids integrity while effectively treating aesthetic defects. This type of surgical precision minimizes trauma, therefore making recovery periods shorter as well as providing improved overall aesthetic outcomes for patients. With advancements in rhinoplasty, it becomes increasingly pertinent to integrate holistic principles centered on preservation and modulation of form, highlighting the importance of surgeons being up to date with current techniques and technologies within the specialty (Carvalho et al., 2020). The impacts of rhinoplasty go beyond physical appearance modification, reaching into the individual's quality of life and self-esteem. Studies demonstrate that these procedures have a positive impact on patients self-esteem and interpersonal relationships, but the intricate relationship between aesthetic objectives and psychological health requires special consideration. Consumerism and beauty standards are frequently complicating factors in patients' motivations for elective rhinoplasty. The expense of this surgery and the risk of unrealistic expectations further highlight the necessity for educational activity and ethical practice in the specialty. A multidisciplinary collaborative strategy between surgeons, psychologists, and health authorities can devise a better-informed and nurturing environment for prospective patients navigating through their cosmetic desires and health-related needs (Manole et al., 2023) (Figure 6.1).

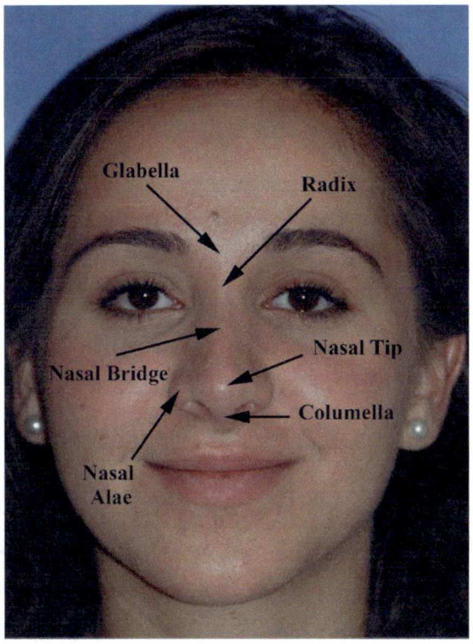

Figure 6.1. The rhinoplasty, commonly referred to as nose surgery.

Source: https://external-content.duckduckgo.com/iu/?u=http%3A%2F%2Fwww.ayoungyou.com%2Fwp-content%2Fuploads%2F2015%2F03%2FRhinoplasty-Anatomy-1.jpg&f=1&nofb=1&ipt=d40686827b64e6d939adca97b14ba9b0e6409844162984ed85a492ec16d7ae7e.

Nose Surgery's Historical Background

Nose surgery, particularly rhinoplasty, has its roots thousands of years old. Nasal surgical manipulation can be traced back to ancient times, where simple procedures were done on injuries or birth defects. The earliest reference to surgical reconstruction procedures of the nose has been quoted through ancient Indian texts, specifically in the Sushruta Samhita around 600 BCE. The classic text mentions several surgical procedures among which is the nasal reconstruction. These early rhinoplasty pioneers set out the role of aesthetics and functional restoration, setting the stage that resonates in modern-day practice. Throughout the centuries, nasal surgery knowledge expanded, driven by cultural and medical advancements in the Arab and European civilizations, which eventually influenced modern practices. Anesthesia and antiseptic treatment in the 19th century introduced a milestone in rhinoplasty practice. Significantly, the operations of surgeons Joseph and Jacques Reverdin served as a starting point for further advanced nasal surgeries. Developments such as the application of skin grafting increased procedure complexity, and surgeons could subsequently achieve better cosmetic and functional outcomes. Furthermore, rhinoplasty began to be considered not only as reconstructive surgery for trauma victims but even as cosmetic treatment for those patients who wanted to enhance their appearance. Facial aesthetics came to be better understood, and surgeons began paying more attention to proportions and harmony among facial elements in their operations. Consequently, by the beginning of the 20th century, rhinoplasty had become well-established as a necessary, two-fold field of surgery treating reconstructive and aesthetic purposes. In modern practice, rhinoplasty has progressed immensely with the use of sophisticated technologies and methods. Surgeons today look to the past while using technology such as computer imaging and minimally invasive methods to enhance outcomes for patients. The techniques have become more individualized, directed against the patient anatomy and desired end result. More recent studies have demonstrated efficacy in a number of grafting methods, such as those utilizing acellular matrices for repair of the nasal septum, which testify to the ongoing evolution of the discipline. Researchers continue to investigate the determinants of surgical success, highlighting the evolution from traditional approaches towards more sophisticated methodologies, and thereby ensuring that the heritage of nasal surgery not only honors its historical past but also ensures a bright future (Saša et al., 2011; Greywoode et al., 2012).

Role of Rhinoplasty in Modern Medicine

The role of rhinoplasty in modern medicine exceeds cosmetic beautification; it is a significant component of reconstructive surgery, particularly for individuals born with conditions, traumatic deformities, or cancer. Rhinoplasty not only restores facial balance and improves looks but also corrects functional imperfections such as impaired breathing. A study refers to how postoperative complications and actual prognostication of such complications can improve patient outcomes, specifically referring to how important it is to have thorough preoperative counseling for potential risks and benefits.

The establishment of the two-faced nature of rhinoplasty as both a cosmetic and reconstructive procedure provides support for its inclusion in existing practices, thereby enhancing patient satisfaction and quality of life among recipients of the procedure (Katatbeh, 2025). Besides, advances in surgical techniques and postoperative care have significantly improved the effectiveness and safety of rhinoplasty. Utilization of minimally invasive techniques, including endonasal techniques, reduces recovery time and improves patient comfort. Furthermore, the utilization of medications such as tranexamic acid and dexamethasone during the perioperative period has been noted to reduce bleeding and accelerate recovery, thus reducing complications following surgery. Importantly, research indicates that routine multivitamin consumption can counteract risks associated with surgery, which suggests the importance of preoperative preparation (Katatbeh, 2025). These technologies provide surgeons with better tools for achieving optimal results and minimizing possible complications, demonstrating the value of rhinoplasty in the grand scheme of modern medicine. With its multifaceted contributions, rhinoplasty can be accurately assessed to be a part of reconstructive and aesthetic surgery in the practice of medicine. The process not only Beautifies the physical shape but also improves nasal function, and therefore overall well-being and health.

The ability to control and prevent postoperative complications using information and preparation is a hallmark of rhinoplasty's evolving face as a surgical discipline. With research keeping techniques and procedures continually current, rhinoplasty remains a mainstay of contemporary medicine, treating an increasingly diverse patient population. As surgical methods evolve, the contribution of rhinoplasty to complete health and quality of life only further solidifies its place in modern medical ideology (Katatbeh, 2025) (Figure 6.2).

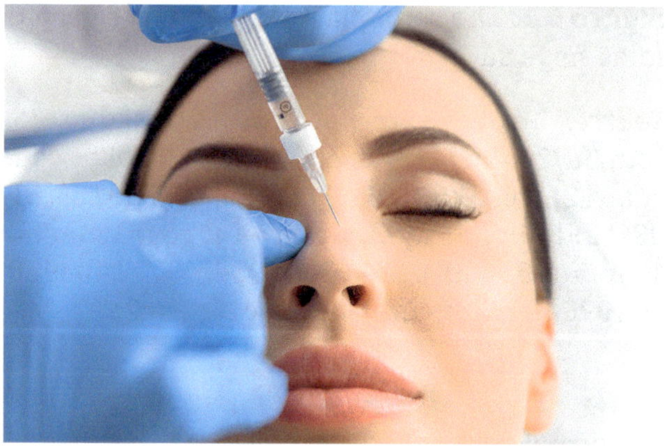

Figure 6.2. Importance of rhinoplasty in modern medicine.

Source: https://www.medicaim.com/uploads/f28beda0-5a45-11e8-8fc5-bf61b50ce761/rhinoplastiemedicale.jpg.

6.1. Types of Rhinoplasty

Learning Outcome

1. Explain the Primary vs. Secondary Rhinoplasty
2. Focus on Open vs. Closed Rhinoplasty Techniques
3. Differentiate Cosmetic vs. Functional Rhinoplasty

Rhinoplasty is composed of a variety of surgical procedures and operations specific to addressing both functional and cosmetic problems of the nose, which can be generalized into two types: cosmetic and reconstructive rhinoplasty. Cosmetic rhinoplasty is simply for enhancing the appearance of the nose, patients being capable of achieving their ideal look through modifications such as the alteration of the nose tip, its bridge, or the correction of asymmetry. In contrast, reconstructive rhinoplasty is typically performed to restore form and function after traumatic injury, congenital deformity, or previous surgical misfortune. Such cases may involve complex structural reconstruction, underscoring the absolute correlation between accurate assessment of nasal anatomy and execution of surgical maneuvers. Surgeons should be aware of these distinctions, as they directly influence preoperative planning and optimal results in rhinoplasty procedures. Challenging rhinoplasty cases, such as those of facial cleft patients, require handling with a highly meticulous approach to planning and operation, given the unpredictability of involved anatomical structures. Deployment of new technologies, such as three-dimensional imaging, has revolutionized practice by allowing greater preoperative evaluation and strategy planning. With a bottom-up approach, starting with the restoration of the basic osseous framework before addressing the soft tissue, surgeons are able to produce more uniform outcomes. With this novel approach, the ability to combine various advanced techniques is facilitated to produce a wholesome workflow that utilizes computer-aided planning along with intraoperative navigation. Therefore, these innovations not only enhance the precision of surgical interventions but also ensure that patients are treated with a tailored approach that caters to their specific anatomical requirements, with the overall outcome being more satisfying outcomes in complex cases (Codazzi et al., 2019). Aesthetic reasoning constitutes a significant component of rhinoplasty, where harmony of the face and overall beauty are pursued.

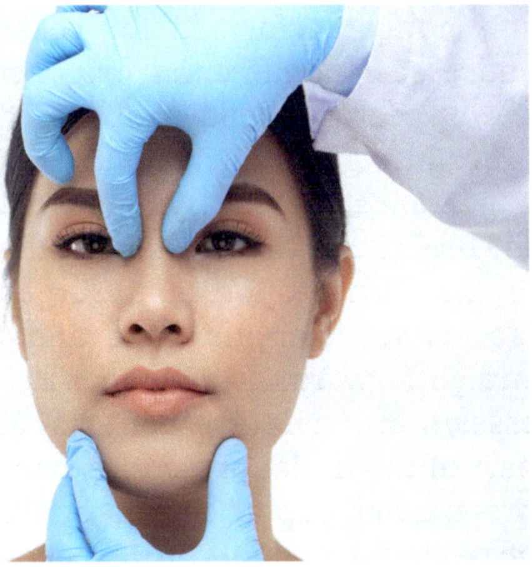

Figure 6.3. Rhinoplasty encompasses a variety of surgical techniques.

Source: https://www.drmarco.com/wp-content/uploads/2024/09/blog-rhinoplasty-c-2048x1389.jpg.

The most recent advances in surgical planning technology have added quantitative analysis to help evaluate and enhance facial attractiveness through comparison to a good facial features database. The new technology allows for data-based decision-making regarding the alterations needed to improve a patient's nose profile in proportion to their face as a whole. By applying morphing technology to implant features of beautiful noses onto patients, surgeons are able to create solutions that promote facial symmetry and proportion.

Inclusion of these aesthetic concerns in rhinoplasty elicits a patient-centered response, allowing for results to address individual desires as well as more general ideas about beauty and attractiveness (Bottino et al., 2008) (Figure 6.3).

6.1.1. Primary vs. Secondary Rhinoplasty

It is important to understand the distinction between primary and secondary rhinoplasty in order to fully realize the complexities of nose surgery. Primary rhinoplasty, which is most commonly performed for cosmetic reasons, addresses fundamental problems concerning the appearance and shape of the nose. The procedure generally aims to enhance the nasal appearance, correct asymmetries, or reestablish the bridge and tip. Because primary rhinoplasty is the initial operation, surgeons generally face fewer complications and have a more straightforward aesthetic goal. However, in some cases, functional corrections may also form a vital part of the initial procedure, particularly when pre-existing septal defects or difficulties with breathing are found on inspection. Secondary rhinoplasty, however, is the repair of issues from a previous nasal procedure. This type of surgery is even more difficult since the anatomy has been altered due to prior surgery. The secondary rhinoplasty poses many challenges, often encompassing scar tissue, structurally altered cartilage, or damaged functions that were not adequately addressed in the initial surgery. As discussed in more recent literature, techniques of functional rhinoplasty have since broadened to include certain corrections of nasal valve collapse, possibly compounded or even caused by prior surgeries (Chan & Shipchandler, 2015). Such intricacies therefore, demonstrate the importance of an exceedingly skilled surgeon capable of addressing the nuances of the nasal complex while maintaining both cosmetic and functional outcomes. The combination of artistic and functional goals is particularly relevant in secondary rhinoplasty patients, which not only aims to repair an aesthetically pleasing look but also functional respiration. Studies show that secondary patients tend to have a higher risk of complications and less consistent outcomes (Cuomo et al., 2024). Surgeons will need to utilize thorough assessment methods to assess both aesthetic outcomes and satisfaction in such patients. Objective evaluation and proven assessment scales have been touted as valuable tools for measuring postoperative changes, especially in functional rhinoplasty environments. With these considerations in mind, secondary rhinoplasty continues to be a dynamic entity that requires advanced techniques and customized approaches in order to realize the optimal outcome with minimal complications (Figure 6.4).

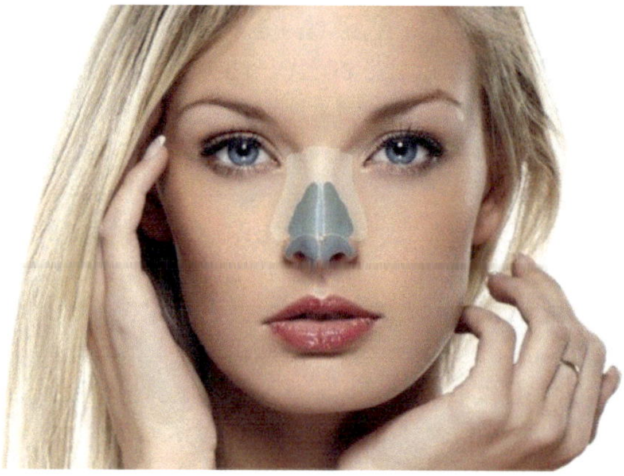

Figure 6.4. The distinctions between primary and secondary rhinoplasty.

Source: https://southdelhicosmeticclinic.net/wp-content/uploads/2017/05/The-Perfect-Nose-Shape-with-Rhinoplasty-Surgery-in-Delhi.jpg.

6.1.2. Open vs. Closed Rhinoplasty Techniques

The controversy over open vs closed rhinoplasty techniques is at the heart of nasal surgery practice, not only defining surgical outcomes but also patient satisfaction. Open rhinoplasty is characterized by an external cut, often along the columella, to offer greater visibility and access to the nasal internal structures. This technique gives the surgeon the freedom to perform overall readjustments and fine-tunings exactly, so it is better suited for complex deformities. There are inherent risks to this method, including scarring and potential nerve damage, that can cause postoperative complications and have negative effects on aesthetic results. The choice between the methods often is dependent upon the surgeon's experience and patient-specific anatomical factors, underscoring the importance of custom surgical planning to maximize outcomes most effectively. Closed rhinoplasty employs incisions inside the nostrils, which lead to less visible scarring and a shorter recovery time. This approach is typically chosen for simpler procedures since there is visibility to the nasal structures to be manipulated without significant dissection. Nevertheless, the disadvantages of closed rhinoplasty are very real; visibility is poor, which can make it difficult to have a whole new set of changes and lead to undesirable outcomes in complex cases. Anatomical accuracy becomes hard to achieve, and this reinforces skepticism regarding the effectiveness of this technique in extreme cases of corrections required. Recent studies have revealed that while closed techniques can reduce recovery and scarring, they generally fail to offer the same level of anatomical information as open techniques, particularly in difficult nasal reconstruction cases. The growing emphasis on outcomes in rhinoplasty surgery measures the performance of such techniques valuable. Recent research has looked towards the Rhinoplasty Outcome Evaluation (ROE) as it systematically assesses patient satisfaction and surgical outcome using different methods. Systematic review information suggests that open rhinoplasty tends to produce superior results where complex procedures are involved, noting a significant difference between preoperative and postoperative measurements. The research takes into consideration how a given surgical technique might influence not only anatomical precision but subjective patient satisfaction following surgery. As the field continues to evolve, the strengths and limitations of open versus closed approaches must be understood, eventually enhancing the practice of rhinoplasty surgery in the future and aligning with patient needs (Bertossi et al., 2022).

6.1.3. Cosmetic vs. Functional Rhinoplasty

Nose surgery or rhinoplasty has both cosmetic and functional indications. Cosmetic rhinoplasty is primarily concerned with altering the aesthetic appearance of the nose to create facial harmony. Patients are typically subjected to this operation for repairing perceived imperfections such as unevenly sized noses, nasal bumps, or other deviations that compromise self-esteem and body image.

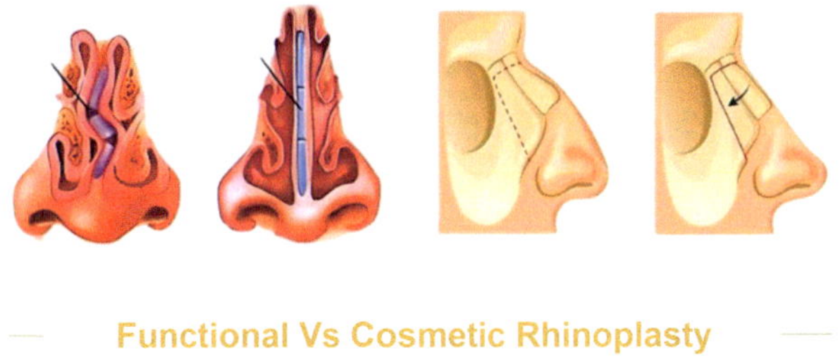

Figure 6.5. Cosmetic vs. functional rhinoplasty.

Source: https://ethnic-rhinoplasty.com/wp-content/uploads/2025/01/Functional-Rhinoplasty-Vs-Cosmetic-Rhinoplasty.webp.

The psychological effect of cosmetic rhinoplasty may be considerable in that patients' self-confidence and contentment with appearance increase following surgery. Plastic surgeons need to address patient expectations, ensuring individuals have realistic hopes concerning the results of surgery (Kalaskar et al., 2016). Conversely, functional rhinoplasty aims to fix structural issues that disrupt normal breathing. Nasal obstruction, chronic sinusitis, or a deviated septum are conditions that could necessitate surgery to improve airflow and alleviate pain. Such surgery is typically performed by patients who want symptom improvement for relief from breathing discomfort as opposed to cosmetic enhancement. Functional rhinoplasty surgeons must be competent in nasal anatomy and form-function relationship. Success in functional rhinoplasty relies heavily on the restoration of optimal airway mechanics with minimal aesthetic alteration. The clinician thus has to be both a skilled surgeon and anatomist so that patients have both functional and acceptable results (Anesi et al., 2014). The distinction between cosmetic and functional rhinoplasty highlights the multidisciplinary nature of nasal surgery, stressing the importance of careful patient assessment as well as individualized treatment plans. Certain patients may be seeking both functional and cosmetic improvement, but surgeons also need to examine why the surgery is being done. In the majority of cases, the combination of cosmetic augmentation and functional return will yield superior outcomes, maximizing patient satisfaction in both aspects. Multi-disciplinary surgeries, with the combined efforts of plastic surgeons and otolaryngologists, can also enhance the surgical outcome by addressing any inherent functional complications while simultaneously achieving cosmetic goals (Kalaskar et al., 2016). This holistic approach to rhinoplasty not only mirrors the complex nature of nose surgery but also ensures that patients receive holistic treatment designed to their specific needs (Figure 6.5).

Test Your Knowledge

1. How does primary rhinoplasty differ from secondary (revision) rhinoplasty in terms of purpose and complexity?
2. What are the main differences between open and closed rhinoplasty techniques, and when might each be preferred?
3. How do the goals of cosmetic rhinoplasty differ from those of functional rhinoplasty?

6.2. Indications for Rhinoplasty

Learning Outcome

1. Discuss the Aesthetic Concerns and Personal Preferences
2. Explain the Medical Reasons, Such as Breathing Difficulties
3. Focus on Trauma or Injury to the Nose

The decision to undergo rhinoplasty, or reconstruction of the nose, is largely based on aesthetic and functional indications. Aesthetic considerations are usually the primary concern, as most individuals desire to enhance the appearance of the nose for the purposes of having a more harmonious face. The most commonly seen aesthetic problems are width, length, and nasal profile abnormalities that may result in facial asymmetry. Moreover, desired adjustments can range from subtleties to as much as reconstructions, up to as much as patients' diverse tastes and wishes permit. Lastly, the extent to which a person's self-esteem and self-assurance are influenced by his or her nasal shape highlights the psychological nature of such aesthetic reasons for rhinoplasty, putting the procedure not merely as a bodily transformation but as a move toward improving self-esteem and quality of life (Tasman, 2008). Apart from aesthetic purposes, there are also functional purposes that play a significant role in the consideration of rhinoplasty. Most patients present with structural abnormalities such as a deviated septum or nasal obstructions that compromise breathing efficiency. These functional impairments can lead to ongoing sinusitis, sleep apnea, or snoring, which can significantly alter one's lifestyle. Rhinoplasty can correct these functional issues along with cosmetic corrections, making it feasible to treat the conditions in two ways. For instance, the use of surgical techniques that repair both anatomic abnormality and cosmetic deformity is used to treat a holistic understanding of the patient's needs. Research has yielded favorable results in terms of both aesthetics and function, as evidenced by significant improvements in quality of life indicators after surgery (Bashir et al., 2023). The varied indications for rhinoplasty reflect the intricacy of the procedure, and it necessitates careful preoperative evaluation and patient counseling. Surgeons must take a thoughtful approach to each patient's personalized goals, anatomical considerations, and history to ideally tailor the surgical plan. The significance of thoughtful planning and surgical precision is underscored by the challenges that are present in achieving acceptable results that can be highly variable depending on individual circumstances (Tasman, 2008). As patients become increasingly enabled to pursue individualized solutions for nasal problems, the popularity of rhinoplasty continues to skyrocket. This change emphasizes the need for ongoing research and development in techniques that take into consideration both the functional need and cosmetic demand of patients who need rhinoplasty in order to develop an overall understanding of their treatment objectives (Figure 6.6).

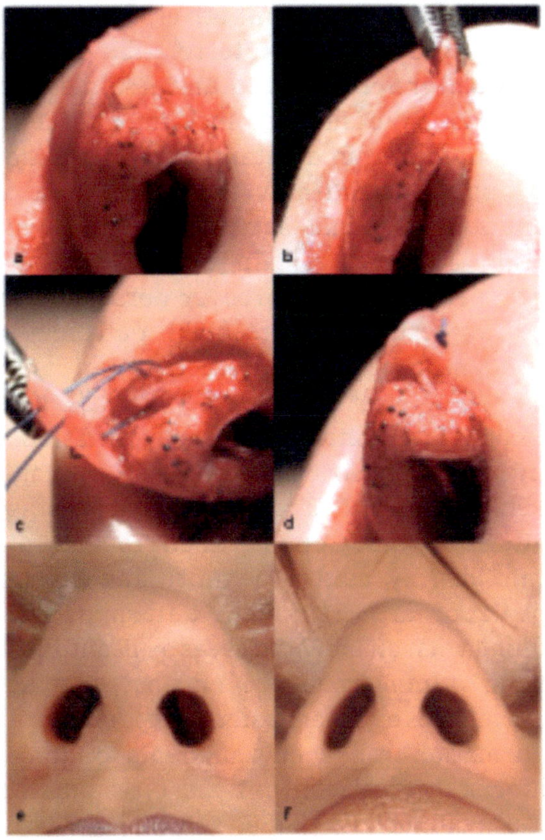

Figure 6.6. The decision to undergo rhinoplasty.

Source: https://www.scienceopen.com/document_file/39df1cd1-d07c-4953-9c68-25d0dff5d8f8/PubMedCentral/large.png.

6.2.1. Aesthetic Concerns and Personal Preferences

The intersection of individual preferences and aesthetic considerations is also a key consideration in whether a person decides to get rhinoplasty. Individuals who get this procedure also generally say that they wish to achieve societal beauty norms, which are generally established by media presentation and cultural expectations. Such standards can define what is beautiful, and hence, the patients undergo the enhancements that can boost their self-esteem and social status. Research has shown that beauty is largely founded on objective attributes that are quantitatively measurable, suggesting a complex interrelation between individual preferences and universal aesthetic standards. By examining such an interaction, one can better understand the motivations of rhinoplasty and how the motivations are shaped by external societal factors, which in turn reaffirm certain beauty standards (Kagian et al., 2010). Moreover, personal tastes regarding aesthetically acceptable outcomes can vary significantly from person to person, so consultation is critical in rhinoplasty. Surgeons prefer to have patients express expectations in words by emphasizing shared decision-making to achieve results that satisfy personal aesthetic goals. As the study of body changes illustrates, ethnic identity, cultural identity, and personal experience are significant determinants in defining what an individual sees as beautiful and desirable. Immigrants, for instance, may seek some changes as a manifestation of identification confirmation in new environments, seeking to conform to local conventions or claim their cultural uniqueness (Ennes et al., 2018). This is an illustration of the multi-dimensional nature of beauty as an individual experience, necessitating practitioners to tread these subtleties with caution while counseling potential procedural impacts. The expansion of aesthetic surgery, including rhinoplasty, signals a more pervasive shift toward consumerism in society, wherein appearance has become a significant commodity. Patients view rhinoplasty as an investment in their own appearance, and desire to develop a sophisticated aesthetic that approaches contemporary ideals. The integration of newer technologies and techniques in cosmetic surgery has further augmented these options, allowing greater degrees of customization of surgical outcomes based on personal preference. But this commercialization of beauty is problematic in terms of implications for authenticity and pressures of conformity to a perpetually shifting definition of beauty. Critics argue that such dynamics may be used to perpetuate unrealistic beauty ideals, challenging the notion of self-acceptance and the forces driving individuals into surgery (Kagian et al., 2010). Consequently, the landscape of rhinoplasty must be carefully examined in order to gain an understanding of the impact of cosmetic problems in a consumerist society.

6.2.2. Medical Reasons, Such as Breathing Difficulties

Medical reasons for rhinoplasty extend past cosmetic improvements, and one prominent driver of rhinoplasty is the alleviation of respiratory issues. Patients with obstructive conditions, such as a deviated septum or other nasal passage structural defects, frequently complain of chronic airflow issues. These structural issues can create a variety of complications, such as chronic sinusitis, sleep apnea, and overall compromised respiratory function. By undergoing rhinoplasty, individuals not only achieve cosmetic benefits but also restore and increase their respiratory health. This dual benefit emphasizes the importance of rhinoplasty in treating medical issues that truly affect the patient's health. A study that examined the nasal deformity procedures shows the necessity of tackling medical requirements alongside cosmetic requirements. For instance, the study indicated that several patients with septal deviation considerably improved in terms of nasal function after receiving rhinoplasty. This shows the effectiveness and necessity of the surgical procedure, particularly when applied in redemptive cases with patients who experience allied conditions. The open rhinoplasty approach, as it has been examined in research in recent years, is an example of greater sensibility for the connection between aesthetics and functional reconstruction, both the physical and psychological dimensions of patient care (Včeva et al., 2019). Rhinoplasty, in other words, can be an anchor procedure for both aesthetic and airway enhancement. Moreover, advancements in rhinoplasty surgery and an understanding of the physiology of the nose have enabled surgeons to now treat more complex sleep breathing disorders. Modern surgical procedures now include a broader scope of considerations, such as medical reasoning in aesthetic treatment. For instance, extensive study of nasal anatomy has revealed correlations of nasal anomalies with conditions such as sleep apnea, and rhinoplasty can thus act as an appropriate type of relief for symptoms (Kalaskar et al., 2016). This collision of the aesthetic and the medical necessity keeps the case strong for rhinoplasty as a multifaceted procedure, beneficial not only for beauty but also for evening out the physiological activity of the nasal passages, ultimately leading to improved overall health outcomes. Thus, the worth of rhinoplasty cannot be overstated for restoring function as well as quality of life enhancement (Figure 6.7).

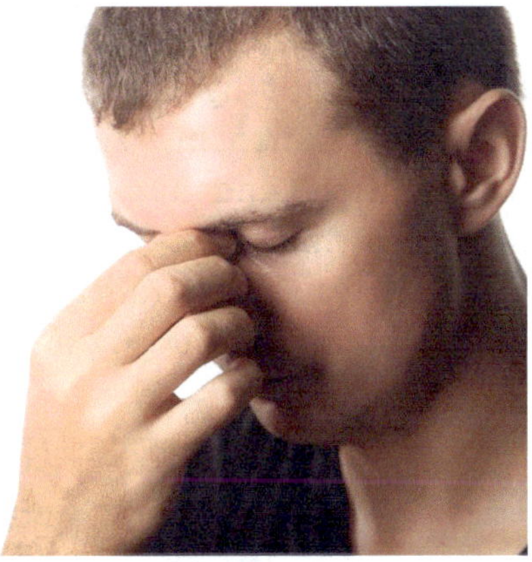

Figure 6.7. Medical reasons for rhinoplasty extend beyond aesthetic improvements.

Source: https://external-content.duckduckgo.com/iu/?u=https%3A%2F%2Fwww.impressionschicago.com%2Fhs-fs%2Fhubfs%2FImported_Blog_Media%2FConsultation-and-Considerations-for-Rhinoplasty-for-Breathing-Problems.jpg%3Fwidth%3D1500%26height%3D1001%26name%3DConsultation-and-Considerations-for-Rhinoplasty-for-Breathing-Problems.jpg&f=1&nofb=1&ipt=999c3396c5b785470bd9d0eef260b6482f01f00afa5d3b22b55ff8f23dbae15d.

6.2.3. Trauma or Injury to the Nose

Trauma or injury to the nose is a frequent clinical problem, most frequently resulting from accidents, sports, or violent crimes. The trauma can range in severity, leading not only to physical impairment but also to immense psychological impact on individuals subjected to it. Specifically, nasal trauma mainly appears as fractures, cuts, or bruises, all of which need personalized treatment. The incidence is also very common among youth, where their lifestyle exposes them to more vulnerability. A study has indicated that foreign bodies are the cause of most nose trauma, along with road traffic injuries, and this needs more public education and protective gear (Okoye et al., 2013).

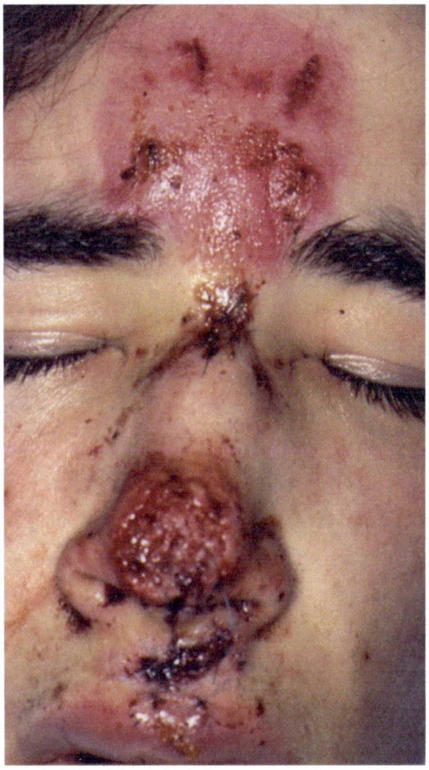

Figure 6.8. Trauma or injury to the nose.

Source: https://media.springernature.com/lw685/springer-static/image/chp%3A10.1007%2F978-3-031-14915-3_6/MediaObjects/525286_1_En_6_Fig5_HTML.jpg.

Identification and early management of the traumas are crucial, since late treatment can lead to complications such as chronic pain, respiratory distress, or cosmetic deformity and could even require the application of surgical procedures like rhinoplasty. Rhinoplasty not only serves as a corrective procedure for aesthetic purposes, but it is also a significant intervention to address nasal function in the case of trauma. Surgical techniques have advanced to the point where subtlety and care in addressing both structural and aesthetic details of nasal reconstruction are accommodated. With extensive trauma, rhinoplasty can be combined with other operations to correct underlying lesions like airway obstruction or collapse of the structure. The reconstruction aims to recreate the nasal anatomy to the original position and shape, along with maximum function. Notably, grafts and biomaterial integration in contemporary rhinoplasty have enhanced the possibility for functional and aesthetically pleasing results in instances of severe trauma, restoring function, as well as beauty (Lazim et al., 2019). As a therapy, both functionally and aesthetically driven, it not only promotes physical recovery but enables the patient to become psychologically whole again with the elimination of fear over appearance after trauma. An appreciation of the impact of nasal trauma reveals the importance of multifaceted management plans in rhinoplasty. Apart from the physical injury, the impacts of the trauma carry over to social and emotional fronts, affecting the quality of one's living. Moreover, such patients with severe nasal injuries also suffer from breathing, speaking, or even sleeping difficulties, necessitating multidimensional treatment plans. The operations are not solely cosmetic reconstruction; they are about enhancing general welfare by restoring normalcy and confidence in individuals after traumatic experiences (Okoye et al., 2013). To this end, rhinoplasty emerges as a central intervention that marries medical expertise with psychological finesse to help patients navigate through the adversity brought about by their trauma. Finally, the intricate relationship among trauma, surgical intervention, and healing proves the strong impact of rhinoplasty in enhancing the impact of nasal trauma, guiding patients towards a better quality of life (Figure 6.8).

Test Your Knowledge

1. What aesthetic concerns or personal preferences might lead someone to consider rhinoplasty?
2. Which medical conditions, such as breathing difficulties, can indicate the need for rhinoplasty?
3. How can trauma or injury to the nose serve as a reason for undergoing rhinoplasty?

6.3. The Rhinoplasty Procedure

Learning Outcome

1. Discuss the Pre-Operative Consultation and Assessment
2. Explain the Surgical Techniques and Anesthesia Options
3. Focus on Post-Operative Care and Recovery Process

Rhinoplasty or nose surgery consists of both aesthetic and reconstructive objectives that aim to enhance facial harmony. This operation fixes a range of problems, from strictly cosmetic advantages such as size and shape adjustments to more medically useful improvements that can fix breathing issues. The most difficult thing about rhinoplasty is that it's a two-for-one operation: not only must surgeons fix the external appearance of the nose, but they also have to make sure its internal function remains or is improved upon. As highlighted by various surgical texts, a successful rhinoplasty requires advanced understanding of nasal attractiveness and human anatomy, with an emphasis on the role played by individualized treatment schemes that accommodate the unique facial structure and desire of every patient (Bottino et al., 2012). The most advanced technologies have also transformed the approach to rhinoplasty. New techniques, such as 3D simulation, allow surgeons to visualize the potential result before the operation and ensure better planning. Advanced systems that compare patients' characteristics with a database of harmonious faces aid surgeons in recommending changes that would create aesthetically pleasing results while preserving function (Bottino et al., 2012). Such technology offers a basis for knowledgeable interaction between patient and surgeon, so that expectations are harmonized. Thus, contemporary rhinoplasty is not so much a surgical makeover but an interactive process based on art and science. In dealing with the subtleties of rhinoplasty, surgeons also need to be well-informed in handling complications and post-treatment care. Every surgery has inherent risks, and meticulous preoperative evaluations are crucial in determining potential difficulties. Immaculate comprehension of the numerous tissues—like cartilage and skin—is critical to a successful outcome, as is the expertise to tackle difficulties such as saddle nose deformity and other conditions that go with it (Kalaskar et al., 2016). Post-operative follow-up is crucial to monitor the progress of recovery and ensure the desired outcome is attained over time. Therefore, rhinoplasty surgery is the culmination of technical skill and understanding of patient needs, emphasizing the need for ongoing education and adaptation in this ever-evolving subspecialty of plastic surgery (Figure 6.9).

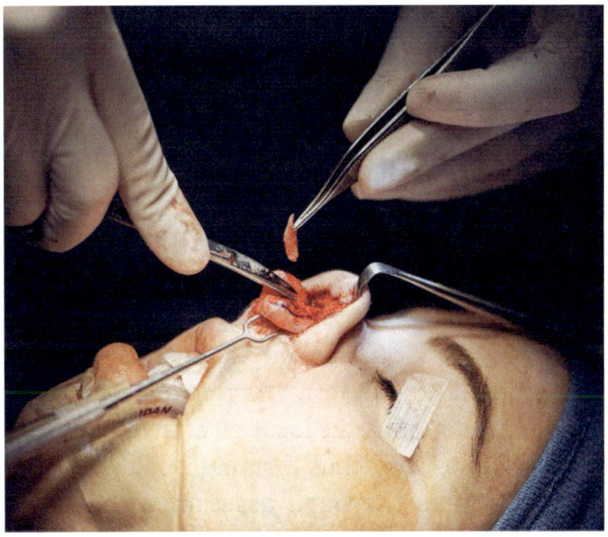

Figure 6.9. The rhinoplasty procedure.

Source: https://media.allure.com/photos/5b58d3e0f85b921a2ff2edda/master/w_1600%2Cc_limit/life-in-plastic-rhinoplasty-first-person-12.jpg.

6.3.1. Pre-Operative Consultation and Assessment

Pre-operative consultation is an essential part of the rhinoplasty process, being the foundation for both operative outcomes and patient satisfaction. In the initial consultation, surgeons engage in thorough discussions with patients regarding the indication for surgery, as well as their expectations and objectives. This is an important conversation, as it acts to reconcile the patient's desires with the ability of the surgeon, ultimately establishing realistic expectations of outcome. Further, the consultation allows one to consider the patient's history, thereby addressing any pre-existing medical issues. Pre-operative management of these expectations has been found to significantly affect post-operative satisfaction and emphasizes the significance of the step in the surgical procedure (Hummelink et al., 2024).

A physical exam and imaging studies are also typically included in the pre-operative assessment and help in gaining valuable information about the patient's nasal anatomy. These findings allow the surgeon to create an individualized surgery plan considering the unique structural characteristics of the nose. For instance, some factors such as cartilage thickness and nasal bone shape may have direct implications for surgical approaches and desired outcomes. With prior knowledge, surgeons can estimate complications and make recommendations. It is imperative that the patients understand the location of their anatomy during the surgery, thus forming a collaborative approach. This thorough assessment not only enables the surgeon to be more accurate with surgical interventions but also enhances the confidence level of the patient as well as the surgeon (Hummelink et al., 2024). There is also the contribution of psychosocial factors to the pre-operative consultation because they can influence the choice of operation and the patient's expectations of the outcome. Surgeons will typically employ validated questionnaires to assess the psychological readiness of the patient and the patient's overall satisfaction with how they look. Studies indicate that patients with previous cosmetic surgery or those above the age of 30 might achieve different levels of satisfaction than younger individuals or those with no past surgical history. The understanding of such demographic factors is important for surgeons in order to effectively manage expectations throughout the consultation process. With these psychosocial considerations, healthcare providers can help patients make proper decisions, thus leading to higher rates of satisfaction following surgery (Hummelink et al., 2024).

6.3.2. Surgical Techniques and Anesthesia Options

In choosing rhinoplasty, it is extremely necessary to learn about the various surgical techniques to achieve maximum aesthetic as well as functional outcomes. For rhinoplasty, surgeons can choose open or closed rhinoplasty techniques, and both have various advantages. Open rhinoplasty entails making a small cut across the columella, allowing better visibility and access to intricate nasal structures. This is particularly beneficial for very complex cases where there is extensive sculpting of the nose tip or structural deformities. Closed rhinoplasty offers incisions that are limited to the nasal passages' interior and may result in minimal scarring.

This approach is usually the better one for less complex cases, having the advantage of quicker recovery times while maintaining the potential for good results. The choice of surgical technique, in the end, is based on a person's specific anatomical needs and objectives, with preoperative consultation of greatest importance to determine the best approach. The choice of anesthesia for rhinoplasty also influences patient comfort and safety during the procedure. Local anesthesia with sedation is commonly applied by surgeons to less invasive techniques, which provide adequate pain management without the risk associated with general anesthesia. This technique is most attractive to patients opting for in-office treatments because it has the possibility of avoiding the risk associated with complications with deeper sedation and the need for an operating room setting. On the other hand, general anesthesia is usually recommended for more complex surgeries, where the control of pain in general and immobility is necessary. This method usually involves an anesthesiologist who keeps a close eye on the patient's vital parameters throughout the process, thereby establishing a higher level of security while operating. The growing need for in-office procedures also reflects a change in patient preferences, where they want efficient treatment without compromising their comfort and safety (Kao et al., 2019). Further, advancements in minimally invasive techniques have made rhinoplasty more popular among various groups, particularly women who require aesthetic enhancement (King et al., 2013). This trend is an indication of the importance of molding both surgery and anesthesia techniques to the individual needs of patients, as well as responding to their cosmetic desires.

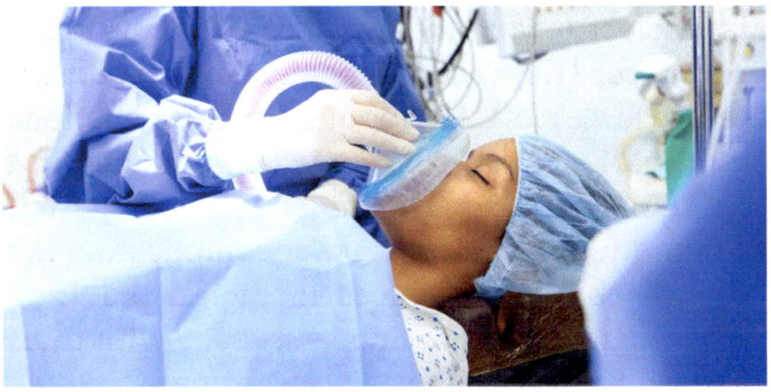

Figure 6.10. Surgical techniques and anesthesia options.

Source: https://ethnic-rhinoplasty.com/wp-content/uploads/2024/09/png-1.webp.

With the emergence of more advanced surgical techniques, such as ultrasound-augmented techniques, surgeons are now able to create extremely precise outcomes that preserve nasal integrity and cosmetics. Additionally, the presence of digital imaging modalities aids the surgeon in preoperative planning such that there is harmonious communication between the physician and patient regarding the expected results. With rhinoplasty as a specialty advancing, the synergy of advanced surgical expertise and differing modalities of anesthesia ensures improved patient outcome and satisfaction, highlighting the need for ongoing education and research in nasal surgery (Figure 6.10).

6.3.3. Post-Operative Care and Recovery Process

Successful post-operative therapy is crucial for complete recovery following rhinoplasty, a procedure to enhance both functional and aesthetic characteristics of the nose. Following surgery, patients typically experience swelling, bruising, and pain, which can be managed using the prescribed drugs and cold compresses. The initial days following surgery are critical as they set the tone for recovery.

Patients need to maintain their head in an elevated position to reduce swelling and should shun intense physical exertions that might complicate the recovery process. Avoiding such demands plays a large role in patient outcomes and satisfaction with the recovery outcome. Follow-up with the surgeon is undertaken routinely to check on healing and any complications that may have arisen. It is during such follow-up visits that the surgeon will check the area of surgery for infection, test the integrity of the nasal structure, and modify post-surgery instructions as may be necessary.

Patients must also report any unusual symptoms they experience, such as bleeding or pain, so intervention can be made before complications set in. A well-planned follow-up increases openness in the healing process, allowing patients to be constantly informed and active in their recovery after rhinoplasty. Emotional rehabilitation after rhinoplasty cannot be downplayed, as psychological satisfaction has a great effect on how patients perceive post-operative results. Support from friends and family during this time can maximize emotional strength and manage anticipated anxiety over physical alteration. Further still, education about the potential for early dissatisfaction from swelling and the gradual maturing of outcomes is also able to temper expectation. Human psychological preparedness is improved by pre-operative consultations, where realistic presentations of post-surgical outcomes are discussed. As recovery unfolds, patients can find solace in the fact that patience is the key, and that final results will gradually reveal themselves over the course of a given time, to lead to higher satisfaction rates in the end (Giorgi et al., 1987; Kalaskar et al., 2016).

Test Your Knowledge

1. What key factors are assessed during the pre-operative consultation for rhinoplasty?
2. What are the main surgical techniques and anesthesia options used in rhinoplasty?
3. What are the essential post-operative care steps and typical recovery milestones following rhinoplasty?

6.4. Risks and Complications

Learning Outcome

1. Discuss the Common Risks Associated with Surgery
2. Explain the Potential Complications Specific to Rhinoplasty
3. Focus on Importance of Choosing a Qualified Surgeon

The process of rhinoplasty, while often sought after for cosmetic or functional enhancement, inherently carries no risks and complications. Many variables are involved in the unpredictable outcomes of surgery, including the surgeon's experience, patient anatomy, and individualized healing patterns. Postoperative deformities are among the great concerns where patients' preoperative expectations for the surgery are not elicited by the resulting result. This indicates the need for extensive preoperative consultation and realistic expectations to avoid dissatisfaction and the possibility for corrective procedures (Hernandez et al., 2010). In addition, the psychological impact of such complications on the patient's self-concept is profound because complications lead to a longer recovery period and emotional distress, further complicating the surgical course. Advances in digital planning technologies have provided surgeons with tools to enhance preoperative assessment, which ultimately affects the risk of complications for the surgery. One study indicated that the application of a three-dimensional radiologic viewer during consultations resulted in improved decision-making for surgery among patients, and consequently, postoperative reinterventions were reduced (Hernandez et al., 2010). The inclusion of technology facilitates visualization of the intricate anatomy of nasal structures and improves patient-surgeon communication. Consequently, these technologies have not only improved levels of patient satisfaction but also minimized the stress of surgery, thereby leading to fewer complications in the postoperative period. Nonetheless, despite all these breakthroughs, there are still risks that are intrinsic in surgery, necessitating that thorough surgical planning be adhered to. Complications following rhinoplasty can range from as mild as nasal congestion and swelling to as severe as infection, scarring, or disturbance in skin texture. While most patients would experience only acceptable side effects, others would experience long-term effects that significantly alter their results. Furthermore, the risk of functional complications, such as airway obstruction due to nasal passage alteration, can act inversely on the outcome and on the quality of life of the patient. Surgeons and patients must engage in lengthy dialogue regarding these risks prior to surgery, thus reinforcing the importance of informed consent. Appreciation of the intricate character of rhinoplasty complications and their importance highlights the importance of thorough operative planning and realistic expectations towards results, thereby ensuring that patients are adequately prepared for the adversity encountered post-surgery (Rettinger, 2008).

6.4.1. Common Risks Associated with Surgery

Surgery, and indeed rhinoplasty, is mostly followed by several risks to be carefully considered by potential patients. One of the biggest concerns is infection, which may occur after surgery and may necessitate additional treatment or longer recovery times. Aggressive methods of sterilization and antibiotics will minimize the risk, but even so, the risk of an infection is still a risk to all surgeries. Furthermore, patients may also experience problems with anesthesia, ranging from small reactions to severe allergic responses. These risks illustrate the necessity for appropriate preoperative screening and patient communication with the surgical team to ensure that patients are adequately informed about outcomes and prepared in the event of contingencies. Ultimately, understanding these risks allows patients to make informed decisions about rhinoplasty to ensure their overall safety and satisfaction with the procedure. Besides infection and anesthetic complications, rhinoplasty has special risks such as less than ideal aesthetic result or the necessity. Surgeons may not deliver the ideal outcome and thus create patient dissatisfaction and potential desire for corrective surgeries. This is more applicable in aesthetic surgery when expectations are subjective in nature. Moreover, the healing process is not always guaranteed; patients can experience complications like scarring, asymmetry, or nasal function deviation. All these outcomes serve to emphasize the role of patient-surgeon communication, in which creating realistic expectations is paramount. Clear descriptions of the risk of revisional surgery or the probability of needing other procedures are likely to prevent disappointment and orient decision-making for those considering rhinoplasty. Another major aspect of rhinoplasty is vascular complication risk, particularly when it comes to nonsurgical approaches like nonsurgical rhinoplasty (NSR). While NSR may seem less aggressive, it still has its own associated risks, including necrosis of the skin and, in very rare cases, blindness due to vascular occlusion. These severe complications demand an intimate understanding of facial anatomy on the practitioner's part because mistakes in procedure during injection can lead to devastating outcomes. As indicated by research, the level of experience and anatomical familiarity on the practitioner's part determine the extent to which risks are mitigated while performing the procedure. Awareness of such serious complications not only serves potential patients with the full range of risks involved but also highlights the importance of selecting a qualified and experienced practitioner for any form of rhinoplasty, surgical or nonsurgical, to ensure patient safety and efficacy of results (Czach et al., 2024) (Figure 6.11).

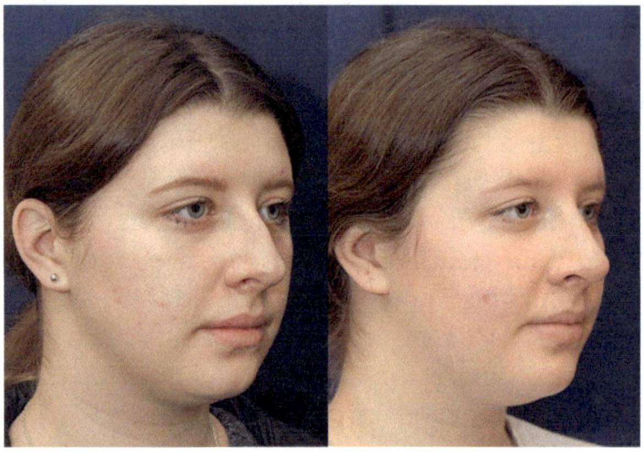

Figure 6.11. Common risks associated with surgery.

Source: https://www.washingtonplasticsurg.com/wp-content/gallery/rhinoplasty/rhino4c_3_8_24.jpg.

6.4.2. Potential Complications Specific to Rhinoplasty

Both patients and medical practitioners need to be aware of the possible rhinoplasty-specific complications. While rhinoplasty is a frequently performed procedure, it entails a multitude of risks that can unfavorably impact outcomes. Some of the typical complications are postoperative deformity, brought about by inadequate technique or aberrant healing response. Displacement of the nasal structure might lead to displeasure with the look, necessitating supplementary corrective surgeries. Besides, the psychological impact of dashed hopes tends to make the emotional impacts on patients even worse because they will end up grappling with frustration and disappointment after undergoing surgery. As highlighted by the literature at hand, there is a need to harmonize the patient's and the physician's expectations in order to prevent such impacts (Rettinger, 2008). Proper pre-operative consultations can help in setting realistic expectations and thereby reduce the risk of dissatisfaction with the cosmetic results of the procedure.

Besides cosmetic problems, rhinoplasty can lead to serious medical complications. One of the serious risks is the formation of vascular obstruction, which can be caused by improper injection techniques used in nonsurgical rhinoplasty. This is a complication that may result in skin necrosis or even blindness in severe cases. Practitioner experience is paramount, with skills from an experienced surgeon being critical to minimizing such risks. Based on a systematic review of nonsurgical rhinoplasty, vascular anatomy knowledge must be imparted to practitioners to recognize and treat potential complications (Czach et al., 2024).

The implications of such complications underscore the value of precise technique and good patient selection, thereby paving the way for safer surgical procedures and improved results in rhinoplasty. A third key consideration to bear in mind under the rheumatology of complications relates to the risk of infection. Following nasal surgery, the nose's anatomical closeness to numerous facial structures leaves it more susceptible to bacterial contamination.

Infection can manifest itself in the form of persistent pain, redness, and the presence of discharge at the site operated on, which not only threatens the success of the procedures but also demands additional interventions. Scarring would also be a long-term consequence if the healing of the wound is not properly monitored and controlled. In some cases, prophylactic antibiotics may be given to prevent this condition. Last but not least, there needs to be a comprehensive plan for the care of the patient that involves careful post-operative follow-up and education on recognizing signs of complications, thus allowing patients to seek timely medical consultation if problems arise in the course of their recovery process. The integration of such information into pre- and post-operative care can ensure improved patient outcomes and patient satisfaction with rhinoplasty procedures.

6.4.3. Importance of Choosing a Qualified Surgeon

The decision to undergo rhinoplasty, which is a popular cosmetic procedure, involves careful examination of the surgeons qualifications. Not only should an experienced surgeon possess technical proficiency but also a complete understanding of the noses delicate anatomy necessary to create balanced aesthetic results. Patients must carefully screen potential surgeons by examining their educational credentials, board certification, and history of past surgeries.

This diligence ensures not only that one is investing in creativity but also in safety. Choosing a surgeon who has done many rhinoplasty operations significantly enhances the possibility of a good outcome, compensating for surgery risks and complications post-surgery.

A master surgeon's service can also be an expression of serious interest in patient education to help individuals create realistic expectations about the outcome and emotional impact of the surgery. In addition, it can be pointed out that understanding psychological motivations for rhinoplasty can stress the importance of choosing a qualified surgeon.

Based on research, patients perform this surgery due to various extrinsic and intrinsic reasons, such as societal pressure and personal body image issues (Auer, 2018). A properly qualified surgeon is attuned to such factors and discusses patients' motivations with them to ensure that their desire is harmonious with realistic surgical possibilities. This patient-centered attitude establishes an environment for educated decision-making and emotional health, reinforcing the surgeon's role as not simply a technician, but a vital component of the patient's care system.

By doing so, selecting a surgeon dedicated to empathy and familiar with the patient can lead to enhanced satisfaction with the surgery experience and its outcome. In addition, rhinoplasty complications are usually ascribed to the surgeon's expertise, which again supports the significance of making the decision. As debated in many works, patients' experiences, both cisgender and transgender, highlight the significance of an expert surgeon who may also solve the complexities of personal goals and perception of body while undergoing surgery (Windsor, 2011).

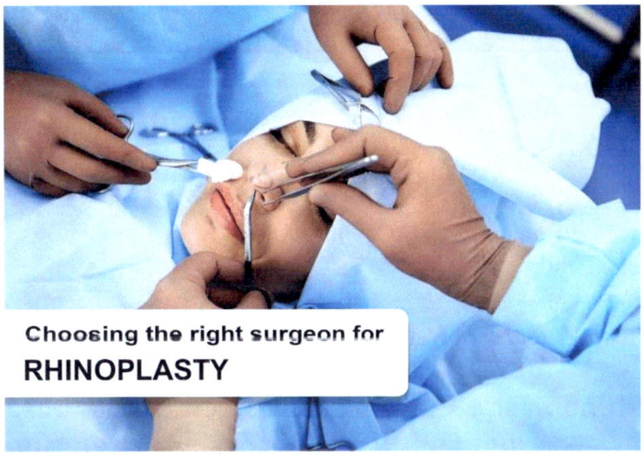

Figure 6.12. Importance of choosing a qualified surgeon.

Source: https://www.doctorsapp.in/uploads/treatment_image/choosing%20the%20right%20surgeon%20for%20rhinoplasty.jpg.

An able surgeon can easily manage such complications, and procedural decisions are not just cosmetically pleasing but also medically appropriate. By entrusting their care in the hands of a skilled surgeon, patients can minimize the possibility of adverse effects and psychological upset and hence make a more pleasant experience overall. Lastly, the skill of the surgeon, experience, and understanding towards the patient are the most important ingredients in guaranteeing not just physical outcomes but also emotional resilience, and therefore the selection process becomes one of the most vital phases in the rhinoplasty procedure (Figure 6.12).

Test Your Knowledge

1. What common risks are associated with any surgical procedure that patients should be aware of?
2. What are some potential complications specific to rhinoplasty procedures?
3. Why is selecting a qualified and experienced surgeon particularly important for rhinoplasty outcomes?

6.5. Psychological Impact of Rhinoplasty

Learning Outcome

1. Explain the Effects on Self-Esteem and Body Image
2. Discuss the Patient Expectations and Satisfaction Rates
3. Focus on Role of Counseling in the Decision-Making Process

Rhinoplasty, otherwise referred to as nose surgery, not only entails physical alteration but also has tremendous psychological impacts. The desire to undergo a rhinoplasty will most likely stem from an earlier history of teasing or bullying regarding the shape of one's nose. In scientific research, nearly half of patients who seek cosmetic enhancement have social teasing experiences contributing to body dissatisfaction. This teasing is known to trigger much distress, depression, and concern about one's looks. These psychological stresses overshadow social functioning and self-image and eventually force people to seek surgical repair as a means to relieve their distress. The decision to undergo rhinoplasty can then be viewed not merely as a pursuit of visual enhancement, but as a regaining of one's mental well-being, suggesting a direct correlation between psychological health and getting beauty treatments. The consequences of rhinoplasty extend to psychological alterations following surgery. Postoperative patients generally describe improvements in self-esteem and overall quality of life. These advantages can be attributed to the elimination of the social stigmas that previously plagued them. Patients following rhinoplasty have been reported to experience increased confidence, which subsequently contributes to increased socialization and overall satisfaction with life. However, it should be noted that while many patients do experience positive psychological adjustment, many will struggle with unachievable expectations about how they will look after surgery. Hopes and realities can lead to disappointment or regret. As observed in more general cosmetic surgery research, for instance, in the analysis of facial feminization surgery, psychological outcomes are extremely variable, and as such, rigid pre-operative psychological evaluations must be performed to identify areas of potential dissatisfaction risk and to manage expectations. In addition, the psychological effects of rhinoplasty also intersect with more general societal pressures around beauty and appearance ideals. The quest for surgical enhancements is indicative not only of individual wants but also of the internalization of social norms that tend to regard certain physical attributes as desirable. This process can only serve to reinforce the feelings of insufficiency that many individuals already experience, particularly those in marginal groups.

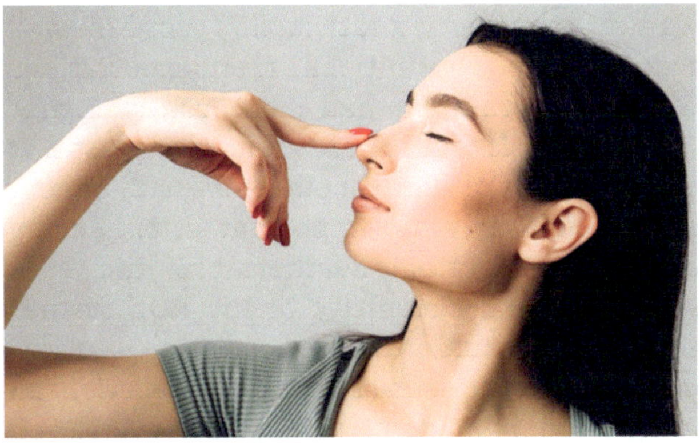

Figure 6.13. Psychological impact of rhinoplasty.

Source: https://cdn.rememore.com/PSYCHOLOGICAL%20EFFECTS%20OF%20RHINOPLASTY.jpg.

For instance, transgender individuals may particularly feel compelled to have operations like rhinoplasty as a means of aligning their physical appearance with gender identity, as a measure to offset minority stress brought about by discrimination and prejudice. As studies highlight, process treatments such as rhinoplasty are also of significant importance in relieving inner distress by enabling people to navigate more securely and independently within their social worlds, ultimately to establish a more positive self-image and life quality subsequent to the operation (Figure 6.13).

6.5.1. Effects on Self-Esteem and Body Image

The reason for rhinoplasty is often a consequence of a desire to improve one's looks and, therefore, self-esteem. For most, the nose is a standout facial characteristic that has a significant influence on one's sense of beauty as well as identity. When individuals believe their nose to be unattractive by societal or personal standards, the outcome may be low self-esteem and feelings of inadequacy. Surgical intervention, therefore, is imagined as a bridge not only to beautification but also to emotional alleviation. It endorses the view that physical appearance can play an important role in personal confidence because those who are satisfied with their facial appearance usually depict greater confidence in social functions. Lastly, rhinoplasty may be life-altering, bringing about an increased feeling of self-worth and an enhanced perception of the self, consequently remitting the maladies of self and societal beauty standards. Moreover, the relationship between body image and rhinoplasty extends further than mere beauty. It involves worldwide societal perceptions of health and beauty, particularly in different societies. For instance, in Brazil, the convergence of beauty ideals and norms of aging is underscored by rising popularity of plastic surgeries like rhinoplasty. The discourse surrounding such interventions embodies a tension in aging to be seen and addressed, especially when it concerns women. Patients typically have rhinoplasty not necessarily for strictly cosmetic gratification but as a means to adapt their appearance to culturally approved ideals of health and youth. This is part of a broader trend of women experiencing pressure from society's beauty mandates, which further elevates the emphasis on appearance as a component of identity and well-being. On this account, surgically enhanced nose reshaping can stand in for a struggle against societal pressure to reclaim control over personal standards of beauty (Edmonds, 2014). In addition, the new research indicates how technology affects beauty concepts, presenting a different angle to the debate regarding the effects of rhinoplasty on self-esteem and body image. With greater advancements in the analysis and processing of images, research indicates that beauty as perceived can be less subjective and more akin to measurements based on quantifiable features identified by the majority of cultures. This objective standard can influence individuals' desires for specific aesthetic results, lending credence to the argument that individuals undergo rhinoplasty with the intention of increasing conformity to such new beauty standards. Individuals can thus seek rhinoplasty in hopes of not only enhancing their physical appearance but also gaining an expected image that aligns with broader metrics of beauty derived from algorithmic appraisals. This combination of social and technological factors contributes to motivations for cosmetic surgery being multifaceted, illustrating how self-image and self-esteem become intertwined with individual wants alongside overall societal norms (Kagian et al., 2010).

6.5.2. Patient Expectations and Satisfaction Rates

Patient expectations play a central role in the rhinoplasty world in determining the level of postoperative satisfaction. Possible patients may possess some ideas regarding what they would like to attain, based on personal beauty ideals, cultural, and social norms. These may significantly impact their psychological well-being and overall level of satisfaction with the procedure. One of the components that ensures patient satisfaction is the pre-operative consultation, where surgeons must fully inform patients about the realistic potential and limitations of rhinoplasty. This process serves not only to reconcile patient expectations with achievable outcomes but also serves the secondary function of diminishing potential post-operative dissatisfaction. As such, understanding of the interdependent nature between patient expectation and satisfaction draws attention to the importance of intentional pre-operative counseling in the formation of positive surgical results. Patient satisfaction following rhinoplasty is commonly measured using tools like the Rhinoplasty Outcome Evaluation (ROE) questionnaire, which assesses a number of factors influencing patient satisfaction with their surgery. For example, the standard normality ratings of this survey provide a consistent method for evaluating subjective patient experiences of patients who receive the procedure. In a sample of patients waiting for surgery, a satisfaction score showed that patients who felt that their expectations were being fulfilled had significantly higher levels of satisfaction. These findings suggest that the alignment of surgical outcomes with patient expectations is most important in enhancing overall satisfaction. Furthermore, the 95% sensitivity and specificity of the ROE further set it as a reliable measure of surgical success, proving that patient-reported information an integral component of rhinoplasty evaluation (Brandão et al., 2012). Aside from this, mental health considerations are the foundation of rhinoplasty outcomes. Studies have indicated that while the degree of anxiety is actually the same post-surgery, symptoms of depression notably diminish after rhinoplasty, again shedding light on the psychological impact of the procedure. The evidence has a compelling narrative: with their nasal cosmetic problem rectified, patients experience enhanced self-esteem and higher mood, elements that by necessity combine with levels of satisfaction. With more and more patients opting for rhinoplasty for cosmetic reasons, healthcare providers need to be sensitive to the physical side but also to the emotional impact. Having an integrated model of patient care that includes mental health and realistic expectations is essential to achieving optimal levels of satisfaction in rhinoplasty units (Bazgir et al., 2023) (Figure 6.14).

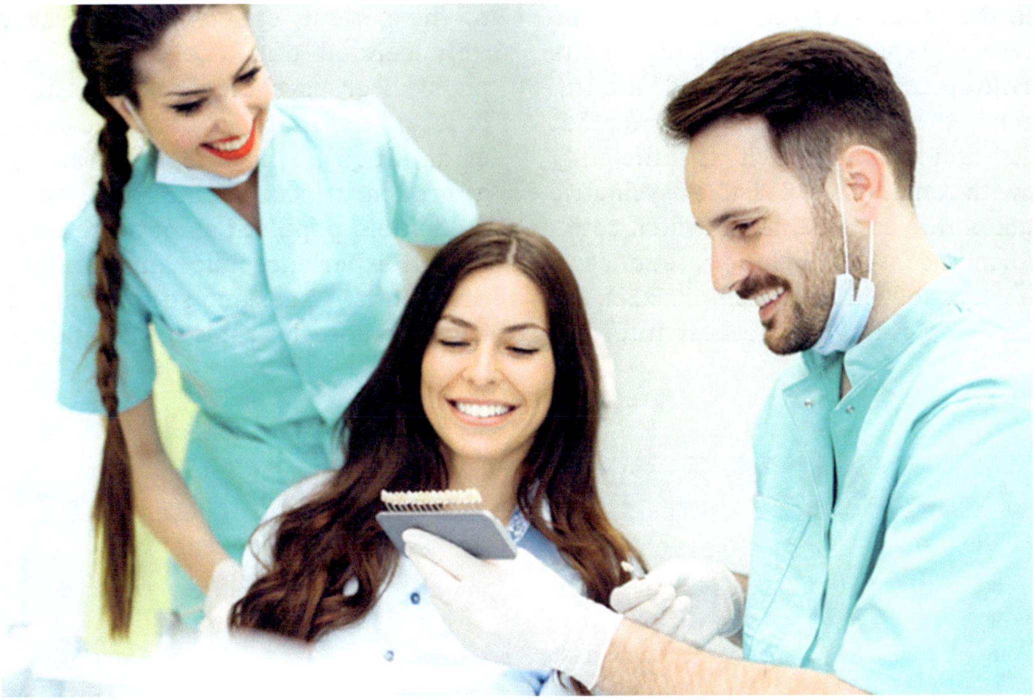

Figure 6.14. Patient expectations and satisfaction rates in cosmetic.

Source: https://cdn.prod.website-files.com/679b67a43a568394e3ce7fb5/67a2101126bad6c7e090379b_65f9f22baa70b179badb48b6_641887b22cfa0ec2d15e043a_Dental%252520Patient%252520Expectations%252520and%252520Experience.png.

6.5.3. Role Of Counseling in the Decision-Making Process

The decision-making process of rhinoplasty is intrinsically woven with counseling, which is part of ensuring patients understand what motivates them and what can ensue. Accurate counseling can aid in helping individuals identify the psychological underpinnings of their requirement for aesthetic surgery, especially in cases where there is a presence of societal pressures. The majority would view rhinoplasty as a means of conforming to perceived beauty ideals, which may preclude natural individual motivation. By engaging in extensive counseling, the patients are able to analyze the primary motivation for seeking the surgery, resulting in greater self-awareness and guiding them to make educated decisions based on individual values and objectives. This process of self-reflection eventually results in a more rational approach to decision-making that prioritizes patient well-being at the top of the aesthetic pursuit. Counseling is also most critical in the area of rhinoplasty among adolescents and young adults, those most likely to be susceptible to external pressures and possibly harmful body ideals. Against this vulnerability, it is the duty of mental health practitioners to evaluate the psychological and emotional state of such patients before any surgical intervention. Since issues such as appearance anxiety can significantly influence social adjustment and quality of life, as seen in the case of facial feminization surgery (Katides et al., 2018), there arises a need for a systematic approach towards measuring the same through the process of counseling. Use of tools like the DAS-59 can give clear-cut indications of psychological problems facing patients, facilitating a clear understanding of motivational reasons and potential risk of operation. Furthermore, ethical issues involved in the process of guidance cannot be overemphasized, especially in younger patients seeking rhinoplasty. Surgeons and mental health specialists need to work together so that patients' decision-making capacity is sufficiently evaluated, with conditions of possible psychiatric disorder taken into consideration, which could impair informed consent. Giving precedence to the ethical aspect of counseling emphasizes the importance of operating in the best interests of the patient, ensuring that procedures are only carried out where there is a certain physical or psychological necessity, as in the case of the ethics of cosmetic surgery (Luca et al., 2018). This integrated and supportive approach to counseling not only protects vulnerable populations but also enriches their overall experience, allowing them to deal with the identity issues and social demands that can lead to a more desirable result following surgery.

Test Your Knowledge

1. How can rhinoplasty affect a patient's self-esteem and body image?
2. Why is it important to manage patient expectations, and how do expectations relate to satisfaction rates after surgery?
3. What role can counseling play in the decision-making process for patients considering rhinoplasty?

6.6. Cultural Perspectives on Rhinoplasty

Learning Outcome

1. Discuss the Rhinoplasty Trends in Different Cultures
2. Focus on Societal Pressures and Beauty Standards
3. Explain Ethical Considerations in Cosmetic Surgery

With rhinoplasty growing in popularity across the world, its cultural influences become increasingly pertinent. Within cultures like urban China, the pursuit of an idealized appearance is deeply interwoven with prevailing socio-economic aspirations. Such women tend to do rhinoplasty to ensure their physical appearance conforms to cultural ideals of beauty as a proxy for success. The desired appearance includes a high-bridged nose, which is a marker of modern femininity and economic achievement. It is not a superficial change but reflective of a wider cultural conversation in which beauty is a tool for individualization and competition in society. These dynamics reveal the ways in which ideologies in society affect the personal decisions on cosmetic surgery, with women navigating identities amidst shifting beauty norms and revealing the tension between old values and new hopes (Lotti et al., 2022). Tension between cultural beliefs and rhinoplasty also manifests in the ways that societies differently embrace cosmetic surgeries. Some societies are highly accommodating to normative surgeries, seeing them as methods of empowerment and self-expression. However, operations that are considered non-normative, such as drastic alteration or ethnic reductions, typically come with heavy social censure. This distinction suggests an essentialist definition of beauty that impacts the perception of individuals who choose to undergo surgical augmentation. It is reflective of social norms of authenticity and conformity, in which some physical attributes are valued, whereas others are diminished. Therefore, the cultural sentiments towards rhinoplasty are an instructive area of focus for exploring the subtleties of gender and beauty standards under a social context, signaling more general social concerns with authenticity, individual choice, and collective beauty standards (Mayeux et al., 2009). The cultural sentiments towards rhinoplasty have implications for how individuals experience the outcomes of their procedures emotionally and socially. For many, the process of undergoing rhinoplasty is merged with hopes for acceptance and approval within their cultures. The postoperative experience may thus bring about a transformation in social capital, influencing interaction with others and self-worth. Narratives around beauty ideals not only decide on the decision to have surgery done but also how these transformations are integrated into identity. As individuals transition through these altered identities, they will seek to express their cultures, which can reinforce or prolong discrimination. Hence, the cultural significance of rhinoplasty surpasses beauty issues and highlights the profound interrelation of identity, social pressures, and the aspiration for self-improvement in multicultural environments (Lotti et al., 2022).

6.6.1. Rhinoplasty Trends in Different Cultures

Rhinoplasty, surgical operations largely aimed at altering the shape and functioning of the nose, has trends that are distinctly different in varying cultures that are more likely to reflect deeper societal values and also aesthetic values. In the majority of Western nations, there is a prevalent aspiration for achieving a desirable nose, which is narrow and symmetrical. The media and celebrity culture go on to reinforce such values, with specific forms of noses being favored. This cultural narrative creates a robust market for rhinoplasty, with individuals turning to surgical intervention as a means of enhancing appearance and social acceptance. Contrarily, cultures that place value on uniqueness and particular characteristics can embrace an alternative ethos, viewing rhinoplasty as an unnecessary alteration of one's identity, thus affecting patient motivations and outcomes significantly (Ahmed et al., 2019). Rhinoplasty trends among the majority of Asian societies today combine a combination of cosmetic enhancement and cultural elements. The desire for a higher nasal bridge, typically associated with Western notions of beauty, is in direct contrast to traditionally prominence-based features that respond to the distinctiveness of each person's heritage. This conflict creates a sophisticated setting in which cosmetic surgery and cultural identity can coexist. Research has revealed that women in some Asian nations increasingly seek rhinoplasty to achieve a look that is a mix of Western influences and indigenous looks, thus reconstituting their identity. These developments reveal a complex relationship between cultural demands and individual desires, in which the two fit into each other as people balance societal influence and their inherent values (Ujam, 2020). This case illustrates the way in which rhinoplasty functions not only as a medical procedure but as a culturally embedded practice. Furthermore, Middle Eastern cultures' application of rhinoplasty further highlights the regional variation of criteria for beauty. In some Middle Eastern cultures, rhinoplasty is a rite of passage with associations to socioeconomic status and personal achievement. The surgery is not aesthetic; it often symbolizes family honor and a social signal. Thus, rhinoplasty could be highly influenced by cultural pressure and family expectations, obscuring personal choices with popular opinions. Minimally invasive procedures are also on the increase among this group, which shows a desire for natural results that straighten one's nose but do not fundamentally change one's nasal features. These cultural nuances highlight the importance of being sensitive to the appreciation of rhinoplasty fashions within specific social contexts, revealing how notions of beauty can manifest in hugely dissimilar forms across global populations (Ahmed et al., 2019) (Figure 6.15).

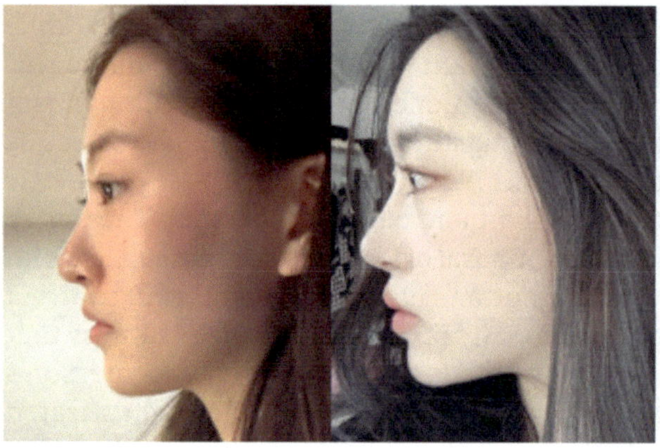

Figure 6.15. Rhinoplasty, a surgical procedure primarily focused on altering the shape and function of the nose.

Source: https://encrypted-tbn0.gstatic.com/images?q=tbn:ANd9GcRCaRMUEy5a62CSi7L7P4p1bLzF1-0X_MxUlA&s.

6.6.2. Societal Pressures and Beauty Standards

Social beauty pressures have been revolutionized during the social media generation, strongly influencing how one views beauty. Social media such as Instagram and TikTok spread ideals that have a tendency to prefer idealized and restrictive views of beauty. Overexposure to airbrushed pictures of stars and influencers can lead to more dissatisfaction with one's appearance, pushing many people into cosmetic augmentation, such as rhinoplasty. Systematic review suggests that high proportions of individuals believe social media affects their self-image, so there is considerable interest in procedures to try and achieve conformity with such unrealistic ideals. Most notably, rhinoplasty is a popular option among individuals who wish to reshape their noses in accordance with prevailing standards offered online, part of a broader trend wherein social pressures inversely correlate with demand for cosmetic surgery (Felimban et al., 2025). The impact of globalization further complicates the global beauty standards environment, particularly in regions like East Asia and Latin America. In countries such as South Korea and Brazil, beauty is frequently culturally determined by localized ideals as opposed to merely adopting Western ideals. Research has shown that women within these countries pursue cosmetic surgery, such as rhinoplasty, in an attempt to attain a homogenized ideal that takes on meaning within their culture. While westernization is at play, it is not the only driving force for increasing demands for cosmetic surgery. This trend illustrates the way that social pressures manifest differently across various regions, with individuals being able to maneuver complicated cultural narratives but nonetheless feeling pressure to conform to evolving ideals of beauty (Vorisek, 2017). Greater popularity for rhinoplasty as a corrective measure to perceived shortcomings marks the site where individual agency intersects with social pressures. As many individuals see cosmetic surgery as an option to enhance their social standing or self-esteem, the implications of such choices need closer examination. The psychological implications of seeking these enhancements include elements of body dysmorphic disorder and long-term satisfaction. The outside guarantee that so many seek through cosmetic surgery can provide temporary comfort; however, it does not necessarily translate into long-term satisfaction. This social relationship then creates significant questions about the relationship between beauty, identity, and self-worth, necessitating in-depth exploration of the means by which beauty norms shape personal choice and the morality of cosmetic surgery (Vorisek, 2017; Felimban et al., 2025) (Figure 6.16).

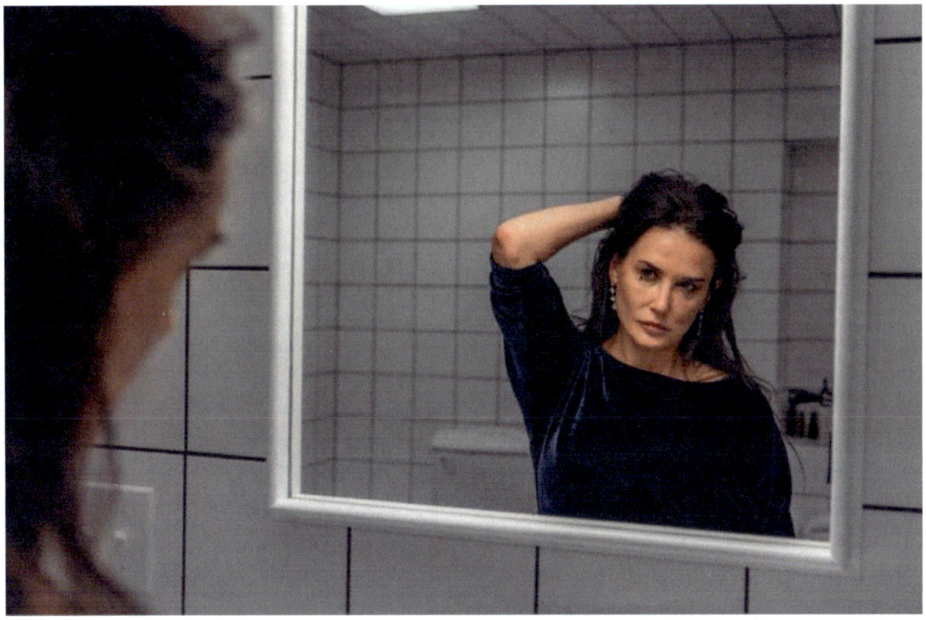

Figure 6.16. Societal pressures regarding beauty standards.

Source: https://www.thehawk.in/_next/image?url=https%3A%2F%2Fd2py10ayqu2jji.cloudfront.net%2Ff8ea9f37-ba9b-4682-9ac0-454442334579%2Fdemi-moore-89a2a987-edc2-4487-a2a6-19a2ac2e2dbc.jpg&w=3840&q=75.

6.6.3. Ethical Considerations in Cosmetic Surgery

The procedure of cosmetic surgery, particularly rhinoplasty, poses special ethical challenges that need to be addressed by clinicians with extreme care. Central to these matters is the doctrine of patient autonomy that requires the surgeon and patient to communicate openly with each other. Informed consent must be given; patients need to be thoroughly informed of the risks, benefits, and realistic results of the procedure. Surgeons must provide clear information regarding potential complications so that informed decisions can be made by patients. Furthermore, the ethics of appearances in cosmetic surgery can be multifaceted because the patients can have unrealistic expectations with regard to celebrity culture and social media. The surgeons are responsible for reorienting patients to a concept of the self that aligns with their true self and not subjective ideals, so that there is a better attitude towards cosmetic change. Another ethical aspect of rhinoplasty is the patient psychological health before and after surgery. Evidence has suggested significant changes in mental health measures among rhinoplasty patients, such as the decrease in depression post-surgery, as per findings from various studies (Bazgir et al., 2023). The figure indicates the urgent yet fragile intersection of cosmetic surgery and mental health. While others might experience enhanced self-esteem and reduced depression symptoms, other individuals may potentially have underlying psychopathology, such as body dysmorphic disorder, that would make their candidacy for the procedure problematic.

Therefore, it is imperative that surgeons conduct thorough psychological assessments in order to identify patients who could be at risk. Ethical surgical practice not only hinges on aesthetic outcomes but also on the preservation of the emotional and psychological stability of treated patients. Additionally, the use of artificial intelligence in cosmetic surgery raises ethical issues of representation and inclusion in the process of patient education and surgical outcomes. With technology inseparable from surgical interventions, AI models can generate treatment pictures that allow patients to see potential outcomes without relying on actual patient images. This innovation enhances patient education by providing combined scenarios drawn from varied anatomical characteristics. However, the innovation discussed here creates an ethical concern: present biases in AI-generated images. It has been found that images created are predisposed to having lighter skin and female facial appearance, excluding a vast portion of the population (Cuomo et al., 2023). Such a gap could lead to myths surrounding what can be achieved for underrepresented groups and thus the significance of the ethical adoption of AI technology in surgery to promote inclusivity and representation in cosmetic surgery (Figure 6.17).

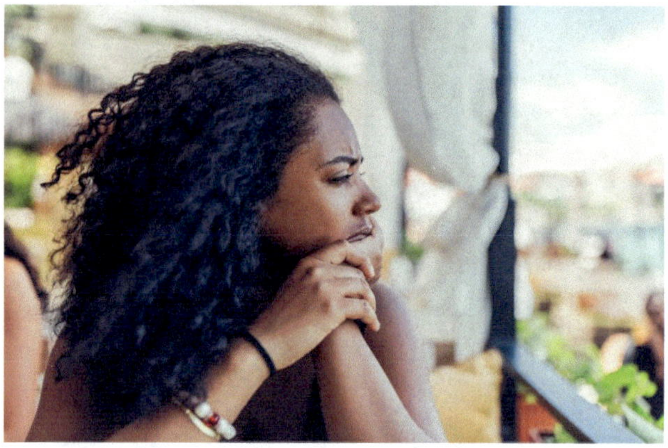

Figure 6.17. Ethical considerations in cosmetics.

Source: https://facialcosmeticsurgery.ca/media/images/iStock-654715244-min.width-800.jpg.

Test Your Knowledge

1. How do rhinoplasty trends vary across different cultures, and what factors influence these trends?
2. In what ways do societal pressures and cultural beauty standards impact the decision to undergo rhinoplasty?
3. What ethical considerations should be taken into account when performing cosmetic surgery in diverse cultural contexts?

SUMMARY

To conclude, rhinoplasty not only looks like a sought-after cosmetic surgery but also a necessary procedure for individuals experiencing psychological anguish over their nose. Enhancement of facial beauty through rhinoplasty can lead to dramatic recovery of social function and self-esteem. Psychological recovery is especially important for the majority of patients, as evidenced in many publications that correlate postoperative outcome with enhanced mental well-being. This interaction emphasizes the necessity of integrating aesthetic and psychological factors when reporting rhinoplasty's role in patient care, particularly in situations involving those affected by minority stress due to discrimination against their appearance (Katides et al., 2018). Furthermore, the measurement of rhinoplasty success with tools such as the Rhinoplasty Outcome Evaluation (ROE) also supports the procedure's effect on patient satisfaction. Detailed evaluations provide useful information about post-operative patient experience and attitudes. By establishing normality and satisfaction standards, as in recent studies, the success of rhinoplasty can be quantified (Brandão et al., 2012). Quantifiable data assist in developing deeper insights into how surgery can be tailored to fit particular requirements, enhancing the quality of the patient experience and levels of satisfaction. In summary, the multifaceted nature of rhinoplasty highlights its significance in contemporary medical practice. It is not only a cosmetic treatment but also an entry to greater mental well-being and personal empowerment for numerous individuals. The symbiotic nature of aesthetic augmentation and mental health underscores the importance of healthcare professionals embracing an inclusive approach in treating patients seeking such procedures. Thus, the future research must continue studying these areas so that rhinoplasty remains a good option to enhance looks as well as life quality.

The controversy surrounding rhinoplasty is really on the twin function of both cosmetic enhancement and functional restoration. The cosmetic concern is about facial contour alignment, where a conformingly pleasing nose is the characteristic most patients desire. Modern developments have made sophisticated systems available that employ 3D technology to generate images of possible surgical results. These systems couple the patient's unique facial structure to a comprehensive database of beautiful facial features to allow the surgeon to model numerous possible changes. This method not only enhances patient satisfaction by providing the patient with a more definitive expectation of outcome but also assists in directing surgical decisions, as is in line with the overall goal of achieving an even and aesthetically best result in nose surgery (Bottino et al., 2012). As a further aesthetic consideration, rhinoplasty also has significant functional components, particularly in the improvement of nasal obstructions. Functional rhinoplasty is the accurate definition for the processes involved in nasal valve collapse correction.

Nasal valve collapse can occur due to a variety of reasons, including trauma or prior surgery that collapses the nasal cartilage. As literature grows, so does the requirement for personalized practices, as functional success is really dependent on the patient's anatomy and specific problems. Improvements also need objective measures and validated scales to improve postoperative evaluations so that the chosen techniques best enhance nasal breathing and overall quality of life (Chan & Shipchandler, 2015). Lastly, the rigorous assessment of rhinoplasty illuminates its complex nature in which form is united with function. The development of aesthetic and functional rhinoplasty tracks broader trends in surgery, where patient-centered outcomes become increasingly highlighted. The use of high-level technology and custom surgical techniques demonstrates a commitment to improving the rhinoplasty process, ensuring patient goals are met and aesthetic standards are achieved. As rhinoplasty becomes more prevalent in both the medical and cosmetic communities, ongoing research and development will be essential to address issues and advance surgical techniques, ultimately producing enhanced patient satisfaction and surgical results that accomplish both functional and aesthetic objectives.

KEY TERMS FROM THIS CHAPTER

Nasal Anatomy
Nasal Septum
Nasal Valve
Closed Approach
Spreader Graft
Dorsal Preservation
Dorsal Hump
Nasal Bridge
Open Approach
Osteotomy
Functional Rhinoplasty

CRITICAL THINKING QUESTIONS

1. **The primary goal of functional rhinoplasty is to:**
   a. Improve nasal shape only
   b. Enhance breathing and airway function
   c. Remove the nasal bones
   d. Reduce skin thickness
2. **The open rhinoplasty approach is characterized by:**
   a. Incisions made only inside the nostrils
   b. A trans-columellar incision allowing full visualization of nasal structures
   c. Using endoscopic guidance
   d. No access to the nasal tip
3. **The most important structure for nasal airway support is the:**
   a. Alar lobule
   b. Nasal septum
   c. Upper lateral cartilage
   d. Nasal skin
4. **A common indication for dorsal hump reduction is:**
   a. Wide alar base
   b. Convex nasal profile
   c. Tip ptosis
   d. Deviated septum
5. **Spreader grafts are primarily used to:**
   a. Reduce nasal width
   b. Improve internal nasal valve function
   c. Strengthen the alar rim
   d. Raise the nasal tip

Short Answer Questions

1. What are the main aesthetic indications for performing rhinoplasty?
2. Differentiate between open and closed rhinoplasty approaches.
3. What is the role of the nasal septum in both cosmetic and functional rhinoplasty?
4. What anatomical structures must be evaluated during nasal tip analysis?
5. What are common complications associated with rhinoplasty?
6. How does skin thickness influence rhinoplasty outcomes?

Answers to Critical Thinking Questions

1. (b) 2. (b) 3. (b) 4. (b) 5. (b)

REFERENCES

1. Czach, M., Kamińska, M. A., Do, M. K., Gonciarz, M. J., Paduszyńska, N., Dąbrowska, A., ... Czach, Z. (2024). Beyond the Aesthetics: Understanding Risks in Nonsurgical Rhinoplasty. Journal of Education, Health and Sport, 74, 52559. https://doi.org/10.12775/JEHS.2024.74.52559(accessed on 14th July 2025).
2. Ahmed, M., Fatima, F., Fida, M., Kamal, et al. (2019). Adjunctive surgical procedures enhancing treatment outcome: A literature review. https://core.ac.uk/download/212885885.pdf (accessed on 14th July 2025).
3. Al Katatbeh, M. (2025). Anthropometrical and nutritional associations with intraoperatively dexamethasone and tranexamic acid in risk propensity for post-rhinoplastic subconjunctival hemorrhages. https://core.ac.uk/download/640071257.pdf (accessed on 14th July 2025).
4. Al Katatbeh, M. (2025). Prognostic model for predicting the probability of post-rhinoplastic complications, accounting for patients' potential confounding factors. https://core.ac.uk/download/640071258.pdf (accessed on 14th July 2025).
5. Moataz Felimban1 , Ayesha Hanin Shaikh2 , Ayesha Jamal2 , Jumana H. Timraz2 , Amjad Ali Khan2 , Wafa Rashid2 , Shahista Raniya Mazher Sultan2 , Saleha Khan2 , Syeda Nafeesa Hashim2 , Husna Irfan Thalib2*, Syed Fouzaan Albeez2 , Faisal Makki2 , Altaf Khan2 The Impact of Social Media on Beauty Standards: A Systematic Review and Meta-Analysis of Patient and Cosmetic Provider Perspectives SEEJPH Volume XXVI, S2,2025, ISSN: 2197-5248 https://core.ac.uk/download/647976468.pdf (accessed on 14th July 2025).
6. Anesi, A., Cavani, F., Chiarini, L., Ferretti, et al. (2014). Preliminary findings of a potenziated piezosurgical device at the rabbit skull. https://core.ac.uk/download/80171725.pdf (accessed on 14th July 2025).
7. Auer, D. (2018). The experience of female patients seeking elective rhinoplasty surgery: A narrative inquiry. https://core.ac.uk/download/573849320.pdf (accessed on 14th July 2025).
8. Bashir, D., Qadri, M. S., & Rather, R. H. (2023). Exploring satisfaction and outcomes in rhinoplasty: Experience from a tertiary care hospital in Kashmir Valley, India. https://core.ac.uk/download/570905641.docx (accessed on 14th July 2025).
9. Bazgir, N., Fazli, M., Gachkar, L., & Ghazizadeh Hashemi, et al. (2023). Comparison of depression and anxiety levels before and after rhinoplasty: A longitudinal study. https://core.ac.uk/download/643598101.pdf (accessed on 14th July 2025).
10. Bertossi, D., Caliskan, G., Chirumbolo, S., Kapoor, et al. (2022). A systematic review and meta-analysis of rhinoplasty using the rhinoplasty outcome evaluation scale. https://core.ac.uk/download/543577334.pdf (accessed on 14th July 2025).
11. Bottino, A. G., De Simone, M., Laurentini, A., & Sforza, et al. (2012). A New 3D Tool for Planning Plastic Surgery. https://core.ac.uk/download/pdf/11429366.pdf (accessed on 14th July 2025).
12. Bottino, A. G., Laurentini, A., & Rosano, L. (2008). A new computer-aided technique for planning the aesthetic outcome of plastic surgery. https://core.ac.uk/download/pdf/11398829.pdf (accessed on 14th July 2025).
13. Brandão, K. V., Garcia, L. B. S., Gregório, L. C., Izu, et al. (2012). Normal values for the rhinoplasty outcome evaluation (ROE) questionnaire. https://core.ac.uk/download/37710575.pdf (accessed on 14th July 2025).

14. Carreno Hernandez, E., Gonzalez Ballester, L., Herrero Jover, J., Moscatiello, F., & Piombino, P. (2010). Preoperative digital three-dimensional planning for rhinoplasty. https://core.ac.uk/download/55042537.pdf (accessed on 14th July 2025).

15. Carvalho, G., Milicic, D., Sousa Vieira, A., Torrão Pinheiro, et al. (2020). Extended dorsal preservation in a new concept of preservational rhinoplasty. https://core.ac.uk/download/334530812.pdf (accessed on 14th July 2025).

16. Chan, D., & Shipchandler, T. Z. (2015). Update on the evidence for functional rhinoplasty techniques. https://core.ac.uk/download/46963024.pdf (accessed on 14th July 2025).

17. Cho Lee, G. Y., González García, R., Muñoz Guerra, M. F., Naval Gias, et al. (2008). Endoscopically-assisted transoral approach for the treatment of subcondylar fractures of the mandible. https://core.ac.uk/download/93038745.pdf (accessed on 14th July 2025).

18. Codazzi, H., Hierl, I., Inanli, K., Koc, O., Ogino, M., Ong, et al. (2019). New technologies in rhinoplasty: A comprehensive workflow for computer-assisted planning and execution. https://core.ac.uk/download/323232725.pdf (accessed on 14th July 2025).

19. Cuomo, R., di Secli, D., Grimaldi, L., Pozzi, M., Roxo, C. W., Schettino, M., & Susini, P. (2024). Augmentation rhinoplasty and centrofacial lipofilling: Our experience (ARCL). https://core.ac.uk/download/622823687.pdf (accessed on 14th July 2025).

20. Cuomo, R., Kah, S., Lim, B., Ross, R. J., Rozen, W. M., Seth, I., & Sofiadellis, F. (2023). Using generative artificial intelligence tools in cosmetic surgery: A study on rhinoplasty, facelifts, and blepharoplasty procedures. https://core.ac.uk/download/643629878.pdf (accessed on 14th July 2025).

21. Di Luca, N. M., Marinelli, E., Napoletano, S., & Vergallo, et al. (2018). Ethics and/or aesthetics? Reflections on cosmetic surgery for adolescents. https://core.ac.uk/download/188823836.pdf (accessed on 14th July 2025).

22. Dowling, N. A., Francis, K. L., Honigman, R. J., Jackson, et al. (2012). The experience of teasing in elective cosmetic surgery patients. http://hdl.handle.net/10536/DRO/DU:30059350 (accessed on 14th July 2025).

23. Edmonds, A. (2014). Surgery-for-life: Aging, sexual fitness and self-management in Brazil. Anthropology & Aging Quarterly 2014: 34 (4) https://core.ac.uk/download/28979727.pdf (accessed on 14th July 2025).

24. Ennes, M., & Ramos, N. (2018). Immigrants and Body Modifications in the Consumer Society. https://core.ac.uk/download/196575527.pdf (accessed on 14th July 2025).

25. Giorgi, G. (1987). Barnes Hospital Bulletin. https://core.ac.uk/download/70381137.pdf (accessed on 14th July 2025).

26. Greywoode, J., Hamilton, J., Malhotra, et al. (2012). Repair of nasal septal perforation with porcine small intestinal submucosa xenograft. https://core.ac.uk/download/46971846.pdf (accessed on 14th July 2025).

27. Hummelink, S., Luong, K. P., Slijper, H. P., & Stubenitsky, et al. (2024). Changes in patient-reported satisfaction and quality-of-life 6 months after rhinoplasty. https://core.ac.uk/download/610639069.pdf (accessed on 14th July 2025).

28. Kagian, A. J., O'Toole, B., Fasel, B., Fink, B., Jones, B. W., Baker, B., et al. (2010). The analysis of facial beauty: An emerging area of research in pattern analysis. https://core.ac.uk/download/pdf/11414133.pdf (accessed on 14th July 2025).

29. Kao, R., Rabbani, C. C., Shipchandler, T. Z., Ting, et al. (2019). In-office functional nasal surgery. https://core.ac.uk/download/286317763.pdf (accessed on 14th July 2025).

30. Katides, K. (2018). Facial feminization surgery and perceived workplace bias in transgender individuals. https://open.bu.edu/bitstream/2144/32970/5/Katides_bu_0017N_14039.pdf (accessed on 14th July 2025).

31. King, K. K., Merianos, A. L., & Vidourek, R. A. (2013). Medicalization of female beauty: A content analysis of cosmetic procedures. https://core.ac.uk/download/51087636.pdf (accessed on 14th July 2025).

32. Lazim, N. M., Rizzo, P. B., & Spinato, G. (2019). Rhinoplasty in context of head and neck malignancy. https://core.ac.uk/download/322443573.pdf (accessed on 14th July 2025).

33. Lotti, V. (2022). What women want: An analysis of cosmetic surgery and social achievements in contemporary urban China. https://core.ac.uk/download/614350451.pdf (accessed on 14th July 2025).

34. Manole, A., Manole, F., Căiță, G. A., & Voiță, N. C. (2023). A review of the effect of rhinoplasty surgery on quality of life. https://core.ac.uk/download/603897998.pdf (accessed on 14th July 2025).

35. Torres, S., & Marianetti, T. (2016). Management of Common Complications in Rhinoplasty and Medical Rhinoplasty. InTech. doi: 10.5772/63130 https://core.ac.uk/download/322427236.pdf (accessed on 14th July 2025).

36. Mayeux, C. (2009). Stigma, surgery and social identity: Attitudes towards cosmetic and sexual reassignment surgeries. https://core.ac.uk/download/216836759.pdf (accessed on 14th July 2025).

37. Milićević, S., Pavlović, A., Piščević, B., Stepić, N., & Vulović, D. (2011). Reconstruction of the columella and the tip of the nose with an island-shaped forehead flap. https://core.ac.uk/download/pdf/27188125.pdf (accessed on 14th July 2025).

38. Deepak M. Kalaskar, Peter E. Butler, Shadi Ghali. (2016). Textbook of Plastic and Reconstructive Surgery. ISBN: 978-1-910634-37-0 (Hbk.) https://core.ac.uk/download/79526588.pdf

39. Okoye, B. C., Bugando Medical Centre, Trunkey, D., Kang, E. G., Orji, F. T., Matilda, I., et al. (2013). Ear, nose and throat injuries at Bugando Medical Centre in northwestern Tanzania: A five-year prospective review of 456 cases. https://core.ac.uk/download/pdf/11307767.pdf (accessed on 14th July 2025).

40. Rettinger, G. (2008). Risks and Complications in Rhinoplasty. https://core.ac.uk/download/pdf/8632770.pdf (accessed on 14th July 2025).

41. Tasman, A J. (2008). Rhinoplasty – Indications and Techniques. https://core.ac.uk/download/pdf/8632778.pdf (accessed on 14th July 2025).

42. Ujam, A. B. (2020). Cartilage Tissue Engineering for Rhinoplasty. https://core.ac.uk/download/341794117.pdf (accessed on 14th July 2025).

43. Včeva, A., Mihalj, H., Maleš, J., Mihalj, M., Grebenar, M., Milanković, S. G., Mendeš, T., et al. (2019). Open Approach Rhinoplasty. https://core.ac.uk/download/286446915.pdf (accessed on 14th July 2025).

44. Vorisek, R. (2017). Cross-cultural comparison of cosmetic procedures in Latin America and East Asia. https://core.ac.uk/download/148696179.pdf (accessed on 14th July 2025).

45. Windsor, E. J. (2011). Regulating healthy gender: Surgical body modification among transgender and cisgender consumers. https://core.ac.uk/download/71423075.pdf (accessed on 14th July 2025).

BROW LIFT AND FOREHEAD REJUVENATION IN FACIAL COSMETIC

7

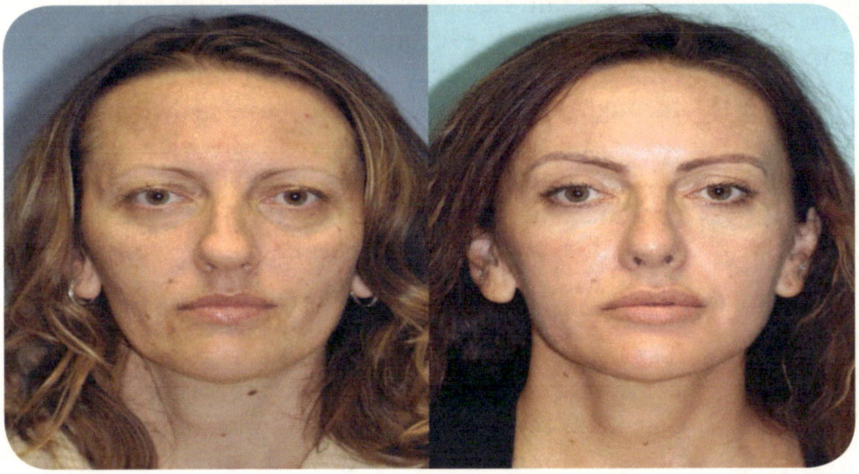

LEARNING OBJECTIVES

After studying this chapter, you will be able to:

1. Describe the historical background;
2. Explain the anatomy of the forehead and brow area;
3. Understand the indications for brow lift and forehead rejuvenation;
4. Focus on surgical techniques;
5. Discuss the risks and complications in facial cosmetic;
6. Evaluate non-surgical alternatives.

Introduction

The human face is a palette for expression and identity, and the perceptions of beauty are highly influenced by cultural standards and individual preferences. Between cosmetic procedures, brow lift and forehead rejuvenation have been extremely sought after because they cannot only change physical appearances but also influence emotional expression. Surgical procedures under this practice aim to restore a youthful look by addressing common problems like sagging skin, deep furrows, and brow sag. With advances in these procedures, their relevance needs to be understood within the general realm of facial cosmetic surgery, which encompasses an array of methods and tendencies individual to different patients' needs. Thorough evaluation of brow lift surgical techniques, to minimize complications and maximize aesthetic outcomes, is most important for practitioners wanting to excel in this intricate field, as reviewed in research focusing on the unique interaction between certain anatomical structures (Keyhan et al., 2016). Even though facial aesthetic treatments receive much attention in both lay and clinical literature, the nuances of upper facial rejuvenation warrant critical analysis. A brow lift, particularly, is a milestone surgery in treating obvious signs of aging with a profound impact on self-perception and social acceptability. The operation can be performed via various techniques, including endoscopic and classical, each of which has its benefits and associated risks. The outcome is often a function of the skill of the surgeon and an accurate comprehension of the underlying anatomy, enabling personalized interventions that are adapted to the unique characteristics of each patient. With popularity comes recognition of potential complications, as in literature indicating dangers to cosmetic procedures such as those posed by Botulinum neurotoxin type A injections (Kąpa et al., 2025). This growing body of research confirms the significance of cosmetic surgeons to evolve and appreciate the safety of patients in brow lifts. With growing demand for facial rejuvenation, particularly from aging demographics who want to keep looking youthful, there emerges a tale that intertwines personal ambitions with new advances in surgery. The increasing use of minimally invasive methods combined with more traditional brow lifts reflects a drift toward more patient-focused practice in cosmetic surgery. Aesthetic balance within the context of forehead rejuvenation also needs to be stressed, since it is a significant factor in facial attractiveness. The cultural and psychological forces that drive such cosmetic desires add depth of understanding to the discussion of brow lifts. Therefore, a multidisciplinary approach encompassing procedural techniques, potential complications, and patient benefits will provide a holistic perspective on brow lift and forehead rejuvenation operations. Such an in-depth examination also attempts to comment on the impact of developments in cosmetic surgery on individual self-concept and societal standards of beauty.

Definition of Brow Lift and Forehead Rejuvenation

A brow lift, also referred to as a forehead lift, is a cosmetic surgical procedure aimed at lifting and recreating the youthful contour of the brow and forehead area. The procedure offers correction for typical aging signs such as sagging skin, frown lines, and forehead wrinkles that may form and give an impression of tiredness or unhappiness. With repositioning of the deeper muscles and tissues, a brow lift can result in a smoother forehead and an older, more rested look to the face. Brow lift surgery can be done through a number of methods, one of which is the endoscopic brow lift that involves smaller incisions and gives quicker recovery and thus remains one of the patient's favorite options even for successful forehead rejuvenation. With these advances in surgical technique, patients can optimize aesthetic outcome with less intrusiveness, thus offering greater patient comfort and satisfaction with the procedure. Forehead rejuvenation entails a broader range of techniques directed towards shaping the upper face as well as improving the look of the forehead and brow region. While brow lifts are a key part of this facelift, augmenting treatments like Botox injections, fillers, and lasers are also done to restore the skin's tone, texture, and flexibility. Non-surgical methods like neuromodulators temporarily weaken the muscles behind wrinkles, providing a less invasive option for patients who don't have time to devote to surgery. As a component of the cosmetic facial environment, forehead rejuvenation addresses the evolving needs of individuals preferring natural-looking results. Both surgical and nonsurgical techniques are used specifically for individual facial goals of each patient, therefore guaranteeing each person's appearance as accurately and creatively defined. The inclusion of brow lifts and forehead rejuvenation under cosmetic facial surgery reflects the importance of multidisciplinary facial aesthetics. Through grasping the relationship between reconstructive principles and aesthetics, clinicians are able to provide well-balanced care that reconciles both functional and aesthetic demands. As demonstrated by the 10 latest studies, advancements in facial plastic surgery have introduced sophisticated techniques that are harmonized with alternatively diverse ethnic and regional preferences, thus improving standards of care and patient satisfaction (Keyhan et al., 2016). As a result, these innovations not only include traditional surgical methods but also integrate new technologies and minimally invasive approaches that have changed the cosmetic landscape. This combined method emphasizes the significance of brow lifts and forehead rejuvenation; not as isolated surgical procedures but as part of a larger paradigm to achieve overall facial harmony and renewal (Chuang et al., 2016) (Figure 7.1).

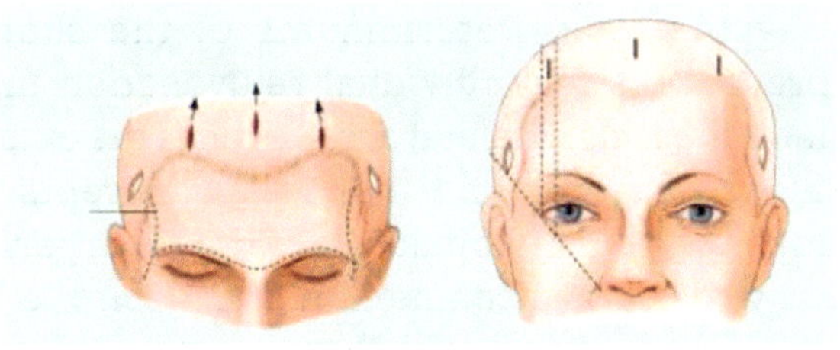

Figure 7.1. The brow lift and forehead rejuvenation.

Source: https://external-content.duckduckgo.com/iu/?u=https%3A%2F%2Fkbeautye.com%2Fwp-content%2Fuploads%2F2024%2F11%2Fghjkhl-optimized.jpg&f=1&nofb=1&ipt=1aea8b900b28a63686238464190e0cc7b06eb98999cce90afc07bdbb285e5040.

Importance of Facial Aesthetics in Modern Society

Facial aesthetics are key to contemporary society, for our sense of self is frequently inextricably tied up with the notions we hold about beauty and attractiveness. Physical appearance is on the increase and pervasive, apparent throughout the mediasphere, wherein our visions of beauty are constantly informed by cultural forces and social standards. For instance, social media has set specific beauty standards, which can put pressure on people to look a certain way, including the case of the Instagram Face phenomenon. This standardization of beauty, like high cheekbones and silky skin, can make people seek cosmetic surgery like brow lifts and forehead rejuvenation in a bid to achieve these standards. As a result, individuals who undergo such treatments more often have improved self-esteem and satisfaction with appearance, which supports a strong association between facial beauty and psychological well-being. The growing popularity of minimally invasive cosmetic procedures also reflects growing social acceptance of augmentation and thus highlights the importance of facial aesthetics. The popularity of procedures like brow lifts speaks volumes about the universal desire to appear young and vibrant, particularly as the signs of aging become more obvious on the face. It has been observed that people who opt for facial rejuvenation surgeries often report wide-ranging advantages for aspects beyond physical transformation; enhanced social lives and enhanced professional prospects are regularly cited, indicating how aesthetics can influence one's varied facets of existence. As noted in the literature, the shift towards more conservative facial aesthetic surgery practices focuses on a balance between maintaining natural appearance and addressing aesthetic concerns so that individuals can restore their looks without compromising individual authenticity or identity (Filippo et al., 2024). Despite being confronted with the benefits of facial aesthetics, the increased popularity of idealized standards of beauty poses concerns about potential negative effects on mental health. The ubiquity of idealized traditional public figures' images on platforms like Instagram can have the ability to create an environment of self-comparison and body dissatisfaction amongst witnesses. Girls and young women, in particular, may be susceptible to self-objectification and affective distress while they incorporate these ideals into their sense of worth (McGinty, 2021). It should be recognized that there is a double-edged quality to beauty standards in modern society, namely the confidence-boosting potential of cosmetic enhancement and the risk to mental health represented by unachievable physical ideals. To this end, while facial beauty has the potential to be a self- and confidence-builder, critical examination of the effect of such social phenomena on individual well-being must take place (Figure 7.2).

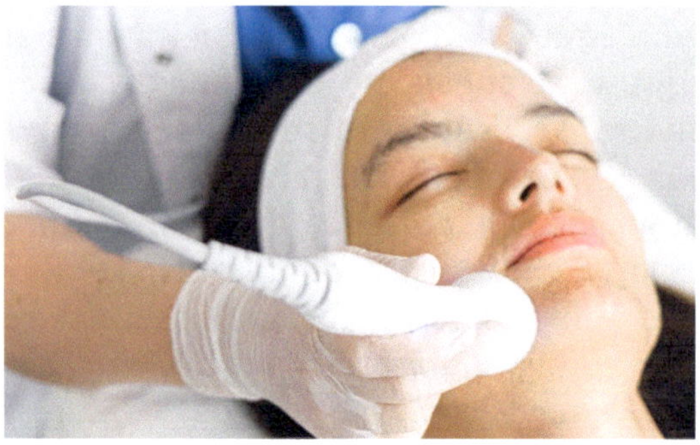

Figure 7.2. Importance of facial aesthetics in modern society.

Source: https://external-content.duckduckgo.com/iu/?u=https%3A%2F%2Fwomenfitnessmag.com%2Fwp-content%2Fuploads%2F2023%2F04%2FBenefits-Of-Facial-Aestheti.jpg&f=1&nofb=1&ipt=ff2909622a6c5e2de6158eef1b131a3cd54c9ff4173f320239d21a7ed5adbe6e.

7.1. Historical Background

Learning Outcome

1. Evolution of Cosmetic Surgery Techniques
2. Discuss the Milestones in Brow Lift Procedures
3. Explain the Cultural Perceptions of Beauty and Aging

The evolution of facial cosmetic surgery, especially brow lifts and forehead rejuvenations, parallels the progression of societal values surrounding beauty and aging. Beauty throughout history has been conditioned by various cultural, social, and technological factors. As aesthetic surgical methods came into being during the 20th century, the demand for non-surgical and surgical treatments increased significantly. Notably, growth in facial plastic surgery coincided with growing societal acceptance of cosmetic surgery, usually associated with personal and business objectives. Facial plastic and reconstructive surgery is a diverse specialty and has followed society trends regarding aesthetic results, representing a growing demand for procedures like brow lifts that restore facial beauty and youth (Keyhan et al., 2016). In an examination of the anatomical underpinnings of brow lifts, it is evident that understanding facial aging is central to successful rejuvenation. Aging causes changes in the texture of the skin, elasticity, and muscle tone, together producing a tired or sagging look. Determinants of the choice of procedures for individual rejuvenation may include the facial skeletal architecture, the extent of aging changes, and individual concepts of beauty. The global popularity of these surgeries bears witness to a common human desire to be youthful and luminous that transcends cultural boundaries. As has been noted (Pourdanesh et al., 2016), there are certain factors to be taken into consideration in selecting the rejuvenation techniques, with particular focus on the necessity of determining the patient's personal anatomy for the best results. Procedures of facial rejuvenation, such as brow lifting, have had significant developments in technique and safety, thus making it increasingly popular. The earlier systems were prone to complications and had long recovery times; however, contemporary techniques brought forth less invasive options that ensured quicker recovery and more natural results. Advances in operating techniques, coupled with the implementation of minimally invasive procedures, have enabled practitioners to tailor interventions based on specific requirements. This change illustrates a high level of aesthetic understanding, supported by copious research and cutting-edge technology that focuses on both results and patient safety. Due to the fact that such operations continue to be in demand, they are an important overlap of art and medicine, ideally aligned to current ambitions for individualized facial rejuvenation procedures.

7.1.1. Evolution of Cosmetic Surgery Techniques

The evolution of cosmetic surgery procedures has significantly influenced facial rejuvenation procedures, particularly in procedures such as brow lifts and forehead rejuvenation. The market has evolved from aggressive procedures to less invasive procedures with time, in a bid to facilitate faster recovery times and better patient satisfaction. Techniques such as endoscopic brow lifts have been developed, with smaller incisions and more advanced camera systems to minimize scarring while offering greater precision. This shift is part of a broader trend in cosmetic surgery to reduce unnatural results while addressing the complex needs of patient populations with diverse desires, emphasizing a more personalized method of aesthetic enhancement. Advances in non-surgical therapies have also transformed face lifts, as experts adopt new approaches to supplement traditional surgical techniques. Techniques such as the administration of botulinum toxin (BT) injections are now widely accepted because of their ability to reduce the appearance of fine lines and wrinkles without the use of traditional incisions. The introduction of BT in 1992 marked the benchmark, with aesthetic practitioners utilizing it as a standalone treatment method for glabellar lines, going on later to realize its worth as part of a combination with other minimally invasive treatments, shortly thereafter. The innovative exchange between various treatment modalities, reflective of the industry's innovative approach and growing patient demands for more holistic aesthetic procedures that prioritize patient comfort and safety (Bouzouaya et al., 2018). Also, the specialty of facial plastic and reconstructive surgery is characterized by cultural sensitivity to change and changing society's ideals of beauty. The surgeons must work in a complex setting where ideals of beauty can vary greatly based on geographic and ethnic factors, according to literature. Therefore, cosmetic treatments have become diversified not just in the surgical interventions but also regarding patient backgrounds. Understanding these preferences offers the ability to develop tailored procedures that resonate with different populations, fostering a more inclusive facial rejuvenation strategy (Keyhan et al., 2016). Ultimately, the ongoing evolution of cosmetic surgery techniques underscores the value of flexibility and sensitivity in this ever-evolving science (Figure 7.3).

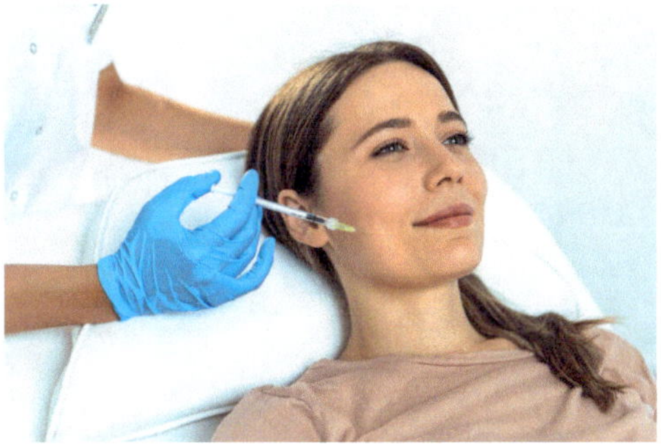

Figure 7.3. The evolution of cosmetic surgery techniques.

Source: https://external-content.duckduckgo.com/iu/?u=https%3A%2F%2Fwww.vargasfaceandskin.com%2Fwp-content%2Fuploads%2F2024%2F05%2Fevolution-in-cosmetics--768x512.jpg&f=1&nofb=1&ipt=cc967cf5c91ceb5c75509cbc58149568b75385089cedc9ebb9545f389a3f12f1.

7.1.2. Milestones in Brow Lift Procedures

The evolution of brow lifts shows significant advancement in surgical methods and patient satisfaction over the past decades. Originally characterized by traditional approaches with extensive incisions and longer recovery, brow lifts have progressed toward minimal-invasive technologies. The introduction of endoscopic methods in the late 1990s was a turning point, which allowed surgeons to perform brow lifts through tiny, hidden incisions along the hairline. This modification not only provided for lesser scarring but also provided more accurate lifting of the brow and reduction of forehead wrinkles. Further, with shifting patient preferences towards natural-looking results with less downtime, the introduction of non-invasive and less traumatic options was a requirement. These landmarks illustrate a steady optimization in techniques with emphasis placed upon both aesthetic outcomes as well as patient safety, projecting brow lift as an essential component of facial rejuvenation. Another important advancement in brow lift procedures lies in the inclusion of technologies that are optimized to deliver better surgical outcomes.

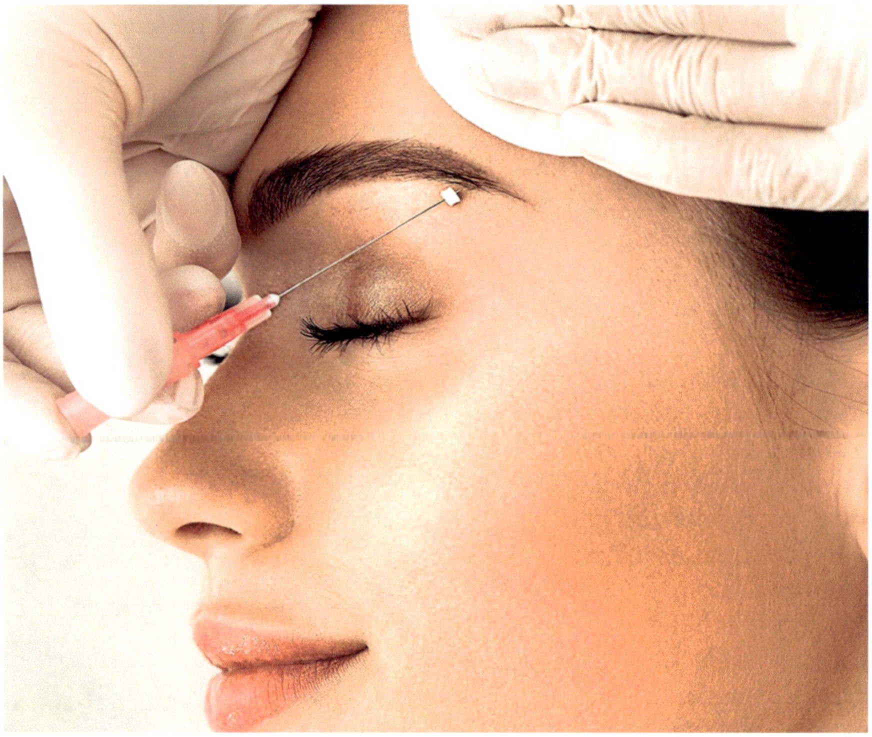

Figure 7.4. Milestones in brow lift procedures.

Source: https://external-content.duckduckgo.com/iu/?u=https%3A%2F%2Fnatural.clinic%2Fwp-content%2Fuploads%2F2023%2F09%2FAn-Overview-of-Eyebrow-lift.webp&f=1&nofb=1&ipt=4d163e9ec81ff10694d1845701fbc88cefd7cfe6178895492357e215d41b1def.

The use of laser-based methods has emerged as an adjunctive technique in brow lifts with better accuracy and recovery. This innovation allows selective tissue excision and coagulation, reducing bleeding and allowing faster healing times. Other procedures, such as Rhytidoplasty Through Minimal Incisions (Rhythmic), have also brought about alternatives with reduced surgery without sacrificing effectiveness. By employing a minimally invasive transcutaneous technique, surgeons can experience significant brow positioning benefits with well-defined cosmetic results, as evidenced by the heightening of eyebrows and reduction in forehead wrinkles, as reported by recent clinical studies (Castillo-Campos et al., 2022). These practices not only simplify the procedure but also demonstrate the growing demand for long-term procedures with fewer invasive treatments. The cumulative progress of brow lift techniques has led to an increasingly sophisticated understanding of aesthetic and reconstructive facial surgery. As the focus changes from requests for aesthetic improvement to requests for uniqueness and personalized surgical treatment, it becomes increasingly important to recognize the importance of patient education in these treatments. Contemporary trends observe an improved understanding of available procedures so that patients can make decisions that uphold their aesthetic goals. In addition, the emphasis on minimally invasive surgery persists to attract a growing number of individuals, even younger patients who want preventive measures against aging. As such, the practice of brow lifts will continue to evolve further, using newer technologies and techniques to offer greater personalization and satisfaction. Milestones in brow lift procedures reflect not only surgical developments but also emphasize the shift toward more integrated patient-centered approaches in the domain of facial cosmetic surgery (Araujo, 2025) (Figure 7.4).

7.1.3. Cultural Perceptions of Beauty and Aging

Cultural notions of aging and beauty have evolved dramatically, influenced by a myriad of social, technological, and aesthetic trends. Beauty is no longer a personal choice in contemporary society but is often mediated by technologies that standardize and distort beauty ideals. For younger generations, especially in Western societies, one of the most widespread trends is celebrity culture and social media influencer worship, where figures like Kim Kardashian West and Kylie Jenner embody a highly stage-managed and homogenized look. This Face phenomenon on Instagram demonstrates the desire to fit into a particular standard of beauty, in which one may develop an increased desire for cosmetic procedures such as brow lifts and forehead reconstructive surgery that will make someone look healthier and reverse signs of aging. Social expectations are the key to shaping individual choices regarding beauty interventions that also reflect more profound cultural issues regarding age and worth. While cosmetic surgery is more and more sought after as a way to combat the visible signs of aging, the cultural narratives around beauty center on a flawed dichotomy: youth is beauty and aging is bad. This cultural narrative encourages people to pursue interventions that can reverse or maintain a youth appearance. Research has determined that when females engage with websites perpetuating beauty standards and perpetuating youthfulness, they tend to internalize a relentless pursuit of such standards, leading to self-objectification and constant discontentment over their natural aging.

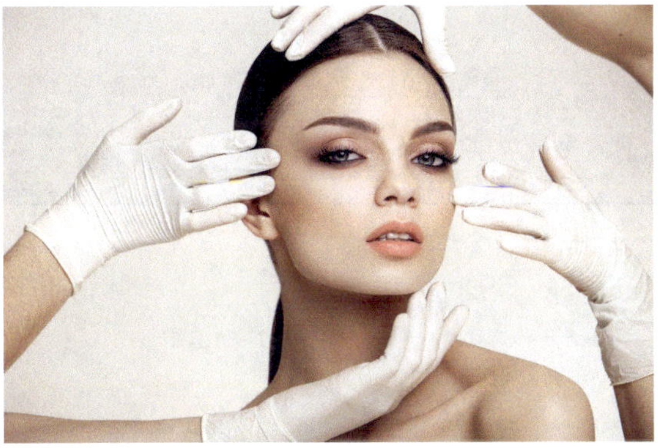

Figure 7.5. Cultural perceptions of beauty and aging.

Source: https://ameorganic.com/cdn/shop/articles/shutterstock_207094993.jpg?v=1706092126&width=3000.

The normalization of aesthetic treatments, fueled by endorsements of nonsurgical procedures by influencers, has led to the normalization of youth-based appearances in public as well as private life, thereby generating very fundamental questions about self-acceptance and identity in the cultural aesthetics of beauty. The implications of these cultural norms are profound, particularly since they relate to identity, femininity and attractiveness as societal constructs. In cultures where one uniform, youth-oriented beauty ideal dominates, the drive to fit in can take many forms, most typically involving physical changes to attain a look that is perhaps impossible for most. This cultural fixation serves not only to market cosmetic procedures such as brow lifts and forehead rejuvenation as the answer to aging but also to create a cycle of comparison and discontentment in women. Furthermore, since the conversation about beauty continues to evolve, there also comes a crucial debate about the ethics and availability of cosmetic procedures, especially in terms of diverse cultural identity and individual experience. The conundrum continues to exist: how to navigate the measures of beauty that construct popular culture without perpetuating harmful norms that belittle the natural aging process (Figure 7.5).

Test Your Knowledge

1. What have been key milestones in the development of brow lift procedures over time?
2. How have cultural perceptions of beauty and aging influenced the evolution of cosmetic surgery techniques?

7.2. Anatomy of the Forehead and Brow Area

Learning Outcome

1. Discuss the Key Facial Muscles Involved in Expression
2. Explain the Skin Structure and Aging Effects
3. Focus on Importance of Understanding Anatomy for Surgical Outcomes

The anatomy of the forehead and brow consists of a complex interplay of tissues, muscles, and vascular structures that are at the core of facial beauty. The forehead, composed mostly of the frontalis muscle, extends from the hairline to the brow ridges. This is the facial expression muscle, which makes functions such as raising the eyebrows, which assist in nonverbal communication. Beneath the skin is a more compact network of vessels that includes arteries such as the supra-orbital and angular arteries, which provide a critical blood supply to the forehead region. They are especially crucial for recognition during surgical operations, such as brow lifts, where precision is essential not to jeopardize the blood supply and optimal healing outcomes (Kleintjes et al., 2007). Understanding the intricate anatomy of this area allows for comprehensive surgical planning and increases the likelihood of successful cosmetic results. In addition to the vascular structures, the forehead and brow region is densely populated with sensory and motor nerves that are vital for maintaining facial functionality and aesthetics.

The supra-orbital and the supratrochlear nerves, arising from the ophthalmic branch of the trigeminal nerve, innervate the forehead and scalp. Damage to these nerves during cosmetic procedures can lead to complications such as sensory neuropraxia, which manifests as altered sensation and could impact the patient's satisfaction with the procedure. Recent studies promote the importance of meticulous anatomical dissection to accurately map these neural tracts to avoid post-operative deficits (Ju et al., 2024). This information can be used by surgeons to maximize results, tailoring interventions to the unique anatomical variation that exists between patients—factors critical in the instance of brow lifts and forehead rejuvenation surgery.

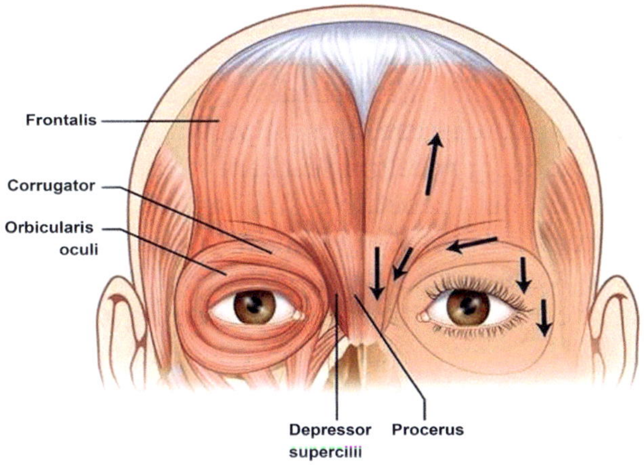

Figure 7.6. The anatomy of the forehead and brow area encompasses a complex interplay of tissues.

Source: https://media.springernature.com/lw685/springer-static/image/chp%3A10.1007%2F978-1-4939-1544-6_83/MediaObjects/82185_2_En_83_Fig2_HTML.jpg.

Also, the cosmetic significance of the forehead and brow anatomy extends into ethnic and age-based variations that influence surgical outcomes. Research has demonstrated that morphometric characteristics such as brow position, shape of eyebrows, and forehead width vary significantly between ethnic groups. Asians, for instance, typically have more superiorly positioned eyebrows than Caucasians, and this needs to be considered when planning cosmetic surgery (Ju et al., 2024). Age is also a determinant, as the increase in age causes changes in skin thickness, fat distribution under the skin, and muscle tone, all of which influence the brow and forehead's look. By balancing a subliminal understanding of these differences in anatomy, cosmetic surgeons then are able to more effectively plan and execute brow lifts and facelifts guided not only by the patient's appreciation for their ideal look but also by their anatomical facts (Figure 7.6).

7.2.1. Key Facial Muscles Involved in Expression

The intricate function of facial muscles is crucial to the expressions conveyed through the visage, playing a wide role in interpretations of intent and emotion. Among all the muscles, the frontalis plays a significant role in the elevation of eyebrows and the creation of horizontal lines on the forehead and hence conveys surprise or interest. Its dominance in the forehead region draws attention to its need for surgical interventions, such as brow lifts, to soften these lines and achieve a fresher appearance. Furthermore, the corrugator supercilii muscles, just above the eyebrows, are in charge of frowning and scowling facial movements. Contraction of these muscles can be the cause of the formation of deep glabellar lines, which have a tendency to give a tired or old appearance and highlight the need to be aware of muscle function in facial rejuvenation surgery, such as treatment with injectable fillers and neuromodulators (Chuang et al., 2016). Brow lifts and forehead rejuvenation surgery treat not only the overlying skin but also the musculature beneath, changing the very dynamics of facial expression. The orbicularis oculi muscle that surrounds the eyes is responsible for both blinking and squinting movements, which are a necessity for many emotional expressions ranging from happiness to astonishment. The interaction of this muscle with other muscles on the face is something that requires consideration in cosmetic assessments, especially in patients with aging, where excess skin due to loss of muscle tone with time may be observed. As the brow drops, there can be a functional deficit in the upper eyelid's ability to completely open, affecting vision. Consequently, cosmetic surgery such as blepharoplasty can then be performed in conjunction with brow lifts to both restore aesthetic beauty and functional capability, leading to a refreshed appearance fitting youthfulness and clarity (Li et al., 2024). Achieving balanced facial beauty relies on a deep knowledge of the key facial muscles involved in expression and how they contribute to aging. The depressor anguli oris muscle that draws the corners of the mouth downwards, contributes to a sad or disapproving facial look. With age, gravity, coupled with continuous loss of subcutaneous fat, may exacerbate this appearance, necessitating even more invasive procedures like a brow lift to revive an uplifting facial shape. Moreover, a comprehensive facial rejuvenation plan must incorporate assessment of other factors, such as skin elasticity and subcutaneous bulk, to complement the outcome generated by surgical procedures targeting muscle dynamics. The holistic approach values the significance of facial muscle function within the broader framework of aesthetic enhancement, ultimately achieving emotionally expressive and aesthetically pleasing outcomes (Chuang et al., 2016).

7.2.2. Skin Structure and Aging Effects

Skin, being the largest organ of the body, consists of a number of layers, each with differing functions essential to the overall health and look. Its outer covering, epidermis, is a protective layer and the dermis below consists of collagen and elastin fibers that provide it with structural strength and elasticity. But with growing age, this intricate structure undergoes enormous changes. The production of collagen reduces, leading to loosening, and the elastin fibers start breaking down, resulting in further laxity and sag. The combination of these factors brings about the characteristic wrinkling and fine lines that develop over time, particularly in sites that come into frequent contact with environmental agents such as the eyes and the forehead. An understanding of them is important when addressing cosmetic concerns because they provide the foundation for treatments like brow lifts and forehead rejuvenation, which are aimed at restoring fresh contours. Apart from intrinsic aging, external factors also play an important role when it comes to skin degeneration. Sun exposure, pollution, and lifestyle choices such as smoking and diet all contribute to accelerating the aging process. External stressors like these tend to amplify the breakdown of collagen and elastin, which results in apparent premature signs of aging appearing earlier than anticipated. For instance, repetitive sun exposure causes photoaging, with pigmentation changes and deep lines. Apart from that, dehydration, in most cases supplemented by extreme weather or by inadequate skincare, may cause a dull appearance of the skin and enhancement of fine lines. A complete approach to facial rejuvenation should consequently consider intrinsic and extrinsic factors equally, pointing to the importance of preventive as well as corrective treatments like brow lifts for optimal cosmetic outcomes. The physiological changes of aging not only affect the appearance of the skin but also necessitate an individualized response to cosmetic treatment. Improvements in surgical technique have enabled cosmetic treatments like facelifts and brow lifts to successfully compensate for structural loss due to aging. The use of subcutaneous dissection enables surgeons to reposition tissue and remove excess skin, thus restoring a youthful appearance. According to research, esthetically acceptable outcomes of these operations are contingent on having good knowledge of the basic structure of the skin and how aging affects the muscle tone and subcutaneous fat. The changing anatomy of the skin demands careful planning and technique when performing surgical procedures to maintain harmony between aesthetic goals and the modified potentials of the skin, highlighting the need for expert practitioners who know the intricacies involved in facial rejuvenation surgeries (Pourdanesh et al., 2016) (Figure 7.7).

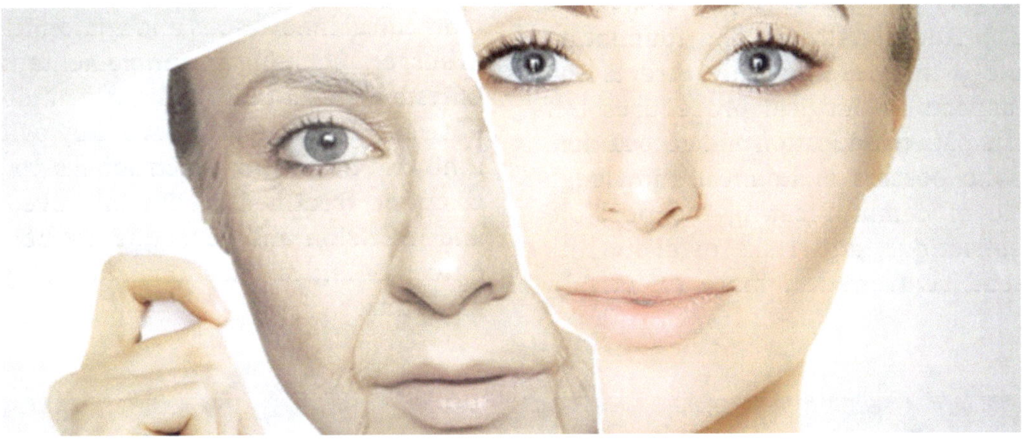

Figure 7.7. Skin structure and aging effects.

Source: https://1.bp.blogspot.com/-q-vf_gQCsxU/XSMRseSpzeI/AAAAAAAAC9Q/iCy5naCuRvslqzq9qXlZ-31jJhCEGaV4QCLcBGAs/s1600/Desired%2Beffect%2Bof%2Banti-aging%2Btreatment.jpg.

7.2.3. Importance of Understanding Anatomy for Surgical Outcomes

Anatomy has a fundamental function to provide optimal post-surgical outcomes, particularly in procedures like brow lifts and forehead rejuvenation. The anatomy of the face is intricate, with the involvement of muscles, nerves, and vascular structures, all of which the surgeon must comprehend. Comprehending these facts not just makes incision precise but also prevents complications such as nerve damage and excessive bleeding. For instance, the facial nerves and superficial temporal artery are key landmarks for brow lift. Omitting these anatomical features can result in suboptimal aesthetic results and prolonged recovery times. Therefore, a good grasp of anatomy can enhance the success of surgery, enabling patients to achieve desired rejuvenating effects with natural facial contours and expressions. Further, the availability of new technologies and materials in cosmetic treatments brings into focus the need for a deep understanding of anatomy, as brought about by the formulation of hyaluronic acid fillers.

The fillers have transformed the practice of facial aesthetic treatments because they make space for a more delicate technique of enhancing facial contours. The skill of a practitioner to analyze facial aging as a total phenomenon depends on their knowledge of anatomy, which enables them to select the correct filler products and techniques for each individual patient. As noted in recent literature, the entire-face approach encourages practitioners to consider the interaction of different facial structures more than addressing discrete features.

This perspective emphasizes the importance of anatomic information in carrying out procedures that result in harmonious and aesthetically pleasing results, further validating the critical contribution of education towards cosmetic surgery procedures (Lipko-Godlewska et al., 2021). Additionally, a solid foundation of anatomic principles not only directs the technical aspects of surgical procedures but also supports patient education and expectation. Surgeons who possess anatomical knowledge are capable of communicating the possible results, restrictions, and risks of brow lifts and forehead rejuvenation more effectively. Such openness builds patient confidence and satisfaction, both of which are paramount in the cosmetic surgery environment. In addition, utilization of sophisticated materials, including polycaprolactone-based fillers, also underscores the interaction between sophisticated biomedical innovations and anatomical prowess in surgery planning and implementation (Marie-Christen et al., 2020). Greater understanding of tissue dynamics, supported by evidence and innovation, allows practitioners to approach cosmetic treatments with improved accuracy and precision and subsequently boost patient outcomes and satisfaction in facial rejuvenation procedures.

Test Your Knowledge

1. Which key facial muscles are involved in forehead and brow movements, and how do they affect facial expression?
2. How does the structure of the skin in the forehead and brow area change with aging?
3. Why is a thorough understanding of forehead and brow anatomy essential for achieving successful surgical outcomes

7.3. Indications for Brow Lift and Forehead Rejuvenation

Learning Outcome

1. Discuss the Common Aesthetic Concerns Addressed
2. Explain the Psychological Impact of Aging on Self-Esteem
3. Focus on Patient Demographics and Trends

Facial cosmetic surgeries, among others, include brow lifting and forehead rejuvenation as pivotal techniques designed to correct the age signs, namely in the upper third of the face. These procedures are specifically aimed at addressing issues such as sagging eyebrows, wrinkled forehead furrows, and facial asymmetry that can make a face appear tired or older. The typical candidates for brow lifts typically include individuals who demonstrate droopy eyebrows and prominent frown lines because these features have the potential to detract significantly from otherwise youthful-looking faces. Moreover, the psychological effects of such aesthetic problems cannot be overemphasized; improving brow aesthetics can potentially boost self-esteem and emotional health. As such, a thorough preoperative evaluation is essential to align patient expectations with desired results, setting the stage for successful surgical results (Różycka et al., 2023). The choice of brow lift or forehead rejuvenation is typically motivated by a set of indications, both aesthetically desired and functionally necessary. A majority of patients are troubled by the tired appearance provided by the sagging brows, diminishing the overall facial harmony. Furthermore, functional indications can be pending when the redundant skin on the forehead presents itself to obstructed vision. In such instances, a brow lift not only enhances cosmetic results but also mitigates functional issues regarding everyday functions. A thorough evaluation that takes into account anatomical elements, facial balance, and patient desires is crucial to ascertain the appropriateness of the procedure. Generally, the synergy among surgical techniques allows for a tailored technique that targets particular needs, thereby maximizing brow lifts' aesthetic and functional benefits (Steenen et al., 2023). Another factor to consider in talking about brow lift and forehead rejuvenation is the growing trend of undertaking these surgical procedures together with other cosmetic procedures. Patients all want total revitalization, which gives a boost in the simultaneous undergoing of brow lifts, eyelid surgery, and other facial enhancements. The intricate beauty of the aesthetic goal highlights the variety and effectiveness of brow rejuvenation in achieving facial harmony all over. Moreover, the psychological benefit of pursuing such enhancement can largely outweigh surgical fears, tending to bring in improved quality of life. But patients must be warned of potential risks, such as scarring or the complications of underlying health. Ultimately, the sustained popularity of brow lifts as a fundamental element in facial rejuvenation is a testament to their relevance in modern cosmetic surgery (Różycka et al., 2023; Steenen et al., 2023) (Figure 7.8).

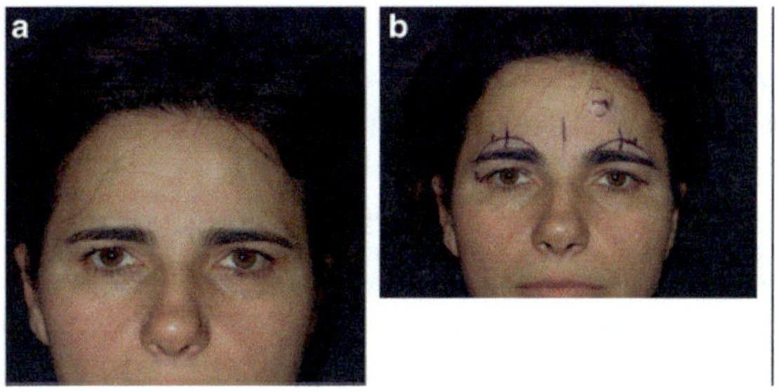

Figure 7.8. Indications for brow lift and forehead rejuvenation.

Source: https://media.springernature.com/lw1200/springer-static/image/art%3A10.1007%2Fs00238-017-1355-2/MediaObjects/238_2017_1355_Fig3_HTML.gif.

7.3.1. Common Aesthetic Concerns Addressed

The forehead rejuvenation and brow lift surgeries address a multitude of cosmetic problems that afflict individuals with progressive age. A first issue that arises is the development of sagging skin and wrinkles on the forehead, which results in a tired or unfulfilling facial look. This is largely a function of the aging process, including loss of muscle tone and elasticity of the skin, causing a puffy face that detracts from otherwise youthful appearance. With the procedure of a brow lift, doctors can reposition the skin and smooth out the wrinkles and thereby making a person more alert and refreshed-looking. This rehabilitation not only lifts the physical appearance of the patients but also can lead to greater self-esteem and improved emotional health, demonstrating the very considerable impact of aesthetic procedures on the overall quality of life, as described in Pourdanesh et al. (2016). A further very significant aesthetic issue alleviated by brow lift surgery is the drooping skin or deep creases, usually referred to as worry lines. These lines can deepen and become more prominent, becoming a constant frown or scowl that may not be an expression of the person's true emotions. These facial expressions can influence how individuals perceive a person in the workplace and society. A brow lift corrects these problems by addressing the source of lax skin, providing a smoother forehead and minimizing the depth of these lines. The result of such a young appearance can improve not only self-confidence but also interpersonal relationships, revealing the affective dimensions surrounding beauty preferences. Such an alteration exemplifies the mutual relationship between facial attractiveness and human interaction during social interactions, as emphasized in Chuang et al. (2016). Besides elevating falling facial skin, brow lifts are also performed for the functional advantage of improving peripheral vision obstructed by sagging eyebrows. This particular case serves to stress the need for addressing aesthetic issues holistically, particularly in both appearance and function. Such patients do report an improved quality of life post-surgery, not so much because a superior aesthetics has been attained but rather because of the return of functional capacities. The psychological impacts of this cannot be underestimated either; the person who perceives himself or herself as being aesthetically pleasing is bound to engage others positively. Thus, the brow lift extends beyond cosmetic augmentation, effectively fusing appearance improvement with functional benefits, hence cementing its position in the greater debate of facial rejuvenation procedures as articulated in Chuang et al. (2016).

7.3.2. Psychological Impact of Aging on Self-Esteem

The psychological impact of aging on self-esteem is a critical consideration in the discipline of facial cosmetic surgeries, particularly that of brow lift and forehead rejuvenation. As people get older, the normal changes in facial contour—i.e., decreased skin elasticity and wrinkles—can profoundly affect one's perception of oneself and one's self-confidence. Studies indicate that these physical changes tend to create a declining sense of self-esteem, specifically among those who associate youthfulness with vigor and attractiveness. The creation of facial signs of oculofacial aging, such as eyebrows sagging and forehead lines, could prompt individuals to turn to cosmetic procedures as a means of reclaiming not just their physical but also mental well-being. This dynamic correlation of body shape and mood reinforces the intricate correlation of aging, self-esteem, and rationale for the use of aesthetic treatments, as attested to by the growing demand for minimally invasive aesthetic treatments intended to reverse these changes (Tao et al., 2025).

Moreover, requests for cosmetic treatments like brow lifts and forehead rejuvenation are typically precipitated by a desire to reacquire a lost identity or enhance interpersonal relationships. Patients who experience the psychological impact of aging can develop an increasing dissonance between their sense of age and their sense of self. It can leave them feeling less than adequate, particularly when faced with societal definitions of beauty that prioritize youthfulness. Improved and enhanced self-esteem is indicated by many patients following cosmetic surgery, as they express that they are restored to their public self and feel more self-assured. Indeed, the outcomes in terms of psychological well-being following aesthetic procedures are significant, with patients experiencing an appreciable improvement in quality of life as they return to social environments more self-assured (Tao et al., 2025).

It is thus crucial for clinicians in this area to know why these types of cosmetic choices are made. The effects of alterations in self-esteem across life are subject to sensitivity to the practice of aesthetic medicine, patient-specific care, and ethics. Practitioners must take into account the psychological underpinnings of an individual's choice for brow lift surgery, as unrealistic expectations can lead to dissatisfaction and negative mental health results. By encouraging an atmosphere of open communication, the practitioner can assist with realistic goal-setting on the part of the patient and a better understanding of the aesthetic options available. The function of education programs is also emphasized at events such as the Italian Association of Plastic Aesthetic Surgery (AICPE) annual congress, where expert discussion emphasizes the psychological considerations of aesthetic surgery.

These encounters not only highlight the necessity of taking on a holistic modality for patient treatment but also shed light on the surgeon's responsibility to address the more pervasive effects of aging on self-esteem and mental well-being. Ultimately, the integration of psychological sensitivity into esthetic practice has the potential to enhance patient satisfaction and promote healthier self-imaginings in the elderly (Figure 7.9).

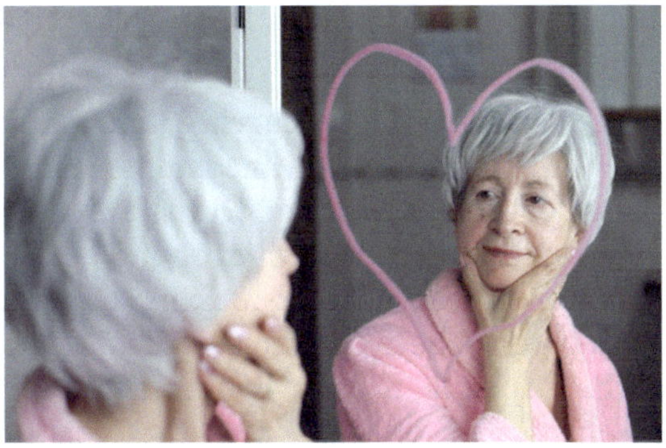

Figure 7.9. Psychological impact of aging on self-esteem.

Source: https://bluemoonseniorcounseling.com/wp-content/uploads/2023/09/Shutterstock_2294517913.jpg.

7.3.3. Patient Demographics and Trends

Patient demographic trends for brow lift and forehead rejuvenation reflect prevailing patterns characteristic of the evolving face of aesthetic plastic surgery. The patient demographic most often undergoing these procedures is predominantly female, accounting for nearly 85% of all patients. Also, there is a considerable age range between the ages of 40 and 60 years, an age range that is most usually found to show considerable signs of aging, such as forehead lines and eyebrow sagging.

Brow lifts have seen an impressive trend surge, particularly in the backdrop of increased self-consciousness amid the COVID-19 pandemic, when facial appearances, especially the upper face region, were emphasized. This demographic change points to a heightened demand for surgical procedures that ensure rejuvenation of the upper face in order to facilitate a youthful appearance aligned with societal expectations of beauty (Roider et al., 2024). In putting patient trends into context, existing evidence indicates that demographic factors are essentially linked with procedural choice and consequent satisfaction rates. Among patients offered brow lifting, a significant percentage were offered preoperative brow aesthetics deemed unfavorable, fewer than 40% of these actually underwent operative treatment, even though they were optimal candidates for brow lifts. Curiously, those who did seek medical attention had larger postoperative improvement in aesthetic outcome, suggesting on the part of patients an awareness of the potential benefits of combined procedures. In this context, the role of preoperative evaluations is increasingly applicable, with the knowledge of patient profiles as individuals being able to make radically profound differences in surgery results and return on aesthetic investment (Kreh et al., 2024). The clear-cut data that reveal an uptick in brow lift procedures has the potential to highlight not just the popularity of the treatment but also an altered sense of value among patients for aesthetic enhancement. The

60% growth in brow lifts in the post-pandemic era is indicative of a shift in patient mindset that prioritizes facial rejuvenation as a component of overall health. Cosmetic procedures like brow lifts have come to be increasingly recognized as more than cosmetic procedures but as positive steps towards rejuvenation, reflective of a larger cultural trend towards self-care. As patient needs become coordinated with options that exist, physicians need to adapt practice styles so that changing expectations can be incorporated into practice in a way that patient-centered surgical planning is directed by demographic shifts and maximizes sustained progress in perceived facial age (Kreh et al., 2024; Roider et al., 2024).

Test Your Knowledge

1. What common aesthetic concerns are typically addressed by brow lift and forehead rejuvenation procedures?
2. How can aging of the forehead and brow area impact a patient's self-esteem and psychological well-being?
3. What are the typical patient demographics and trends for individuals seeking brow lift or forehead rejuvenation procedures?

7.4. Surgical Techniques

Learning Outcome

1. Discuss the Traditional vs. Endoscopic Brow Lift Methods
2. Explain the Anesthesia Options and Considerations
3. Focus on Post-Operative Care and Recovery

The evolution of surgical techniques in facial rejuvenation, particularly in brow lift surgery, has come a long way along the route to achieving subtle aesthetic outcomes. Brow lifts were traditionally performed via a coronal incision, from the midline of the scalp, for repositioning the forehead and brow soft tissue. However, the strides taken in minimally invasive surgery, such as through the employment of endoscopic brow lift, have transformed the technique of rejuvenation of the forehead. This method involves smaller incisions hidden in the hairline, creating less scarring and shorter recovery times. These advancements not only maximize patient satisfaction with more discreet procedures but also fit with evolving aesthetic wants that prefer natural-looking outcomes. This is a balance between technique and patient care that speaks to the dynamic aspect of facial plastic surgery, in which the artistry of surgery must be in concert with the anatomy of the individual, since the differing practices within the discipline make emphatic (Keyhan et al., 2016). The combination of adjunctive treatment with surgical techniques speaks to the complexity of brow lift and forehead rejuvenation. Non-invasive alternatives, such as injectables, are a critical component in complementing surgical treatments, offering a full facial aesthetics system. An example involves the usage of Botulinum toxin (BT), which will effectively diminish the prominence of glabellar lines to smooth out the region and render it more youthful, supporting the structural treatment with surgery. Whereas BT provides an interim solution, its complementarity with surgical procedures has the possibility of enabling a more complete enhancement of aesthetic outcomes. This complex strategy encourages practitioners to see brow lifts not in isolation but as part of an holistic treatment strategy that will yield superior outcomes when integrated with other rejuvenating strategies (Bouzouaya et al., 2018).

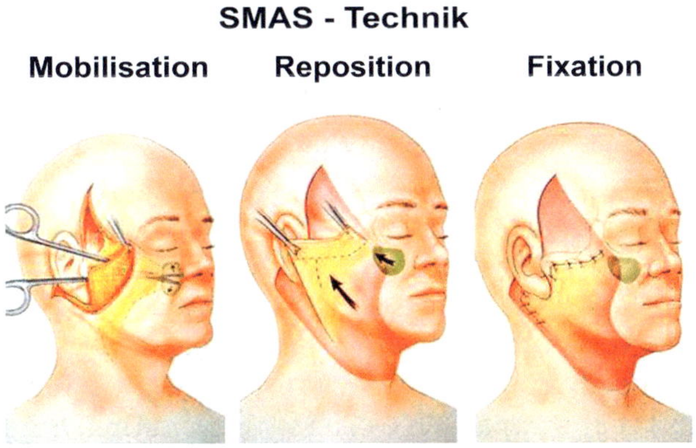

Figure 7.10. The evolution of surgical techniques in facial rejuvenation.

Source: https://static.wixstatic.com/media/f6412e_6938c7e2c27f422f878ea5624ba67688~mv2.png/v1/fill/w_495,h_350,al_c,q_85,enc_avif,quality_auto/f6412e_6938c7e2c27f422f878ea5624ba67688~mv2.png.

Moreover, understanding the patient's unique anatomical features and personal preferences is crucial in tailoring surgical techniques for brow lift and forehead rejuvenation. Each patient presents a distinct combination of facial contours and aging patterns, necessitating a customizable approach to surgical intervention. Surgeons must therefore assess characteristics such as skin elasticity, forehead height, and brow position to devise the most effective surgical strategy. This individualized approach not only enhances the likelihood of achieving expected aesthetic outcomes but also optimizes patient satisfaction and trust through mutual decision-making. With advances in facial plastic surgery, the incorporation of individualized procedures grounded both in art and science will further enhance the standard of care in brow lift and forehead rejuvenation (Keyhan et al., 2016) (Figure 7.10).

7.4.1. Traditional vs. Endoscopic Brow Lift Methods

Brow lift is a significant operation in facial cosmetic surgery for forehead and brow rejuvenation. Out of the two, the primary techniques at hand—traditional and endoscopic procedures—there is a considerable difference between their way of attaining esthetic goals. Traditional brow lift surgeries involve a broad incision across the forehead, offering direct visibility to the underlying tissues. The surgery allows one to easily reposition muscles and remove excess skin, thereby creating a dramatic and immediate result. However, the operation may cause more noticeable scarring and longer healing time, which may deter some people from getting this procedure done. With facial beauty still a focal point of cosmetic surgery, understanding the implications of the traditional method is significant to surgeons and patients alike, especially with the increasing popularity of less invasive methods of facial rejuvenation (Pourdanesh et al., 2016). On the contrary, the endoscopic brow lift method is well-liked due to the fact that it is less invasive. This modern approach employs high-tech techniques, with small incisions hidden in the hairline and an endoscope that allows surgeons to visualize the structures below without creating large, conspicuous scars. With the specialized instruments for the manipulating the brow tissues, the endoscopic method minimizes damage to surrounding tissues, resulting in quicker healing and fewer postoperative aches. The delicacy offered through this method is in accord with the contemporary aesthetic preference for natural outcomes, as patients are now more concerned with enhancing their look without much alteration. Nevertheless, while the endoscopic brow lift has numerous advantages, the requirement of a very skilled surgeon ranks first to get optimal outcomes, which means that the choice of method should be in accord with the needs of patients and the skillfulness of the surgeon (Pourdanesh et al., 2016). Ultimately, the decision between endoscopic and traditional brow lift techniques rests with a complex interaction of factors that include patient anatomy, personal preference, and desired outcome.

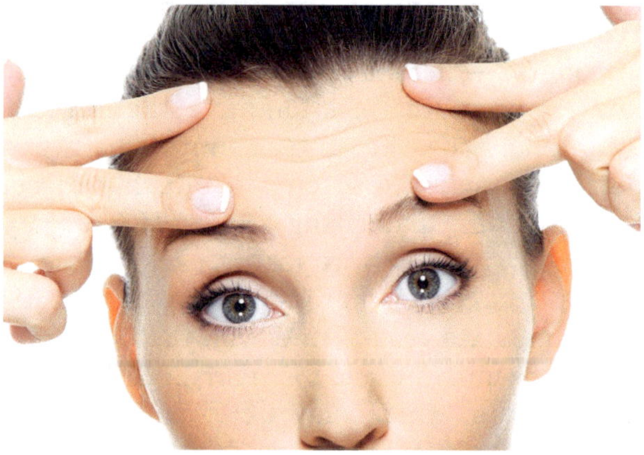

Figure 7.11. The brow lift is a critical procedure in facial cosmetic surgery.

Source: https://d3b3by4navws1f.cloudfront.net/iStock-147308544.jpg.

Both techniques have been successful in treating facial aging, yet the respective methods make candidacy for each procedure vary. Traditional brow lifts can be considered in those patients who desire more elevation or have excess skin that must be excised, while endoscopic methods can be desired by patients seeking a less aggressive intervention. A thorough consultation process involving determining the laxity of the skin, the patient's facial structure overall, and any pre-existing medical conditions is critically important in making this decision. With evolving facial rejuvenation procedures, the surgeons have to be familiar with both methods in order to make recommendations suited to the aesthetic as well as functional needs of the patients (Chuang et al., 2016) (Figure 7.11).

7.4.2. Anesthesia Options and Considerations

In brow lift and forehead rejuvenation procedures, the selection of anesthesia is a critical choice that has a direct bearing on outcomes and satisfaction in the patient. Anesthesiologic options are typically based on patient history, complexity of the procedure, and patient preference by the recommending surgeon. Local anesthesia with sedation is applied most frequently in brow lift procedures due to its effective pain management and quick recovery. Alternatively, general anesthesia can be used for longer procedures, allowing for a full scope approach to facial rejuvenation. Both types of anesthesia offer unique advantages and disadvantages, requiring extensive conversations between the patient and surgical team to customize a strategy ensuring safety and comfort throughout the procedure. In choosing the anesthesia, it is most important to keep in mind the complexity of facial anatomy. The brow and forehead area contains a rich vascular plexus, requiring precise deposition of anesthetics to prevent complications. With the advent of aging changes prompting patients to undergo surgical correction, surgeons must also take into account tissue flexibility differences and skin thickness typical of aging populations. As mentioned, anatomical variation between individuals as well as the severity of aging changes influence surgery, which is attributable to anesthesia choice (Pourdanesh et al., 2016). This confirms the connection between anatomical considerations and anesthesia, solidifying their position in optimizing the surgical process and resultant aesthetic result. Post-operative treatment is also an area influenced by the type of anesthesia used in forehead and brow lift. Local anesthesia and sedation tend to have quicker recovery, allowing mobilization for the patient a short while after surgery and potentially the duration of hospitalization. On the other hand, patients undergoing general anesthesia may have a longer recovery depending on the more pronounced sedative actions and monitoring requirements. Through this knowledge of the anesthetic effect of postoperative care, patient education and guidelines for pain management can be set accordingly to create realistic expectations of recovery. Besides, with the development of cosmetic surgery, inclusion of developments in anesthesia, for example, minimally invasive technology and energy-based devices, further increases patient comfort and safety, thus improving the overall surgical process (Kalaskar et al., 2016).

7.4.3. Post-Operative Care and Recovery

Recovery after the operation is important in ensuring successful recovery and best results following a brow lift and forehead rejuvenation procedure. The initial healing phase normally involves managing swelling and pain, for which relief can be guaranteed by proper rest, icing, and medication. Proper dressing of the wound also contributes significantly to preventing infection and healing. The surgeon would usually provide special advice on how to clean the operative site and when normal activity should resume, an element that is crucial in avoiding complications. This focus on post-op care is founded on the knowledge that the effect of aging on the skin and muscle tone can significantly influence recovery results and aesthetic outcomes, thereby making diligent postoperative care essential to rejuvenation (Pourdanesh et al., 2016). During the recovery process, the emotional component cannot be overruled. There may be expected improved aesthetic results, leading to overplayed emotional responses during healing. In the case of the majority of patients, the convalescence time following a brow lift can cause apprehension in terms of appearance as well as healing. Therefore, paying attention to psychological care and open communication is necessary. The patients must be educated by the surgeons and healthcare teams about the anticipated length of swelling, bruising, and healing. Open communication in such a manner creates reassurance, eliminating fear and enhancing compliance with post-operative care.

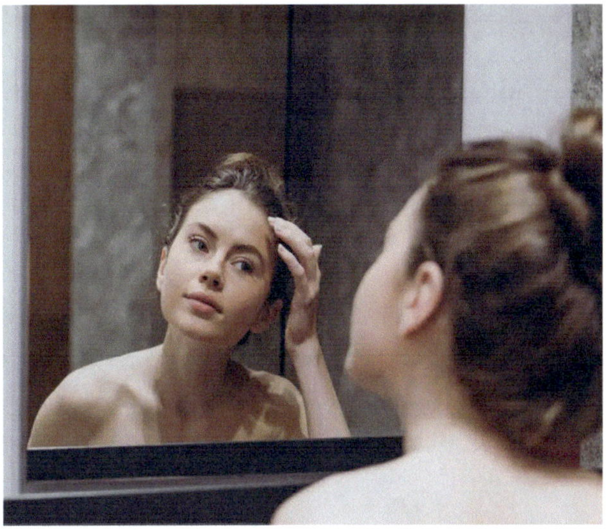

Figure 7.12. Post-operative care and recovery.

Source: https://www.kamfacialplasticsurgery.com/wp-content/uploads/2023/08/endoscopic-brow-lift-dr-kam-new-jersey-02-1024x768.jpg.

This is particularly pertinent in facial cosmetic surgery, where notions of physical and social attractiveness may play a powerful role in patient satisfaction with outcome after recovery (Keyhan et al., 2016). Finally, provision of follow-up visits is a critical component of post-operative care for brow lifting and forehead rejuvenation surgery. This allows health care professionals to monitor healing, assess the aesthetic outcome, and address any patient issues. Follow-up appointments not only facilitate the early detection of complications but also enable greater patient confidence in the surgical outcome. Furthermore, educational conversation during these visits often centers around how to maintain skin quality and cope with long-term skincare needs, issues equally essential after facial rejuvenation surgery. Lastly, a focused effort towards post-operative care—i.e., patient teaching, psychological therapy, and strict follow-up—typically optimizes both the physical and mental aspects of recovery, playing significantly towards patients' overall satisfaction (Keyhan et al., 2016; Pourdanesh et al., 2016) (Figure 7.12).

Test Your Knowledge

1. What are the main differences between traditional and endoscopic brow lift methods?
2. What anesthesia options are available for brow lift procedures, and what factors influence the choice?
3. What are the key post-operative care steps and typical recovery milestones following a brow lift?

7.5. Risks and Complications

Learning Outcome

1. Discuss the Common Surgical Risks Associated with Brow Lifts
2. Explain the Long-Term Effects and Potential Complications
3. Focus on Importance of Choosing a Qualified Surgeon

The brow lift and forehead rejuvenation surgery, although often yielding significant aesthetic improvement, is not without the associated risks and complications. The surgeries have the potential to result in a range of postoperative complications, including bruising, swelling, and pain in the surgical areas that are quite common but temporary. More challenging are permanent complications such as scarring, which affect the overall aesthetics and satisfaction of the result. Anesthesia-related risks are also an important consideration, from minor, transient side effects to major adverse reactions requiring urgent medical intervention. A thorough pre-operative assessment and informed consent process are thus of the greatest importance in maintaining patient safety and expectation management. In addition, the nuances of facial anatomy present unique challenges to brow lift and forehead rejuvenation surgery. According to recent studies, unexpected damage to important structures like nerves and vessels will result in complications like facial asymmetry or eyelid ptosis. Even with optimal procedures, anatomical variations among individuals may not be addressed, and these variations may have a significant impact on outcomes. The significance of injector competencies becomes obvious when one puts into perspective the need for precise techniques to minimize the risk of complications from the administration of botulinum neurotoxin type A (BoNT-A) for the upper face, thereby making a consideration of anatomy and injection protocols important for optimal results (Kąpa et al., 2025). In addition, differential cultural values in relation to aesthetic results complicate the landscape of facial cosmetic surgery. Different regional and ethnic tendencies could decide what is being seen as beautiful, therefore necessitating individualization of every procedure. Such a difference in patient needs should be approached with care because it could determine the extent of satisfaction after surgery. The evolving trends in facial plastic and reconstructive surgery oblige practitioners to keep themselves abreast with new methods and patient needs to be able to reduce risks effectively (Keyhan et al., 2016). Last, acknowledging the inherent risks and complications of brow lift and forehead rejuvenation operations is paramount to enhancing patient outcomes and aligning aesthetic goals with appropriate expectations.

7.5.1. Common Surgical Risks Associated with Brow Lifts

As a cosmetic surgery procedure, brow lifts, or forehead lifts, are increasingly popular to rejuvenate the upper one-third of the face. Despite being highly sought after, these procedures carry risks that are inherent in surgery and must be considered by the patient. These include the most frequently encountered risks such as complications from anesthesia, bleeding, and infection. Complications of anesthesia, though generally rare, may lead to serious complications that are potentially dangerous to patient safety. Excessive blood loss either during or after the surgery can necessitate further medical intervention, complicating the recovery process. Infection, although rare, can influence the healing of the operated sites and, in severe cases, may require antibiotic treatment or further surgical procedures to correct. Knowing these risks is an essential consideration before patients have a brow lift and serves to emphasize the importance of thorough consultation with capable specialists. Scarring and nerve damage are other significant risks that brow lifts are associated with, and relate to surgical complications. While surgeons employ techniques aimed at minimizing visible scarring, hypertrophic or keloid scarring still can develop, especially in persons with a history of abnormal scarring. Facial nerve damage from surgical handling can also lead to transient or, rarely, permanent alteration in facial animation. This may range from minimal asymmetry to not being able to close the eyelids or raise the eyebrows, significantly impacting the patient's quality of life. These are a reminder that facial change is subtle and accuracy is crucial. Therefore, anyone who is contemplating a brow lift should be very sensitive to such risks and have a conversation regarding potential outcomes with their doctor. Lastly, psychological effects post-surgery are an essential element in the brow lift process. While as much as possible the primary objective is to enhance aesthetics and patient satisfaction, there are also patients who may end up disappointed with unrealized expectations or surprise complications. The inconsistency may make the patient depressed or anxious, which contributes to the recuperation problems. In addition, the social pressures that come with cosmetic surgery can enhance inadequacy if the result does not fit society's standard of beauty. As attested in cosmetic surgery advertising practices, there is a pervasive culture under which surgical repair and improved self-esteem and acceptance coincide (King et al., 2013). It is critical that patients have realistic expectations and an adequate pre-operative consultation wherein both the physical and emotional implications of the procedure are addressed in order to ensure a better experience and outcome (Giorgi et al., 1987).

7.5.2. Long-Term Effects and Potential Complications

The long-term effects of brow lift and forehead rejuvenation surgery are critical considerations for probable candidates. As patients attempt to fight the outward signs of aging, they tend to concentrate on short-term aesthetic benefits. But the maintenance of results and potential complications needs to be assessed with caution. Interestingly, skin characteristics can vary with time, impacting the sustainability of surgical results. As one grows older, the skin will even lose some of its thickness and elasticity, and in this way, wrinkles or a sag could reappear even if a procedure has been perfectly successful. It is crucial that patients understand that although initial outcomes may be satisfactory, the relentless effect of aging will persist, meaning that further intervention will still be necessary. These results emphasize the importance of having realistic expectations and teaching patients about the kind of changes that happen on the skin as a result of aging (Goldust et al., 2022). Complications of brow lift and forehead rejuvenation can be temporary or permanent. In the immediate postoperative period after surgery, the patient can present with swelling, bruising, and pain, which are most often bearable. However, long-term complications are more severe and could include scarring, asymmetry, or even complications related to nerve damage. In a few patients, some feel numbness or altered sensation in the forehead region lasting after surgery. The anatomical intricacies of such procedures make it extremely important to possess an extensive understanding of facial anatomy to minimize risks (Pourdanesh et al., 2016). Secondly, underlying medical conditions or poor technique may aggravate such complications, leading to longer recovery times or unsatisfactory aesthetic results. Therefore, the surgeon's skill and adherence to established surgical procedures are necessary in order to prevent possible complications. Furthermore, the psychological impacts of having cosmetic surgery like brow lift and forehead rejuvenation need to be factored into discussions about long-term effects. Patients also develop unrealistic expectations regarding what they will look like following the operation, which may make them dissatisfied even if clinical results meet medical standards. This then leads to a vicious cycle where multiple operations are undertaken as a way to get an ideal look that is unattainable due to physiological restraints. Additionally, the psychological effect of postoperative complications such as scarring or unhappiness can lead to increased anxiety and lower self-esteem upon surgery. It is necessary for surgeons to address these psychological factors through preoperative consultations directed toward not only the aesthetic goals but also the emotional well-being of their patients. Educating prospects about the complexity of their desired goals is instrumental in ensuring proper insight into cosmetic surgery (Pourdanesh et al., 2016).

7.5.3. Importance of Choosing a Qualified Surgeon

Selecting a suitable surgeon to carry out forehead rejuvenation and brow lift operations is the determining factor for satisfactory outcomes. Sophistication of these surgeries demands a surgeon who not only possesses advanced technical skills but also an ample understanding of facial anatomy and aesthetic concepts. A good surgeon, who is generally certified by medical boards, has undergone rigorous training and experience that prepares him/her to deal with the nuances of facial cosmetic surgery. This professionalism reduces the chances of complications from surgery and increases the opportunities for achieving aesthetically pleasing outcomes. Hence, patients are encouraged to investigate potential surgeons thoroughly, focusing on their credentials, experience, and patient reviews, as these factors are closely connected with the quality of treatment provided. Furthermore, the history of a surgeon cannot be overstated, particularly within a field as constantly changing as plastic surgery, where practice and technology are being developed continually. As advances change the environment of the operation, a competent surgeon remains up-to-date with contemporary practice that can improve proceedings to be safer and more efficient. The shared facilities available to veteran surgeons, highlighted in the literature, are instrumental. Surgeons prefer to work together with a multidisciplinary team of professionals, like aestheticians, for the best preoperative and postoperative care, as has been experienced in Costeloe et al. (2023). This wholistic treatment is a clear pointer to commitment to the well-being of the patient, with a further implication of selecting a surgeon who is equipped with the latest knowledge and technology.

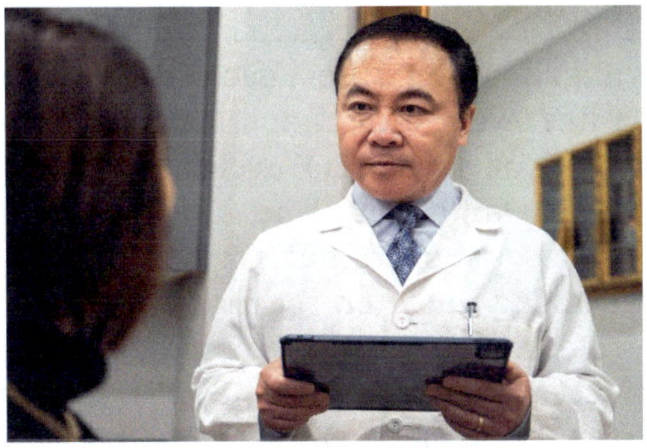

Figure 7.13. Importance of choosing a qualified surgeon.

Source: https://external-content.duckduckgo.com/iu/?u=https%3A%2F%2Fpremiercosmeticla.com%2Fwp-content%2Fuploads%2F2024%2F04%2Ffacelift-why-choose.webp&f=1&nofb=1&ipt=b32fe48a778a6fbebfe07f7e6f08051082416ce46d4cee49ae13bf66ea6f3965.

Further, the informed decision-making process to choose a qualified surgeon is more than mere qualifications; it touches upon the sense of art and the sensitivity of a surgeon and his/her sensitivity to what a patient specifically desires and requires.

The success of brow lifts and forehead rejuvenations, although based on technical ability, also hinges on the surgeon's ability to translate a patient's vision into a harmonious aesthetic result.

Engagement in thorough consultations allows individuals to assess whether a surgeon's method is appropriate for their goal and build a trusting doctor-patient relationship. An interaction like this can illuminate essential factors of care, as well as the extensive guidance an educated professional can provide. Finally, all the time just for this important choice can really make a significant impact on the quality of the surgical outcome, as clearly stated by the very significant observations from Farhadieh et al. (2015), emphasizing the importance of continuous advancement in surgery (Figure 7.13).

Test Your Knowledge

1. What are the main differences between traditional and endoscopic brow lift methods?
2. What anesthesia options are available for brow lift procedures, and what factors influence the choice?
3. What are the key post-operative care steps and typical recovery milestones following a brow lift?

7.6. Non-Surgical Alternatives

Learning Outcome

1. Discuss the Botox and Fillers for Brow and Forehead Rejuvenation
2. Explain the Laser Treatments and Their Effectiveness
3. Understand Comparison of Non-Surgical vs. Surgical Options

Based on patients ever more seeking to feel more beautiful in their faces, non-surgical alternatives to traditional brow lifts have received lots of attention. These alternatives are less invasive options for those resistant to surgery, with generally shorter recovery times and lower risks of complications. Perhaps the most famous of these is the use of botulinum neurotoxin type A (BoNT-A), aimed at dynamic forehead and brow lines with great effectiveness. By causing temporary paralysis of muscles that create such wrinkles, the patients have a smoother and younger appearance without undergoing surgery. The growing popularity of BoNT-A has also transformed the practice of aesthetic medicine by making patients able to achieve visible outcomes with minimal downtime while enjoying the procedural versatility that non-surgical interventions have in store. Apart from BoNT-A, the market has witnessed growing demand for dermal fillers as alternative methods of non-surgical brow lift and forehead rejuvenation. Fillers, employed to restore lost volume and enhance facial contours, can complement the effect of the neurotoxin, thereby resulting in a more defined and rejuvenated appearance. The marriage of both treatments allows the practitioner to maximize the cosmetic outcomes by addressing various concerns at once. Furthermore, the flexibility of fillers enables the potential of being tailor-made for specific patients' needs, so treatment is personalized. With the much-discussed public popularity of non-surgical treatments, as aforementioned, the business has experienced unprecedented growth, enabling more experts to offer these treatments, thereby improving the overall level of access to aesthetic enhancement (Bowler, 2009). In view of the widespread use of non-surgical interventions, clinicians need to know about potential complications associated with these procedures. The intricate upper face anatomy provides unique challenges in the administration of injectable treatments, e.g., BoNT-A. Complications can range from local injection-site side effects to devastating effects like eyelid ptosis and facial asymmetry, which can occur in the event of inadequate anatomical familiarity and experience-based procedures. A systematic review calls for standardizing injection regimens and ensuring that professionals possess the skills required to minimize risks (Kąpa et al., 2025). Even with persistent demand for non-surgical treatments, safety and efficacy will be top priority in providing maximum aesthetic benefits while safeguarding patient satisfaction.

7.6.1. Botox and Fillers for Brow and Forehead Rejuvenation

The utilization of Botox and dermal fillers has revolutionized brow and forehead renewal, with the offering of non-surgical treatments for conventional lifting techniques. Botox is a neurotoxin solution derived from botulinum toxin and is most frequently utilized to diminish dynamic wrinkles resulting from involuntary muscle spasms, particularly in the areas of the brow and forehead. By temporarily paralyzing the muscles, Botox not only softens existing lines, but also elevates the brow slightly, creating a youthful appearance. The non-surgical treatment has no downtime, so patients can get back to their lives almost immediately. Increased use of Botox for brow renewal reflects a general aesthetic medicine trend towards less aggressive interventions rather than surgical ones, thus addressing the varied needs and demands of patients (Goldust et al., 2022). Coupled with Botox, dermal fillers are also essential in the rehabilitation of brow and forehead aesthetics by filling out and defining the lost elasticity and plumpness of the areas over time. Fillers are typically composed of hyaluronic acid, an ingredient that is naturally found within the body and holds water to create a full, fat appearance. Strategically injected into the brow and forehead region, fillers are capable of lifting droopy brows and filling in deep lines, basically restoring a younger face. With both operations done together, there is also an appropriate balance, treating dynamic and static wrinkles.

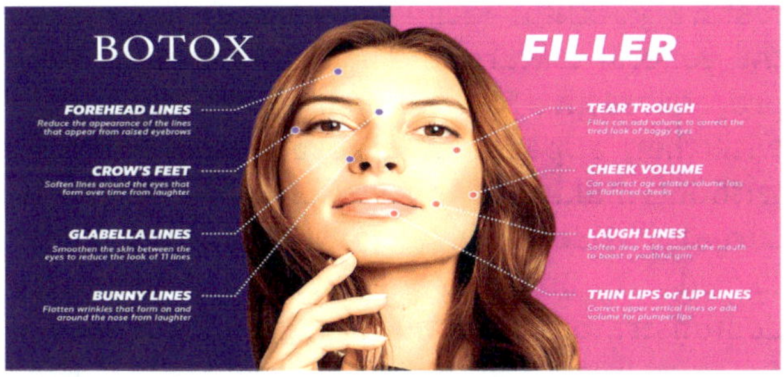

Figure 7.14. Botox and fillers for brow and forehead rejuvenation.

Source: https://dranmolchugh.com/wp-content/uploads/2025/03/Comparison-between-fillers-and-Botox-for-facial-rejuvenation-and-wrinkle-reduction.png.

The harmonious blend of Botox and fillers not just enhances facial aesthetics but also assists in overall rejuvenation, making it possible for a more rested and luminous appearance (Chuang et al., 2016). And with the progress made in the vocation of facial cosmetic treatment, the blend of Botox and fillers keeps evolving, with improved techniques and outcomes for brow and forehead rejuvenation. The non-invasive nature of these treatments appeals to a wide demographic, making them accessible to individuals seeking aesthetic enhancement without the commitment of surgical procedures. The recent surge in requests for these treatments reflects a cultural shift toward preventive aesthetics, with individuals seeking to maintain a youthful appearance before significant aging sets in. With practitioners perfecting their skills and accepting new technologies, the efficacy and safety of these treatments are becoming more solidified, so that Botox and fillers are here to stay in the center of facial rejuvenation (Goldust et al., 2022) (Figure 7.14).

7.6.2. Laser Treatments and Their Effectiveness

The effectiveness of laser treatments in brow lifting and forehead rejuvenation is augmented by growing technological advancements, allowing for more extensive and varied usage. Laser treatment stands out due to its low-invasive nature and ability to stimulate the synthesis of collagen, which is instrumental in the elasticity of the skin and complete rejuvenation. Through these treatments, the patient can achieve visible improvements in skin firmness, tone, and texture with the benefits of quicker recovery times than with conventional surgery. Also, lasers like fractional CO_2 and Erbium:YAG have been noted for having a focused action in the reduction of fine lines and wrinkles, thus further improving the outcome of a brow lift. This convergence of technology and cosmetic intervention has generated a top choice in facial rejuvenation, with laser treatments becoming a favorite complement to facial rejuvenation methods, yielding to patients a highly diverse strategy for attaining optimal aesthetic results. Additionally, the incorporation of laser therapy into cosmetic treatment underscores the need for an all-encompassing knowledge of facial anatomy and the multiplicity of methodologies utilized within aesthetic medicine. The intricate anatomy of the upper face creates unique challenges that emphasize the importance of precision in any treatment modality, particularly in those involving lasers. As hinted by recent research, the application of botulinum neurotoxin type A (BoNT-A) to the upper face is not complication-free, emphasizing the importance of precise anatomical knowledge and adherence to evidence-based practices in esthetic treatments (Kąpa et al., 2025). This backdrop emphasizes the ability of lasers to be utilized as a complete plan in relation to countering certain issues faced during brow lifts, such as asymmetry or irregular contours, therefore yielding superior results for patients. Lastly, with facial rejuvenation ongoing, the role of laser treatments increasingly becomes more pivotal to counteracting diverse patient needs.

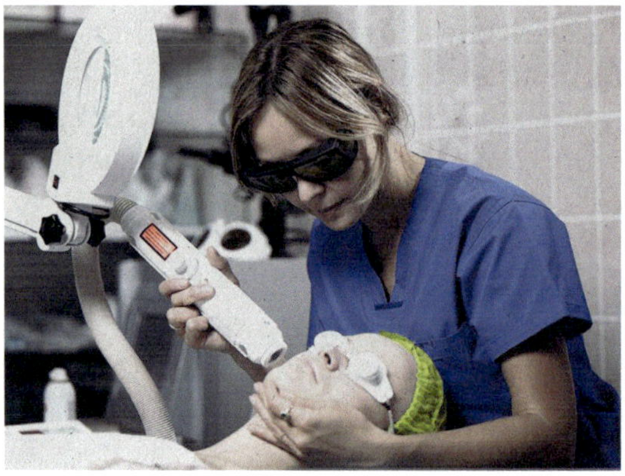

Figure 7.15. Laser treatments and their effectiveness.

Source: https://media.post.rvohealth.io/wp-content/uploads/sites/3/2022/01/laser-skin-resurfacing-procedure-thumb-732x549.jpg.

The selection of a suitable laser modality is often made based on considerations such as the patient's skin type, cosmetic goals, and individual characteristics of his or her facial anatomy (Keyhan et al., 2016). Additionally, the continued progress in laser technologies has yielded enhanced safety profiles and increased efficacy for more extended applications. As medical practitioners adopt laser techniques in overall treatment regimens, they must be aware of the shifting patterns of aesthetic desire so that treatment is tailored and culturally appropriate. This combined approach will eventually result in improved outcomes in brow lift and forehead rejuvenation, aligning with patient expectations and improving satisfaction (Figure 7.15).

7.6.3. Comparison of Non-Surgical vs. Surgical Options

Surgery versus non-surgical options for forehead rejuvenation and brow lift are decided by multiple factors like the patient's expectation, degree of facial aging, and the amount of downtime needed. The demand for non-surgical treatments such as skin-tightening devices and injectables has increased due to these procedures being less invasive. They help to treat mild signs of aging with lower risk and less downtime. For instance, procedures like botulinum toxin and fillers can restore youthful facial contours and enhance the general texture and tone of the skin. Such procedures give patients a chance to experiment with their appearance and see gradual results without making a long-term commitment to surgery. Also, advances in techniques like thread lifts and radiofrequency rhytidectomy demonstrate that non-surgical solutions can achieve drastic changes in facial beauty, thus broadening the range of possibilities for patients seeking rejuvenation therapy (Li et al., 2022). Conversely, procedures like brow lifts provide a more long-term solution for people with severe manifestations of aging, like severe skin sagging and deep lines. Surgical operations can be long-lasting in their outcomes by addressing the tissues directly underneath, like muscle and fat repositioning. While these operations tend to have longer recovery times and potential side effects, they are best for individuals who desire drastic changes in the shape of their faces. Furthermore, surgical techniques can create a stronger and immediate visual impact that cannot be attained with non-surgical means, especially for individuals with extreme signs of aging. The commitment to surgical recovery has the advantage of longer longevity in results compared to non-surgical methods, which often need constant maintenance and repeated sessions throughout life (Khan et al., 2021). Thus, the choice is reflective of the patient's lifestyle and personal aesthetic ideals. Lastly, a comparison between both non-surgical and surgical treatments allows for a tailored approach in brow lift and forehead rejuvenation procedures. The majority of patients are able to go for a synergistic treatment protocol that engages non-invasively and invasively with a purpose of achieving the optimal result. For example, using non-surgical treatments as an initiation step can delay subsequent surgical treatment as a transitional phase allowing the patient to assess satisfaction with results. Moreover, the advancement of sophisticated technologies, such as micro-focused ultrasound therapy, also enhances the efficiency of non-surgical procedures, making them an increasingly appealing choice for those that desire facial rejuvenation (Khan et al., 2021). Hence, the facial cosmetic surgery scene today requires discussions between practitioners and patients on an informed basis for the benefits, drawbacks, and realistic expectations of outcomes from each modality, ultimately culminating in customized and satisfying treatment experiences.

Test Your Knowledge

1. How do Botox and dermal fillers work to rejuvenate the brow and forehead area, and what results can patients expect?
2. What types of laser treatments are used for forehead and brow rejuvenation, and how effective are they?
3. What are the main differences in outcomes, risks, and longevity between non-surgical and surgical brow/forehead rejuvenation options?

SUMMARY

In conclusion, brow lift and forehead rejuvenation procedures are significant breakthroughs in facial cosmetic surgery with enhanced aesthetic outcomes for patients worried about combating evidence of aging. The complex nature of these procedures requires intimate knowledge of the anatomical and physiologic changes with aging and the various techniques with which the surgeon is familiar. An effective brow lift not only eliminates sagging skin and diminishes the visibility of wrinkles but also improves the overall balance of facial structure. Hence, when done competently, these procedures are capable of changing one's life with improved confidence and self-esteem and thus demonstrate their importance in cosmetic surgery. In addition, safety and efficacy for brow lifts largely rely on the experience of the practitioner and the technique selected. As highlighted in recent literature, side effects of BoNT-A injections in the upper face also highlight the necessity for a proper understanding of facial anatomy and potential risk factors (Kąpa et al., 2025). Adhering to recent best practices and embracing novel approaches, facial plastic surgeons can avert risks as well as improve aesthetic benefits. This commitment to safety and precision lies at the center of achieving maximum outcomes for patients, emphasizing the absolute necessity of ongoing education and training in this rapidly evolving field of facial rejuvenation. Furthermore, the increasing diversity of modalities within facial plastic surgery is redefining the boundaries of the brow lift and forehead rejuvenation. The integration of non-invasive options, including injectable fillers and modulators of neural influence, complements traditional surgical interventions and offers patients a range of choices that best address their individual needs (Chuang et al., 2016). As such, this interprofessional use not only enhances facial rejuvenation outcomes but also meets the varied desires of patients, making rejuvenation treatments more accessible and less intimidating. Lastly, as technology and technique continue to advance, the future of forehead rejuvenation and brow lifting looks promising, paving the way to an era of increased personalization and sophistication in facial cosmetic surgery.

During analysis of the advancements involving brow lift and forehead rejuvenation, great attention is given to the efficacy of various techniques employed in this field of aesthetic surgery. The brow lift, for instance, is a surgery aimed at fixing sagging brows, which are usually exacerbated by the natural aging process and external pressure. As patients are now more keen on obtaining youthful appearances, facial anatomy aspects have to be understood. Clinical data support that targeted interventions, including strategic incision placement and manipulation of underlying anatomy, can provide substantial gains in aesthetic improvement and satisfaction. Utilization of injectables, like Botulinum neurotoxin type A (BoNT-A), is also critical in maximizing surgical skills and providing combined rejuvenation of the upper face, minimizing risks for suboptimal technique, as referenced in the literature. Furthermore, the effect of aging on skin, particularly over facial anatomy, is exaggerated. As has been written in more recent descriptions, the combination of thinning epidermis and diminished muscle tone not only creates a cosmetically unappealing face but also impacts self-esteem and social relationships among patients. This aging process necessitates inclusion of a multidisciplinary plan when one considers rejuvenating procedures, with emphasis on both operative and nonoperative measures. Contemporary methods highlight the value of individualized treatment plans that take into account anatomical variations and patient-specific characteristics, such as skin texture and economics. With these personalized modalities, surgeons can better address patients' diverse expectations, ensuring the outcome is what they are seeking in a more youthful look. Lastly, brow lift and forehead rejuvenation are topics that include safety and potential complications of the procedures. The literature gives utmost importance to thorough anatomical knowledge and injector experience to avoid unwanted results, which can range from subtle bruising to severe complications like facial asymmetry. With the ongoing need for aesthetic procedures, maintaining equilibrium between effective rejuvenation and safety is a key consideration in practice. Compliance with standard protocols and ongoing education among practitioners is key to minimizing risks associated with procedures such as BoNT-A injections and facelifts. In this way, the science of facial cosmetic surgery can enhance not only aesthetic outcomes but also patient satisfaction and confidence, encouraging an improved, educated method of facial rejuvenation.

KEY TERMS FROM THIS CHAPTER

- Brow Ptosis
- Lateral Brow Elevation
- Endoscopic Brow Lift
- Temporal Brow Lift
- Pretrichial Incision
- Subgaleal Dissection
- Frontalis Muscle
- Forehead Rhytids
- Medial Brow Elevation
- Coronal Brow Lift
- Direct Brow Lift
- Hairline Incision
- Subperiosteal Dissection
- Corrugator Supercilii

CRITICAL THINKING QUESTIONS

1. **The primary goal of a brow lift is to:**
   a. Elevate ptotic eyebrows and smooth forehead lines
   b. Reduce nasal width
   c. Reshape eyelids
   d. Increase hair density
2. **Which muscle is mainly responsible for horizontal forehead lines?**
   a. Orbicularis oculi
   b. Frontalis
   c. Corrugator supercilii
   d. Procerus
3. **Vertical glabellar lines (frown lines) are primarily caused by overactivity of the:**
   a. Frontalis muscle
   b. Corrugator and procerus muscles
   c. Masseter muscle
   d. Temporalis muscle
4. **Which brow lift technique uses small scalp incisions and an endoscope?**
   a. Direct brow lift
   b. Endoscopic brow lift
   c. Coronal brow lift
   d. Temporal brow lift
5. **A coronal brow lift incision is usually placed:**
   a. Along the upper eyelid crease
   b. Under the jawline
   c. Inside the nostril
   d. At the hairline or within the scalp

Short Answer Questions

1. What are the main aesthetic indications for performing a brow lift?
2. How does the frontalis muscle contribute to forehead aging?
3. What is the difference between a coronal brow lift and an endoscopic brow lift?
4. Which muscles are primarily responsible for glabellar frown lines?
5. What are common complications associated with brow lift procedures?
6. How does Botox contribute to nonsurgical forehead rejuvenation?

Answers to Critical Thinking Questions

1. (a) 2. (b) 3. (b) 4. (b) 5. (d)

REFERENCES

1. Araujo, M. J. (2025). *New minimally invasive technique for the treatment of labia minora hypertrophy: Vulvar endolifting*. https://www.amwc-conference.com/content/dam/markets/aest/amwc-conference/2025/pdf/AMWC2025-Abstratcs.pdf (accessed on 14th July 2025).
2. Keyhan, S. O., Asayesh, M. A., Khojasteh, A., & Iranaq, M. H. A. (2016). Complications in Esthetic Surgery. InTech. doi: 10.5772/63371 (accessed on 14th July 2025).
3. Chuang, J., Barnes, C., & Wong, B. J. F. (2016). Overview of Facial Plastic Surgery and Current Developments. *Surgery journal (New York, N.Y.)*, *2*(1), e17–e28. https://doi.org/10.1055/s-0036-1572360 (accessed on 14th July 2025).
4. Kąpa, M., Szepietowski, B., Szustak, J., Wijata, M., Wijata, A. M., Przybyłek-Stępień, Z. A., ... Pasek, P. (2025). Complications and Anatomical Considerations in Botulinum Neurotoxin Type A Injections for Upper Face Rejuvenation: A Systematic Review. *Quality in Sport*, *39*, 58445. https://doi.org/10.12775/QS.2025.39.58445(accessed on 14th July 2025).
5. Bouzouaya, C., & Feiner, R. (2018). *Adjuvant botulinum toxin harmonization in minimally invasive facial aesthetic surgery*. https://core.ac.uk/download/322438270.pdf (accessed on 14th July 2025).
6. Bowler P. J. (2009). Impact on facial rejuvenation with dermatological preparations. *Clinical interventions in aging*, *4*, 81–89. https://doi.org/10.2147/cia.s3524(accessed on 14th July 2025).
7. Castillo-Campos, P. (2022). Rhytidoplasty through minimal incisions (rhythmic). *Aesthetic Surgery Journal Open Forum*. https://doi.org/10.1093/asjof/ojac059 (accessed on 14th July 2025).
8. Christen, M. O., & Vercesi, F. (2020). Polycaprolactone: How a well-known and futuristic polymer has become an innovative collagen-stimulator in esthetics. *Clinical Cosmetic and Investigational Dermatology*, *13*, 31–48. https://doi.org/10.2147/ccid.s229054 (accessed on 14th July 2025).
9. Costeloe, A., & Newman, J. (2023). Aesthetician role in facial plastic surgery and systemic therapy for healthy skin. *Facial Plastic Surgery Clinics of North America*, *31*(4), 557–566. https://doi.org/10.1016/j.fsc.2023.05.007 (accessed on 14th July 2025).
10. Di Filippo, J., Gagliano, C., Grando, M., Miotti, et al. (2024). *Fat management in upper blepharoplasty: Addition or subtraction blepharoplasties, how and when*. https://core.ac.uk/download/614033783.pdf (accessed on 14th July 2025).
11. Pourdanesh, F., Esmaeelinejad, M., Jafari, S. M., & Nematollahi, Z. (2016). Facelift: Current Concepts, Techniques, and Principles. InTech. doi: 10.5772/63150(accessed on 14th July 2025).
12. Farhadieh, R. D., Bulstrode, N. W., & Cugno, S. (2015). *Plastic and Reconstructive Surgery: Approaches and Techniques*. https://www.ceydeli.com/files/2016/06/Plastic-Reconstive-Surgery.pdf (accessed on 14th July 2025).
13. Giorgi, G. (1987). *Barnes Hospital Bulletin*. https://core.ac.uk/download/70381137.pdf (accessed on 14th July 2025).
14. Goldust, M., Gupta, M., Kassir, M., Kroumpouzos, et al. (2022). *Complications of Botulinum Toxin A: An Update Review*. https://core.ac.uk/download/621756021.pdf (accessed on 14th July 2025).

15. Ju, S. (2024). *Three-Dimensional Periocular Morphometry of Populations in the European region*. https://core.ac.uk/download/638448205.pdf (accessed on 14th July 2025).

16. Khan, U. U., & Khalid, N. (2021). A systematic review of the clinical efficacy of micro-focused ultrasound treatment for skin rejuvenation and tightening. *Cureus*. https://doi.org/10.7759/cureus.20163 (accessed on 14th July 2025).

17. King, K. K., Merianos, A. L., & Vidourek, R. A. (2013). *Medicalization of female beauty: A content analysis of cosmetic procedures*. https://core.ac.uk/download/51087636.pdf (accessed on 14th July 2025).

18. Kleintjes, W. G. (2007). *The vascular anatomy of the forehead related to forehead flaps and its application in plastic and reconstructive surgery*. https://core.ac.uk/download/37319075.pdf (accessed on 14th July 2025).

19. Kreh, C. C., Roider, L. A., Firouzbakht, P. K., Nathan, C., Prada, C. A., Lund, H. G., Sarhaddi, D., et al. (2024). Artificial intelligence analysis of periorbital rejuvenation. *Aesthetic Surgery Journal*. https://www.semanticscholar.org/paper/02d9b50399228324977b8e1009d66b4efdc3f459 (accessed on 14th July 2025).

20. Kumar, N. (2021). *Design, development and implementation framework for a postgraduate non-surgical aesthetics curriculum*. https://core.ac.uk/download/480391006.pdf (accessed on 14th July 2025).

21. Li, K., Meng, F., Li, Y. R., Tian, Y., Chen, H., Jia, Q., Cai, H. X., et al. (2022). Application of nonsurgical modalities in improving facial aging. *International Journal of Dentistry, 2022*, 1–18. https://doi.org/10.1155/2022/8332631 (accessed on 14th July 2025).

22. Li, X. (2024). *Quantifying Dermatochalasis Using 3-Dimensional Photogrammetry*. https://core.ac.uk/download/621205163.pdf (accessed on 14th July 2025).

23. Lin, L. (1996). *Facial Rejuvenation with Aesthetic Surgeries*. https://core.ac.uk/download/232135231.pdf (accessed on 14th July 2025).

24. Lipko-Godlewska, S., Bolanča, Ž., Kalinová, L., Kermen, I., Onisak, B., Papp, I., Rebrov, M., et al. (2021). Whole-face approach with hyaluronic acid fillers. *Clinical Cosmetic and Investigational Dermatology, 14*, 169–178. https://doi.org/10.2147/ccid.s292501 (accessed on 14th July 2025).

25. McGinty, K. (2021). *You all look like @wolfiecindy: The homogeny of facial self-presentation among female Instagram users*. https://core.ac.uk/download/478652031.pdf (accessed on 14th July 2025).

26. Deepak M. Kalaskar, Peter E. Butler, Shadi Ghali. (2016). *Textbook of Plastic and Reconstructive Surgery*. ISBN: 978-1-910634-37-0 (Hbk.) https://core.ac.uk/download/79526588.pdf

27. (accessed on 14th July 2025).

28. Roider, L. A., Firouzbakht, P. K., Kreh, C. C., Nathan, C., Prada, C. A., Lund, H. G., Sarhaddi, D., et al. (2024). Periorbital rejuvenation: Artificial intelligence highlights the importance of brow lift. *Aesthetic Surgery Journal Open Forum, 6*. https://www.semanticscholar.org/paper/288cb79b7e53c47693629e45b15eac66481b6f52 (accessed on 14th July 2025).

FACIAL IMPLANTS AND CONTOURING: CHIN, CHEEK, AND JAW IMPLANTS; FAT GRAFTING AND LIPOSCULPTURE

8

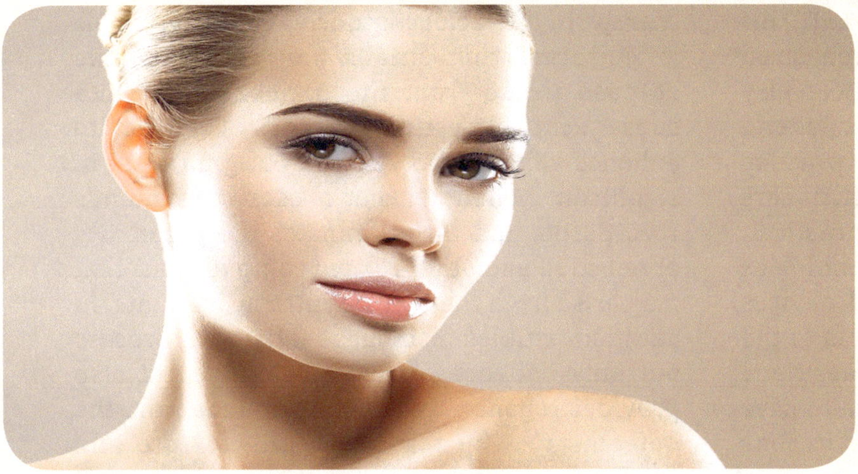

LEARNING OBJECTIVES

After studying this chapter, you will be able to:

1. List the types of facial implants;
2. Explain the benefits of facial implants;
3. Understand risks and considerations in facial implants and contouring;
4. Identify fat grafting;
5. Highlight liposculpture;
6. Understand combining procedures.

Introduction

The search for a facial look pleasing to the eye has prompted many surgical and nonsurgical interventions, particularly in facial implants and facial contouring. Most vital driving force behind this has been the search for greater confidence and self-esteem, and appearance is highly capable of affecting this. The United States accounted for an estimated 15.5 million cosmetic procedures in 2020, which reflects heightened acceptance and demand for facial enhancement treatments, including chin, cheek, and jaw implants. Not only do these advanced technologies promote aesthetic improvements, but they also are used to treat patients who have issues with facial volume loss or asymmetry. The mounting evidence surrounding these techniques emphasizes their success and the worth of individualized treatment plans, with patient preference and anatomy taken into account to gain optimum benefits (Garcia et al., 2022). Fat grafting and liposculpture, in addition to conventional implants, have also emerged as key components of modern facial aesthetic surgeries. Liposuction, once a basic fat-reduction device, is currently a high-tech procedure that involves the use of various techniques based on unique patient needs. Of these, cervicofacial liposuction offers a less disruptive approach to facial and neck sculpting, allowing for exact mold-like shaping of fatty tissue accumulation. The systematic review of clinical outcomes indicates high-density fat transfer, using the application of stromal vascular fraction gel, not only replaces facial volume but also with improved patient satisfaction scores (Kalaskar et al., 2016). This evolution of liposuction techniques emphasized the value of the role aesthetic procedures play in progressing patients' self-esteem and general well-being. With advancements in the practice of facial contouring, it is vital that practitioners are in line with current protocols and practices. Specialized training in emerging technologies and techniques, such as energy-based devices or combination therapy, also contributes to the necessity for a multidisciplinary facial aesthetic approach. For this reason, it is important to have knowledge of the limitations and complications of various procedures to ensure effective and safe care. Evidence from different research studies and clinical outcomes shows that patients who undergo facial augmentation are likely to show significant improvements not only on their faces but also in their lifestyle. Ongoing practice of facial implants, fat grafting, and liposculpture is thus central to influencing aesthetic surgical techniques and attaining patient satisfaction (Garcia et al., 2022).

Definition of Facial Implants and Contouring

Facial contouring theory and facial implants are a wide variety of facial procedures intended to reshape and redefine the facial structure and beauty. Facial implants are artificial bodies that are surgically implanted in an effort to support or redefine portions of the facial structure, primarily the jawline, cheek, and chin. The implants offer a permanent solution for individuals seeking a more harmonious profile or structural flaw correction. Surgeons evaluate each patient's unique anatomical attributes and aesthetic preferences to determine implant size, shape, and material. Rising demand for these surgeries is a symptom of a broader societal trend toward individualized cosmetic enhancement, wherein interest fluctuates away from abstract beauty and towards individualized aesthetic gratification and expression of self. Fat grafting has expanded in the last 10 years as an adjunct therapy in the facial contouring repertoire. This is a process that entails the removal of the adipose tissue from the patient's body and subsequent reinjection into sites of the face to enhance volume and contour. Fat grafting is of significant benefit in that it uses the patient's own tissue, and this eliminates the possibility of rejection and other related complications that may arise from the use of synthetic implants. In addition, studies also suggest that the process not only enhances facial appearance but also provides regenerative benefits for the skin, the outcome of which is a youthful texture and appearance. The dual function of aesthetic enhancement along with stimulation of the skin care makes fat grafting a universal tool for modern facial sculpting. Liposculpture, on the other hand, is a development of the traditional method of liposuction specifically adapted for facial applications. This method uses negative pressure through a cannula to carefully suction out excess fat in targeted areas of the face and neck while shaping the contours to yield a slimmer profile. Recent clinical studies indicate that liposculpture has emerged as the forefront choice due to its minimally invasive nature and maximum patient satisfaction. As listed in certain research, including that viewed from substantial databases, patients who have undergone cervicofacial liposculpture have reported admirable improvement in facial contour in addition to increased emotional satisfaction and self-esteem following the procedure (Garcia et al., 2022). Moreover, advancements in energy devices and combination therapy have also increased contouring potential, consistent with the increased sophistication of these aesthetic treatments (Kalaskar et al., 2016) (Figure 8.1).

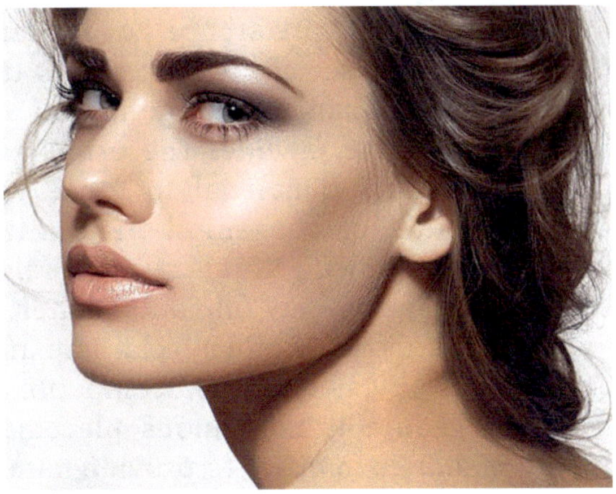

Figure 8.1. The concept of facial implants and contouring.

Source: https://greatyou.com/wp-content/uploads/2016/05/Cheekbone-Contour.jpg.

Facial Aesthetics Role in Modern Society

The role of facial aesthetics in modern society cannot be overstated, as physical appearance plays an important role in private and social life. Clean and defined facial features have a tendency to suggest perceived traits like confidence, health, and beauty and influence anything from career opportunities to social relationships. In a time of increasingly visual stimulation, initial impressions are often made based on facial beauty. As people navigate the spheres of social existence, those who are seen to have such aesthetics may have higher self-esteem and improved social standing. Beauty being emphasized in culture can drive the motivation of individuals to seek out many avenues of augmentation, such as facial implants and the practice of contouring, to achieve what society deems attractive. Consequently, the growing popularity of treatments aimed at beautifying the face is a larger social movement toward valuing looks as part of assessing personal worth. Additionally, cosmetic technologies have made facial aesthetic improvements more accessible, thereby normalizing such behaviors in contemporary society. Techniques such as chin, cheek, and jaw implants, fat grafting, and liposculpture have gone far in offering individuals more effective and less damaging methods for reaching their desired look. That these techniques progressed from specialty clinics to mainstream choices indicates a great deal about cultural values when it comes to beauty and physical appearance. With best medical experts continually refining procedural techniques and outcomes, cosmetic surgery can now address more aesthetic concerns while decreasing recovery times and risks. As encapsulated in recent literature, innovation in minimally invasive techniques allows patients to try out their desired appearance without subjecting themselves to the long recovery long typical of these interventions (Kalaskar et al., 2016). The additional convenience and security are contributing factors to rising acceptance of body modification procedures. Facial aesthetic beautification is also catching on in educational institutional environments. As discussed in comprehensive treatises on reconstructive and plastic surgery, there is a clear commitment among medical practitioners to train professionals in reconstructive as well as aesthetic applications. This dual emphasis assures that advances in facial aesthetics are underpinned by strict medical standards and ethical strategies, balancing artistic imagination with patient welfare (Kalaskar et al., 2016). As long as society insists on being concerned with desiring and appreciating idealized facial aesthetics, then the intersection of medical innovation and cultural desire remains a significant site for discussion. This transformation represents not only a change in looks but also marks wider societal perspectives on self-worth, identity, and acceptance within contemporary society, energizing the debate on the role of aesthetics in human experience (Figure 8.2).

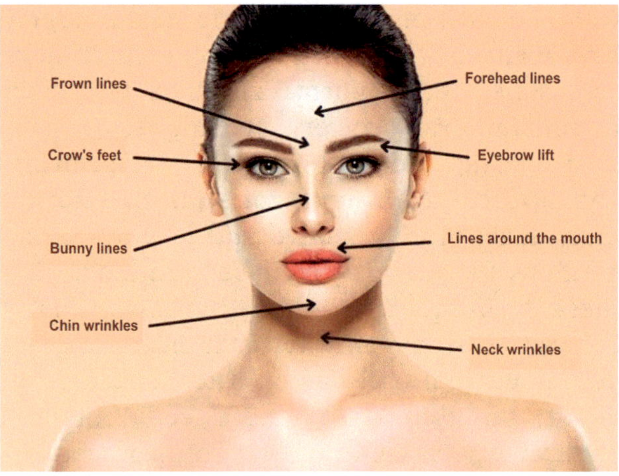

Figure 8.2. The significance of facial aesthetics in modern society.

Source: https://www.optidentdentalclinic.co.uk/wp-content/uploads/2025/01/facial-aesthetics-picture-768x576.webp.

8.1. Types of Facial Implants

Learning Outcome

1. Discuss the Chin Implants
2. Explain Cheek Implants
3. Explain Jaw Implants

The range of facial implants available today allows for multiple aesthetic goals, and some of the most prominent include chin, cheek, and jaw implants. Chin implants, typically composed of materials like silicone or porous polyethylene, are designed to increase projection and definition to the chin and, consequently, improve overall facial harmony. By augmenting the underlying bone structure, these implants can make a dramatic alteration to the look of the face, offering balance to the nose, forehead, and jawline ratios. Cheek implants, on the other hand, are intended to reestablish volume and definition to the mid-face that might recede with age or be underdeveloped. The placement of these implants can lead to subtle enhancements or dramatic alterations, which are reliant on patient desire and anatomy. The last, the choice of implants, is well-balanced and has to be established through thorough preoperative evaluation and patient preference. Jaw implants are the second key set of facial implants that are dedicated to enhancing the definition and strengthening of the jawline. These implants can be particularly beneficial to those who desire correction of congenital deformities, reconstruction following trauma, or merely a more defined jawline. Jaw implants' materials are identical to those of other facial implants, with emphasis on safety and biocompatibility. Surgical procedure is meticulous placement along the mandible in order to provide natural results while maintaining functionality. The incorporation of jaw implants into overall facial aesthetics can yield a more balanced and proportionate facial structure. In facial contouring, the synergistic or combined effect of multiple implants, with chin and jaw implants used together, usually yields improved aesthetic outcomes by addressing many areas of concern simultaneously, thereby yielding a concordant profile. With the current age of facial aesthetics, one is required to recognize both the use of non-surgical and minimally invasive treatments and traditional facial implants. Fat grafting and liposculpture are some of the methods that have evolved to enhance the effects achieved through implants. Fat grafting, in particular, utilizes the body's own fat, being a natural alternative to unnatural materials and enhancing volume and form where needed, such as under the eyes and along the cheeks. While simultaneously, liposuction enables the elimination of unwanted fat, carving facial shape and enhancing the overall aesthetic result. As documented in literature, a full facial aesthetic treatment typically integrates these procedures into one, with less invasive interventions such as Botulinum toxin treatments, to maximize outcomes and address various issues at once (Bouzouaya et al., 2018). This diversity-oriented treatment serves to highlight the importance of individualized treatment protocols considering the various tools of Facial Beautification at hand and ensuring that each patient reaches his/her desired result effectively (Kalaskar et al., 2016) (Figure 8.3).

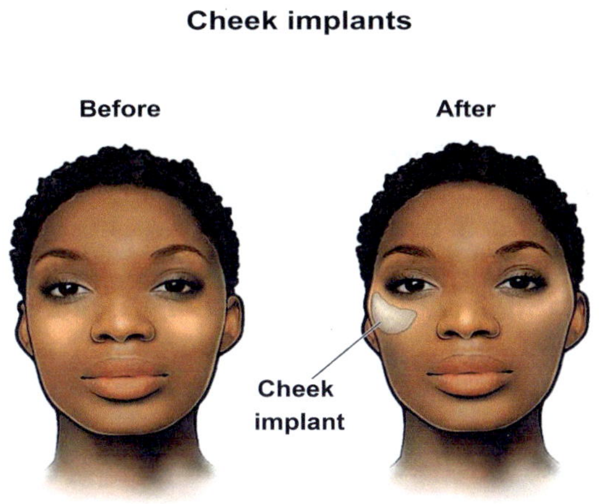

Figure 8.3. Types of facial implants.

Source: https://my.clevelandclinic.org/-/scassets/images/org/health/articles/cheek-implants.

8.1.1. Chin Implants

A search for beauty in facial looks most likely prompts one to reflect on chin implants, which are designed to expand or reform the jaw shape and outline. Chin augmentation is a surgery that aims at fixing a recessed or deficient chin so that the overall facial proportion can be enhanced. Patients typically seek chin implants for individual esthetic needs, congenital deformity corrections, or merely post-traumatic repair. The innovation in various materials and shapes for implants has further popularized the procedure, with some level of customization being most appropriate for individual anatomical needs. As in the instance of other contemporary surgical trends, chin implants are nowadays often synergistically combined with other facial contouring operations, i.e., cheek and jaw implants, to provide a complete, aesthetically pleasing outcome that enhances facial symmetry and definition, thereby triggering greater self-confidence in patients. In addition to the aesthetic outcome, the psychological impact of chin augmentation cannot be overemphasized. Research has indicated that individuals who have received cosmetic surgery frequently report higher levels of self-esteem and improved mental health post-surgery. The life-changing nature of chin implants may create dramatic changes in the manner in which individuals perceive themselves and interact with their world. This is particularly relevant for social engagement, where the visual appearance of the face can influence first impressions. Also, enhanced surgical methods, as reported in the literature today, have provided high satisfaction levels among patients following chin implant surgery. Such satisfaction is typically linked with the customized approach of selection and placement of implants, which ensures that each individual's special facial structure is catered to so that a more natural and balanced appearance is achieved. The combination of chin implants with other facial cosmetic surgery is a paradigm change in facial contouring. The combination of implants, fat grafting and liposculpture enhances aesthetic value for more facial morphology. For instance, the incorporation of liposculpture in the neck area can improve the new prominence of the chin with a chin implant to create a streamlined jawline. These combined techniques have been confirmed by clinical studies highlighting their effectiveness in yielding improved aesthetic results. Moreover, application of technologies like VASER liposculpture has introduced new aspects to harvesting and fat extraction contouring, to provide effective and safe procedures (Garcia et al., 2022). By addressing multiple areas of concern simultaneously via one surgery, patients can receive a more complete transformation, and chin implants become a crucial component of modern facial aesthetic surgery (Davies et al., 2023) (Figure 8.4).

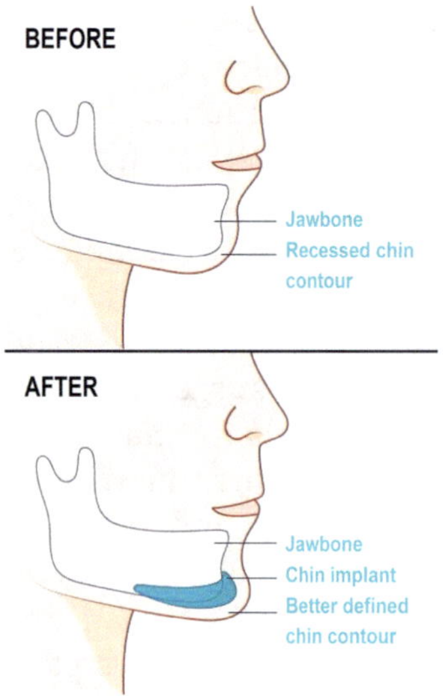

Figure 8.4. Chin implants.

Source: https://www.americanboardcosmeticsurgery.org/wp-content/uploads/2017/03/3057-0ad0a28560.jpg.webp.

8.1.2. Cheek Implants

Cheek implants have emerged as a vital component within the world of aesthetic augmentation, allowing individuals to contour their facial profiles for a clearer shape. Ancient ideals of beauty have changed, with current society being so concerned with youthful, angular facial contours. This is perpetuated by the influence of mass and social media, where certain facial features have become normative of beauty and sex appeal. Cheek implants provide a perfect option for people looking to enhance the midface, providing volume and structure that can significantly enhance facial harmony and proportion. Further, studies show that cheek augmentation surgeries could restore self-confidence and satisfaction, making them all the more essential in the burgeoning cosmetic surgery industry, especially as a response to social pressures and aesthetic expectations fueled by social exposure (Skrynnyk, 2024). The cheek implant surgery typically involves implanting a silicone or other biocompatible material in the cheek area, giving it a fuller and more defined appearance. Surgeons are inclined to personalize implant shape and size to suit the individual requirements of patients, realizing that facial anatomy presents great variability among populations. This customization is the hallmark of natural-looking results and fewer complications. Recovery is generally rapid from cheek implant surgery, and the minimally invasive approach embraced by contemporary plastic surgeons is in compliance with patient requests for less downtime and lower risk. As patient populations shift, with increasing numbers of teenagers and young adults undergoing cosmetic enhancements, there is an increasing demand for safe, quality services like cheek implants, which drives R&D in surgery and postoperative care (Kamal et al., 2019). In facial aesthetics, cheek implants are being most predominantly used alongside other treatments like chin and jaw implants, providing a comprehensive approach to facial contouring. The combination of various implants can lead to a harmonious augmentation of the overall facial appearance, allowing for three-dimensional reconstruction that addresses a particular issue. Furthermore, due to the waning social stigma regarding cosmetic procedures, more and more individuals are receptive towards availing themselves of treatments that enormously improve their confidence and self-esteem levels. The inclusion of cheek implants in the broad umbrella of aesthetic surgery represents a new frontier of individualized beauty, with fat grafting and liposculpture possibly augmenting or replacing implant surgery. Aesthetic medicine improves with time, and understanding the significance of these developments on self-esteem and social conduct is still important (Skrynnyk, 2024).

8.1.3. Jaw Implants

The application of jaw implants as a contouring procedure for the face is now quite common in contemporary cosmetic surgery, reflecting a broader societal trend towards improving looks. The implants, usually made from biocompatible materials such as silicone or porous polyethylene, aim to augment the jawline to achieve a more defined profile that enhances facial balance. The procedure not only enhances the physical appearance but also has a significant psychological effect, giving individuals increased self-esteem and self-confidence. Furthermore, advancement in surgical techniques allows for more precise positioning of the implants, thus lessening complications and healing time. Since patients now look for individualized aesthetic treatment, jaw implants provide an effective way that can accommodate personal facial structure and desired outcome. In addition to jaw implants, combined with fat grafting and liposculpture, facial contouring is further refined. Fat grafting allows for artistic utilization of a patient's own fat, which can be reshaped to restore the facial beauty, actually restoring the lost volume due to aging or birth. This procedure introduces a pleasant balance between the jawline and the surrounding features, rectifying localized flaws that cannot be fully treated by implants. Liposculpture also assists in achieving a reduced profile through the removal of excess fat deposits, thereby making the jawline more evident. This integrated strategy emphasizes the use of more than one modality in aesthetic treatments, behind the increasing trend of synergistic facial enhancement that prioritizes individuals' facial harmony (Kalaskar et al., 2016). The impact of these operations extends beyond appearance and into the greater issue of patient satisfaction and quality of life. Jaw implants, used in conjunction with other therapies like botulinum toxin injections, represent a multi-dimensional approach to facial enhancement whereby long-term results can be obtained. Practitioners, as they address the complexities of facial contouring, need to remember that patient education and realistic expectations about outcomes are of utmost importance. This awareness aids in promoting informed decision-making and encourages a positive relationship between practitioner and patient. Ultimately, the purpose is not just to alter appearance but to establish identity and sense of well-being, and facial implants, therefore, like jaw implants, are not merely surgeries; they are vehicles for life-altering experiences (Bouzouaya et al., 2018) (Figure 8.5).

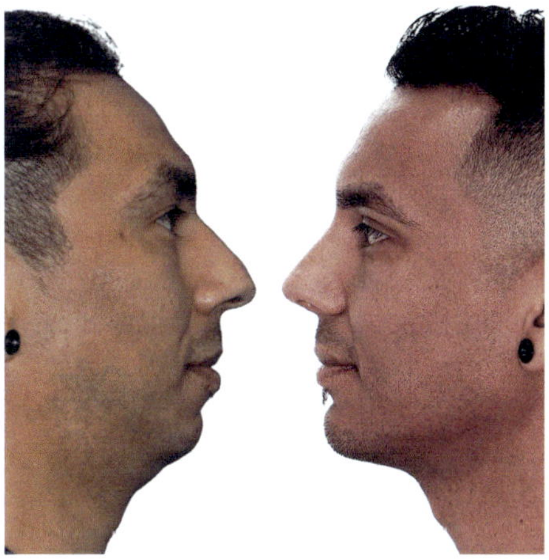

Figure 8.5. The utilization of jaw implants as a form of facial contouring.

Source: https://drdhir.com/wp-content/uploads/How-a-Custom-Jaw-is-Made.jpg.

Test Your Knowledge

1. What aesthetic concerns are commonly addressed using chin implants, and how do they improve facial balance?
2. How do cheek implants enhance midface volume, and what anatomical areas do they primarily target?
3. What functional and aesthetic benefits can jaw implants provide, and how do they influence lower facial contouring?

8.2. Benefits of Facial Implants

Learning Outcome

1. Discuss the Enhanced Facial Symmetry
2. Explain the Improved Self-Esteem and Confidence
3. Focus on Long-Lasting Results Compared to Non-Surgical Options

Facial implants have caused considerable popularity in aesthetic surgery due to their ability to enhance and reshape facial contours. Through the strategic positioning of chin, cheek, and jaw implants, patients are able to exhibit a more harmonious and balanced facial profile, consequently correcting asymmetries or volume deficits. The surgery provides aesthetic improvement as well as psychological benefit as most patients report enhanced self-esteem and overall confidence upon improvement. Notably, facial implants are a long-lasting answer compared to other non-surgical procedures, such as dermal fillers, which tend to have to be treated repeatedly. Moreover, the technique of facial implants has evolved significantly, adopting advances in material and technology to attain biocompatibility and durability, ultimately providing results for patients that conform to their desired aesthetic goal. In addition to enhanced facial appearances, facial implants can also be applied to functional augmentation. Chin implants, for instance, can enhance jawline definition, which results in enhanced facial proportions as well as assist in occlusion and overall dental alignment. In keeping with the discussion in the Textbook of Plastic and Reconstructive Surgery, various aesthetic procedures intersect with reconstructive procedures, and the importance of individualizing treatment options cannot be overstated. This blend of interest in both form and function is critical to holistic patient care. A patient is enhanced by a system of interdepartmental cooperation that unites anatomical understanding and surgical expertise to offer them safety and satisfaction. This intense focus on both aesthetic shape and functional employment emphasizes the significance of facial implants in contemporary plastic surgery, as they can greatly improve both visual appearance and anatomical functioning. Moreover, the ability of facial implants to be altered to fit a patient's diverse facial anatomy and need for appearance makes it extremely versatile.

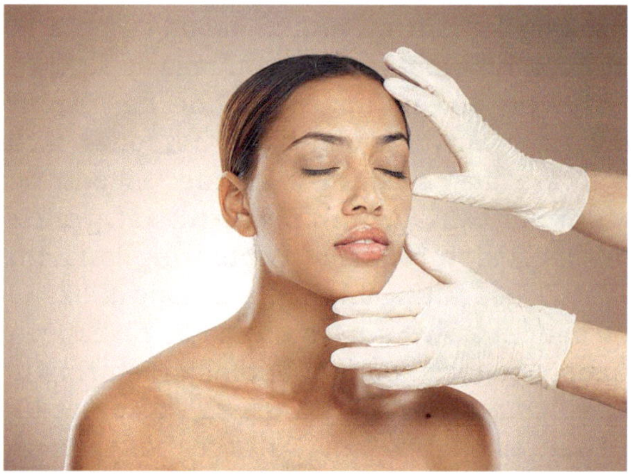

Figure 8.6. Facial implants have gained considerable traction in aesthetic surgery.

Source: https://associatesplasticsurgery.com/wp-content/uploads/facial-implants-benefits.jpg.

Surgeons have the option of selecting among shapes, sizes, and materials so that they can end up with aesthetically pleasing results that not only look attractive but also meet the needs of the patient. As theorized in the writings of advances in cosmetic surgeries, such as the vivid accounts in various authoritative books, the procedural options are ongoing to improve in terms of becoming safer and more effective. The integration of facial implants with supportive procedures such as fat grafting and liposculpture also enhances the potential of customized contouring to deliver more natural-looking and appealing outcomes. In general, facial implants are a complementary response to both aesthetic enhancement and reconstruction of facial harmony, solidifying their place in surgical aesthetics (Figure 8.6).

8.2.1. Enhanced Facial Symmetry

The pursuit of enhanced facial symmetry has long tantalized the scientific community, as well as aesthetic practitioners, particularly regarding beauty and attractiveness. This goal remains achievable with the newer techniques of facial contouring and augmentation, including strategic placement of implants to the chin, cheeks, and jawline. Enhanced facial symmetry not only adds to facial harmony but also can serve as a corrective measure for congenital asymmetries and age-related changes. With varying modalities such as facial implants, patients can achieve a more proportionate facial appearance that is aesthetically pleasing in addition to youthful. Through the correction of asymmetries in facial structure, these treatments have a significant role in one's confidence and social life, upholding the link between body appearance and mental wellness. The role of fat grafting and liposculpture cannot be underestimated, either, for enhanced facial symmetry. By obtaining and re-injecting fat from other areas of the body, surgeons can sculpt and design the face into more symmetrical contours. This procedure, in addition to giving bulk where required, also allows more natural integration of tissue, supporting bone with soft tissue. Improvements with fat grafting can create dramatic improvements in terms of symmetry, but in order to achieve maximum results, knowledge of facial anatomy and customized planning is required. The ability to manipulate different facial elements with these techniques is a sign of evolving strategies in aesthetic surgery, which aim to enhance facial harmony and symmetry overall, as discussed in works such as (Kalaskar et al., 2016). In addition to surgical interventions, the advancement of non-surgical treatments forms part of the quest for facial harmony. Techniques such as fillers and neuromodulators have subtle modifications to address patients' demands for additional symmetry without requiring significant recovery or operative risks. Practitioners can offer individualized care plans that connect patients with facial targets by considering temporary as well as long-term results. Moreover, the arrival of energy-based devices has allowed practitioners to leverage new technologies to offer contours that enhance facial harmony while minimizing the chances of complications. As the debate regarding aesthetic surgery progresses, understanding the concepts of enhanced facial symmetry continues to be at the heart of practitioners and patients alike, eventually leading to more gratifying results in facial rejuvenation and facial augmentation procedures (Figure 8.7).

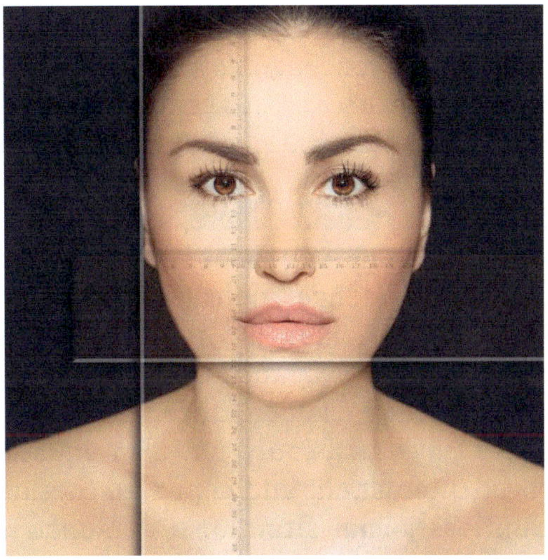

Figure 8.7. The pursuit of enhanced facial symmetry.

Source: https://www.lhochsteinmd.com/wp-content/uploads/2021/09/woman-with-rulers-on-face.jpg.

8.2.2. Improved Self-Esteem and Confidence

The journey towards increased self-esteem and confidence often overlaps significantly with cosmetic treatments such as facial implants and contouring. Most individuals seek these procedures in hopes of not only enhancing their physical appearance but also their image. The psychological impacts of altered facial contours, particularly in areas like the chin, cheeks, and jawline, have been documented in a number of studies. These enhancements can lead to a more harmonious appearance, conveying a sense of attractiveness that translates into increased confidence levels within social as well as professional environments. Besides, as patients observe desirable changes in the shape of their face, they also exhibit higher self-confidence and readiness to more actively engage in many aspects of their life. Plastic facial contouring, like with surgeries such as liposculpture or fat grafting, is imperative in order to achieve desired beauty outcomes. The ability to improve one's appearance can lead to a change in self-concept, allowing individuals to overcome their insecurities concerning specific facial features. As posited in research, patients also experience a significant boost in satisfaction levels following the procedure, which is directly attributed to high self-esteem and emotional health. The evidence indicates a firm trend towards better mental health whenever patients feel more beautiful. Studies suggest that successful facial enhancement not only increases physical beauty but also equates to improved interactions and improved confidence in countless social situations, demonstrating the significant psychological benefits of such cosmetic treatments (Garcia et al., 2022). Moreover, the evolution of procedures, such as high-density fat transfer and emerging contouring techniques, has been vital in overall patient satisfaction, further enhancing their confidence. The evolution of liposuction and its advanced applications in facial reconstruction has rendered the procedures safe and effective, but also personalized to achieve definite needs and desires (Kalaskar et al., 2016). Such personalization of aesthetic enhancements allows patients to take charge of how they perceive themselves, developing a positive self-image that can have long-lasting impacts on their psychological and emotional health. Generally, the blending of physical alteration via facial implants and patient self-confidence highlights the broader value of cosmetic surgery as an agent of change, ultimately to result in increased self-esteem and socialization across populations (Figure 8.8).

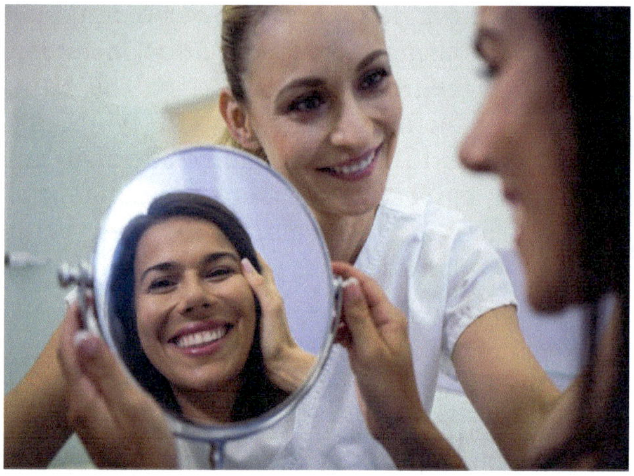

Figure 8.8. Improved self-esteem and confidence.

Source: https://drvsrathore.com/wp-content/uploads/2021/06/CS-1.jpg.

8.2.3. Long-Lasting Results Compared to Non-Surgical Options

The desire for aesthetic enhancement in facial contouring also naturally leads patients to choose between surgical and non-surgical options. Whereas non-surgical procedures, like Botox and dermal fillers, offer instant gratification with limited downtime, they do not last long. They usually last a few months only, requiring regular touch-ups to achieve the desired look. Surgical procedures, such as jaw, cheek, and chin implants, offer longer-lasting results that fundamentally change facial proportions. The long-term nature of these outcomes makes them extremely valuable to those seeking a long-term fix to facial contouring, despite the more extensive recovery time associated with surgical intervention. In an age of instant gratification, the promise of long-lasting outcomes offers many the allure of seeking out surgical intervention as a more realistic, though more comprehensive in nature, option in facial augmentation. Facial aesthetics, fat grafting is also a viable alternative for individuals who want long-term results without implantation. Fat grafting is focused on harvesting fat from areas of the body that have too much fat and transplanting it to areas of the face, such as the cheek or chin, for enhanced volume and contour. As compared to other non-surgical methods that require multiple procedures, fat grafting is capable of yielding long-term results as fat cells being transplanted can become a permanent component of the recipient tissues, providing a more natural and permanent augmentation. However, it should be noted here that the longevity of fat grafting results will vary based on various factors like the patients individual physiology and the precise technique employed in the treatment. Thus, while fat grafting presents a natural option for patients seeking long-term results, patient analysis and technique refinement are the secrets. With an aesthetic twist, comparison between surgical implants and non-surgical options enters well into the realms of effectiveness and satisfaction with the result. Textbook of Plastic and Reconstructive Surgery provides a comprehensive review of how prospective patients might be helped by having knowledge of these techniques (Kalaskar et al., 2016). The long-term consequences with regard to surgical implants encourage higher patient satisfaction due to the durability of cosmetic results, giving individuals the confidence they seek without constant upkeep. While non-surgical treatments may at first look more attractive due to their immediate satisfaction and lower up-front cost, the relatively shorter lifespan of their results has a tendency to make patients discontent in the end. Lastly, for the daring who are ready to change drastically in their facial feature and appearance, surgical options tend to be the more durable and outcome-guaranteed option, one which is a salient consideration in the decision-making process of aesthetic improvement.

Test Your Knowledge

1. How do facial implants contribute to enhanced facial symmetry, and which areas benefit the most from this improvement?
2. In what ways can facial implants positively influence a patient's self-esteem and confidence?
3. Why are facial implants considered longer-lasting compared to non-surgical volumizing treatments such as fillers?

8.3. Risks and Considerations

Learning Outcome

1. Discuss the Potential Complications and Side Effects
2. Focus on Importance of Choosing a Qualified Surgeon
3. Explain the Psychological Considerations before Undergoing Surgery

The pursuit of facial beauty through contouring and implant surgery, while often offering radical alterations, entails an entire spectrum of risks and considerations that potential patients must carefully balance in. One of the most critical concerns is whether or not there are any complications of the surgeries themselves, e.g., infection, scarring, and dislocation of the implants. The latter can cause not only physical disabilities but also psychological disappointment as the patients usually are incapable of accepting the outcome in terms of their initial expectations.

Therefore, it is advisable for those who are considering treatments like chin, cheek, or jaw implants to receive intensive consultations with experienced specialists to make them well conversant with the dangers surrounding the interventions of their choice. Besides surgical risks, patients who are considering fat grafting and liposculpture should be made aware of the unique complications surrounding these procedures. Fat grafting, for instance, takes adipose tissue from one region of the body and reinjects it into another region for the purpose of contouring. The process is capable of producing complications such as uneven outcome or resorption of grafted fat in the long term. Similarly, liposculpture can change body contours but is capable of producing major irregularities or even damage to nearby structures in the event of an error in technique. As argued in recent literature, even less invasive procedures carry inherent risks and complications, which are hotly debated among expert surgeons, as a reason why patients ought to properly weigh the pros and cons before proceeding with surgery (Kalaskar et al., 2016). Appreciation of the broader context of facial plastic surgery also necessitates deliberate consideration of one's psychological and emotional readiness. Negative outcomes, although rare, can affect self-esteem and mental well-being significantly. Also, social pressures and unrealistic expectations regarding the results of facial surgery may lead individuals to have surgery without obvious reasons. It is necessary to conduct a thorough pre-surgical assessment, including mental health and body image discussions, to form an ethical surgical plan. In order to realize that aesthetic outcomes are subjective and vary from person to person, it is crucial; therefore, debates on the aesthetic expectations should be made depending on realistic assessments of what may be achieved by such procedures (Kalaskar et al., 2016). They contribute to establishing a means for informed decision-making, finally targeting patient health alongside aesthetic enhancement (Figure 8.9).

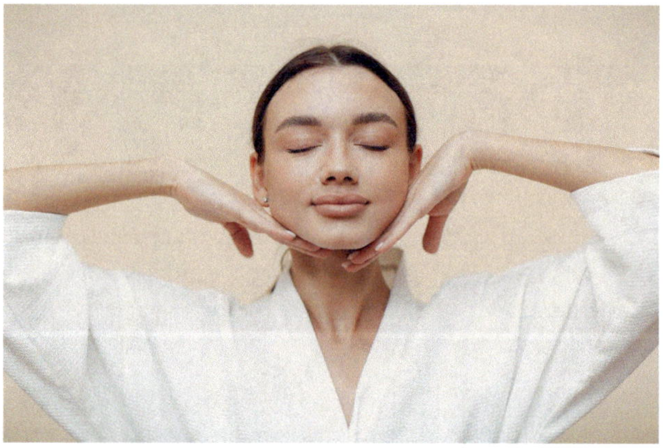

Figure 8.9. The pursuit of facial beauty through implants and contouring procedures.

Source: https://www.applebaummd.com/wp-content/uploads/2022/08/Facial-Contouring.jpg.

8.3.1. Potential Complications and Side Effects

When facial implants and contouring are being considered, potential side effects and complications are essential considerations for both surgeons and patients. Infection, hematoma, and asymmetry are some of the common problems that may arise from chin, cheek, and jaw implants. Infection along the surgical area may result in delayed healing or even further procedures. Hematomas, which are collections of blood outside the blood vessels, may take the form of swelling and bruising and may need to be drained. Asymmetry resulting from uneven implant positioning or birth defects in anatomical structure can render patients dissatisfied with their result. Such complications are capable of affecting patients' cosmetic outcomes significantly, and therefore detailed preoperative evaluation and realistic expectation (Kalaskar et al., 2016). Where fat grafting and liposculpture are concerned, additional complications may result depending on the unique nature of these procedures. For instance, fat transfer can lead to asymmetrical outcomes when the transferred fat cells do not survive in the recipient site and, as a result, they produce contour abnormalities. Also, necrosis or tissue death can result if the transferred fat is poorly vascularized. Another complication of liposculpture includes the development of seroma, which is a fluid collection under the skin that may have to be drained surgically. Identification of these outcomes is significant to both patients and practitioners since this data promotes wise decision-making and enhances the overall safety of such treatments (Kalaskar et al., 2016). Besides that, psychological impacts cannot be overlooked while examining facial contouring's potential side effects and complications. The risk of undergoing a procedure evokes worry and tension, particularly where patients are misinformed regarding the risk of the procedure and realistic expectations. Complications after surgery can prolong these feelings, leading to unhappiness with the cosmetic result. In extreme cases, this discontent can lead to conditions like body dysmorphic disorder, where individuals become preoccupied with what they perceive as their own flaws. Thus, the preoperative procedure has a crucial component to make sure that counseling is conducted in depth to handle patients' expectations and psychosocial problems and to foster a deep understanding of facial implant and contouring complications (Kalaskar et al., 2016) (Figure 8.10).

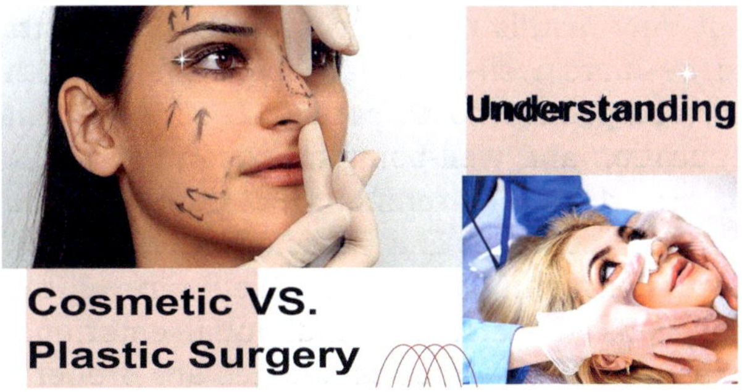

Figure 8.10. Potential complications and side effects.

Source: https://www.clinikally.com/cdn/shop/articles/Khushi_Banner_Blog_50.jpg?v=1705919295&width=1024.

8.3.2. Importance of Choosing a Qualified Surgeon

Choosing an experienced surgeon is the most crucial aspect in facial implant and contouring procedures, i.e., chin, cheek, and jaw implants, as well as fat grafting and liposculpture. Individuals underestimate the delicacy of such operations, which require a sensitive understanding of facial aesthetics and anatomy. A skilled and specially trained surgeon, beyond demonstrating technical proficiency, helps ensure a safer operating room. Skilled surgeons can better anticipate complications and manage unforeseen problems that arise with recovery after surgery. Additionally, an experienced surgeon will conduct a thorough preoperative workup and develop individualized treatment plans based on the patient's own facial structure and desired outcomes. Lastly, letting the appearance fall into the hands of a professional establishes trust in the surgery process and, therefore, the result achieved. Apart from technical competence, the worth of an experienced surgeon also resides in the comprehensive care and communication they provide patients throughout their stay in treatment. A seasoned surgeon has frank conversation about the expected results, risks entailed, and healing processes associated with facial contouring procedures. This openness not only instills trust but also allows patients to be more well-informed about their health care. Surgeons who are passionate about patient education and well-being are also more likely to provide an environment that addresses the patients' concerns and expectations efficiently. By emphasizing patient-focused care, gifted surgeons can also test individual emotional preparedness, so that candidates are properly prepared for the life-changing implications of facial implants and contouring. Moreover, the selection of an experienced surgeon is directly correlated with long-term aesthetic outcomes. Surgeons with higher levels of expertise are better equipped to carry out new technologies and methods, which can significantly enhance both the safety and effectiveness of operations carried out. A poorly performed operation may result in poor results, protracted recuperation, or even irreversible facial disfigurement, thus emphasizing the significance of expert know-how in surgical operations. Additionally, a seasoned surgeon is likely to be involved in ongoing learning and training and stay up to date with developments in cosmetic surgery." Ongoing professional development not only develops his competencies but also reinforces best practice safety. So, investing the time and effort in selecting an experienced surgeon actually serves to protect and enhance the result of facial implants and contouring surgery (Steinbacher, 2019) (Figure 8.11).

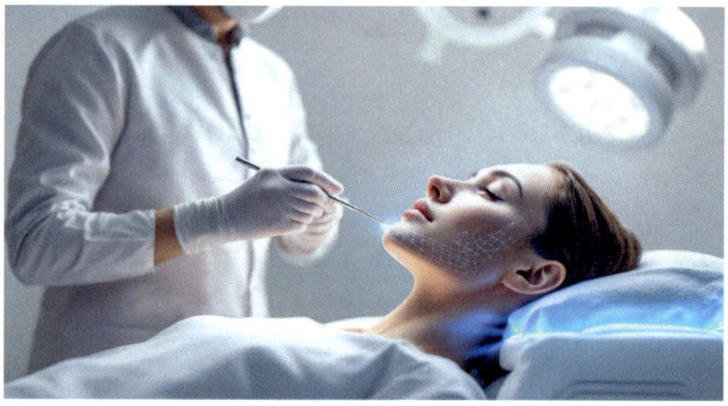

Figure 8.11. The choice of a qualified surgeon is paramount when considering facial implants and contouring procedures.

Source: https://images.surferseo.art/c0f0c9a8-9c7c-4e4a-9bf0-a97d0dc02856.png.

8.3.3. Psychological Considerations before Undergoing Surgery

Before patients have procedures such as facial implants and contouring, they will have to go through a complete psychological evaluation to identify their motivations and expectations. This preoperative evaluation is significant in the process of determining whether or not there exist mental health issues, like body dysmorphic disorder, that will distort a patient's perception of their appearance. A clear understanding of the psychological self will guarantee sounder judgment when selecting cosmetic surgery. For instance, individuals can undergo these procedures as a solution to personal fears, but exaggerated expectations may lead to dissatisfaction and complications post-surgery. Thus, open communication between the patient and the surgeon is important to obtain a clear evaluation of the outcome and limitations of procedures like fat grafting and liposculpture. In addition, psychological support should not be overemphasized throughout the surgical process—preoperatively, intraoperatively, and postoperatively. Having an effective support system at hand would minimize anxiety with regard to surgery, hence enhancing overall patient satisfaction. Mental health professionals should be consulted to advise patients on the emotional process involved in cosmetic surgery, including the challenges of post-operative difficulty such as adjustment disorders. Therapy also addresses navigating healing time expectations and the gradual nature of aesthetic improvement. Through robust mental preparation, patients can establish their mental health, which is a significant factor in their satisfaction with the procedure. This factor is particularly relevant to procedures such as chin, cheek, and jaw implants, where beauty transformation can muster more emotional responses. Last but not least, general awareness of the psychological aspect of surgery can lead to better informed consent procedures. Aesthetic professionals and surgeons alike need to treat counseling as a matter of utmost urgency so that patients not only stand physically ready for surgery but are also ready mentally. Such preparation involves discussing the physical and emotional impact of procedures, in which the impact can be highly variable, as one can deduce from the variable applications of surgical procedures discussed in texts like the Textbook of Plastic and Reconstructive Surgery. These resources provide useful information regarding patient outcomes and psychological effects related to different surgical techniques, including the latest developments in body contouring and facial aesthetic treatment, eventually forming a platform for improved patient satisfaction and mental health literacy (Kalaskar et al., 2016).

Test Your Knowledge

1. What are the common potential complications and side effects associated with facial implant surgery?
2. Why is choosing a qualified and experienced surgeon essential for ensuring safe and successful facial implant outcomes?
3. What psychological factors should be evaluated before a patient proceeds with facial implant surgery?

8.4. Fat Grafting

Learning Outcome

1. Definition and Process of Fat Grafting
2. Focus on Advantages of Using Body Fat for Contouring
3. Explain Areas Commonly Treated with Fat Grafting

Fat grafting, or autologous fat transfer, is now a more sought-after, safe procedure for facial sculpting as a solution for volume loss in the chin, cheek, and jaw areas. The procedure involves taking fat from donor sites, often the abdomen or thighs, and injecting it into specific areas of the face in a very controlled process to give the area a fuller, more defined look. The technique not only provides cosmetic improvements but also smoothes the texture and quality of the skin, typically rendering the skin younger. Of significance, with the enhanced techniques in liposculpture, fat grafting as a process has become a safer and more effective procedure that renders it simpler to achieve standard results and higher patient satisfaction rates, especially for individuals with major volume loss of the face (Garcia et al., 2022). The effectiveness of fat grafting is also supported by more recent research that indicates its role in promoting facial aesthetics and patient satisfaction. Through research, it has been demonstrated that high-density fat transfer techniques can offer superior results, particularly in patients who have facial volume deficiency due to aging or other conditions. Studies have found that the patients receiving this therapy report more confidence and better quality of life, demonstrating the psychological benefit of aesthetic improvement. Besides, the application of techniques such as the use of Stem Cell-Enriched Fat (SVF-gel) has been noted to provide additional benefits in facial rejuvenation, ultimately leading to enhanced clinical outcomes and patient satisfaction among those desiring the enhancement of the appearance of their face (Garcia et al., 2022).

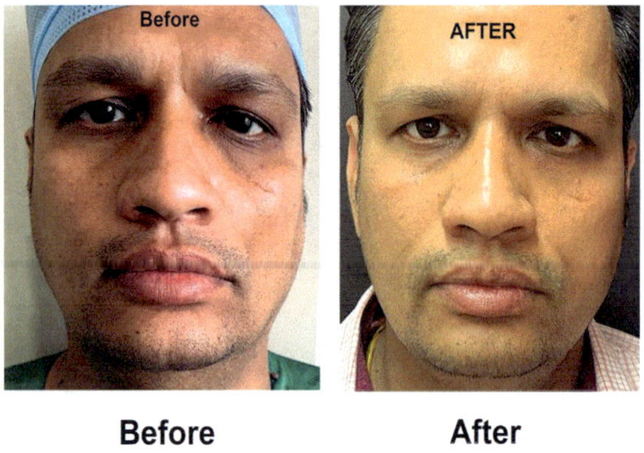

Figure 8.12. Fat grafting, also known as autologous fat transfer.

Source: https://sandipjain.com/wp-content/uploads/2022/06/front-1-injection.jpg.

In tandem with the evolution in fat grafting, the advances in liposuction techniques have played a significant role in making it work. Originally a no-nonsense method of fat removal, liposuction today uses sophisticated methods that allow for controlled contouring and volume transfer. Several energy-based devices and hybrid therapies are now available, facilitating procedures to be tailored to the patient's needs individually while decreasing complications and increasing efficiency. An example of a growing trend in cosmetic surgery is the combination of liposuction and fat grafting as two-pronged methods are utilized to complement facial rejuvenation methods. As experts continue to refine these procedures, fat grafting is likely to remain one of the cornerstones of facial contouring procedures, offering patients effective treatments for the sought-after facial shapes (Figure 8.12).

8.4.1. Definition and Process of Fat Grafting

Fat grafting, also known as autologous fat transfer, is a two-stage cosmetic treatment that employs the removal of fat from one area of the body to provide bulk and shape to another. The procedure has gained universal popularity in facial aesthetic applications, particularly for the contouring of the chin, cheek, and jawline. The procedure begins with liposuction, wherein fat is removed through a minimally invasive technique. The extracted fat is then treated to isolate healthy fat cells from other tissues so that only the best quality tissue will be used in the injection into the treatment area. Not only does this procedure enable facial rejuvenation, but it also treats volume loss, which frequently accompanies aging, making the entire face look more harmonious. Thus, fat grafting seems to be a groundbreaking option in cosmetic surgery with aesthetically rewarding outcomes, less scarring, and quicker recovery compared with traditional implants. Fat cell survival following harvesting is critical to the success of the grafting procedure, with most grafted fat typically lost from the recipient site. Techniques such as centrifugation can also be employed to further cleanse fat before injection, ensuring graft survival. Surgeons inject the treated fat in multiple thin layers in order for it to be spread evenly and lumpiness or imperfections are not created. The technical nature of the process ensures that there is a demand for professionals because facial anatomy varies immensely from individual to individual. Successful fat grafting can lead to improved contouring outcomes, which satisfy the patients' cosmetic expectations of chin, cheek, and jaw augmentations. Ultimately, fat grafting is a varied technique that can complement other surgical procedures, thereby satisfying the facial rejuvenation's varied demands. The outcome of fat grafting is more than superficial aesthetic enhancement; it allows for a better understanding of the relationship between functional and cosmetic aspects of facial surgery.

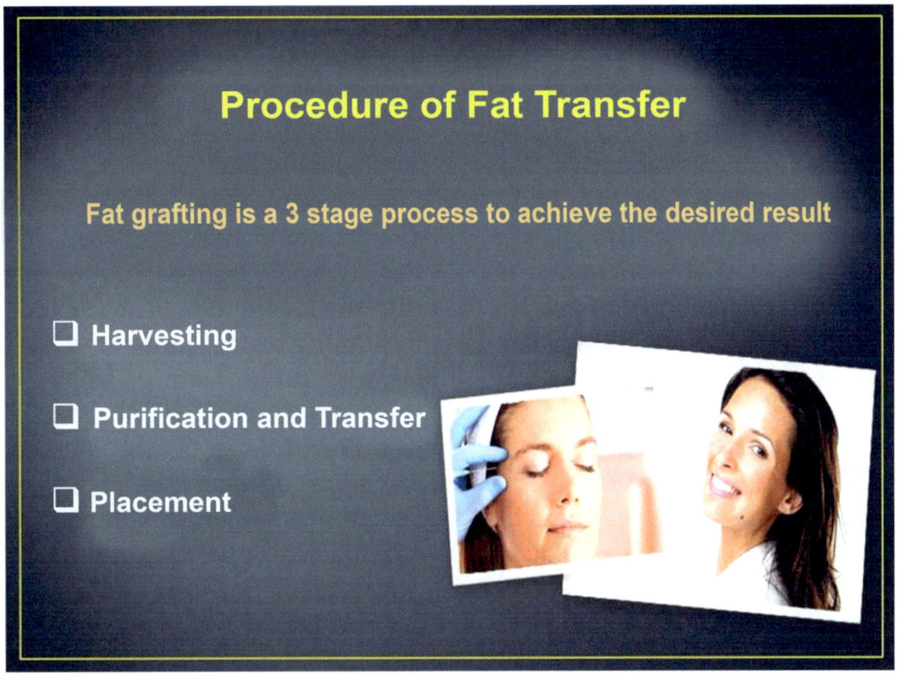

Figure 8.13. Fat grafting is a dual-process cosmetic procedure.

Source: https://image4.slideserve.com/7281697/slide6-l.jpg.

For instance, in oral and maxillofacial surgery, enhancement of facial appearance by fat grafting can optimize patient satisfaction and quality of life. This factor underscores the importance of an integrated approach that values both functional and aesthetic outcomes at the planning stage for surgery. With advancing technology and methods, fat grafting continues to evolve, yielding innovative solutions for complex facial asymmetry and volume loss. The expanding body of evidence underscores the imperative for formal training and compliance with best practices by the surgeons to maximize the advantage of this new technique. Hence, the integration of fat grafting in the series of treatments for facial contouring shows its place as a component of aesthetic enhancement (Kalaskar et al., 2016; Ahmed et al., 2019) (Figure 8.13).

8.4.2. Advantages of Using Body Fat for Contouring

The advantages of contouring with body fat in facial aesthetic procedures are three-dimensional in nature, thus contributing to benefits in outcomes and patient experience. One of the greatest benefits is that fat grafting utilizes the patient's own fat, thus removing the potential for allergic reactions or rejection with the use of synthetic implants. This autologous fat transfer provides a natural texture and look that is preferred by patients who want the more natural route of restoring facial volume, particularly in the cheeks and chin. In addition, fat grafting is also capable of more gradual and subtly enhanced contours, with the ability to make adjustments for variation in individual anatomy and for cosmetic objectives, leading to a harmonious result consistent with facial beauty. This degree of personalization is sometimes difficult to achieve with rigid implants, so body fat presents as a welcome alternative. Moreover, fat grafting is also unique in that it serves both contouring and rejuvenation purposes simultaneously. Excess fat is removed during the liposculpture procedure from regions of the body where it is not desirable, like the abdomen or thighs, thus improving the body proportion and contour overall. Not only does this procedure offer an avenue for sculpting the face, but it also plays a role in body shaping, creating an artistic balance between facial and body looks. In addition, the process promotes survival of the transplanted fat cells, which can bring long-term impacts as they integrate into the host tissue. Such global advantages are illustrated in literature accounts of developing such procedures and applying them to facial surgery (Kalaskar et al., 2016). This integration benefits patient satisfaction and longevity of the aesthetic effect. In addition to cosmetic advantage, body contouring by the transfer of fat has the benefit of a faster recovery period compared to more invasive surgery. The minimally invasive process of fat grafting tends to result in less postoperative discomfort and fewer complications, allowing patients to return to normal activities sooner. This is most attractive for people who desire facial enhancement with less downtime since the procedure is usually performed under local anesthesia, which minimizes the danger of systemic complications. As demonstrated by detailed books on reconstructive and plastic surgery, the new technology in fat grafting is consistent with today's themes of aesthetic treatments with a focus on safety and efficacy (Kalaskar et al., 2016). Overall, body fat contouring boasts an array of persuasive benefits for both practitioners and patients alike within the evolving framework of cosmetic surgery.

8.4.3. Areas Commonly Treated with Fat Grafting

Fat grafting has been a widely used technique of restoring volume and enhancing contours on much of the face. One of the most frequent applications of fat grafting is facial volume loss treatment, which can happen in regions such as the cheeks, temples, and in front of the eyes. During aging, natural stores of fat may diminish, and the face can get hollowed out, impacting beauty and self-esteem. By removing adipose tissue from other regions of the body through liposuction, cosmetic surgeons are capable of re-injecting such fat into targeted locations on the face strategically, effectively reviving the overall beauty of the face without compromising its original look. The procedure not only adds volume but also improves the tone and texture of the skin, thus resulting in a more youthful look, as noticed by improved scores of improvement and satisfaction of the patients in recent studies (Garcia et al., 2022). Another significant region treated using fat grafting is the chin and the jawline. With evolving contouring techniques, fat transfer offers an option that is less invasive than implants for the definition of the jaw and augmentation of the chin projection. This technique is especially helpful for individuals who wish to enhance the facial structure without exposing themselves to the risks of implant surgery. A well-defined jaw and chin can contribute immensely towards enhancing an individual's profile as well as the overall facial balance. In addition to beautifying the appearance of aesthetics, fat grafting in this region can even make the skin appear more elastic, fine-tuning problems that have arisen due to aging, such as sagging or loss of tautness. Fat grafting's twin benefit of adding volume and reviving the skin has made it a favorite of patients seeking facial contouring procedures (Kalaskar et al., 2016). Moreover, fat grafting is also integral to enlarging the lips and restoring facial symmetry. With the proper injection of fat on the lips, surgeons can bring back a fuller, plumper appearance that complements other facial elements. The surgery is also advantageous because it utilizes the patient's own tissue for a secure and more natural texture without triggering allergic reactions, since artificial fillers were not utilized. Additionally, fat grafting can effectively correct asymmetry in the lip area to achieve a proportionate and aesthetically pleasing outcome. Overall performance and safety of the treatment have been emphasized in various studies, highlighting its ability to be of great importance to enhance a patient's facial beauty and satisfy the patient's perception of self (Garcia et al., 2022). By these many applications, fat grafting has emerged as a valuable and versatile tool in contemporary facial contouring procedures.

Test Your Knowledge

1. What are the key steps involved in the process of fat grafting, from harvesting to injection?
2. Why is autologous body fat considered advantageous for facial contouring compared to synthetic fillers?
3. Which facial areas are most commonly treated using fat grafting procedures?

8.5. Liposculpture

Learning Outcome

1. Definition and Techniques of Liposculpture
2. Differences Between Liposuction and Liposculpture
3. Focus on Ideal Candidates for Liposculpture

Liposculpture represents the next evolution of the traditional liposuction procedure, with even finer body contouring and beauty refinement achievable. Initially applied as a method of localized fat bulge removal, liposculpture now encompasses techniques that enhance the natural contours of the face and body. Such a process utilizes advanced technologies, such as tumescent liposuction and ultrasonic-assisted liposuction, to extract fat effectively with minimal damage to adjacent tissues, thereby preventing trauma and ensuring quicker recovery. Ironically, utilization of liposculpture in facial beauty gives the patient the option to achieve a more angular and elongated jawline, sharp cheekbones, and proportionate facial contour, which suits the trend of subtle but deep effect in cosmetic therapy. With the combination of these processes, practitioners may tailor outcomes to meet the individual needs of patients who want to restore greater facial symmetry and contour. The combination of fat grafting with liposculpture complements its utility in facial aesthetic surgery. Fat grafting, which is the transfer of fat tissue from one region of the body to another, is an adjunct to liposculpture in volumizing areas that are more hollowed or deficient. This combination offers the ability to address facial rejuvenation in an integrated way, both contouring defects and loss of volume. As proposed in the literature today, utilization of these procedures together not only increases the degree of aesthetic achievement but also the quality and consistency of the treated skin (Kalaskar et al., 2016). In addition, with experience in these methods, practitioners learn to manage potential complications as well, so that all patients can have personalized treatment in which safety takes top precedence and desired results in facial contouring and augmentation are achieved as well. Liposculpture overall indicates a direction towards the application of minimally invasive approaches, prioritizing patient satisfaction and safety in plastic surgery.

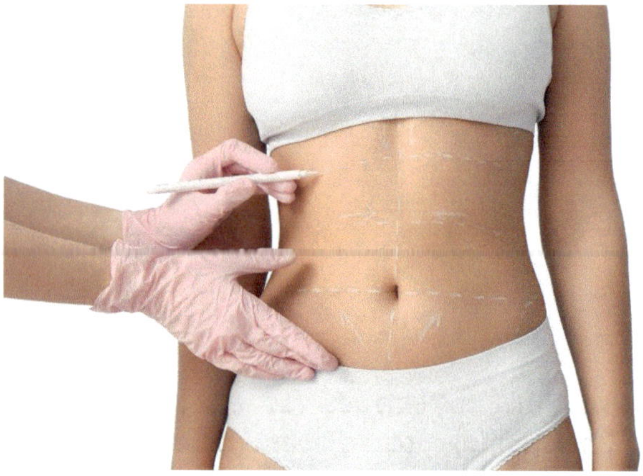

Figure 8.14. Liposculpture represents an advanced evolution of traditional liposuction.

Source: https://www.lydianclinic.com/wp-content/uploads/2025/02/how-much-does-liposculpture-cost-1.jpg.

The comprehensive description of liposculpture's development in the field of aesthetic surgery illustrates its relevance in contemporary practice (Kalaskar et al., 2016). With more individuals searching for alternatives to intrusive surgical procedures, demand for less invasive contouring treatments is likely to grow. Liposculpture offers patients a choice of creating extreme changes with fewer risks and less downtime compared to traditional surgical treatments. With facial uses, the procedure is an excellent example of the innovation being explored by plastic surgery to fulfill the patient's desire for natural-looking outcomes with less strain on recovery. Therefore, it is a very promising procedure as a standard addition to the arsenal of aesthetic procedures reserved for facial enhancement (Figure 8.14).

8.5.1. Definition and Techniques of Liposculpture

Liposculpture, an advanced technique of body sculpture, is one definition of the technique of removal of localized fat pads to enhance facial and body contours. With the employment of techniques that involve various types of liposuction, surgeons are able to contour the chin, cheeks, and jawline and achieve a proportionate and harmonious facial outline. In recent years, this procedure has seen massive popularity, fueled by technological advances that offer minimally invasive alternatives to traditional surgical procedures. According to observations made by research, cervicofacial liposuction tackles the redundant fat of the face and neck using negative pressure and a cannula in order to avulse soft fat cells. This detailed manipulation allows for proper sculpting, enhancing the natural contours without infringing on patient safety and satisfaction, as evidenced by data related to high-density fat transfer procedures yielding meaningful facial aesthetic and quality of life improvements (Garcia et al., 2022). The technique applied in liposculpture has been developed and modified widely, applying various methodologies to achieve optimal results. A simple procedure for local fat reduction in its initial stages, liposuction has grown into a highly advanced operation with different types of treatment tailored to cosmetic needs. Contemporary practitioners use energy-based devices and minimally invasive techniques to ensure maximum success with the least threat from traditional approaches. These advances focus not just on reducing fat but also on solving issues such as skin laxity and contour irregularities. Additionally, the precision in technique offers tailored solutions that take into account specific patient anatomy, hence developing ultimate outcomes that deliver anticipated aesthetic goals (Kalaskar et al., 2016). Similarly, the enhanced understanding and application of such techniques have placed liposculpture at the center of facial implants and contouring discussions. Safety and efficacy remain paramount in the practice of liposculpture, highlighted by clinical practice that attests to its efficacy. A systematic review highlighted that most patients experience significant facial contour and augmentation improvement after the procedure. Patients who manifest volume loss in the face exhibit substantially improved outcomes from the more contemporary methods, such as high-density fat transfer and stromal vascular fraction gel injection, which notably enhance patient satisfaction scores. With advancing surgical methods, complications have been minimized by far, and the patient's overall experience has become better with enhanced confidence and psychological health. This development in liposculpture not only highlights its prowess as a procedure itself but also supports other modalities, including facial implants, to develop holistic and individualized treatment plans for facial cosmetic improvement (Garcia et al., 2022).

8.5.2. Differences Between Liposuction and Liposculpture

The distinctions between liposuction and liposculpture are of critical significance in today's cosmetic surgery, particularly for facial contouring. Liposuction typically deals with the elimination of excess fat from the various regions of the body, allowing patients to reduce localized fat deposits efficiently. Although the procedure is most commonly utilitarian, it tends to cause a generalized reduction in size in order to form smoother contours. Liposculpture, by comparison, emphasizes the art of body shaping. It is achieved by meticulously extracting fat to provide enhancements to a specific area, sculpting not only the volume but also the overall appearance of the enhanced area. From the literature, as noted, modern surgical methods have evolved to enhance these procedures from what they were originally meant for, offering refined methods of body sculpting that enable meeting cosmetic requests in a more in-depth manner (Kalaskar et al., 2016). While both procedures have comparable technology advancements and surgery techniques, they have significantly different goals. Liposuction tends to target fat volume reduction, often employing suction-assisted devices to treat extensive areas of the abdomen or thighs. The procedure tends to leave an unchanged skin surface, which may create varying degrees of skin tightness and contour. On the other hand, liposculpture is more of an artful method to redistribute and mold fat reservoirs in such a manner as to produce an attractive silhouette. Such procedures may involve aspiration and also injection of fat into zones of strategic distribution, thereby enhancing volume and contour where desired. It is important that practitioners and patients alike are aware of such differences because these define expectation and results while going through the body contouring process (Kalaskar et al., 2016). Between liposuction and liposculpture, the difference is a lot. There is much influence on facial aesthetic results, particularly when there are implants and fat grafting involved. Patients requesting facial implants, like chin, cheek, and jaw implants, can be content with liposculpture as a complement to the implants that enhances the surrounding fat tissue of the sites of augmentation. This procedure has more harmony between the implants and facial contours that look natural. In contrast, however, patients who are more interested in fat elimination than contour redrawing may find standard liposuction techniques to their taste. Of particular interest, changing technological advances in surgical methods are continually rewriting what is possible in facial recontouring, making an understanding of these distinctions a prerequisite for successful patient assessment and treatment planning (Kalaskar et al., 2016) (Figure 8.15).

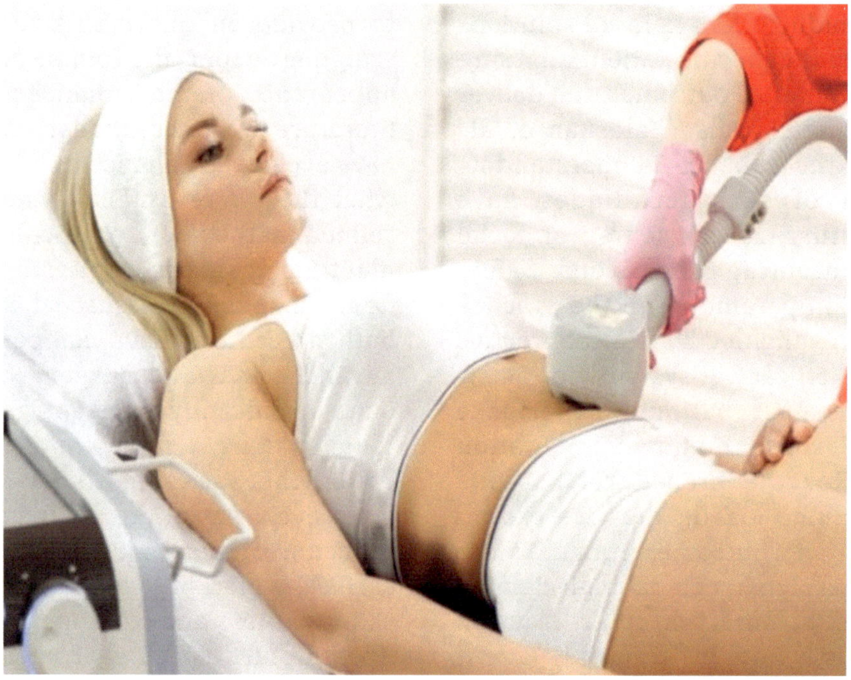

Figure 8.15. The distinctions between liposuction and liposculpture hold significant relevance in contemporary cosmetic surgery.

Source: https://hws.raadinahealth.com/images/user_upload/blog/en-liposuction/Liposculpture-vs-Liposuction12_1707550496_large.webp.

8.5.3. Ideal Candidates for Liposculpture

With respect to the ideal liposculpture candidates, there are various elements that have to be assessed in order to achieve the best possible outcome. A primary requirement is the patient's health; the candidate must be healthy with no medical issues that can hinder the process. Ideal candidates should have localized fat deposits that do not respond to diet and exercise, as this shows the need for focal body contouring measures. The procedure is especially beneficial to those who want to redefine the face by removing excess fat in regions of their own choice, thereby achieving a cleaner appearance. By being consistent with these cosmetic and health standards, surgeons can ensure that the process of liposculpture is as productive as possible in fulfilling the targets and expectations of the patients, and finally bestowing them with a successful transformation. In addition to physical health, mental readiness is an important component of candidate selection for liposculpture. Successful candidates typically entertain realistic expectations of their potential outcomes, aware that while liposculpture can enhance looks to a significant degree, it isn't a reward for practicing good habits. Candidates need to enter the treatment with a clear idea of what they desire from the procedure and be willing to maintain healthy habits after that. Emotional regulation and positive disposition toward undergoing the surgical process are also important because these factors may influence healing and satisfaction with the final outcome. Surgeons usually evaluate these psychological attributes in consultations to gauge candidates' readiness and willingness to embrace the alterations liposculpture brings into their bodies and lives. Moreover, timing is also a key aspect to be taken into account in becoming a possible candidate for liposculpture. The optimal candidates are usually 18 to 65 years old since younger patients possess optimal skin elasticity and overall resilience, which allows them to heal and shape postoperatively. Age is not an absolute contraindication, however, since even older patients can be optimally managed by experienced surgeons using proper techniques to accommodate their needs, as well as achieve satisfactory aesthetic outcomes. Candidates must not smoke at all, preferably, since smoking has a negative impact on healing and subverts surgical outcomes. Having this knowledge of the age and lifestyle considerations, in addition to professional guidance provided by highly educated practitioners, is important for patients who contemplate liposculpture. This means that surgery not only serves to meet their beauty ambitions but can also have a positive long-term effect on their health and confidence (Kalaskar et al., 2016).

Test Your Knowledge

1. How does liposculpture differ from traditional liposuction in terms of technique and aesthetic goals?
2. What characteristics define an ideal candidate for liposculpture procedures?

8.6. Combining Procedures

Learning Outcome

1. Discuss the Benefits of Combining Implants with Fat Grafting
2. Identify Case Studies of Successful Combined Procedures
3. Focus on Considerations for Recovery and Aftercare

Combination procedures in facial aesthetics are driven by a desire to achieve total outcomes that optimize the facial balance and contour. Techniques such as cheek, chin, and jaw implants can successfully enhance the bony structure to produce a more defined appearance. However, these types of procedures usually lead to even higher satisfaction when complemented by reinforcing techniques such as fat grafting and liposculpture. Fat grafting, apart from reestablishing lost volume as a result of aging, also sculpts transition points between augmented areas, thereby producing a smoother, natural contour. This complementarity results in personalized treatment programs according to the specific needs of the patients and synthesizing various aesthetic goals into a single coordinated plan. Moreover, technology supporting the combined procedures has developed immensely and therefore plastic surgeons are in a position to benefit from sophisticated instruments and methods. High-level sculpting outcomes, for instance, can be provided by cutting-edge liposuction techniques, ensuring the removal of fat from targeted areas. An understanding of intricate facial anatomy allows surgeons to create a harmonious aesthetic outline. With energy devices becoming a part of the surgical arsenal, and traditional techniques, practitioners are able to not only correct superficial outlines but also deeper structural rearrangements, thus enhancing rejuvenation outcomes. All such holistic techniques not only make the surgery process more streamlined but also enhance the range of treatment options available to patients, offering them increased satisfaction rates. The addition of a multidisciplinary strategy also allows improved regulation of any complications that could arise, as asserted by combined expertise in the field. Practitioners recognize that the combination of these procedures necessitates careful planning and execution to guarantee minimized risks while obtaining maximal aesthetic outcomes. As discussed in the literature, this informed type of plastic surgery, spanning a spectrum of subspecialties, ensures surgeons are sufficiently prepared to deal with complications arising during such sophisticated procedures. The integration of advanced techniques serves to reinforce the general purpose of combined procedures: achieving harmonious results that extend beyond aesthetic purposes to encompass patient health and satisfaction, a fundamental aspect of modern facial aesthetic surgery (Kalaskar et al., 2016).

8.6.1. Benefits of Combining Implants with Fat Grafting

Within the ever-evolving field of aesthetic facial contouring, the combination of using implants alongside fat grafting has been a wonderful advance in providing a naturally appearing result. Chin, cheek, and jaw implants provide the foundation to create the implant's shape, while fat grafting provides volume and enhances the softness of the contours. This strategic mix gives a superior concordant ratio among the hard and soft tissues of the face, ultimately achieving a renewed appearance. Facial proportion improvement not only makes facial beauty more excellent but also renews the confidence of those who receive facial enhancement, thereby addressing physical and psychophysical aspects of beauty. The dual method can also help minimize the possibility of complications normally associated with implants by creating an encapsulating layer of fat that can possibly protect the implants and assist in the integration of the material with the tissue. In addition, the integration of fat grafting and implants can significantly improve overall aesthetic outcomes by encouraging the sustainability of the outcomes. While silicone implants offer durability and structural support, fat grafting offers the additional advantage of bioactive cells that will help in tissue regeneration. The bioactive components will stimulate local blood supply and promote a normal healing environment, which is crucial in achieving the desired aesthetic outcome. Studies show that the microenvironment created by transplanted fat can indirectly contribute to the healing processes of the corresponding implants and thus potentially advance their integration and longevity in the craniofacial complex (Anesi et al., 2014). Moreover, the possibility of achieving a better aesthetic outcome is a sufficient reason for patients to embrace the combined procedure, as it comes with fewer revisions and an overall better facial reshaping solution. In addition to the cosmetic enhancement, the harmony of the procedure also decreases the implant sizes needed, making it a less painful process for the patient. Since surgeons use fat grafting to enlarge certain areas, they can use smaller or improved-shaped implants, which minimizes complications and makes recovery more comfortable. This technique is especially useful for instances of limited bone or soft tissue health, where large implants are extremely risky. Furthermore, combining these methods is consistent with a greater emphasis in oral and maxillofacial surgery to apply treatment strategies that maximize outcomes while minimizing risks and recovery time (Kalaskar et al., 2016). Generally speaking, the benefits of using implants in combination with fat grafting emphasize the expansion of aesthetic surgery towards a more extended and patient-tailored approach to facial contouring.

8.6.2. Case Studies of Successful Combined Procedures

Facial implants in combination with fat grafting provide a strong model for aesthetic improvement, as some case studies of successful combined procedures illustrate. A notable example comprises patients who are subjected to simultaneous chin and cheek implant surgery, augmented by fat grafting to reconstitute facial volume and form. Coupling the procedures serves to create a synergy that optimizes the overall aesthetic outcome, producing a harmonious balance that promotes both tissue enhancement and structural support. Surgeons have reported increased patient satisfaction as the combined process facilitates well-planned augmentation according to individual facial anatomy. Moreover, fat grafting not only provides volume but also contributes to the natural feel and appearance of the postoperative result, reducing the risk of complications in rigid implantation (Kalaskar et al., 2016). Other liposculpture and jaw implant combinations have also produced promising outcomes in a clinical review, attesting to the efficacy of these treatments. Case reports illustrate how a combination of jawline augmentation with implants and precise liposculpture can redesign the lower third of the face with considerable aesthetic improvement. Of interest is that the selection of these combined treatments allows for complete contouring, both skeletal and soft tissue characteristics, simultaneously. Surgeons also underscore the importance of individualized treatment planning in order to achieve successful outcomes, as optimal outcomes in most instances hinge on careful consideration of patient-specific facial measurements and aesthetic goals. The corroborative function of liposculpture and jaw implants additionally attests to the appropriateness of a multidisciplinary treatment in facial aesthetic surgery (Kalaskar et al., 2016). Lastly, patient healing experiences similarly reveal the efficacy of simultaneous facial procedures. Notable case studies have indicated a reduced total downtime when multiple aesthetic improvements are performed at once, as opposed to spreading out the surgeries over many months. With advancements in surgery techniques and post-surgery care, patients have reported greater comfort levels and satisfaction with results. Success using these multi-modalities depends primarily on the all-encompassing evaluation capacity of practitioners who are competent in both contouring and implant technologies. This improved postoperative course allows for a smoother recovery process, eventually resulting in a satisfactory patient experience and earlier return to normal functions, thus identifying the benefit of combined surgical methods in aesthetic practice (Kalaskar et al., 2016).

8.6.3. Considerations for Recovery and Aftercare

Facial implant operations, such as chin, cheek, and jaw implants, recovery and aftercare demand meticulous attention to detail in order to maximize healing and aesthetic outcomes. The initial postoperative phase typically features swelling, pain, and bruising, which are all normal responses to the surgical trauma. Patients are mostly advised to remain upright and limit physical activities in order to minimize swelling. Also, adherence to medications taken for pain relief and antibiotics is critical to prevent complications such as infection. At this time, follow-ups with the surgeon every now and then are critical to monitor the healing process and manage any problems that arise, so recovery can proceed uninterrupted. Once the initial healing is achieved, the focus is on overall aftercare procedures that can aid in providing the outcome one desires. The importance of good hygiene surrounding the operation sites should be explained to the patients, since this can significantly reduce the rates of infection while enhancing healing. Good nutrition is equally significant; an adequate diet with intensive consumption of vitamins and minerals enhances tissue growth and can maximally enhance overall recovery. Also, certain activities need to be avoided, such as strenuous exercise or sunlight exposure on the places where the cuts were made, to prevent complications and ensure that the implants settle well within the framework of the skin. These subtle adjustments in one's lifestyle bring long-term benefits by maintaining the result of the surgery while optimizing the overall health of the patient. Lastly, considerations for recovery and aftercare extend beyond the clinical, such as psychological adjustment to one's altered shape. Recovery can induce emotional mood swings as the patient adjusts to their new shape, and therefore, emotional counseling by relatives, friends, or expert counselors would be in order. Open discussions concerning body image and self-awareness would help balance feelings of anxiety or discontent during recovery. Apart from that, patients may also be guided to exercise realistic hopes regarding the recovery period and ultimate result, which could take a couple of months to fully manifest. Combining physical as well as emotional rehabilitation in aftercare can work wonders in developing a broad healing experience, and patients would learn to embrace their changed features confidently (Park, 2008).

Test Your Knowledge

1. What aesthetic advantages can be achieved by combining facial implants with fat grafting in a single treatment plan?
2. What key factors should be considered regarding recovery and aftercare when multiple facial procedures are performed together?

SUMMARY

Briefly, the advancement in facial contouring and implants, particularly chin, cheek, and jaw implants and fat grafting and liposculpture, has greatly advanced aesthetic outcomes for patients wishing for facial rejuvenation. The synergy of such treatment not only improves cosmetic deformity but also adds to self-esteem and overall quality of life. As attested by clinical evidence, such as articles reviewed from a systematic review, these techniques are safe and effective, with high levels of patient satisfaction following treatment. Particularly, the revolution in high-density fat transfer methods has been impactful in revolumizing the face and, in turn, redefining the traditional facial aesthetic approaches (Garcia et al., 2022).

Furthermore, the evolution of liposculpture techniques is used to illustrate enhanced refinements in minimally invasive facial contouring procedures. Through the cooperation of expert surgeons and access to advanced energy-based devices, the variety of treatment options is further expanding. Not only is this development improving the precision of fat removal, but also risk and patient downtime are minimized. As in many studies, including those that are concerned with facial augmentation outcomes, the integration of deeper anatomical insight has given rise to innovative practices that resonate with individual needs (Kalaskar et al., 2016). Lastly, practitioners working in facial aesthetics must keep themselves updated about new techniques and technologies. Continuing education will optimize their ability to achieve the best outcomes under the patient's anxiety regarding safety and effectiveness. The reassuring results of recent research are giving the procedures more confidence, supporting a large trend toward tailored treatment protocols that aim for patient satisfaction. By encouraging a holistic appreciation of both the cosmetic and psychological impacts of facial augmentation, practitioners can be confident that they are doing a positive service for their patients' health as they navigate the processes of aesthetic enhancement (Garcia et al., 2022).

The following conversation about facial implants and contouring has enumerated a range of approaches that promote better aesthetic outcomes. Among them, chin, cheek, and jaw implants are particularly significant aspects of face reshaping surgery. These implants hold great significance in changing facial contours to facilitate proportional balance capable of significantly boosting people's self-image. Clinical research has indicated that these types of implants are both safe and effective for different patients, delivering measurable improvements in looks and mental well-being.

The use of new technology and materials has also further enhanced patient outcomes further, upholding the importance of tailored approaches to cosmetic surgery. Fat grafting and liposculpture, aside from implants, are also now integral to reshaping the face. Using methods like cervicofacial liposuction, surgeons can reshape and redefine facial contours by liposuctioning unwanted fat and restoring volume where needed. The technique not only improves the cosmetic effect by evening out the contours but also improves patient satisfaction scores.

Studies have shown excellent success in using fat transfer with high density, particularly in patients with facial volume loss, with higher improvement scores and desirable psychological outcomes. This makes it evident how very important such techniques are towards achieving facial aesthetic outcomes while maintaining the safety and efficacy of patient care. The evolution of liposuction and its application in facial recontouring is a paradigm shift in plastic procedures. It was once a simple procedure for the removal of fat and now has evolved into a complex technique encompassing various innovations and techniques aimed at facial enhancement. The literature on the evolution of liposuction is a complete understanding of the technique, limitations, complications, and indications for the various methods. Expert consultation for combination treatments and energy-based devices is a goldmine for practitioners who are thinking about introducing an additional tool in their practices in facial surgery (Kalaskar et al., 2016). Conscious focus on these innovations ensures that patients obtain useful and well-rounded treatments tailored to their specific facial anatomy and individual goals.

KEY TERMS FROM THIS CHAPTER

- Adipose tissue
- Aesthetic beautification
- Augmentation
- Cervicofacial liposuction
- Contributes
- Energy-based devices
- Facial beauty
- Aesthetic applications
- Aesthetic improvements
- Bone structure
- Combination therapy
- Dramatic alterations
- Ensure effective
- Facial implants

CRITICAL THINKING QUESTIONS

1. **The primary goal of facial implants is to:**
   a. Remove excess skin
   b. Restore or enhance skeletal projection
   c. Tighten facial muscles
   d. Correct pigmentation
2. **Chin augmentation is most useful in improving:**
   a. Vertical midface height
   b. Nasal tip rotation
   c. Lower facial third balance
   d. Forehead symmetry
3. **Which of the following materials is most commonly used for chin and cheek implants?**
   a. PMMA
   b. Silicone
   c. Hydroxyapatite cement
   d. Titanium mesh
4. **Medpor (porous polyethylene) implants are preferred because they:**
   a. Are easily removable
   b. Allow tissue ingrowth
   c. Have high elasticity
   d. Are self-dissolving
5. **The most common complication of silicone implants is:**
   a. Osseointegration
   b. Migration
   c. Tissue ingrowth
   d. Implant hardening

Short Answer Questions

1. What are the primary aesthetic indications for chin augmentation with implants?
2. How does malar (cheek) augmentation enhance mid-face aesthetics?
3. What anatomical landmarks are crucial when planning jaw (mandibular) implant placement?
4. What is the main difference between structural fat grafting and liposculpture?
5. What factors influence long-term fat graft survival after liposuction harvesting?
6. How does chin projection influence facial balance and the perception of nasal size?

Answers to Critical Thinking Questions

1. (b) 2. (c) 3. (b) 4. (b) 5. (b)

REFERENCES

1. Ahmed, M., Fatima, F., Fida, M., Kamal, et al. (2019). *Adjunctive surgical procedures enhancing treatment outcome: A literature review.* https://core.ac.uk/download/212885885.pdf (accessed on 14th July 2025).
2. Anesi, A., Cavani, F., Chiarini, L., Ferretti, et al. (2014). *Preliminary findings of a potenziated piezosurgical device at the rabbit skull.* https://core.ac.uk/download/80171725.pdf (accessed on 14th July 2025).
3. Bouzouaya, C., & Feiner, R. (2018). *Adjuvant botulinum toxin harmonization in minimally invasive facial aesthetic surgery.* https://core.ac.uk/download/322438270.pdf (accessed on 14th July 2025).
4. Davies, S., Hayek, J., & Juma, A. (2023). *Body contouring and VASER technology, the fourth dimension.* https://core.ac.uk/download/553310020.pdf (accessed on 14th July 2025).
5. Garcia, J. L. V. ., Garcia, V. R. do P., & Valente, S. M. de M. (2022). Major clinical outcomes and analysis of the risk of bias of the advances in cervicofacial liposculture: a systematic review. *MedNEXT Journal of Medical and Health Sciences, 3*(3). https://doi.org/10.54448/mdnt22301(accessed on 14th July 2025).
6. Kamal, A. T., Fatima, F., Fida, M., Ahmed, M., & Mehmood, H. T. (2019). Adjunctive surgical procedures enhancing treatment outcome—A literature review. *Journal of Pakistan Medical Association, 69*(5), 705–710. https://ecommons.aku.edu/pakistan_fhs_mc_surg_surg/776 (accessed on 14th July 2025).
7. Deepak M. Kalaskar, Peter E. Butler, Shadi Ghali. (2016). *Textbook of Plastic and Reconstructive Surgery*. ISBN: 978-1-910634-37-0 (Hbk.) https://core.ac.uk/download/79526588.pdf
8. Park, S. S. (2008). *Revision Rhinoplasty*. Thieme. http://books.google.com/books?id=vwHmwB8qSeAC&dq=Facial+implants+recovery+aftercare+chin+cheek+jaw+fat+grafting+liposculpture+considerations&hl=&source=gbs_api (accessed on 14th July 2025).
9. Skrynnyk, S. (2024). *Innovative Approaches to Improving Facial Contours, 1*(1), 22, 23. https://www.eujini.org.pl (accessed on 14th July 2025).
10. Steinbacher, D. M. (2019, March 14). *Aesthetic Orthognathic Surgery and Rhinoplasty*. John Wiley & Sons. https://play.google.com/store/books/details?id=ri6NDwAAQBAJ&source=gbs_api (accessed on 14th July 2025).

BOTULINUM TOXIN AND DERMAL FILLERS IN FACIAL COSMETIC

9

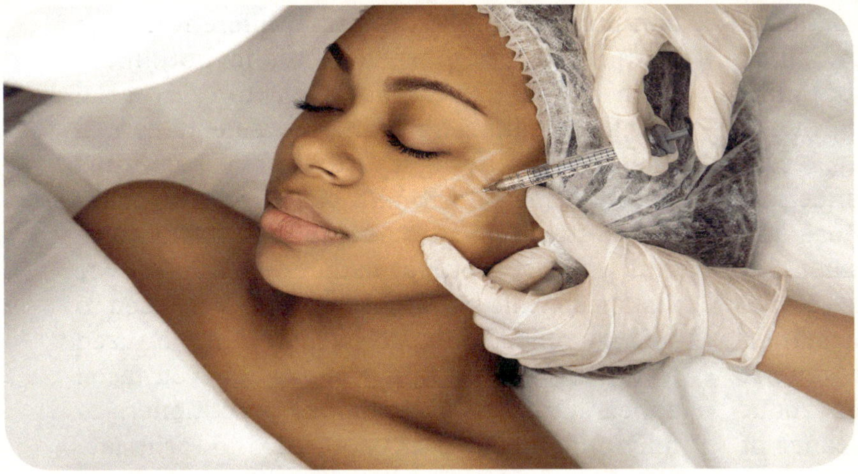

LEARNING OBJECTIVES

After studying this chapter, you will be able to:

1. Describe the history of botulinum toxin in aesthetics;
2. Explain the mechanism of action of botulinum toxin;
3. Discuss the types of dermal fillers;
4. Understand the comparison of botulinum toxin and dermal fillers;
5. Focus on safety and regulatory aspects;
6. Learn about trends in facial cosmetic procedures.

Introduction

The area of facial aesthetics has experienced a radical change over the past couple of decades with the advent of non-surgical cosmetic treatments. Among these developments, botulinum toxin and dermal fillers are two of the most widely used among individuals seeking to enhance the contours of their faces and to reverse the effects of aging. These treatments give patients an alternative that is less invasive than surgery, meeting a growing need for less invasive but effective methods. As society places pressure on looking more youthful, the use of these treatments has increased, drawing in practitioners and potential patients alike. This is a trend that can be seen with the increased number of aesthetic dermatological treatments being performed worldwide, showing the need to pay attention to both mechanisms and implications of the treatments in achieving beneficial outcomes in facial cosmetics (Madnani et al., 2022). As popular as they are, though, a proper full understanding of the benefit and risk frameworks of botulinum toxin and dermal fillers remains relevant. Not only do practitioners have to be technically proficient in the injection of these drugs, but they also have to be informed about pre- and post-procedure care to prevent complications and achieve the maximum results. Most practitioners, however, have complained that they did not feel properly trained as far as the technicalities of such beauty treatments were concerned. These knowledge deficiencies may lead to adverse patient outcomes, taking away from the potential benefit offered by botulinum toxin and dermal fillers (Madnani et al., 2022). It is therefore critical to critically address this educational deficiency, since evidence-based decision-making can optimize patient satisfaction and safety in the growing field of cosmetic dermatology. In addition, recent studies emphasize the psychological effects of botulinum toxin in young patients. More and more people are now seeking such treatments at a younger age, driven by a need to take control of the aging process and prevent the formation of facial wrinkles. This preventive strategy not only demonstrates evolving attitudes about aging but also underscores the significance of taking patient happiness and self-esteem into account when it comes to aesthetic treatments. As younger patients find earlier treatment more satisfactory, the possibility of preventive botulinum toxin therapy is an emerging part of cosmetic procedures. Therefore, both clinical treatments and psychological effects of these treatments should be discussed in the case of botulinum toxin and dermal fillers, given their emphasis on a multidisciplinary strategy in facial cosmetics.

Definition of Botulinum Toxin

Botulinum toxin, a neurotoxic protein excreted by the bacterium *Clostridium botulinum*, is a significant consideration in cosmetic and therapeutic applications. The potent toxin affects the release of acetylcholine at the neuromuscular junction to induce temporary paralysis of the muscles. In facial cosmetology, botulinum toxin is prevalently employed to oppose the appearance of wrinkles and fine lines by temporarily relaxing overactive facial muscles. Thereafter, its popularity has increased, transforming non-surgical facial enhancement. The control of dosage is most appealing to practitioners and patients because it allows individualized treatments to achieve a younger face without the need for any invasive surgical procedures. As an adjunct to its role in the therapy of anti-aging, botulinum toxin is commonly compared with dermal fillers, and they are applied to serve different though complementary purposes. While botulinum toxin targets muscle movement to relax facial wrinkles resulting from facial movements, dermal fillers target filling spaces in the face, thus re-establishing form and contour. This makes it a better choice for combination therapies that produce optimal esthetic outcomes. For instance, while botulinum toxin may be used to soften forehead lines, dermal fillers may be used to fill cheeks and lips, creating an even facial appearance. It is essential for practitioners to fully understand both modalities to formulate effective treatment plans specifically tailored to the requirements of each individual patient. Blending botulinum toxin and dermal fillers in cosmetic treatment has spurred widespread research on optimal application practice. It is essential to understand the anatomical details of the facial region to attain maximum benefit from treatment while reducing complications. Among the noteworthy advances in the field, studies show that new combinations of hyaluronic acid fillers with the addition of amino acids enhance facial volume and appearance when combined with botulinum toxin treatment. Such synergistic approaches have proved effective for the treatment of conditions like eyebrow ptosis, which could have its basis in muscular dysfunction or tissue deflation, as reported in the literature. These observations not only confirm the universality of botulinum toxin but also show how it is pivotal in optimizing the overall beauty landscape in facial aesthetics, where rejuvenation as well as preservation of natural expression are both the objectives (Amuso et al., 2021; de Lima Faria et al., 2025) (Figure 9.1).

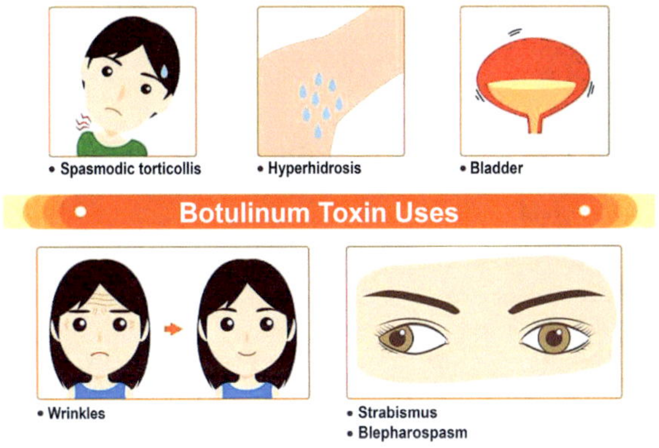

Figure 9.1. Botulinum toxin.

Source: https://biologydictionary.net/wp-content/uploads/2020/10/botoxuses.jpg.

Overview of Dermal Fillers

The popularity of dermal fillers has increased exponentially over the past several years, making them a focal point of non-invasive cosmetic care. They emerge as a way to fill wrinkles, fine lines, and areas of volume loss with an injectable solution, greatly updating the face. Composed of hyaluronic acid, collagen, and other biocompatible materials, dermal fillers offer a means of regaining youthfulness by filling out the skin and augmenting facial contours. The increasing popularity of minimally invasive treatments is a manifestation of the broader cultural trend toward achieving beauty ideals without resorting to surgical intervention. Because trained medical professionals give these cosmetic treatments, it is necessary to know the various types of fillers and what they are used for to ensure patient safety and satisfaction. Besides, ongoing education in the techniques and technology of fillers' administration will enhance the performance of these treatments (Kumar, 2021). Different dermal fillers are formulated for various cosmetic concerns, with each type of formula applied to address different skin properties and aging features. Hyaluronic acid fillers, for instance, are favored as they are water-retentive, restoring facial volume with immediate hydration and enabling natural facial movement.

Conversely, collagen fillers are a lasting repair for the structure and elasticity of the skin. In addition, poly-L-lactic acid and calcium hydroxylapatite fillers stimulate long-term collagen formation, thus depicting a gradual change in the skin's texture. Practitioners need to highlight these distinctions so that they can customize treatments for specific patient needs and outcomes. The dynamic development of dermal fillers continues to drive innovation in cosmetic medicine, with materials and methodologies further elevating patient expectations (Abdel-Sayed et al., 2024). While dermal fillers can significantly enhance aesthetic outcomes, they do not come without risk and consideration. Potential complications, such as allergic reactions, inflammation, and vascular occlusion, necessitate a thorough assessment of every patient before treatment. Furthermore, the utilization of certified and experienced practitioners should not be emphasized sufficiently, as technique is paramount to avoiding side effects. Safety protocols and patient education become focused on building trust and satisfaction on the part of individuals who are obtaining cosmetic augmentation. With the evolution of the non-surgical aesthetics industry, ensuring patient welfare remains the priority, sparking ongoing debates over standardization and regulation within the industry. By prioritizing safety at the forefront, practitioners are able to make the process enjoyable for clients, hence enhancing the overall acceptance and success of dermal fillers in facial cosmetics (Kumar, 2021) (Figure 9.2).

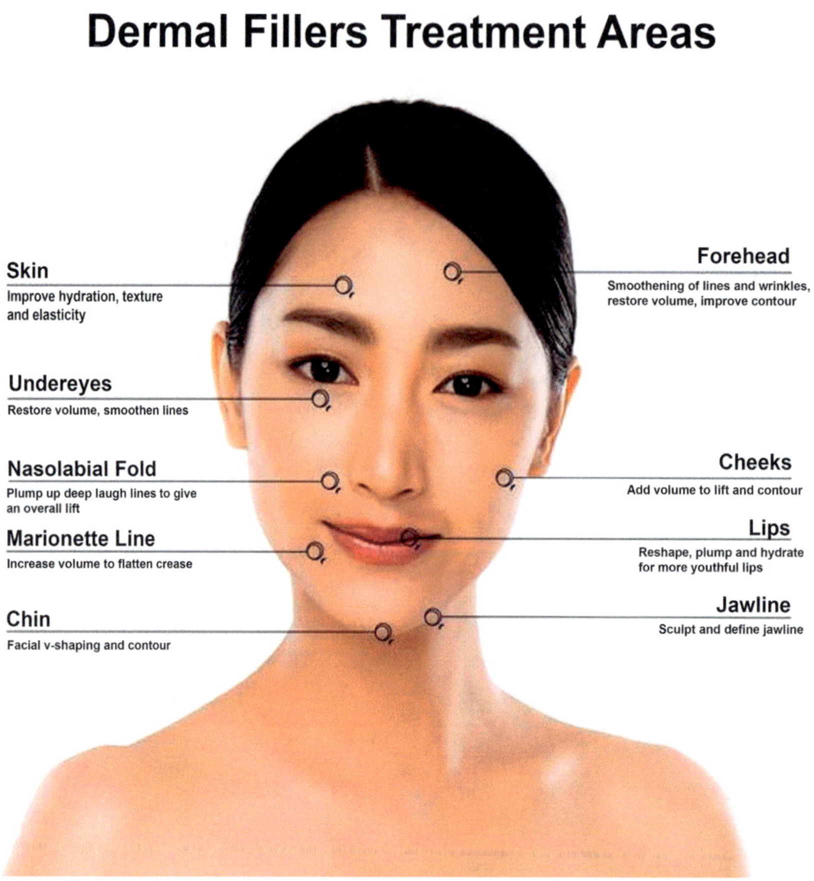

Figure 9.2. The dermal fillers treatment areas.

Source: https://luna.clinic/wp-content/uploads/2022/07/derma-fillers-treatment-areas.jpg.

Role of Facial Cosmetics in the Contemporary World

The contemporary situation of facial cosmetics has experienced a complete transformation, driven largely by the proliferation of non-surgical practices like the use of botulinum toxin and dermal fillers. These technologies have democratized cosmetic treatments to the masses, enabling people with diverse backgrounds to participate in practices that were once exclusive to those with immense spending capacity. Specifically, the popularity of injectables undermined the exclusivity thresholds that otherwise have been the defining characteristic of cosmetic surgery, and it changed the social definition of beauty. As a result, these low-profile procedures have generated a culture where self-enhancement is socially acceptable and trendy. This model prioritizes ongoing education, reflecting the growing need for structured postgraduate training in non-surgical aesthetics, as identified in their delivery and implementation within clinical settings (Kumar, 2021). Also, the relation between facial aesthetics and social pressures determines the psychological importance of cosmetic treatments. Individuals are defining self-worth more and more in terms of body image, so the need for treatments and products that can provide an improvement is growing. These treatments have psychological returns that are not purely vanity; they can increase confidence and self-worth, personally and professionally. Most significantly, beauty stories across cultures are always evolving because gender, race, and economics all affect experiences of diversity. The recent discourse in sociology brings to light the complexities of these narratives, especially those of non-surgical beauty, as it invites researchers to study further the impact of cosmetic habits on social structures and individual identity (Dowrick & Holliday, 2022). Lastly, the ethical concerns involved in facial cosmetics cannot be ignored, with the existence of treatments like botulinum toxin and dermal fillers ushering in possibilities along with challenges. While the democratization of enhancing beauty can be liberating, regulating such practitioners and ensuring treatment safety is a concern. The accessibility of aesthetic providers with minimal complete training calls for strict guidelines guaranteeing ethical practice in this expanding industry. The risks present in the treatments necessitate that the response be cautious to counterbalance consumer protection with stimulating innovation. As growth in the area grows greater by the day, curriculum design for non-surgical aesthetic training is imperative to answer these ethical issues while maintaining professional standards on the pursuit of beauty and improvement (Kumar, 2021) (Figure 9.3).

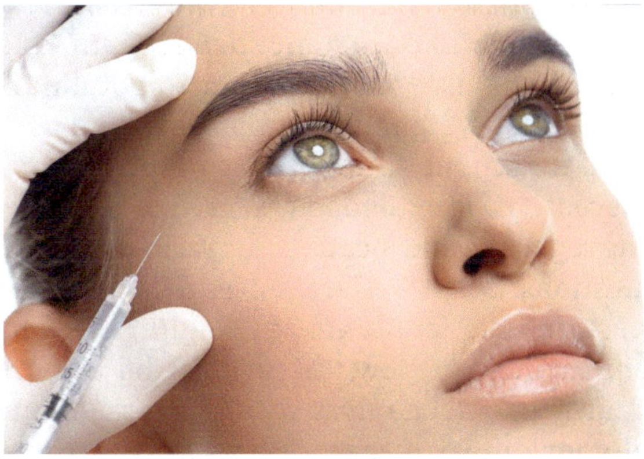

Figure 9.3. The contemporary landscape of facial cosmetics.

Source: https://hedoxclinic.co.uk/wp-content/uploads/2021/02/botox-1024x680.jpg.

9.1. History of Botulinum Toxin in Aesthetics

Learning Outcome

1. Discovery and Medical Uses
2. Introduction to Cosmetic Applications
3. Evolution of Public Perception

The history of botulinum toxin in aesthetics is one of a revolutionary transformation that has reshaped current cosmetic procedures. First found in the late 19th century, botulinum toxin as an extract from the *Clostridium botulinum* bacterium was originally known for its neurotoxic features. Its original switched application in clinical beauty was during the 1980s when eye physicians noted a decrease in eyelid spasms among patients injected with botulinum toxin for strabismus. It was an accidental find that led to the door opening for the substances research in cosmetic applications, targeting its muscle-paralyzing action to minimize facial wrinkles, particularly frown lines. The FDA subsequently licensed botulinum toxin for cosmetic use in 2002, an event that transformed medicine and aesthetics, which resulted in an universal acceptance of the treatment by dermatologists and cosmetic surgeons. As the popularity of procedures based on botulinum toxin grew, it was clear that demand for minimally invasive aesthetic treatments was on the increase among the population. This increase was fueled by cultural pressures to look young and non-surgical procedures, showing the cultural shift toward self-improvement behaviors. Botulinum toxin not only introduced a relatively safe and effective method for the reduction of the cosmetic indicators of aging but also ushered in a new era of aesthetic dermatology where results could be attained by patients with little downtime. This phenomenon is preceded by innovations and diversity of dermal fillers, which are similarly effective in restoring facial volume and contours. As per the literature, understanding the potential benefits and drawbacks of these treatments is essential for providers to optimize patient outcomes and overall satisfaction in aesthetic dermatology (Madnani et al., 2022).

The concurrent rise of dermal fillers with botulinum toxin acts to further affirm the dynamic character of cosmetic treatments. From its humble origins in animal-based materials like bovine collagen, dermal fillers have come a long way in the last two or three decades to give rise to a host of synthetic derivatives like hyaluronic acid and PMMA-based products. These fillers provide a diverse range of applications in soft tissue augmentation, addressing numerous aesthetic concerns such as loss of volume and pronounced wrinkles (Mohamed, 2020). The combination of botulinum toxin and dermal fillers in cosmetic procedures suggests an integrated facial appearance, where the combination of muscle relaxation and volumetric restoration enhances the overall patient experience. As aesthetic innovations continue to unfold, understanding the history of these treatments is crucial to a deeper understanding of the complexities and ethical considerations that underlie today's cosmetic procedures (Figure 9.4).

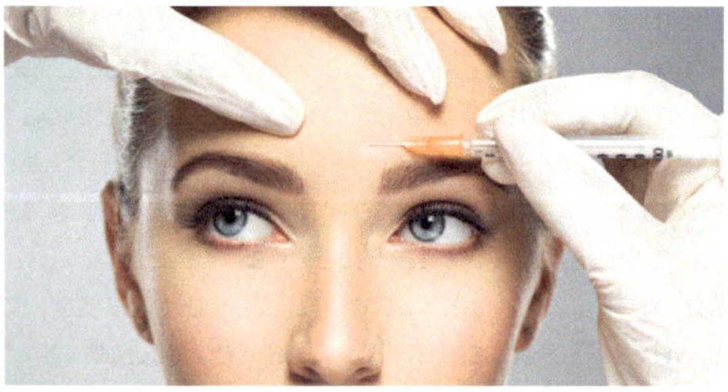

Figure 9.4. The historical journey of botulinum toxin in aesthetics.

Source: https://crstodayeurope.com/wp-content/uploads/sites/5/2020/06/0620CRST_ES_Toxins-600x315.jpg.

9.1.1. Discovery and Medical Uses

The discovery of botulinum toxin, predominantly defined by the bacterium *Clostridium botulinum*, has transformed the realm of therapeutic and cosmetic medicine. Initially recognized to induce food poisoning, scientists later found its therapeutic applications, transforming the substance's profile from a lethal toxin to a beneficial medicinal drug. The ability of botulinum toxin to temporarily paralyze muscles created the prospect of its use in therapy for a wide variety of neuromuscular diseases, such as blepharospasm and cervical dystonia. This groundbreaking finding served as the foundation for further studies into its uses, eventually bringing its utility to aesthetic treatment for reducing facial wrinkles and, thereby, revolutionizing cosmetic dermatology. Understanding this intricate genesis is important to comprehending today's medical procedures and its strong standing in the cosmetic field. Apart from its noted applications in cosmetic surgery, botulinum toxin is also being explored with increasing interest for various medical ailments beyond the realm of cosmetics. Significant advancements have surfaced in urology and gynecology, exhibiting the universality of application to treat a variety of ailments. For instance, recent studies have reported positive results in the treatment of conditions like chronic pelvic pain and vaginismus by using specially aimed botulinum toxin injections, signaling its potential as a non-surgical treatment option. These findings signal the necessity for extended research to optimize dosing regimens and locations for various medical applications. Despite effectiveness demonstrated in certain use contexts, as highlighted by recent medical review, there must be a more standardized mechanism to ensure the same results for different therapeutic cases (Etrusco et al., 2023). Such continued studies not only make the insight into botulinum toxins medical applications easier but also lay a blueprint for other therapy approaches. Furthermore, the evolving face of botulinum toxin medical uses reflects a growing trend toward exploiting its unique qualities to treat an increasing spectrum of diseases. As more research into the promise of botulinum toxin becomes a future possibility, a sincere debate has arisen regarding dosage precision and injection technique within different therapeutic settings. For instance, in gynecology, precise research is now focused on clarifying optimal doses and injection sites needed to achieve maximum therapeutic effectiveness and minimize potential side effects. These are not only theoretical activities but carry real implications for improved patient care and extended treatment availability (Etrusco et al., 2023). As the medical community struggles with these subtleties, robust discussion of best practices is certain to bring about further understanding of botulinum toxin. This progress underscores the importance of continued research and development in medical and cosmetic applications, leading ultimately to the development of interdisciplinary medicine practice.

9.1.2. Introduction to Cosmetic Applications

The beauty industry has undergone a remarkable transformation with the arrival of minimally invasive procedures that utilize products such as botulinum toxin and fillers. Such applications not only enhance the cosmetic appearance but also find therapeutic use since they successfully manage conditions such as facial wrinkles and volume deficiency. Botulinum toxin, first applied in the medical sector, has found its application in cosmetics and is used to temporarily relax muscles to reduce the visibility of dynamic wrinkles. As the popularity of the intervention grows, it is important to recognize the action mechanisms, side effects, and the effectiveness of botulinum toxin in aesthetic treatments, which are of utmost importance for practitioners as well as consumers. Dermal fillers, on the other hand, are volume-inducing substances that restore the lost facial fullness and offer a complementary therapy to botulinum toxin injection. Fillers, which may be composed of various substances like hyaluronic acid, collagen, or synthetic polymers, serve the critical function of keeping the face looking youthful by adding volume to areas such as the cheeks, lips, and nasolabial folds. Extended expertise in filler characteristics, longevity, and facial anatomy appropriate for treatments is required from the practitioners in order for them to produce successful outcomes. Moreover, the integration of such cosmetic applications involves extensive training and adherence to proper safety protocols, highlighting the need for practitioner skill in maintaining aesthetic integrity and avoiding risks associated with these treatments.

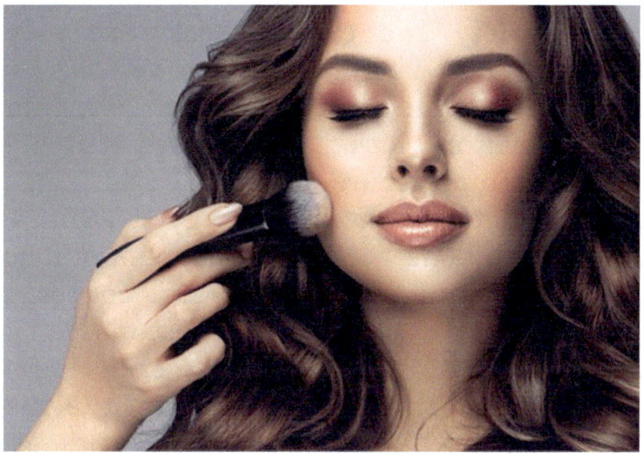

Figure 9.5. Introduction to cosmetic applications.

Source: https://www.shutterstock.com/image-photo/makeup-artist-applies-powder-blush-600nw-1805797540.jpg.

As the size of cosmetic procedures increases, the need for standardized treatment and complete clinical guidelines becomes more distinct. Although several studies have compared the use of botulinum toxin and dermal fillers, variability in method of application and dosage remains a challenge to practitioners. For instance, research has shown that optimal dosage and injection techniques for botulinum toxin remain subjects of debate and research. Hence, further research will be necessary to optimize best practices and the understanding of the anatomical issues of safe and effective cosmetic treatment. This necessitates a multidisciplinary approach that unites empirical research with clinical practice, so that cosmetic application is not only aesthetically desirable but also honors patient safety and satisfaction (Etrusco et al., 2023) (Figure 9.5).

9.1.3. Evolution of Public Perception

Public perception of the use of dermal fillers and botulinum toxin in facial cosmetics has evolved significantly over the past few decades. Initially, the treatments were viewed skeptically and negatively due to misperceptions about safety and effectiveness, but they have gradually become accepted by a larger population. This shift has been owing to various reasons, including increased visibility of cosmetic procedures in mainstream media and the status of endorsement by celebrities. As this aesthetic became mainstream, public discourse shifted away from risk concerns for procedure to the normalization of seeking cosmetic looks as self-care. The sociocultural context in which these products operate has been instrumental in influencing attitudes, manifesting an overriding embracing of beauty ideals involving enhancement and alteration (Kumar, 2021). Further, the establishment of professional standards and regulatory practices has had a significant influence on the confidence of the public in cosmetic procedures. With the launch of specialized training programs focusing on enhancing competency in delivering non-surgical aesthetic treatments, like the evidence-based postgraduate scheme for non-surgical aesthetics (NSA), providers currently demonstrate concern for quality and safety (Kumar, 2021). This has ensured that there is an increasingly educated public that can engage with informed debate regarding the possible benefits and drawbacks of such treatments. As patients continue to learn more about the procedures, more and more of them are making a choice based on sound information, rather than stigma or fear. The dialogue surrounding these enhancements now encompasses broader issues of autonomy and personal choice, shifting toward a healthier and more mature approach. As this positive trend continues, there remain disjunctures between public expectations and the reality of cosmetic procedures, and this sometimes results in confusion and suspicion. Cosmetic dentistry literature shows overarching institutional narratives that are prone to shape the public's attitude toward cosmetic treatment, perpetuating beauty within the health paradigm and removing the profit motive from public knowledge. A rich intertextual connection between social mores and institutional narratives highlights the irony of public perception: in an age of heightened tolerance for cosmetic operations, there are still voids in the perception of quality, safety, and ethics of the processes. As the field advances, instilling transparency and ethical business will be critical in attempting to reverse these disjunctures and establish positive public opinion.

Test Your Knowledge

1. How was botulinum toxin first discovered, and what were its early medical uses before cosmetic applications emerged?
2. What factors contributed to the introduction of botulinum toxin as a cosmetic treatment for facial wrinkles?
3. How has public perception of botulinum toxin evolved from its early medical use to its widespread acceptance in aesthetic practice?

9.2. Mechanism of Action of Botulinum Toxin

Learning Outcome

1. Discuss the Neuromuscular Blockade
2. Explain the Effects on Facial Muscles
3. Focus on Duration of Results

The mechanism of action of botulinum toxin is an extremely intricate process that has a profound impact on the practice of facial cosmetics. When botulinum toxin is injected into targeted regions of muscle, it inhibits the presynaptic release of the neurotransmitter acetylcholine, which plays a role in muscle contraction. This inhibition leads to transient paralysis of the injected muscles, effectively decreasing the ability of the muscles to contract. Relaxation of the muscle induced by this has the effect of minimizing the prominence of fine lines and wrinkles, particularly in moving areas like the forehead and around the eyes. Consequently, this biochemical action yields smoother skin texture and a young-looking appearance, appealing to cosmetic dermatology practitioners and patients alike. Further, the selectivity of botulinum toxins' mechanism holds tremendous promise in various applications outside of cosmetic applications. Its therapeutic possibilities reach beyond the field of medicine into the realms of gynecology, where it has been investigated for the treatment of chronic pelvic pain and vaginismus. Despite the therapeutic applications of these combined uses, however, the specific dosing regimens and best locations for injection of these diverse uses still lack proper standardization. The absence of specificity in implementation refers to an urgent need for further research into botulinum toxin different uses. This highlights not just the potential of botulinum toxin as a treatment agent but also the necessity for consistent guidelines of use among specialties, allowing practitioners to obtain optimal patient results while lessening risks. Of relevance to facial cosmetics is the possible adverse effect of botulinum toxin injection, which needs to be taken into serious consideration. Side effects, while usually minor, may comprise bruising, swelling, and in isolated instances, spontaneous muscle weakness. An appreciation of the exact biological interactions happening after injection is important for practitioners to effectively prevent risks. Clinicians must remain updated on the most recent research summarizing both the efficacy and safety of botulinum toxin in its different applications, including cosmetic enhancement. With the constantly evolving skin care environment of dermatological treatments, it is increasingly important to pair the science of the mechanism of action of the toxin with best cosmetic use practices such that patient safety and satisfaction remain at the forefront of the clinical practice (Etrusco et al., 2023) (Figure 9.6).

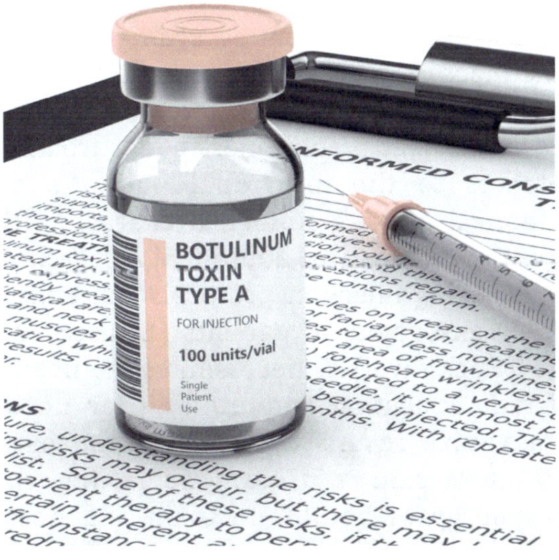

Figure 9.6. Mechanism of action of botulinum toxin.

Source: https://www.thepmfajournal.com/media/31952/pmfa-jj23-botulilium-image-small.jpg.

9.2.1. Neuromuscular Blockade

Neuromuscular blockade is central to the mechanism of action of botulinum toxin in most fields, particularly in aesthetic medicine. Botulinum toxin, derived from *Clostridium botulinum*, achieves its effect through the inhibition of the release of acetylcholine at the neuromuscular junction and resultant temporary muscle paralysis. This activity is critical in its application in facial cosmetics, where it is used to reduce the appearance of dynamic wrinkles. With practitioners seeking maximum aesthetic outcome, awareness of the dynamics of neuromuscular blockade allows precise dosing and precise injection placement. By the realization of this neuromodulation, aesthetic practitioners can achieve a natural outcome with less side effect, making neuromuscular blockade a key part of effective treatment with botulinum toxin. Although botulinum toxin has become universal acceptance in aesthetic practices, variation in patient response presents severe implications in its use. Neuromuscular blockade can be different according to patient-related factors such as muscle bulk, sites to be treated, and overall health status. Therefore, it is essential that practitioners adapt treatment protocols to the individual patient's own anatomical and physiological characteristics. There is evidence that additional research into standardizing injection protocols can enhance efficacy and safety in patients (Etrusco et al., 2023). Such diversity necessitates the need for constant education and training for doctors to maximize results and correct the use of botulinum toxin in a cosmetic setting. Also, the synergy of botulinum toxin and dermal fillers demonstrates the combined possibility of the two treatments to achieve worldwide rejuvenation of the face. As botulinum toxin acts on neuromuscular blockade to soften wrinkles caused by muscle contractions, dermal fillers add volume and structure to areas that may have lost shape due to aging. This synergy permits an interdisciplinary method of facial aesthetic management, in which practitioners can design treatments to address multiple issues at the same time. But still, the challenge lies in identifying the best techniques and dosages for the best results when combined with neuromuscular blockade. Addressing this, research will have to explore the various applications of botulinum toxin beyond aesthetics, e.g., managing diverse conditions, so as to highlight the need for a better understanding of how it acts (Etrusco et al., 2023) (Figure 9.7).

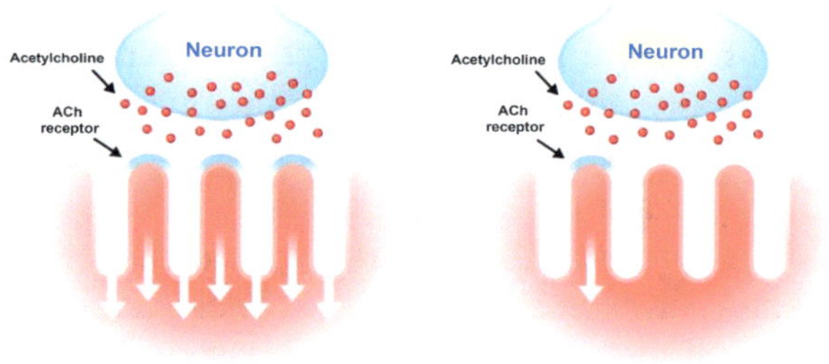

Figure 9.7. Neuromuscular blockade.

Source: https://clinicalview.gehealthcare.com/sites/default/files/styles/paragraph_scaled_picture_fallback/public/Subtypes%20of%20neuromuscular%20blocking%20agents.png?itok=oNo2g1xl.

9.2.2. Effects on Facial Muscles

Botulinum toxin administration in cosmetic therapy has significant effects on facial muscles, with the primary influence being on their functionality and appearance. By causing temporary paralysis of some muscles, botulinum toxin is able to reduce the appearance of wrinkles and thus modify the facial topography to one of youthfulness. The process is through inhibition of acetylcholine release at the neuromuscular junction with consequent diminution in contraction of the affected muscles. This degree of accuracy allows practitioners to create desired cosmetic alterations with a minimal amount of exaggerated movement of the muscles leading to facial aging. But such changes are not cosmetic but potentially affect facial expression dynamics, emotional expression, and muscle coordination needed for effective non-verbal communication. Beyond the cosmetic benefits, effects upon facial muscles extend beyond the cosmetic effects desired. Prolonged treatments with botulinum toxin can cause muscle atrophy and a change in muscle tone, leading to a phenomenon of compensatory recruitment of muscles. This occurs when untreated facial muscles overcorrect immobilized muscles, which can lead to an imbalance of facial symmetry. This implies individuals can notice altered expressions and a general adjustment in facial dynamics. Also, awareness of such unwanted effects highlights the importance of thorough pre- and post-procedure education, as addressed in numerous expert reviews. Such knowledge is crucial for both practitioners and clients in terms of setting realistic expectations as well as understanding the development of their facial musculature following botulinum toxin treatment (Madnani et al., 2022). In addition, the psycho-social implications of botulinum toxin use must be considered, particularly in relation to its impact on facial muscles. The rise in BOTOX for aesthetic use is fueled in part by social media photo ideals, which value younger and unblemished looks. In this regard, the application of botulinum toxin may be interpreted as a reaction to external pressures influencing one's identity and sense of self. As individuals struggle to fulfill these beauty ideals, the effects spread far beyond the body, spilling over into psychological complications, such as body image disturbance and self-esteem problems. Recognition of the double-edged nature of botulinum toxin's effect on facial muscles highlights not only the requirement for fully informed consent but also the ethical implications of its use in cosmetic treatment. Emphasizing these aspects works to ensure responsible use of botulinum toxin, taking into account both therapeutic and potential psychosocial impact (Akuma et al., 2024).

9.2.3. Duration of Results

Duration of results following cosmetic treatments with botulinum toxin (Botox) and dermal fillers is a consideration of significance both for practitioners and patients. Botulinum toxin characteristically results in a reversible suppression of muscle activity, producing a smoother facial appearance. The effect has been shown to last three to six months, varying with a variety of factors, including personal metabolism and the treated site. With time, as the original function of the muscle is regained, wrinkles and lines are reduced. This attribute demands periodic treatments, which are both beneficial for skincare care as well as strategically planned to achieve greater aesthetics. Awareness of this temporary nature promotes realistic expectations and can lead to informed treatment frequency and cost considerations, hence improving patient satisfaction and safety in aesthetic dermatology clinics. Dermal fillers, however, have a different array of outcomes, which vary with their content and injection depth. The longevity of each type of dermal filler varies from six months to two years. Hyaluronic acid fillers, for instance, endure 6–12 months, while longer-acting products like polymethyl methacrylate (PMMA) endure more than a year. This difference underscores the importance of selecting the appropriate type of filler based on desired outcomes and individual factors such as skin type and lifestyle. Producers must be thoroughly familiar with these differences if they are to optimize treatment regimens. Furthermore, the long-term persistence of the effects of dermal fillers underlines the importance of ongoing practitioner education, as innovations in filler technology continue to reshape the limits of aesthetic treatment available (Madnani et al., 2022). The duration of results can also be affected by external factors, e.g., lifestyle and aftercare. Behaviors like smoking, sun exposure, and an unhealthy diet can promote the deterioration of both botulinum toxin effects and dermal fillers, resulting in reduced periods of satisfaction. Also, following the of recommended post-treatment care can play an important role in prolonging the effects. Patient education on these factors is crucial in dermatology practice to maximize procedure outcomes. A reflection on the relationship of lifestyle problems with cosmetic treatment and appropriate pre- and post-procedure management should be the emphasis of consultations to deliver satisfactory results and an active approach to the maintenance of cosmetic enhancement (Mohamed, 2020). Such awareness is attained to have a worldwide outlook on the efficiency of aesthetic treatment and enhances the patient education commitment in aesthetic medicine.

Test Your Knowledge

1. How does botulinum toxin produce neuromuscular blockade at the molecular level?
2. What effects does botulinum toxin have on targeted facial muscles to reduce the appearance of wrinkles?
3. What factors influence the typical duration of results following botulinum toxin injections?

9.3. Types of Dermal Fillers

Learning Outcome

1. Discuss the Hyaluronic Acid Fillers
2. Explain Collagen-based Fillers
3. Focus on Synthetic Fillers

In cosmetic dermatology, the number of dermal fillers available has increased, providing patients with several choices for resolving a variety of aesthetic problems. There are primarily four injectable filler categories: fat, collagen, hyaluronic acid, and microsphere-containing carriers, such as polymethyl methacrylate (PMMA) (Madnani et al., 2022). All of the categories are utilized for various purposes; hyaluronic acid fillers, for example, are highly sought after as they possess the ability to retain water and add bulk to the skin and therefore work best for filling fine lines and adding facial definition. Fat fillers, being derived from the patient's own body, are a natural option, but would entail invasive surgery to remove. Identification of the differences between these classes is significant for practitioners, as each filler can possess specific benefits and shortcomings, which will need to be considered before treatment. Additionally, safe application of dermal fillers necessitates extensive knowledge of both pre- and post-treatment care. Lack of proper comprehension of these factors can lead to unsatisfying results or side effects, and hence, the clinician's skill in conducting aesthetic treatments is very important (Madnani et al., 2022). For instance, there can be specific advice on avoiding anticoagulants or anti-inflammatory medications before the treatment to minimize bruising. Additionally, post-treatment care, like staying away from intense exercise and proper skincare, can positively affect recovery and filler longevity. Thus, success with dermal filler treatments not only relies on the product but on the provider's ability to manage the patient's experience before and after treatment as well. As demands for non-surgical cosmetic enhancements rise, the complexity of dermal filler products and treatments rises as well. Advances in filler technology have resulted in products with longer-lasting duration and improved safety profiles to address concerns regarding complications or dissatisfaction with the early results (Mohamed, 2020). For instance, more recent versions of hyaluronic acid fillers have cross-linking agents that produce a more stable gel so that longer-lasting effects can be expected. In addition, the advent of long-lasting fillers has been accompanied by a simultaneous focus on patient education about what outcomes to expect and what side effects may occur. It is interesting to note that the evolution of dermal fillers reflects broader trends in aesthetic dermatology, where the focus has been on creating natural-looking results and prioritizing safety and patient satisfaction in practice (Figure 9.8).

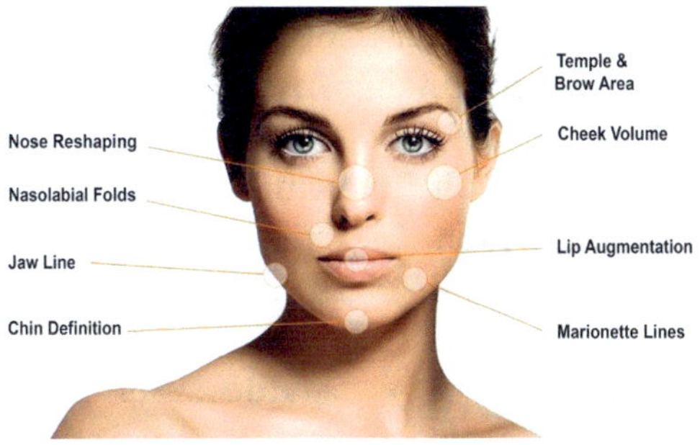

Figure 9.8. The variety of dermal fillers available has expanded significantly.

Source: https://www.aboutfacebrisbane.com.au/wp-content/uploads/2019/08/Filler-image-blog-1.jpg.

9.3.1. Hyaluronic Acid Fillers

The evolution of hyaluronic acid fillers has revolutionized the face of non-surgical facial aesthetics. Being a naturally occurring polysaccharide in connective tissue, hyaluronic acid is vital for maintaining moisture, volume, and structure of the skin. When injected, fillers like these reverse loss of volume, recontour features, and soften the appearance of fine lines and wrinkles. Unlike some of their heritage, hyaluronic acid fillers offer a more biocompatible answer with less likelihood of inducing a major side effect. Furthermore, the flexibility of having the capability to customize filler thickness and density enables personalized treatment for various areas on the face so that patients are given results that appeal to their distinctive looks. This versatility comes hand-in-hand with a bigger trend in the cosmetic industry to have more of a customized treatment regimen, eventually leading to enhanced patient satisfaction and outcomes in facial cosmetic treatments. One strong point of hyaluronic acid fillers is their temporary character, which many patients find preferable as it leaves them free to modify the look over time. As filled tissues slowly metabolize the product, the patients are given the chance to review their satisfaction with outcomes, enabling them to make educated choices about subsequent treatments. On average, hyaluronic acid fillers endure between six months and two years, depending on many factors, including the specific product being injected and the individual's metabolism. This is compatible with contemporary aesthetic practice, where only rapid changes are observed and many modalities, including botulinum toxin, are being used in combination to represent a multifaceted approach to rejuvenating the face. The synergy of these two modalities underscores a dynamic evolution in facial rejuvenation paradigms toward an emphasis on the instant and cumulative aesthetic outcomes, as clinicians begin to adopt increasingly more integrated treatment strategies that encourage long-term patient satisfaction and improved quality of life. As the clinical application of hyaluronic acid fillers has grown exponentially, their integration into the greater paradigm of facial plastic surgery portends a fundamental shift in the cosmetic treatment paradigm. Aesthetic doctors are realizing more and more that they must use a combination of different techniques, such as the utilization of botulinum toxin in combination with fillers, to produce the best results. Not only does this treat dynamic and static rhytides, but it also improves global facial harmony and equilibrium. The ongoing innovation within the field, such as advancements in filler formulations, injection techniques, and the development of combination therapies, continues to push the boundaries of what is achievable in non-invasive facial aesthetics. There are numerous studies that report above 80% satisfaction levels in clients given treatments with hyaluronic acid fillers and adjunctive treatment, indicating a trend towards integrative and more holistic practice in facial aesthetic advice, eventually making the aesthetic options open to patients and clinicians broader (Chuang et al., 2016; Bouzouaya et al., 2018) (Figure 9.9).

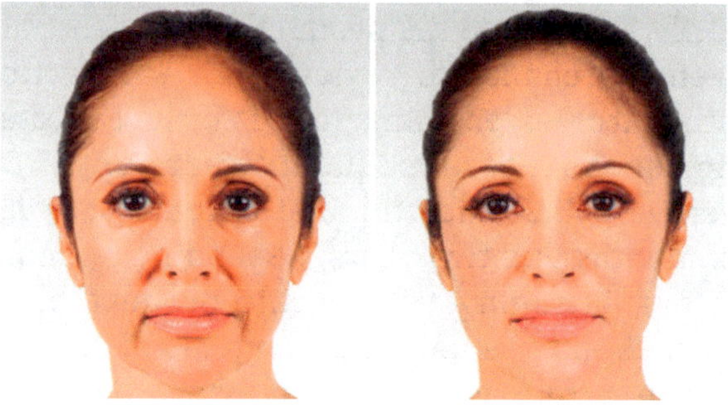

Figure 9.9. The emergence of hyaluronic acid fillers.

Source: https://www.missionplasticsurgery.com/wp-content/uploads/2016/04/Before-and-After-Facial-Fillers.png.

9.3.2. Collagen-based Fillers

Collagen fills have emerged in recent times as a recognized alternative for individuals seeking facial rejuvenation. Collagen fillers are produced from collagen, which is an existing protein found naturally in the skin that provides strength and elasticity to the skin. Collagen depletes as one grows older, resulting in folds and sagging of the skin. Collagen fillers undo these alterations by adding volume, smoothing fine lines, and smoothing overall facial contours. The rejuvenating effect can produce a more youthful look, complementing increased patient self-esteem. Finally, as technology continues to improve, practitioners are increasingly able to optimize filler placement to achieve optimal natural-appearing results with fewer complications, further enhancing the efficacy of such treatment in cosmetic practice. The climbing demand for these treatments reflects their immediacy in the current era of aesthetic dermatology, especially one in which physical looks are increasingly important (Madnani et al., 2022). Secondly, the use of collagen fillers indicates a greater cultural movement toward non-surgical cosmetic procedures characterized by ease and minimal downtime. Patients are drawn to such options because they bring significant aesthetic transformation without operating risk and convalescence. Social media, as a matter of fact, has had a significant influence in transforming public attitudes towards beauty and self-image, in that there is more tolerance for cosmetic enhancements. With individuals wanting to be as good as they can be online, demand for such treatments as fillers of collagen has risen, altering the landscape of cosmetic operations. This trend is assisted by technological advancements in the medical field, which not only provide safer modes of application but also more satisfaction overall for the patient in terms of better outcomes. Thus, collaborations among physicians, beauty influencers, and technology entrepreneurs are reshaping facial beauty, and collagen fillers are at the center of this new narrative (Fedorchenko, 2024). Although popular, physicians and patients need to recognize the potential risks associated with collagen-based fillers. While the treatments are, in most instances, safe, complications can arise, including allergic reactions, infection, or inadequate aesthetic outcomes. The significance of proper training and understanding of pre- and post-procedure care cannot be overestimated since these factors are responsible for the success of collagen filler procedures. Doctors possessing extensive information are capable of dealing with such intricacies to make sure proper precautions are exercised to avoid complications and react suitably to any issues of patients. Also, with the increased use of newer techniques and higher technologies in the field, there will have to be a focus on patient education and realistic expectations. Balancing the champagne-sippers' optimism of cosmetic innovation with a down-to-earth awareness of underlying hazards will be necessary to hone not only the safety but also the efficacy of collagen-based fillers in the new practice of aesthetic dermatology and realizing their full potential for transformation (Madnani et al., 2022) (Figure 9.10).

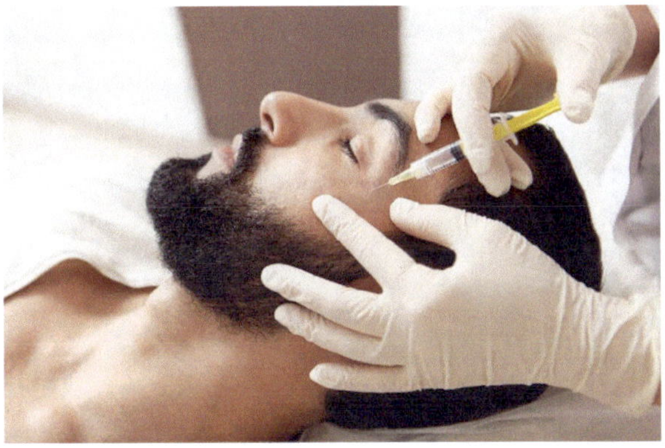

Figure 9.10. Collagen-based fillers.

Source: https://anuaesthetics.com/wp-content/uploads/2021/11/a-e1661575778477.webp.

9.3.3. Synthetic Fillers

Synthetic fillers have become the cornerstone of facial aesthetic practices, and they play a vital role in cosmetic treatments as innovative solutions for rejuvenating the skin. These fillers are produced from different synthetic sources and gain their value through distinct merits such as consistency, predictability, and lower potential for allergic reactions. Unlike traditional fillers, which lean towards utilizing biological material like collagen or fat, synthetic fillers make use of materials like polymethyl methacrylate (PMMA) and poly-L-lactic acid (PLLA). These molecules are capable of duplicating the structural attributes of living tissue, developing facial volume and definition and the look of youthfulness. The rising need for synthetic fillers in aesthetic procedures emphasizes a significant change in the understanding and provision of dermatological procedures, reflecting the advancement of medical technology and the preference of patients for non-invasive care (Mohamed, 2020). A look at the application of synthetic fillers in the big picture of aesthetic medicine reveals their significance in addressing the signs of aging and achieving facial balance. As more individuals seek non-surgical interventions, synthetic fillers have come into favor to provide volume and structure to the area of concern, such as the cheeks and lips. Practitioners can tailor treatments based on the anatomical and aesthetic needs of individual cases with their versatility, which increases satisfaction and outcomes.

Additionally, advancements in technology in terms of formulations have meant longer-lasting outcomes and more natural results, further popularizing the overall aesthetic application of synthetic fillers. By looking at trends and outcomes regarding such products, it is seen that synthetic fillers have had a profound impact on the realm of facial cosmetics and are often utilized instead of other more traditional methods, with a clear indication of an attitude shift between patient and practitioner preferences (Bowler, 2009). Furthermore, the ubiquity of synthetic fillers is reflective of broader cultural beauty and self-presentation trends, indicating how aesthetics coexist with psychological well-being. With the increasing need for non-invasive cosmetic procedures, synthetic filler treatments have become more widespread, transforming the face of aesthetic medicine. The widening acceptance and popularization of these treatments illustrate a deep cultural change toward bringing aesthetic consideration into focus, with increased regard for personal grooming and personal health. These trends necessitate a well-developed comprehension of the consequences associated with synthetic fillers, including potential complications and ethical considerations related to their use. Finally, the prevalence of synthetic fillers within the cosmetic industry is a testament to an ever-present debate of beauty ideals and the importance placed on boosting individual self-esteem through aesthetic yet medicine-based approaches (Mohamed, 2020) (Figure 9.11).

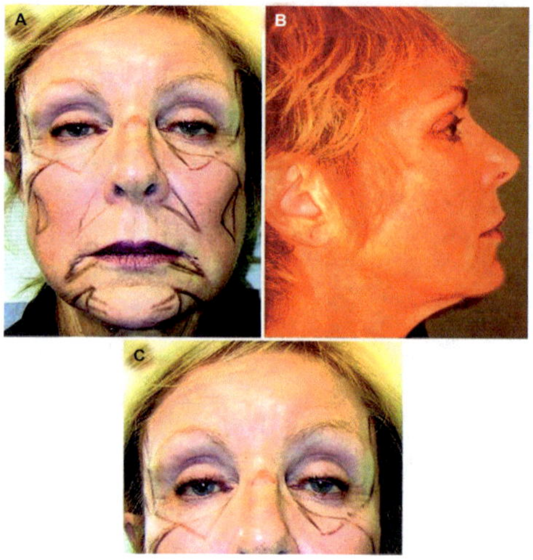

Figure 9.11. The synthetic fillers have emerged as essential components in cosmetic procedures.

Source: https://media.springernature.com/lw685/springer-static/image/chp%3A10.1007%2F978-1-4614-1007-2_12/MediaObjects/188911_1_En_12_Fig1_HTML.jpg.

Test Your Knowledge

1. What properties make hyaluronic acid fillers popular, and how do they function to restore facial volume?
2. How do collagen-based fillers differ in composition and longevity compared to HA fillers?
3. What are synthetic dermal fillers, and in what situations might they be preferred over natural or biodegradable filler options?

9.4. Comparison of Botulinum Toxin and Dermal Fillers

Learning Outcome

1. Discuss the Treatment Areas
2. Explain Results and Longevity
3. Focus on Side Effects and Risks

Botulinum toxin vs. dermal fillers is par for the course in understanding the functions of each in facial cosmetics. Botulinum toxin, arguably better known as a temporo-paralytic muscle agent, actually removes the visible signs of dynamic wrinkles, such as crow's feet and forehead furrows. This process is accomplished by preventing the release of acetylcholine, which eases muscle contractions and forms a smoother skin complexion. Dermal fillers, in contrast, are primarily used to replace lost volume and plumpness on the face as a result of aging, such as on the cheeks and lips. Composed usually of material such as hyaluronic acid, the fillers bring immediate volume and can mold the facial structure contours, giving a youthful appearance. Both treatments have specific indications, and an in-depth understanding of their differences is important for customizing cosmetic therapies according to patient requirements. Although both procedures effectively treat areas of aging, their effects vary in longevity and use. Applications of botulinum toxin generally last three to six months, with frequent follow-up needed to maintain the desired effects. Its application tends to be more directed toward expression lines than toward volumetric losses. On the other hand, dermal fillers provide outcomes of six months to two years, depending on the product and area treated. Fillers also lead to foreign body reaction since the body metabolizes the substance that is injected, which necessitates careful consideration in clinics. Research suggests that although it is rare to have such reactions, clinicians should be particularly vigilant to catch any indication of complications, as in the case of Restylane® injections (Edwards et al., 2006). Therefore, information regarding the maintenance and duration of each process is a significant aspect of planning comprehensive facial cosmetic therapy. The choice between botulinum toxin and dermal fillers is largely a matter of patient preference and desired outcome. Younger patients, in particular, may opt for preventive treatments, such as botulinum toxin, to prevent wrinkles from appearing and preserve their self-esteem in the long term (Cox et al., 2016). Preventive treatment can be most preferable since it is likely to require smaller doses over time as the aging process progresses. Older patients may, however, prefer volumizing, especially where they are experiencing deep lines or facial fat loss. Thus, clinicians must conduct extensive consultation to evaluate the best treatment combination with respect to patient goals and anatomical setting. A compound of the two treatments in a single patient's regimen can also yield synergistic results, attaining a harmonious as well as youthful appearance when properly planned.

9.4.1. Treatment Areas

The application of botulinum toxin and dermal fillers has transformed the practice of facial aesthetics, and a wide range of treatment locations have become very trendy. Forehead, glabellar lines, and crow's feet are among the most focused locations that receive injections of botulinum toxin to relax muscle contractions leading to noticeable wrinkles. Concurrently, areas such as the cheeks, lips, and nasolabial folds are being treated routinely with dermal fillers, which bring volume restoration and youthful contours. Every area presents unique anatomical issues and mandates, necessitating a deep understanding of the facial anatomy in order to get the best outcomes and minimize complications, thus the necessity of skilled practitioners in the aesthetics domain (Madnani et al., 2022). In addition, as popularity grows among the public for cosmetic procedures, knowing about these trendy treatment zones is important to practitioners and potential patients alike. Contributing to their popularity are the minimally invasive nature of the procedure and relatively swift recovery times, which appeal to a wide audience. For instance, patients seeking non-surgical interventions approach the skin's appearance in the long term; thus, procedures like dermal fillers provide immediate results that reverse aging around the face without limiting natural expressions. The strategy of targeting isolated treatment regions necessitates thorough patient assessment, as lifestyle will affect outcomes, thereby guiding personalized treatment strategies (Mohamed, 2020). Therefore, practitioners need to keep up with developments in techniques and also filler materials so that they can adjust methods according to patients' aesthetic intentions as well as protect against inherent risks. Familiarity with treatment sites encompassed by botulinum toxin and dermal fillers is also complicated by changing trends in the field of cosmetology. New technology and products allow for more precise application and more variety in treatment, with products specifically designed to address specific problems such as laxity and volume loss. As more and more procedures on delicate regions, including the periorbital area, are being done, safety measures and post-procedure care must receive the utmost attention so as to achieve maximum patient satisfaction (Madnani et al., 2022). With the expansion of the field of aesthetic dermatology, extensive training and ongoing education will be absolutely critical for providers in order to successfully manage the expanding number of treatment areas, retaining efficacy along with safety in facial cosmetic treatments (Figure 9.12).

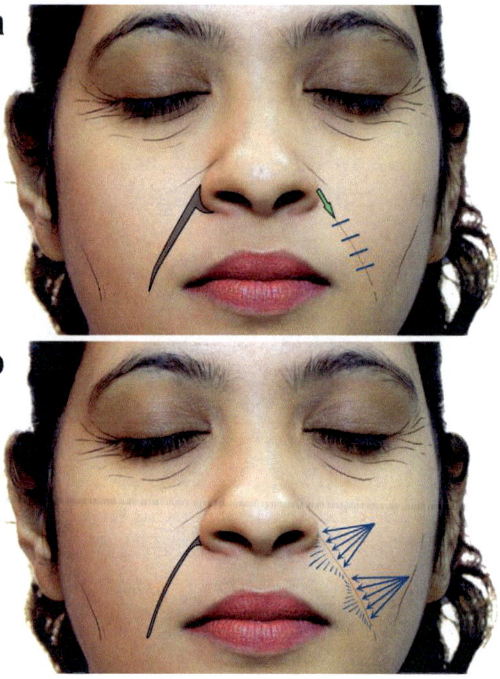

Figure 9.12. Treatment areas.

Source: https://media.springernature.com/lw685/springer-static/image/chp%3A10.1007%2F978-981-15-1346-6_33/MediaObjects/462947_1_En_33_Fig14_HTML.png.

9.4.2. Results and Longevity

The results of botulinum toxin and dermal fillers in facial cosmetics are divided largely between the results to be obtained and the duration. Botulinum toxin is especially valued for its targeted ability to reduce muscular hyperactivity, literally ironing out dynamic wrinkles. The results are temporary, however, lasting anywhere from 12–16 weeks before further treatments must be performed in order to obtain the desired appearance. This involves a commitment to more regular injections for people who seek long-lasting outcomes, a factor that can influence their satisfaction with the treatment procedure overall. Furthermore, the time-dependent quality of botulinum toxin treatments calls for considerations regarding patient compliance and psychological factors, bearing in mind that people will have changes in their appearance within periods between treatments, and therefore will have an influence on self-esteem and perception of aging. On the other hand, dermal fillers offer a longer-term solution to volumetric enhancement with results ranging from a few months to years based on the product used. Not only do these procedures restore lost volume, but they also define facial contours with instant gratification that is considerably more patient-friendly. The longevity of dermal fillers depends on the composition, method of injection, and metabolic factors of the patient. Therefore, even though patients prefer the immediate action and duration of dermal fillers, the interactive dynamics between the fillers and the botulinum toxin is an area that needs improvement for aesthetic practitioners. A synergistic approach, using both modalities, can optimize results by addressing multiple aspects of facial aging and maintaining a more evenly balanced appearance over time. New additions, most significantly the addition of technologies such as ultrasound (US), further improve the effects and safety profiles of botulinum toxin and dermal fillers as well. US allows clinicians to safely navigate facial anatomy while treating, with precise placement and a lower risk of complications. This accuracy not only enhances the quality and lifespan of outcomes but also guarantees higher patient satisfaction by minimizing adverse effect events. The integration of US technology with fillers and botulinum toxin is laying the foundation for a more personalized and powerful treatment regimen, highlighting the importance of safety and competence in aesthetic dermatology. As these developments continue, they promise to refine the aesthetic outcome and longevity associated with these highly desired cosmetic treatments, hence enhancing standard procedures in the practice (Benzaquen et al., 2022).

9.4.3. Side Effects and Risks

The increasing popularity of botulinum toxin and dermal fillers in cosmetic facials has been followed by an increased examination of their associated side effects and risks. While these procedures are heavily marketed as being safe and fairly non-surgical, they are not without potential issues. Patients can have localized bruising, swelling, or tenderness where injections are given, which, while generally short-lived, can be severely discomforting and impact overall satisfaction with the procedure. It is important for both practitioners and patients to have knowledge of these risks, highlighting the importance of proper consultations where possible side effects are properly explained. As mentioned in existing literature, not all practitioners possess adequate awareness of the intricacies of such treatments, inferring the necessity for enhanced education and familiarity with the pre- and post-procedure care required to minimize complications (Madnani et al., 2022). Except for common minor side effects, complications can result from botulinum toxin and dermal fillers. Infection, vascular occlusion, and even permanent damage to the tissue have occurred, making it imperative to choose experienced practitioners familiar with such procedures. Notably, dermal fillers can cause the formation of granulomas, which are inflammatory cells that aggregate to form tender, red cutaneous lesions. Furthermore, lack of coordination in the injection of the filler may place the filler in undesired areas, thereby leading to asymmetry or deformed facial structures. These risks necessitate a cautious deliberation of the products and methods employed, that the best standards of safety and effectiveness are utilized by practitioners (Mohamed, 2020). As patients balance cosmetic enhancement through the application of botulinum toxin and dermal fillers, a well-educated understanding of the potential side effects and risks is crucial. The psychological impact of such procedures also plays a critical role, as patients may have enhanced expectations and consequent disappointment with complications. Counseling and education regarding possible outcomes can minimize anxiety and encourage a more realistic appreciation of the postoperative process. Lastly, to ensure that patients are well informed and supported optimizes their satisfaction and also satisfies the broader professional commitment of practitioners to prioritize safety and ethical practice in aesthetic medicine. These measures can help build a more informed patient population, a key consideration in an industry characterized by rapid advances and novel techniques (Mohamed, 2020).

Test Your Knowledge

1. How do the typical treatment areas differ between botulinum toxin injections and dermal fillers?
2. In what ways do the results and longevity of botulinum toxin compare with those of dermal fillers?
3. What are the key side effects and risks associated with each treatment, and how do they differ?

9.5. Safety and Regulatory Aspects

Learning Outcome

1. Discuss the Food and Drug Administration (FDA) Approval Process
2. Explain Common Adverse Effects
3. Focus on Importance of Qualified Practitioners

The increasing popularity of botulinum toxin. and dermal fillers for facial aesthetic treatment. has brought with it severe safety and regulatory concerns in the aesthetics market. With these. treatments being made more widely available, typically through non-specialized practitioners, the possibility of side effects and malpractice has increased. A cross-sectional survey of practitioners in London reported that a whopping 88% of the clinics were not adhering to the Advertising Standards Authority (ASA) ad rule for advertising prescription-only medication, such as botulinum toxin (Davies et al., 2023). This absence of regulation not only erodes patient security but also suggests a disconcerting disregard for long-established medical procedures, highlighting the need for rigorous regulatory measures that actually protect consumers wanting to purchase cosmetic enhancements. In response to the global boom in aesthetic treatments, the regulatory framework is adjusting to address the issues of practitioner qualifications and procedure standardization. The popularity of noninvasive care has attracted a diverse group of health care professionals who are not all properly trained or experienced (Bowler, 2009). The lack of regulation can cause uneven practices and harm to patients, so it is extremely important to have stringent licensing requirements and education standards in the field. The application of more stringent controls is able to manage risks that involve abuse of products and practitioner incompetence, which will eventually make the environment more secure for patients. With the market continuing to expand, good regulatory systems will be critical in ensuring that safety remains an essential top priority for all. Furthermore, familiarity with the geographical variations of cost and availability of botulinum toxin and dermal fillers could assist in shedding light on broader concerns of safety and regulation. The differences in prices quoted for different areas, with an average cost of treatment at £284.45 per mL of botulinum toxin, reflect not only economic factors but also the potential effect of competition on treatment quality level (Davies et al., 2023). Differences in clinic densities can result in over-saturation by poorly regulated distributors, which ultimately creates a higher risk to consumers. Creating awareness in these fields can drive legislative action towards a more balanced and controlled platform geographically, optimizing availability as well as safety in cosmetic treatments. Through regulatory compliance focus as well as bridging regional gaps, stakeholders can work towards an improved, healthier and safer environment for patients taking cosmetic treatments (Figure 9.13).

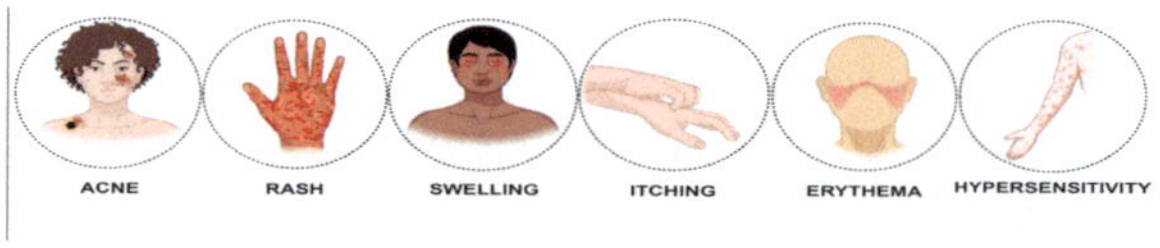

Figure 9.13. Safety and regulatory aspects in cosmetics.

Source: https://www.mdpi.com/cosmetics/cosmetics-11-00184/article_deploy/html/images/cosmetics-11-00184-g005.png.

9.5.1. Food and Drug Administration (FDA) Approval Process

FDA approval of medical products, including botulinum toxin and dermal fillers, is a very sophisticated and rigorous process that ensures the safety and efficacy of the products before they reach the consumer market. Manufacturers initially need to conduct extensive preclinical evaluation to investigate the pharmacodynamics and pharmacokinetics of their products. Once finished with successful preclinical trials, companies submit an Investigational New Drug (IND) application, which outlines their research protocols and seeks permission to begin human tests. This is a very significant step in an effort to find out if any side effects will result and to establish standards for dosages, particularly useful in the application of botulinum toxin to cosmetics. The FDA's review of the IND submission is the first major landmark in the long approval process, followed by significant criticisms that may require months and that may require alterations or additional information from the applicant. The second thing to do following positive clinical trial results is the submission of a New Drug Application (NDA) or Biologics License Application (BLA), which includes all clinical study results. Both include full data on efficacy, safety, manufacturing controls, and labeling. It is also examined by a specialist team of experts, including pharmacologists, biostatisticians, and medical officers, who inspect each part of the application to find compliance with federal regulations. For products like botulinum toxin, formulation details are of paramount significance as minor variations could mean very diverse therapeutic outcomes. So, the history of any licensed product is founded on the thorough documentation and studies submitted at this point, reflecting commitment to public safety and informed medical practice. After FDA review and approval are complete, ongoing surveillance still maintains surveillance over the safety and efficacy of botulinum toxin and dermal fillers postmarketing. This Phase IV clinical trial post-approval typically reveals additional data regarding longer-term consequences and limits of use parameters. For example, while botulinum toxin reflects remarkable success in treating cosmetic concerns like wrinkles, therapeutic potential within other areas, for example, gynecology, remains under investigation. Studies discover patients can benefit from additional research to optimize injection techniques and dosages across environments (Etrusco et al., 2023). Thus, the FDA also plays a crucial role in not just the initial approval but in establishing an atmosphere of constant critique and refinement within the medical cosmetic field to ensure patient safety remains at the top of medical development (Etrusco et al., 2023).

9.5.2. Common Adverse Effects

On the cosmetic side of facial surgery, the use of botulinum toxin and dermal fillers, while universally commended for their aesthetic benefits, is not without an array of possible adverse effects. Awareness of these common complications is imperative to practitioners and patients alike interested in investigating the nuances of such interventions. Proximal responses in the form of condensation or bruising over the area of injection are not unusual; these normally recover over a few days but at times can be uncomfortable. Further caution must then be exercised in observing, even though uncommon, more severe reactions such as allergic response and vascular occlusion leading to skin necrosis. With knowledge of these issues, clinicians can better inform their patients about what to expect and establish proper post-procedure care protocols that allow for minimizing risks in relation to these very common treatments (Madnani et al., 2022). With long-term side effects, patients must also consider the long-term implications of botulinum toxin and dermal fillers. For example, repeated use of botulinum toxin over an extended period causes resistance to the treatment, something that can cause disappointment for the providers and patients alike. Moreover, slow deterioration of dermal fillers results in an unnatural appearance, particularly when touch-up injections are not administered regularly. Though patients do not undergo any subcutaneous scarring during the process of repeated treatment cycles, they are at risk of atrophy of the skin or lumps. These are long-term side effects caused by incorrect technique or product placement, and this reinforces the importance of thorough consultations and careful consideration of both the patients' aesthetic goals and their ability to tolerate potential adverse outcomes (Mohamed, 2020). Furthermore, the psychological consequences can even be created by the injection of botulinum toxin and dermal fillers, creating a multilayered debate over common side effects. Some of the patients may get body dysmorphic problems where the quest for a flawless appearance leads to an endless cycle of procedures and dissatisfaction, no matter what is achieved. This impact is likely to increase the level of anxiety and lower the self-esteem, and as such, there should be sufficient mental health assessment before such procedures. Knowledge about such psychological impacts is also necessary for practitioners, as they are able to enable patients to explore realistic expectations against unattainable ideals. By creating a comprehensive understanding of cosmetic improvement, where physical and psychological impacts interact, healthcare providers are in a position to improve patient satisfaction and quality of life (Madnani et al., 2022).

9.5.3. Importance of Qualified Practitioners

The increasing popularity of botulinum toxin and dermal fillers in facial cosmetics has placed emphasis on the role of trained practitioners in these practices. With greater demand for non-surgical cosmetic procedures, it is crucial that those who administer these procedures have extensive training and education. Trained practitioners not only learn proper usage of these products but also gain valuable skills to assess individual patient needs. This comprehensive training will ultimately create a greater appreciation for the potential complications, allowing better informed consent discussions with patients. A lack of standardized training can lead to negative consequences, thereby emphasizing the need for regulated training programs. Authors complement formal postgraduate curricula based on critical thinking as well as the practice of evidence-based practices in developing procedural skills in implementation through the establishment of a curriculum to educate clinicians for non-surgical aesthetics (Kumar, 2021). In addition, trust between patient and practitioner is essential for cosmetic procedure success. Since botulinum toxin and dermal fillers are linked with aesthetic payback along with inherent risks, the patient must believe that his or her practitioner possesses the capability and professionalism to guide him or her through. Competent practitioner roles extend into ethical practice and patient education, where disclosure about potential risk and realistic expectations is paramount. For instance, as in the case of cosmetic dentistry, these professional-public expectation disjunctures could lead to disillusion and disappointment (Lala et al., 2020). Practitioners openly talking about procedures and results are essentially bridging this gap themselves. In creating an open conversation, skilled practitioners not only facilitate informed decision-making for patients but also enhance their overall experience, which is crucial in this competitive environment. Furthermore, the role of competent practitioners is also important in matters of compliance with regulations as well as safety standards within aesthetics. As the cosmetic procedures market continues to expand, so does the requirement for enforcing regulations that guarantee safety among patients and quality of care. Untrained personnel can cause serious risks, including giving the wrong doses or utilizing inferior products. Graduates from accredited programs are less likely to disregard safety procedures and recognize unforeseen complications. They are also less likely to seek continuous professional growth, which supports their skills in the face of evolving techniques and products. This commitment to excellence ultimately serves the profession at large, making it possible to have higher industry standards and safer interactions with clients. As the market continues to mature, the role of qualifications and formal training increases in importance to maintaining the integrity and trustworthiness of aesthetic practices (Kumar, 2021) (Figure 9.14).

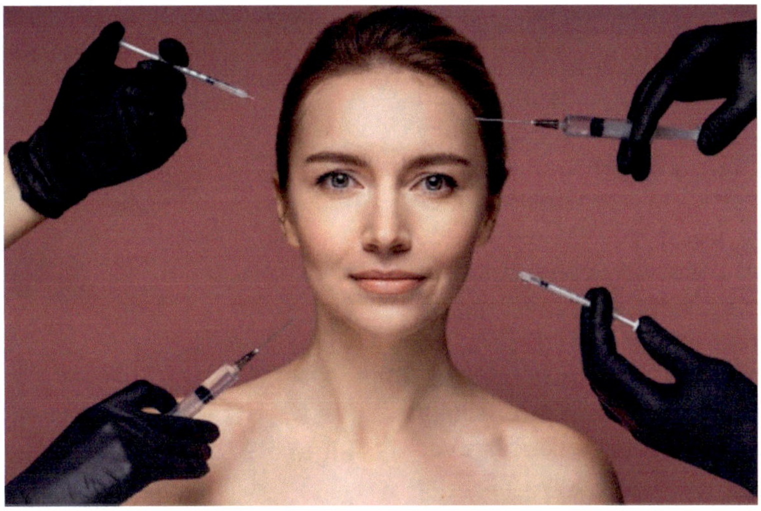

Figure 9.14. Importance of qualified practitioners.

Source: https://www.inurskn.in/wp-content/uploads/2025/02/Botulinum-toxin.jpg.

Test Your Knowledge

1. What key steps are involved in the FDA approval process for botulinum toxin and dermal fillers used in aesthetic procedures?
2. What common adverse effects may occur after injectable aesthetic treatments, and how are they typically managed?
3. Why is it crucial to seek treatment from qualified and trained practitioners when undergoing injectable cosmetic procedures?

9.6. Trends in Facial Cosmetic Procedures

Learning Outcome

1. Discuss Increasing Popularity among Different Age Groups
2. Focus on Cultural Influences on Cosmetic Choices
3. Explain the Innovations in Techniques and Products

The growing popularity of facial cosmetic procedures is evidence of a broader cultural trend towards self-enhancement and wellness. In the last few years, growing social acceptance of cosmetic alteration has driven many patients toward non-surgical means like botulinum toxin and dermal fillers. Both offer patients an opportunity to get back youthful appearances without suffering from long recovery times traditionally associated with surgery. Therefore, demand for the same has gone up exponentially, particularly among youthful populations that are interested in treating indicators of premature aging. This is indicative of a change in attitude to beauty and aging, where the pursuit of perfection still prevails. With such consumer trends being met by practitioners, enhanced techniques and safety are frequently argued, and this will continue to ensure improvement of procedures in facial aesthetics. With increased demand comes the integration of new technology in facial cosmetic treatments, enhancing the effectiveness and safety of treatments. For instance, there has been recent evidence showing that vibration anesthesia can be used to increase pain tolerance in patients undergoing cosmetic facial injections. Evidence that vibration anesthesia significantly alters pain scores, optimizing patients' experience and potentially affecting injectable treatment preferences over surgical treatment, is particularly key in a time when patient comfort and satisfaction are of the utmost priority. Also, improvements in injectable methods and formulas, such as the establishment of dermal fillers that can last longer, have further entrenched the place of non-surgical treatments in the cosmetic industry. These advancements in particular are key to making facial cosmetic treatments continually available, safe, and attractive to an extensive clientele. With the evolving area of facial cosmetic surgery, business professionals are keen on staying aware of current techniques and trends. With its multidisciplinary focus, facial plastic surgery utilizes insights from all types of specialties, including otolaryngology, dermatology, and plastic surgery, further enhancing the realm of cosmetic treatments. Above all, the dominance of social media has also played a role in shaping the appearance of beauty and the beauty of aesthetic treatments. Celebrities and social media influencers are now widely popular, with many openly embracing and affirming their aesthetic inclinations. In such a culture where this environment encourages greater acceptance of cosmetic treatments, clinicians can expect ongoing expansion in the market for botulinum toxin and dermal fillers in facial cosmetics. With ongoing advancements and the overlap of different medical specializations, facial aesthetics' future appears bright and dynamic, eventually resulting in more subtle, customized treatments (Figure 9.15).

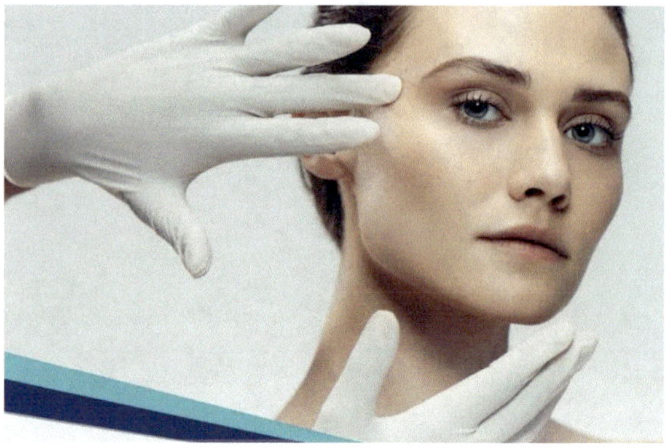

Figure 9.15.

Source: https://lerraclinic.com/wp-content/uploads/2025/01/latest-trends-in-facial-plastic-surgery-2025.jpg.webp.

9.6.1. Increasing Popularity Among Different Age Groups

Increasing popularity of botulinum toxin and fillers with everyone aged shows an amazing transformation in society's attitude towards cosmetic procedures. The youth, particularly in late 20s to early 30s, are increasingly opting for such procedures to stop the process of facial aging and to provide their facial structure with an enhancement before ageing can be seen. With cosmetic treatments more accessible and socially acceptable, individuals within this age group are utilizing these treatments not just for appearance but as a normal component of caring for oneself (Boulle et al., 2010). Increased use of social media and celebrity influences has assisted in fueling this trend, as individuals tend to compare themselves to celebrities who are highly recognized for their youthful looks. In addition, the middle-aged population, typically individuals in their 50s and 40s, demonstrates heightened demand for non-surgical cosmetic treatments. The majority of them seek botulinum toxin as well as dermal fillers for overt signs of aging, such as wrinkles, fine lines, and loss of volume in specific facial regions. These treatments provide such patients with an opportunity to appear younger without undergoing invasive surgical interventions. Educational programs, such as cadaver anatomy courses for aesthetic physicians, recently indicated that there were enhancements in doctors' knowledge, which enhanced their confidence to perform such non-surgical treatments effectively (Boulle et al., 2010). As more people are learning about the safety and efficacy of such treatments, middle-aged individuals are increasingly opting for aesthetic enhancements, which also addresses the trend for cosmetic treatments. And lastly, older adults, particularly those over 60, have embraced cosmetic enhancement as well, consistent with broader acceptance in the marketplace. This demographic views botulinum toxin and fillers for the skin not only as vain weapons but also as means of boosting self-esteem and overall living standards. Many older people seek such interventions in order to become essential once more and become more engaged in society, indicating the importance of appearance on one's health. As more emphasis is being placed on training practitioners in the anatomy and correct administration of such interventions, the age group participating in cosmetic interventions will likely grow, potentially leading to more emphasis on individualized care to address diverse age-related needs (Kumar & Rahman, 2017). The relationship between expanded practitioner training and evolving mindsets regarding cosmetic enhancements across various age groups will continue to shape the area of facial aesthetics.

9.6.2. Cultural Influences on Cosmetic Choices

The evolution of cosmetic treatments is strongly intertwined with a variety of cultural influences, shaping perceptions of beauty and self-representation in society. The standards of beauty have evolved drastically over time in most cultures, depending on the historical conditions as well as the prevailing trends. For instance, in Western societies, the pursuit of youthfulness will govern the demand for cosmetic procedures, including botulinum toxin and fillers, to give way to smoother skin and more-defined facial features. Media portrayal and celebrity culture also influence these demands, making cosmetic enhancement mainstream or even glamorous. This trend is evident through the global popularity of certain standards of beauty that transcend geographical location and influence consumer attitudes and decisions toward cosmetic procedures. Since cultural influences continue to be dynamic and evolving, they have the influential function of dictating what cosmetic procedures are desirable and socially acceptable, or not. Beyond Western standards, cultural environments may interpret their own standards of beauty, providing cosmetic preference attributes that differ. In certain Asian cultures, for example, there is a particular emphasis on the possession of fair skin, large eyes, and a small face, and this has determined which kinds of cosmetic procedures have been sought. Such cultural influences can result in increased use of botulinum toxin and dermal fillers to shape the face, create the appearance of a youthful face, and achieve a desired brow shape. Also, global interconnectedness through social media has enabled the easy sharing of beauty standards at pace, making it possible for people to adopt those employed in other cultures. Cosmetic enhancement is more a reflection of the overall cultural values and societal norms that dictate nearly every step of life, rather than an individual preference. Also, heightened sensitivity towards diversity in beauty perceptions has led to broadened acceptance of diverse cosmetic procedures by multicultural communities. The Orna Face Analysis (OFA) is one such new way of thinking in facial aesthetics research that incorporates ethnic and cultural considerations into aesthetic treatment design.

This tool introduces practitioners' ability to comprehend various notions of beauty as they adapt treatments to meet the unique preferences of patients from various backgrounds, thereby providing inclusivity in cosmetic treatments. All these advancements render culturally aware training and education, particularly in non-surgical aesthetics, even more essential, where the practitioners have to fine-tune themselves with the expectations and aspirations of their diversified patient population. By embracing cultural influences in cosmetics, practitioners can become more individualized and holistic in their approach to facial beauty, ultimately forming patient relationships based on knowledge and respect for individual standards of beauty (Kumar, 2021; Germani et al., 2024) (Figure 9.16).

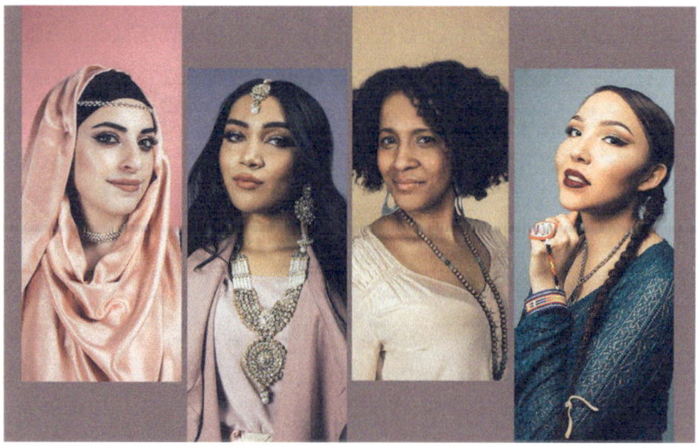

Figure 9.16. Cultural influences on cosmetic choices.

Source: https://www.avenuecalgary.com/wp-content/uploads/2017/05/Cultural_BeautyCOVER.jpg.

9.6.3. Innovations in Techniques and Products

The world of facial cosmetic surgery has been dramatically influenced by recent developments in product and technique, perhaps most significantly in the areas of botulinum toxin and dermal fillers. Non-surgical aesthetics (NSA) are so popular now because they are minimally invasive with quick recovery and are therefore more accessible to the masses. A structured course of postgraduate training is necessary for practitioners carrying out these treatments, thereby providing them with adequate training in up-to-date developments. Development of evidence-based education models, as evolved through systematic reviews of literature and Delphi studies, ensures that the practitioners possess the skills necessary to apply such innovations safely and efficaciously. Such education programs not only support practical implementation but also foster a culture of ongoing learning among healthcare professionals, thus generating upgraded standards of care in the constantly evolving non-surgical aesthetic practice (Kumar, 2021). Innovations have also been key in the creation and application of dermal fillers. More recent studies have highlighted the efficacy and safety of newer products like SilverNovaTM skin cream, which utilizes colloidal nano-silver technology alongside other rejuvenating agents like hyaluronic acid. Not only do these work together to ensure quick recovery, but they also minimize downtime following cosmetic treatments. Clinical trials also offer compelling evidence of symptom improvement with post-treatment erythema and edema, which enhance patient comfort and satisfaction. Furthermore, the ability of such formulations to improve skin texture and tone offers an added incentive for patients seeking the best results from aesthetic treatments. With the changing cosmetics industry, the inclusion of new products like SilverNovaTM underscores the importance of safety and effectiveness in post-procedure care products (Jadhav et al., 2023). Technological developments also encompass techniques employed during non-surgical aesthetic treatments. The use of objective structured clinical examinations (OSCEs) and other types of evaluation in training programs has been highly effective in assessing practitioner competence. This emphasis on evidence-based practice strategies builds critical thinking and problem-solving skills in practitioners, thereby enhancing patient outcomes. Such innovations in the education system and methodology not only build professionals for the demands of today's aesthetic practices but also respond to increasing patient demands for safety and quality. Lastly, innovations on both the financial and product sides operate synergistically to develop a future-oriented culture of facial cosmetics that makes aesthetic treatments more effective and safer than before (Kumar, 2021).

Test Your Knowledge

1. What factors explain the increasing popularity of facial cosmetic procedures among different age groups, including younger patients?
2. How do cultural influences and societal beauty standards affect individuals' choices regarding cosmetic treatments?
3. What recent innovations in techniques or products have contributed to the growth and evolution of facial cosmetic procedures?

SUMMARY

The growing popularity of botulinum toxin and dermal fillers among facial cosmetics is a part of a broader societal shift towards non-invasive aesthetic improvements. These treatments give patients an opportunity to address problems such as fine lines and volume loss with minimal hassle and short recovery time. Nevertheless, the practitioners need to be cautious of the possible risks and complications that are usually linked with these treatments. Continued training and education are imperative, as most practitioners might not possess extensive knowledge about the specifics of effectively injecting botulinum toxin and dermal fillers. As testified by several expert opinions and clinical experience, informed practitioner interaction is key to maximizing patient satisfaction and minimizing unwanted outcomes towards a safe and efficient cosmetic dermatology practice (Madnani et al., 2022). Patient education is also necessary in keeping with realistic expectations and enabling educated decision-making of cosmetic procedures. An understanding of the merits and demerits of treatments such as botulinum toxin and fillers aids the patient's decision-making process more. With an increasingly number of people accessing aesthetic treatments, it is necessary that patients receive extensive consultations from qualified practitioners who can reassure their concerns. The systematic review of safety and satisfaction in abobotulinumtoxinA-treated patients underscores that if performed correctly, interventions can yield outstanding results (Cohen & Scuderi, 2017). A collaboration between practitioners and patients can thus improve the overall experience and efficacy of esthetic treatments. Finally, the future of facial cosmetics is not only in the development of technology but also in the ethical application of aesthetic medicine. Continuous R&D will most likely yield new formulations and approaches; however, the need for practitioner knowledge and sensitivity remains supreme. With changing domains, safety, knowledge, and ethical practice always need to be prioritized by patients and also by clinicians. Continuing innovation in cosmetic dermatology will unavoidably accompany increased recognition of the relationship between various treatments so that patients can be provided with balanced, individualized therapy representative of their unique needs and cosmetic aspirations. Ultimately, commitment to education, practice, and patient engagement excellence may positively affect outcomes that go along with botulinum toxin and dermal fillers in facial cosmetics to create a safety and satisfaction culture for this emerging specialty.

The landscape of cosmetic procedures, particularly with botulinum toxin and dermal fillers, has greatly altered in recent years. The increasing demand for aesthetic procedures that are not surgical has highlighted the importance of core training and education in these specialties. The provision of structured education platforms becomes imperative to ensure that practitioners in these areas possess the requisite skills and knowledge. The said research, but one that sought to develop an evidence-based curriculum for postgraduate training in non-surgical aesthetics, establishes this reality through its emphasis on critical thinking and inquiry-based learning in the development of professionals to handle the complexity of these cosmetic procedures (Kumar, 2021). This curriculum addresses not just the technical but also includes ethical concerns, so practitioners are well equipped to address the complicated interaction between cosmetic enhancement and patient safety. In addition, the influence of societal attitudes and norms strongly affects aesthetic procedure practice and cosmetic dentistry. Institutional ethnography has revealed that higher discourses, such as professional norms and safety concerns, are an integral aspect of how cosmetic interventions are made sense of and translated (Lala, 2020). This social relations mapping of the context of the cosmetic procedure identifies power relations at play, namely that cosmetic practitioners are being positioned as gatekeepers to treatments. These dynamics highlight the imperative on dentists and aesthetic professionals to establish trust with patients as they navigate across the gap between public expectations and professional education reality. These are realities that form the basis of working out ethical benchmarks and codes of practice to secure patient autonomy and protection in this new field. Finally, it is critical to appreciate the all-encompassing implications of the convergence of aesthetic treatments into the arena of healthcare. As botulinum toxin and dermal fillers gain acceptance within medical systems, they increasingly overlap with concepts of beauty and health. This overlap is raising grave ethical issues regarding the commercialization of beauty and the role of health practitioners in this process. The distinction between medical and cosmetic standards can create a gap in public safety because patients may misconstrue the risks involved in these procedures. Through addressing such challenges through proper curriculum development and professional education, the cosmetics industry can offer its customers better service without compromise to patient welfare (Lala, 2020). Overall, this constant debate around education, cultural values, and ethical practice is necessary for the accountable advancement in non-surgical aesthetic treatments.

KEY TERMS FROM THIS CHAPTER

- Botulinum Toxin Type A
- Dynamic Wrinkles
- Injection Units
- Dermal Fillers
- Cross-Linking
- Volumization
- Cannula Technique
- Lip Augmentation
- Neurotoxin Injection
- Muscle Relaxation
- Diffusion
- Hyaluronic Acid
- Viscosity
- Soft Tissue Augmentation
- Injection Plane
- Cheek Volumization

CRITICAL THINKING QUESTIONS

1. **Botulinum toxin acts by blocking:**
   a. Serotonin release
   b. Dopamine receptors
   c. Acetylcholine release at neuromuscular junction
   d. GABA uptake
2. **The most common cosmetic use of botulinum toxin is for:**
   a. Nasal reshaping
   b. Glabellar frown lines
   c. Lip augmentation
   d. Blepharoplasty
3. **The effect of botulinum toxin typically begins in:**
   a. 1–2 hours
   b. 12–24 hours
   c. 3–5 days
   d. 14 days
4. **Duration of botulinum toxin results usually lasts:**
   a. 1–2 weeks
   b. 1 month
   c. 3–4 months
   d. 12 months
5. **The most common dermal Silicone oils**
   a. Collagen fillers
   b. Hyaluronic acid
   c. Gold thread implants
   d. fillers used today are:

Short Answer Questions

1. What is the mechanism of action of botulinum toxin at the neuromuscular junction?
2. Which facial areas are most commonly treated with botulinum toxin for wrinkle reduction?
3. What is the purpose of using hyaluronidase in dermal filler complications?
4. What factors influence the longevity of hyaluronic acid fillers?
5. What is the typical onset and duration of action of botulinum toxin type A?
6. Describe one difference between neurotoxins and dermal fillers in aesthetic practice.

Answers to Critical Thinking Questions

1. (c) 2. (b) 3. (c) 4. (c) 5. (c)

REFERENCES

1. Abdel-Sayed, P., Applegate, L. A., Hadjab, B., Hsin, et al. (2024). *Pilot clinical safety and efficacy evaluation of a topical 3% tranexamic acid cream and serum protocol for managing facial hyperpigmentation in Caucasian patients.* https://core.ac.uk/download/631534027.pdf (accessed on 14th July 2025).
2. Akuma, O. M., Azi, C. I., Carsrud, N. D. V., Chawla, et al. (2024). *BOTOX's mechanism, diversity considerations, and therapeutic potential in cosmetic, medical, and dental practice.* https://core.ac.uk/download/621451720.pdf (accessed on 14th July 2025).
3. Amuso, D., Inchingolo, F., Lorusso, F., Rapone, et al. (2021). *Hyaluronic acid fillers enriched with glycine and proline in eyebrow augmentation procedure.* https://core.ac.uk/download/541256214.pdf (accessed on 14th July 2025).
4. Chuang, J., Barnes, C., & Wong, B. J. F. (2016). Overview of Facial Plastic Surgery and Current Developments. *Surgery journal (New York, N.Y.)*, *2*(1), e17–e28. https://doi.org/10.1055/s-0036-1572360(accessed on 14th July 2025).
5. Benzaquen, M., Cartier, H., Damiani, G., Habib, et al. (2022). *The growing importance of ultrasonography in cosmetic dermatology: An update after the 23rd IMCAS Annual World Congress (2022).* https://core.ac.uk/download/543781798.pdf (accessed on 14th July 2025).
6. Bouzouaya, C., & Feiner, R. (2018). *Adjuvant botulinum toxin harmonization in minimally invasive facial aesthetic surgery.* https://core.ac.uk/download/322438270.pdf (accessed on 14th July 2025).
7. Bowler P. J. (2009). Impact on facial rejuvenation with dermatological preparations. *Clinical interventions in aging*, *4*, 81–89. https://doi.org/10.2147/cia.s3524(accessed on 14th July 2025).
8. Etrusco, A., Geru, M., Laganà, A. S., Chiantera, V., Giannini, A., & Buzzaccarini, G. (2023). Use of botulinum toxin in aesthetic medicine and gynaecology: current approaches, controversies, and future directions. *Przeglad menopauzalny = Menopause review*, *22*(3), 155–160. https://doi.org/10.5114/pm.2023.131457 (accessed on 14th July 2025).
9. Cohen, J. L., & Scuderi, N. (2017). Safety and Patient Satisfaction of AbobotulinumtoxinA for Aesthetic Use: A Systematic Review. *Aesthetic surgery journal*, *37*(suppl_1), S32–S44. https://doi.org/10.1093/asj/sjx010 (accessed on 14th July 2025).
10. Cox, K. A. (2016). *The association between age and long term cosmetic effect of treatment with botulinum toxin.* https://open.bu.edu/bitstream/2144/19172/1/Cox_bu_0017N_12285.pdf (accessed on 14th July 2025).
11. Davies, J., Mosahebi, A., Sousi, S., Weyrich, et al. (2023). *Cosmetic business mechanics in London: A cross-sectional analysis and audit of ASA compliance.* https://core.ac.uk/download/564422122.pdf (accessed on 14th July 2025).
12. De Boulle, K., Fagien, S., Glogau, R., Sommer, et al. (2010). *Treating glabellar lines with botulinum toxin type A-hemagglutinin complex: A review of the science, the clinical data, and patient satisfaction.* https://core.ac.uk/download/pdf/8403709.pdf (accessed on 14th July 2025).
13. Madnani, N., Vedmurthy, M., Parthasarthi, A., Dhawan, S., Kandhari, R., Pillai, R., & Nischal, K. C. (2022). Expert opinion on pre and post procedure care in aesthetic dermatology. *International*

Journal of Research in Medical Sciences, 10(4), 991–1000. https://doi.org/10.18203/2320-6012.ijrms20220999(accessed on 14th July 2025).

14. Dowrick, A., & Holliday, R. (2022). *Tweakments: Non-surgical beauty technologies and future directions for the sociology of the body*. https://core.ac.uk/download/644552916.pdf (accessed on 14th July 2025).

15. Edwards, P. C., Fantasia, J. E., & Iovino, R. (2006). *Foreign body reaction to hyaluronic acid (Restylane®): An adverse outcome of lip augmentation*. https://core.ac.uk/download/46958591.pdf (accessed on 14th July 2025).

16. Faria, G. E. de L., Medina, R. I. S., & Boggio, R. F. (2025). *Eyebrow lift with cosmetic procedures: How to approach it*. https://core.ac.uk/download/655869463.pdf (accessed on 14th July 2025).

17. Fedorchenko, Y. (2024). ANTI-AGING COSMETIC PROCEDURES: BENEFITS AND RISKS. *Anti-Aging Eastern Europe, 3*(3), 135-140. https://doi.org/10.56543/aaeeu.2024.3.3.04(accessed on 14th July 2025).

18. Germani, M., Granjeiro, J. M., & Lopes, A. (2024). *Orna face analysis: Development of a clinical tool for facial aesthetic evaluation*. https://core.ac.uk/download/634328288.pdf (accessed on 14th July 2025).

19. Jadhav, A., Kondadi, P., Mehta, A., Poojary, et al. (2023). *Efficacy and safety of SilverNovaTM skin cream in post-aesthetic skin procedures*. https://core.ac.uk/download/588568165.pdf (accessed on 14th July 2025).

20. Kumar, Narendra; (2021) Design, Development and Implementation Framework for a Postgraduate Non-Surgical Aesthetics Curriculum. Doctoral thesis (Ph.D), UCL (University College London).(accessed on 14th July 2025).

21. Kumar, N., & Rahman, E. (2017). *Effectiveness of teaching facial anatomy through cadaver dissection on aesthetic physicians' knowledge*. https://core.ac.uk/download/157582887.pdf (accessed on 14th July 2025).

22. Lala, R. (2020). *The Great British smile: An institutional ethnography of power in cosmetic dentistry*. https://core.ac.uk/download/363145639.pdf (accessed on 14th July 2025).

23. Mohamed, D. A. (2020). *Dermal filler types, effect on soft tissue and lifestyle correlation*. https://core.ac.uk/download/386340236.pdf (accessed on 14th July 2025).

24. Westerbeck, R. N. (2020). *Does vibration anesthesia improve pain tolerance in patients receiving cosmetic facial injections?* https://core.ac.uk/download/386148674.pdf (accessed on 14th July 2025).

SKIN RESURFACING AND LASER TREATMENTS

10

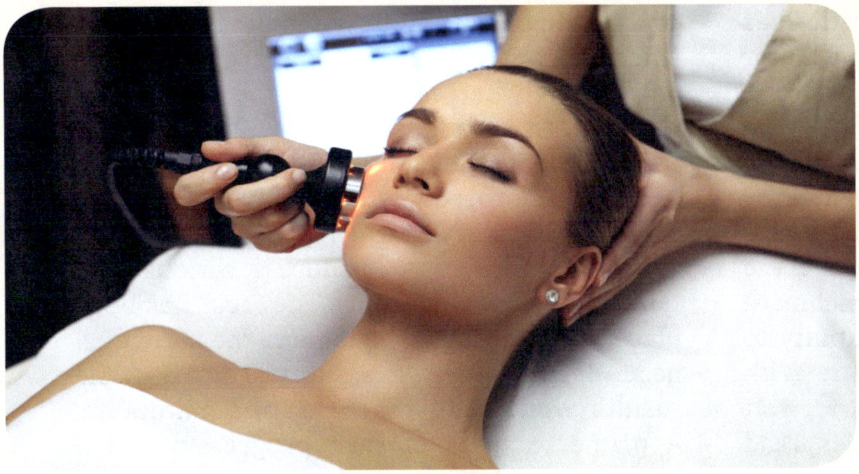

LEARNING OBJECTIVES

After studying this chapter, you will be able to:

1. Outline the types of skin resurfacing treatments;
2. Define laser treatments;
3. Describe the benefits of skin resurfacing treatments and laser treatments;
4. Emphasize risks and side effects;
5. Outline pre-treatment considerations;
6. Evaluate post-treatment care.

Introduction

The recent novelty in the practice of dermatology has been the emergence of immense importance, particularly with the development of skin resurfacing and laser treatments. These technologies have not only changed the practice of doing cosmetic procedures but also the mindsets of the patients regarding skin aesthetics and health. Laser technology has provided dermatologists with extremely versatile tools capable of treating an enormous number of skin conditions, ranging from very superficial imperfections to far more invasive scarring. This essay attempts to scrutinize the mechanisms of skin resurfacing with laser treatments, specifying the assumptions of various laser technologies and their clinical applications. Investigating the mechanisms of action, benefits, and risks of the procedures will pave the way for a complete understanding of their applications in modern cosmetic dermatology, setting the stage for relevant considerations of patient outcomes and industry practices. With the evolution of laser treatment modalities, they have become a common name in the cosmetic industry. Earlier, these modalities were mainly aimed at aesthetic purposes, but studies have only shed more light on their effectiveness for the treatment of dermatological ailments. The regulatory landscape concerning the application of lasers in dermatology has emerged as an important issue in light of the fast-growing nature of this industry. In order to be both safe and effective, critical reviews of existing regulations governing laser therapy treatments must be undertaken. A special focus must be on the potential risks of their application, as described in recent literature. The need for standardization becomes increasingly relevant, emphasizing the importance of notifying practitioners and patients alike about the dangers of laser procedures, as highlighted by the debate on the topical industry concerns (Youngerwood, 2012). Beyond any doubt, the carbon dioxide (CO_2) laser is now the benchmark in dermatological surgery due to its ability to achieve good skin resurfacing results. With extensive past utilization, its potential for soft tissue vaporization has garnered widespread appreciation and admiration across healthcare practitioners. Studies have established that CO_2 laser therapy can result in reduced healing times and complications, thereby enhancing patient satisfaction (Arunachalam et al., 2012). With the continued advancement of laser techniques, balancing development with extensive clinical evaluations and procedural outcomes discussions is paramount. While risks such as erythema and pain still exist, advancements in laser technology have enhanced patient experience and outcome. This essay will continue to analyze the advantages and limitations of CO_2 laser treatments, providing insightful information on their position in contemporary dermatological interventions.

Definition of Skin Resurfacing

Skin resurfacing is defined as a variety of cosmetic procedures aimed at rejuvenating the appearance and sensation of the skin. Most significantly, this technique is designed to improve skin imperfections, such as wrinkles, fine lines, acne scars, and general skin laxity. It achieves these results by stripping the outside layer of skin and causing the formation of new, healthier skin on the inside. Among the techniques employed for skin resurfacing, laser procedures have become particularly prevalent due to their precision and efficacy. These treatments utilize intense light energy to target focal areas of skin, stimulating collagen production and cell turnover. Patients thus have smoother skin with enhanced tone and texture, and this is what underscores the therapeutic potential inherent in skin resurfacing. The improvement in technological devices applied in cosmetic procedures has further diversified the field of skin resurfacing, involving more advanced techniques to address various skin types as well as conditions. The focus has been placed on tailoring treatments to the individual needs of each patient to ensure the best possible results while reducing risks to a minimum. A prime example of such progression from traditional ablative therapy is fractional laser therapy. Fractional laser therapy is a technique that makes use of laser energy in fractionally ablating skin, thereby enabling faster healing and with reduced downtime. Additionally, these developments have led doctors to perform searches for integration of therapies, creating a more well-rounded skincare regimen. This leads to improved patient satisfaction and outcomes. The demand for applying evidence-based medicine and studying the long-term effects of those treatments necessitates staying up to date on current studies in skin resurfacing. Finally, the skin resurfacing discipline, and especially laser therapy, requires an interdisciplinary educational and practice environment. Integrating aesthetics in somatology education has been highlighted in recent research to address changing market requirements and skill deficiencies in the sector (Ambrosio, 2018). With aesthetic procedures becoming more popular, it is extremely important that professionals are well-versed in various methods and equipment to be able to administer successful treatment. Continuing education will not only enable professionals but also equip them with the capability of implementing advanced treatments, such as skin resurfacing and laser therapies. By merging theoretical knowledge with applied skills, the medical and beauty industries have been able to come together in a process that maximizes patient outcomes and experience, thereby creating a holistic approach to skin care that is effective and innovative (Figure 10.1).

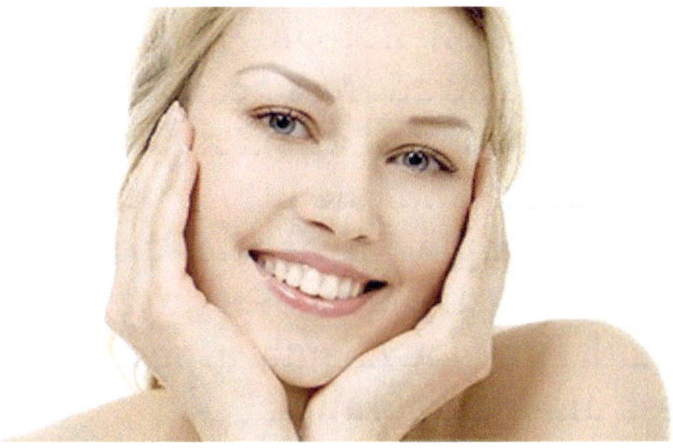

Figure 10.1. Skin resurfacing encompasses a variety of cosmetic procedures.

Source: https://external-content.duckduckgo.com/iu/?u=https%3A%2F%2Fhealthjade.net%2Fwp-content%2Fuploads%2F2019%2F03%2Flaser-skin-resurfacing.jpg&f=1&nofb=1&ipt=f3b87a7e79918aeddcee1927d954dc386b7459cb31425c9871238cceffe0067e.

Overview of Laser Treatments

As a revolutionary advancement in dermatological treatments, laser treatments have significantly transformed the environment of skin resurfacing. The therapy primarily employs intense beams of light that concentrate on specific spots of the skin, removing or restructuring the outer layers of the skin. Ablative lasers such as CO_2 and erbium YAG lasers work by causing dead skin cells to vaporize, thereby encouraging new skin to form. These have played a vital role in the treatment of some of the most common skin ailments, including wrinkles, acne scars, and pigmentation. They have high downtime and potential side effects, such as dyspigmentation and prolonged erythema, that have pushed the development of less invasive methods that minimize these risks, those which are known to affect the patient's acceptability in receiving treatment (Barikbin et al., 2011). Advances in laser treatments have gravitated toward nonablative methods of obtaining optimum results at lower risks. Nonablative lasers, unlike their ablative counterparts, work by traveling into the skin but not removing the surface. This process boosts collagen content and firms up the skin, reacting well to signs of aging with minimal recovery. Though the rate of success might be slightly less than ablative procedures, nonablative procedures are gaining popularity for having fewer side effects, allowing patients to resume normal activities with minimal rest other than a few days. The introduction of fractional laser technology is just one example of this progression, since it draws upon the advantages of both approaches while restricting the skin's overall trauma. The aim of these developments is to maximize cosmetic results with patient safety and comfort (Barikbin et al., 2011). In addition, the incorporation of laser treatment within the field of aesthetic treatments reflects a more general movement away from invasive methods. Many patients are increasingly becoming drawn to these options due to their reduced costs and reduced complication rates compared to traditional surgical procedures. Non-invasive treatments in the form of a range of laser and Intense Pulse Light (IPL) therapies have proven to be favored solutions for issues such as skin discoloration and sagging. They tend to carry minor complications, such as transient erythema and edema, which typically clear spontaneously, making them desirable choices for patients seeking cosmetic enhancements with lower risk. With the rising incidence of demand for less traumatic aesthetic procedures, laser surgery will be guaranteed to be at the leading edge of skin resurfacing modality, with high-volume, high-yield outcomes that reflect patient demand and lifestyle requirements (Figure 10.2).

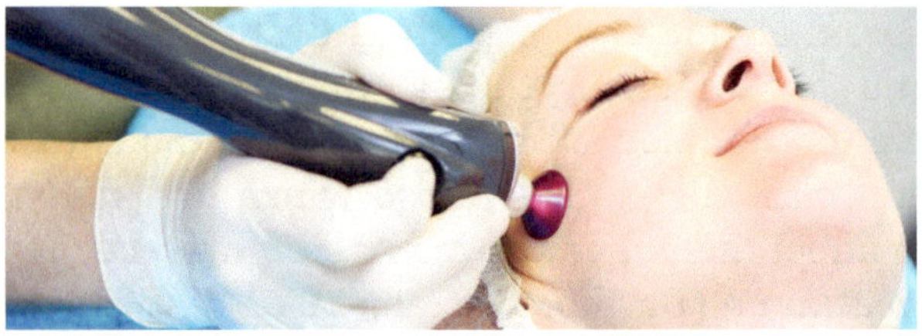

Figure 10.2. An overview of laser treatments.

Source: https://external-content.duckduckgo.com/iu/?u=https%3A%2F%2Fwww.bhrcenter.com%2Fwp-content%2Fuploads%2F2024%2F12%2F6084ca8477a979a0ffef76c6_Medspa-Laser-Treatments-An-Overview.jpg&f=1&nofb=1&ipt=5687d465e115e333571034c370c6594058b05a759dd5c523e86147f8e0763d7d.

Importance of Skin Health and Aesthetics

Beyond aesthetics, the importance of skin health is extremely intertwined with the overall sense of well-being and self-esteem of a person. Healthy skin serves as the body's outer layer of defense against environmental insults from the outside, like pathogens and pollution. Moreover, skin well-being is often a sensory indicator of overall health, reflecting nutritional inadequacies or chronic disease. Skin care protocols are one factor in maintaining this barrier function, which is conducive to preventing complications like infection and inflammation. In the particular instance of skin resurfacing and laser treatments, not only do these enhance cosmetic results but also stimulate healthy skin. By stripping away damaged skin layers, these treatments can stimulate collagen production and improve skin texture overall, resulting in the overall healthier appearance and improved physiological performance of the skin, which can boost an individual's confidence and social life. In recent years, the introduction of new technologies to aesthetic medicine, particularly skin resurfacing and laser treatments, has radically transformed the means by which individuals can acquire and maintain healthier-looking skin. These treatments provide advanced solutions to a variety of skin conditions, such as hyperpigmentation, acne scars, and wrinkles. As witnessed in research, the advantage of both continuous and fractional ablative CO_2 laser treatments over a host of common dermatological conditions attests that effectiveness and aesthetics tend to go together in aesthetics. For instance, in the study, both modal treatments had the highest efficacy rates and equivalent aesthetic outcomes, which suggested an impressive cosmetic enhancement overlap with skin health (Boone et al., 2018). Thus, treatments aimed at surface or targeted skin rejuvenation not only resolve cosmetic problems but also address healing skin integrity and vitality, ensuring both aesthetic satisfaction and improved skin health. The heightened incidence of employing aesthetic treatments in the beauty industry promotes the importance of skin health as a fundamental aspect of individual wellness and recuperation.

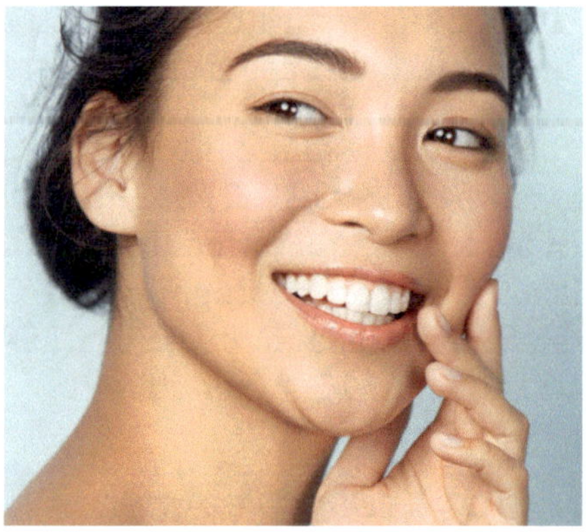

Figure 10.3. Importance of skin health and aesthetics.

Source: https://external-content.duckduckgo.com/iu/?u=https%3A%2F%2Fwww.aestheticsoftheroyalliverbuilding.co.uk%2Fwp-content%2Fuploads%2F2022%2F10%2FImportance-of-Skin-Health.jpg&f=1&nofb=1&ipt=f9a8a7a8281d6bf3dcbf7f55c74b5b220064f49ea11000592eb6f6c71dd6c0fb.

As the consumer now chooses integrated procedures that enhance the beauty of their faces more than ever before, there is also a corresponding surge of demand for experts trained to administer these treatments professionally. The research points to the vast skills gap of the industry, with the need to create more advanced aesthetic somatology educational programs, such as skin care and treatment modalities (Ambrosio, 2018). Filling the gap and making the education requirements uniform will allow beauty professionals to better prepare themselves to meet prevailing needs and offer educated treatment options. With evolving aesthetic modalities, practitioners should make themselves familiar with the correlation between cutaneous wellness and aesthetics so that patients receive both cosmetic and curative results in their skin care therapy (Figure 10.3).

10.1. Types of Skin Resurfacing Techniques

Learning Outcome

1. Discuss the Chemical Peels
2. Explain the Microdermabrasion
3. Focus on Laser Resurfacing

Skin resurfacing treatments are no longer primitive as they have advanced a lot to offer several options to patients who want to rejuvenate their skin. The most common ones are ablative and non-ablative laser treatments. Ablative lasers, such as the carbon dioxide (CO_2) and erbium lasers, work by removing the outer layers of the damaged skin, resulting in sharp tightening of the skin and improved texture. These treatments are most effective in treating deep wrinkles, scars, and hyperpigmentation. The healing process, though, is extensive, with side effects such as increased risk of infection and prolonged erythema and hence warrants serious consideration by patients and practitioners before undergoing treatment (Carniol et al., 2015). While ablative lasers perform their magic by deconstructing the outer layer of the skin, non-ablative lasers operate without damaging the epidermis, a more conservative approach with fewer complications and downtime. Fractional technology is a game-changer in laser resurfacing. Fractional lasers, both ablative and non-ablative, treat only a fraction of the skin's surface, stimulating surrounding tissues to help in healing while leaving as much tissue intact as possible. The most significant benefits are that they cause widespread collagen production and remodeling and possess a faster recovery time, thus being more suitable for a wide range of skin types, including darker complexions (Carniol et al., 2015). Fractional lasers are flexible since they can allow practitioners to adjust treatment parameters, such as pulse duration and microspot density, in an effort to create a tailored method based on the patient's specific needs. The technology has made fractional laser treatments a prime option for those interested in addressing skin issues with less risk than traditional procedures. Ablative and non-ablative lasers are both viable options for resurfacing skin, but trends indicate more usage of non-ablative treatments due to fewer side effects and faster recovery times (Barikbin et al., 2011). Non-ablative fractional resurfacing lasers, in particular, tread that delicate line of safety and efficacy, and their appeal is broad-based to many patients. These lasers induce collagen production without having a significant impact on the epidermal barrier, making the procedure comfortable and allowing return to usual activity in less time. Further research and developments in the future will continue to refine these methods, possibly with greater effectiveness and expansion of indications to non-cosmetic applications. With advancing technology, the future of skin resurfacing is full of promise, striking a balance between safety and efficacy in the pursuit of young, radiant skin (Figure 10.4).

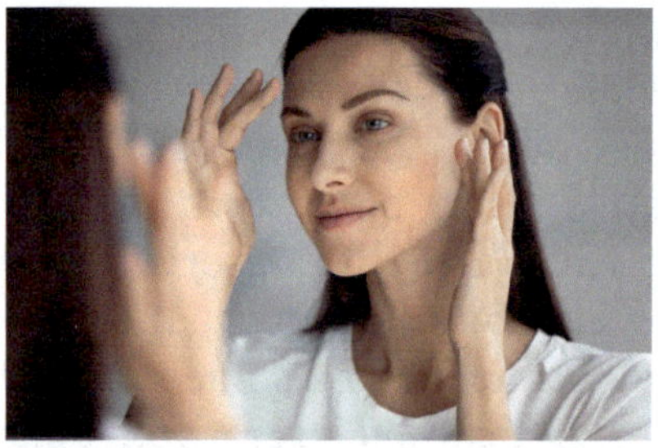

Figure 10.4. Skin resurfacing techniques have evolved significantly.

Source: https://external-content.duckduckgo.com/iu/?u=https%3A%2F%2Fdzgcx8rfb0md3.cloudfront.net%2Fwp-content%2Fuploads%2F2022%2F07%2FiStock-1209020063-scaled.jpg&f=1&nofb=1&ipt=87093619b3dff87de1b1c69e46250de8351e145a0e11f0ae41b36f371a959e9c.

10.1.1. Chemical Peels

Chemical peels constitute a significant segment of skin resurfacing techniques, offering an effective solution for various skin imperfections. These therapies involve the use of chemical solutions to be used on the skin, which brings about controlled exfoliation, leading to the removal of discolored outer layers. By doing so, it is achievable to improve the texture of fine lines, uneven skin tone, and some types of pigmentation disorders. Chemically, chemical peels are able to treat cases of hyperpigmentation of the skin, where a broad range of conditions can vary according to their etiology and treatment outcome. The versatility of chemical peels allows for tailored treatments based on the type and intensity of hyperpigmented lesions, thus making it useful in enhancing clinical results in aesthetic dermatology clinics (Halim et al., 2016). The effectiveness of chemical peels is also established by the fact that it can be given as an adjunctive treatment with other dermatologic interventions, such as laser therapy. With advancements in the field of aesthetic dermatology, the combination of chemical peels and lasers has become a widespread trend, especially when dealing with more difficult cases of hyperpigmentation. For example, while laser treatments can be bolstered by a chemical peel, the latter can also be used as an independent modality for those who want aversive interventions. The use of proper peeling agents, concentrations, and techniques is, however, crucial to avoid possible complications. Clinicians ought to be greatly educated on the pre- and post-procedure care in order to acquire the best healing and aesthetic outcomes, justifying the need for extensive training in the procedures (Madnani et al., 2022). Lastly, the role of chemical peels in resurfacing the skin is multifaceted, with an impact beyond cosmetic improvement.

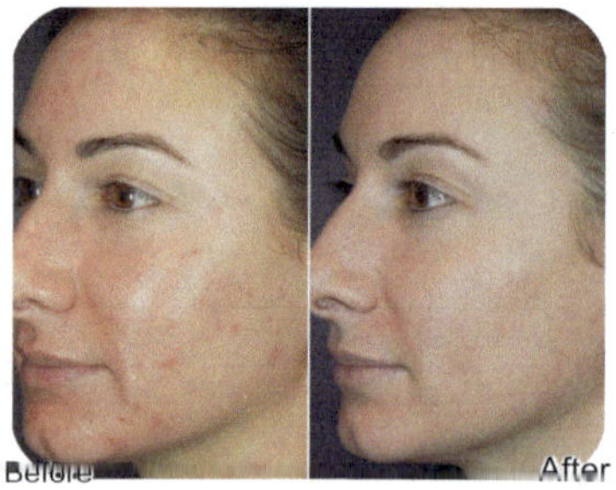

Figure 10.5. Chemical peels constitute a significant segment of skin resurfacing techniques.

Source: https://external-content.duckduckgo.com/iu/?u=http%3A%2F%2Fwww.charmedmedispa.com%2Fwp-content%2Fuploads%2FCharmed-Medispa-3-Step-Peel-ZO-Skin-Health-Results-Face-1024x839.jpg&f=1&nofb=1&ipt=7c747e2abc985829dd7ea456599d91407f6a2dc52a80548acb2f14c090c92e9a.

As dermal procedures advance, the intricacies of chemical peels, such as their indications, contraindications, and possible risk factors, grow more important to understand. Practitioners have to move through these complexities in order to deliver effective and safe treatments, ultimately leading to heightened patient satisfaction. Further, as the demand for these treatments rises, ongoing education on their benefits and limitations will be essential to practitioners to ensure good clinical outcomes and to patients to ensure realistic expectations concerning their treatment pathways (Halim et al., 2016) (Figure 10.5).

10.1.2. Microdermabrasion

Microdermabrasion is a popular non-surgical cosmetic procedure aimed at enhancing the look of the skin by mechanical exfoliation. By the action of mild crystals or a diamond-tipped wand to remove the outermost layer of dead skin cells, the process stimulates cellular turnover, resulting in smoother, more uniform skin texture. Patients prefer to get microdermabrasion done to address a series of problems affecting the skin, such as minute scars, uneven pigmentation, and signs of aging in the form of fine lines. The treatment is so appealing due to its minimal downtime and immediate results, making it a popular choice for the current progressive world of cosmetic treatments. Growing skin health awareness and the pursuit of youthful appearance have placed microdermabrasion as a routine procedure in the majority of dermatology clinics and beauty salons, emphasizing its sustained significance in practice for skin resurfacing procedures. Everything that has been developed in microdermabrasion technology has had a tremendous influence on procedural efficacy and patient satisfaction with practice for skin resurfacing procedures. Over the decade, a number of modalities have been formulated that offer more sophisticated mechanisms of exfoliation and enabling protocols that can be modified to special requirements. As the need for effective, non-surgical rejuvenation of the skin continues to grow, practitioners are employing more microdermabrasion as part of multimodal treatment protocols with concomitant peeling or laser treatment. This multidisciplinary strategy maximizes results while integrating diverse skin concerns within a single treatment paradigm. Furthermore, with ongoing refinement of optimal methods and uses, microdermabrasion remains a center of interest among aesthetic practitioners as well as patients seeking innovative, effective treatments for skin renewal alongside more aggressive treatments (Bowler, 2009). Microdermabrasion integration into training programs of aesthetic practitioners is essential in characterizing the industry's dynamism. Through awareness among practitioners of being current with new technologies and techniques, enhancing education programs within aesthetic modalities is critical.

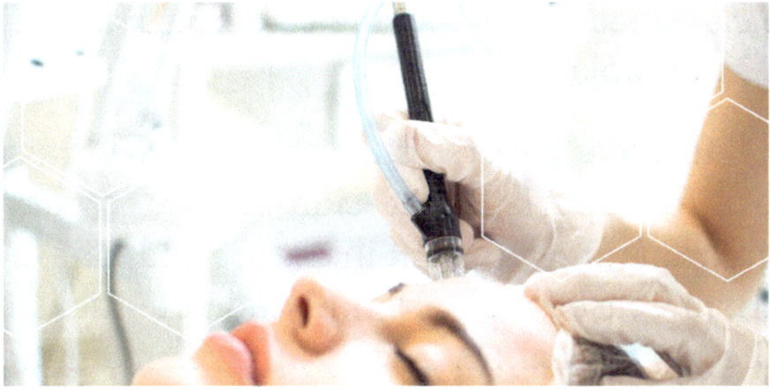

Figure 10.6. Microdermabrasion.

Source: https://external-content.duckduckgo.com/iu/?u=https%3A%2F%2Fcdn.prod.website-files.com%2F5e16b0053c053f77e181e525%2F673d6634a2feea40075523ca_00978_ACHW_BlogPostImage_1200x600_20241114%25201.png&f=1&nofb=1&ipt=cf259af1d64063f8a64e816e10fb01921cfaa644601f7e1de3e559eb643bda5f*Source:*.

For instance, studies stressed the necessity for somatology curricula to include advanced aesthetic procedures, pointing out the rising need for non-surgical procedures like microdermabrasion (Ambrosio, 2018). By providing a rounded learning foundation in somatology and aesthetic areas, practitioners can build a balanced skill set that will increase their capability for delivering innovative solutions in the area of skin resurfacing. Through this, microdermabrasion will not only contribute significantly to the aesthetic industry but also empower professionals to innovate towards increasing consumer demands as well as bridge the knowledge gap between the medical and beauty industries (Figure 10.6).

10.1.3. Laser Resurfacing

Laser resurfacing has emerged as a significant procedure in dermatology, focusing on enhancing the skin through the reduction of imperfections, wrinkles, and signs of aging. The treatment uses focused light energy in scorchedering the surface layers of damaged skin, thus stimulating collagen production in deeper layers. The procedure can be classified into two wide categories: ablative and non-ablative lasers.

Ablative lasers, such as the CO_2 laser, work by vaporizing the skin surface, creating significant improvement in texture and tone, but with increased recovery time and potential side effects of post-inflammatory hyperpigmentation and scarring. Conversely, non-ablative lasers, despite being less effective in causing deep skin changes, have fewer adverse effects and shorter recovery periods, making them more acceptable to more patients who are ready to undergo skin rejuvenation with minimal disruption of daily routines (Barikbin et al., 2011).

The improvement in laser resurfacing technology brought about by the innovation of fractional laser technology has revolutionized the process of treating the skin. Fractional lasers emit energy in a pattern that creates micro-zones of changed skin with relative sparing of the surrounding tissue, thereby contributing to faster healing time and reduced side effects. This new technique capitalizes on the skin's own healing mechanisms, providing dramatic improvement in skin texture and color with minimal downtime. Studies have proven that fractional ablative CO_2 lasers are best used to rejuvenate the face with superior outcomes compared to the outcomes of non-fractional laser treatments through addressing deeper skin layers without requiring extensive recovery periods (Baldin et al., 2023). Fractional laser resurfacing is hence a popular technique among patients and practitioners because of the blend of safety with efficacy to rejuvenate the skin. But selection of patients for laser resurfacing treatments has to be done based on the patient's skin type, problems, and overall health. Skin color, sensitivity, and certain skin conditions significantly influence the selection of the laser and the level of treatment. Darker-skinned patients, for instance, will be more susceptible to pigmentation changes with ablative lasers and thus should need more caution or careful consideration of non-ablative treatment.

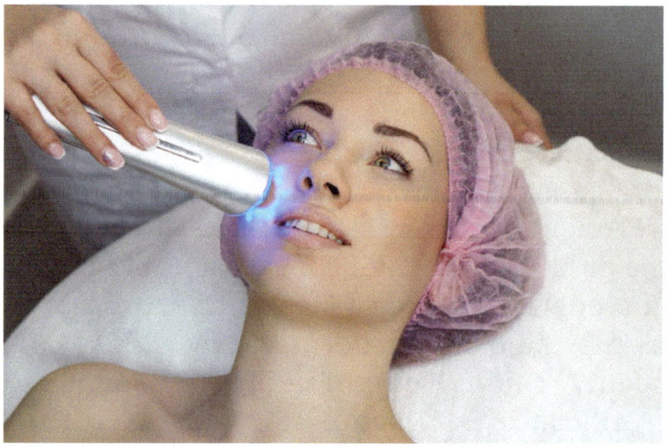

Figure 10.7. Laser resurfacing.

Source: https://external-content.duckduckgo.com/iu/?u=https%3A%2F%2Fi0.wp.com%2Fdermcollective.com%2Fwp-content%2Fuploads%2F2019%2F09%2Flaser-skin-resurfacing-cost-1.jpg%3Ffit%3D1000%252C667%26ssl%3D1&f=1&nofb=1&ipt=6d755fbd38a500ed90ac7ffbd8b681d17e29b007c3fefb3e3134f7bd6a5c156a.

Moreover, combining laser treatment with adjunctive therapies, such as topical retinoids or chemical peels, has the potential to enhance final results and reduce recovery time. Continuous advancements in laser technology and techniques promise enhanced outcomes of cosmetic dermatology and solidify the position of laser resurfacing as a cornerstone of the overall paradigm of skin resurfacing and treatments for keeping skin younger and healthier in appearance (Barikbin et al., 2011) (Figure 10.7).

Test Your Knowledge

1. What are the different depths of chemical peels, and how does each depth affect the type of skin concerns treated?
2. How does microdermabrasion exfoliate the skin, and what makes it a gentler option compared to other resurfacing techniques?
3. What is the difference between ablative and non-ablative laser resurfacing, and how does each impact treatment outcomes and recovery time?

10.2. Understanding Laser Treatments

Learning Outcome

1. Explain the Types of Lasers Used in Dermatology
2. Discuss the Mechanism of Action of Laser Treatments
3. Focus on Comparison of Ablative and Non-Ablative Lasers

For both practitioners and patients, understanding laser treatments is important in aesthetic dermatology. The laser technology has advanced significantly to offer new remedies for resurfacing and revitalizing the skin with less invasiveness. The treatments involve focused light energy applied to treat some problems in the skin, such as pigmentation, wrinkles, and scarring. In contrast to conventional surgical procedures, laser therapy is able to attain significant aesthetic enhancement at the expense of shorter recovery and fewer possible complications. As emphasized in recent research, the switch toward non-invasive treatment has attracted higher levels of patient satisfaction, with prevalence reported at around 74.5% (Timraz et al., 2025). This surge reflects a growing need for aesthetic treatments that offer successful outcomes without long downtime, reflecting the importance of education and technological advancements in the field. In addition to enabling conspicuous skin improvement, laser treatments also provide dermatologists with the opportunity to tailor their approach based on particular skin types and concerns. Tailoring laser parameters to the unique skin characteristics of an individual patient is essential in optimizing outcomes. The range of lasers available, from fractional lasers to pulsed dye lasers, allows technicians to adjust parameters such as wavelength and intensity, thereby optimizing efficacy and minimizing side effects. Such understanding not only helps practitioners make informed choices but also patients through informed consent. As the world continues to need more sophisticated aesthetic solutions, constant education and adaptive procedures by practitioners are highlighted as necessitating the re-examination of the existing curricula employed in the skin care profession around the world (Ambrosio, 2018). Moreover, highly-rated research revealed an ongoing necessity to integrate advanced aesthetic education in somatology studies, which parallels the evolving forces of the aesthetic and beauty industries. The identification of skill deficits among practitioners highlights the imperative of filling education gaps to effectively meet industrial demands. Schools and academies are required to expand curricula to include sophisticated laser technology and skin resurfacing procedures to equip future professionals with the requisite skills in cutting-edge technologies. Collaboration among beauticians and medical specialists can also enhance patient results through safe understanding and skillful application of lasers. Thus, the study of laser therapy in cosmetic training not only enhances professional growth but also enhances the overall quality of treatment to patients who seek good skin renewal programs.

10.2.1. Types of Lasers Used in Dermatology

The field of dermatology has experienced massive expansion with the application of various forms of lasers in treating and resurfacing the skin. Of these, the most commonly employed are ablative lasers, i.e., CO_2 and erbium: YAG lasers, which effectively vaporize the skin surface. Ablative lasers target both the superficial and deeper layers of skin, inducing collagen synthesis and leading to rejuvenation of the skin. Non-ablative lasers, i.e., pulsed dye lasers and Nd:YAG lasers, act by penetrating the skin without damaging the surface. They are particularly valuable in the treatment of vascular lesions, acne scarring, and pigmentation. The specific laser to employ is typically based on the nature of the skin condition to be treated, and consideration of patient safety and desired outcomes. As the popularity of laser procedures increases, the policy climate regarding these technologies has become increasingly important. The swift evolution of lasers in cosmetic dermatology raises fundamental concerns over safety and efficacy. Regulatory agencies, including the Food and Drug Administration (FDA), have the responsibility of determining that devices utilized in dermatology are held to rigorous safety standards before they can be utilized for clinical practice. This regulation is important in light of the dangers the laser treatments can inflict, even as they offer significant benefits to patients seeking skin rejuvenation. While advances in technology for laser therapies have significantly catalyzed therapeutic yields, education on the regulatory space may mitigate the risks associated with their application to make the eventual result safer for patients in dermatologic treatment (Youngerwood, 2012). The psychological and social aspects of skin diseases, particularly acne, contribute additional significance to laser therapy in dermatology. Not only does acne physically bother the individual, but acne also leads to a lot of emotional distress, particularly when scarring occurs.

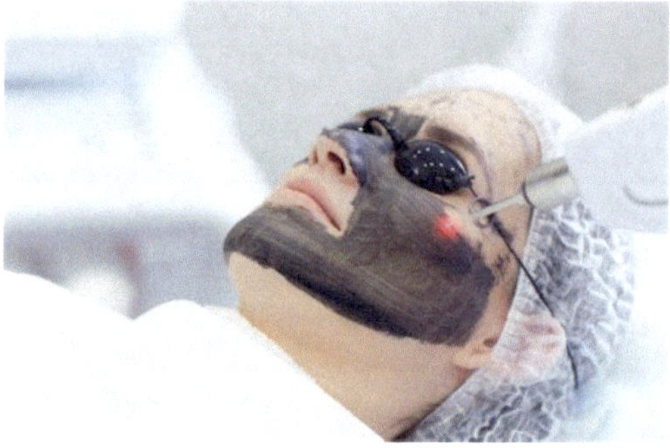

Figure 10.8. Types of lasers used in dermatology.

Source: https://external-content.duckduckgo.com/iu/?u=https%3A%2F%2Ftse4.mm.bing.net%2Fth%2Fid%2FOIP.bDoOSEHnvxbBhBrUbABKSQHaE8%3Fpid %3DApi&f=1&ipt=d5efa4e0713d3c0e4a83c71dd74c816ba2f5f1b582d87ab0a2f307d41a88f99d.

Accurate treatment of acne scarring is essential to improve a patient's self-esteem as well as quality of life; laser treatments have a significant role in fulfilling this purpose. Both ablative and non-ablative lasers have been discovered to be capable of treating different kinds of acne scars, alleviating the pain that these conditions inflict on patients. For example, the CO_2 laser has been shown to lead to extensive improvement of atrophic scars, while non-ablative lasers would be best suited for hypertrophic scars due to their shorter recovery time. As a result, the application of laser treatments is a complex treatment for acne scarring and highlights the broader dermatological therapeutic application of lasers (Annunziata et al., 2010) (Figure 10.8).

10.2.2. Mechanism of Action of Laser Treatments

The mechanism of action for lasers for resurfacing the skin is primarily selective destruction of the skin chromophores, including melanin, hemoglobin, and water. Lasers emit concentrated light beams, which are absorbed and penetrate into the skin at varying depths, depending on the laser source and skin being treated. When the laser light is absorbed by the chromophores, it induces thermal damage localized to the desired areas. Thermal damage results in stimulation of the body's natural healing process, collagen regeneration, and turnover of damaged skin cells. Fine lines, wrinkles, and skin irregularities of pigmentation can consequently reduce gradually, resulting in smoother and more revitalized skin. The effectiveness of this technique is due to the precision with which lasers can be directed onto specific skin layers without causing injury to the adjacent tissue, which is due to their application in dermatological therapies. In addition to the thermal effects, laser techniques also induce photothermal and photochemical reactions that enhance rejuvenation of the skin. Non-ablative lasers, for instance, permit collagen remodeling without significant epidermal removal, causing minimal downtime to patients. The lasers address the layers of the dermis primarily with heat stimulation of fibroblast synthesis of elastin and collagen. Ablative lasers, on the other hand, remove outer layers of the skin efficiently, allowing for more aggressive resurfacing and quicker results in wrinkle and scar reduction. The choice of laser is based on factors such as skin type, the type of treatment outcome desired, and the severity of the skin condition. Understanding the general mechanism helps professionals tailor treatments to the individual requirements of patients and optimize the outcome of laser treatments for skin resurfacing. Laser treatment application, however, is not without issues, primarily with safety and regulatory concerns. The use of lasers in cosmetic dermatology has expanded, and concerns regarding standardization of practice and operator competence have arisen. With the number of laser units available and minimal regulatory oversight, there are inherent hazards from misuse, such as burns or unintended skin damage. To reduce such risks, ongoing training and education are essential for professionals to enable them to be informed about both the manner of actions and the operating processes of the equipment that they work with. As per literature, addressing the regulatory context in the actualization of cosmetic lasers is necessary to enable safe practice in the field and optimize patient safety and treatment results (Youngerwood, 2012). Therefore, as laser treatments continue to develop further, focus on both their mechanisms and everyday application will remain crucial to the future of skin resurfacing.

10.2.3. Comparison of Ablative and Non-Ablative Lasers

Use of laser technology in skin resurfacing has come a long way, particularly with developments in ablative and non-ablative lasers. Ablative lasers such as erbium yttrium aluminum garnet (Er:YAG) and CO_2 lasers produce effects by erasing outer skin layers, thereby stimulating new growth of skin and collagen. The lasers provide a more extreme effect in eliminating wrinkles, acne scars, and other imperfections as they can vaporize the damaged tissue. There is a considerably longer period of recovery, however, compared to non-ablative processes that simply provide less downtime. Non-ablative lasers, on the other hand, bypass the top layer of the skin, treating deeper structures with less significant destruction of the epidermis, and therefore are most suited for milder skin issues with shorter recovery time after the procedure. This side-by-side analysis portrays how laser treatment protocols need to be tailored to meet a patient's specific needs. The recent years have witnessed fractional technology as a breakthrough in both ablative and non-ablative lasers. This new treatment allows the laser to treat part of the skin but spare the surrounding tissues. Leaving intact the untreated tissue, fractional lasers stimulate quicker healing and fewer opportunities for complications compared to traditional ablative and non-ablative systems. The success of this method has been extensively described, and studies have provided significant improvement in the complexion and texture of the skin with maintenance of patient comfort. For instance, the advent of non-ablative fractional photothermolysis, FDA-approved, has revolutionized the treatment of a variety of conditions such as melasma and acne scars. Similarly, ablative fractional technologies like the Er:YAG laser have been highly effective in treating more aggressive skin conditions, illustrating the scope and potential of fractional lasers in therapeutic dermatology (Allemann & Kaufman, 2018). The efficacy and safety profiles of ablative and non-ablative laser treatment are of particular concern in the clinical setting. Research indicates that while both treatments can provide satisfying aesthetic results, patient tolerance for pain and values may be considerable. As an example, non-ablative therapy is often considered less painful with fewer possible side effects, making it attractive to patients with little desired downtime. Studies have found patients who underwent fractional ablative treatments recorded acceptable levels of pain when compared to conventional ablative treatments, and it continues to affect their treatment of choice (Boone et al., 2018). Ultimately, the use of either ablative or non-ablative lasers should be between the patient and clinician through a mutual decision-making process based on skin type, outcome desired, and individual tolerance for various treatments. This subtle balance of patient needs and treatment potential will be improved in skin resurfacing treatments (Figure 10.9).

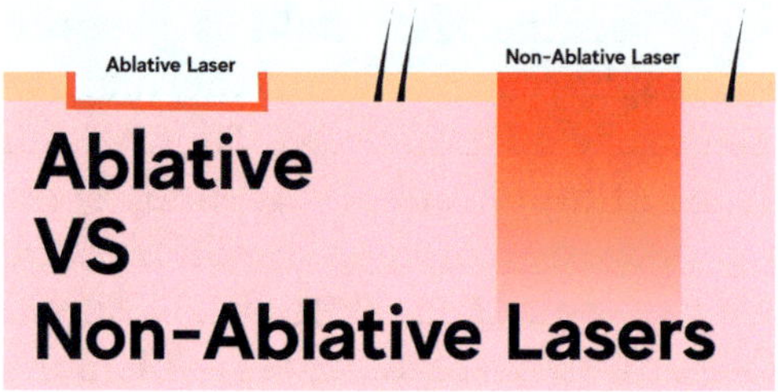

Figure 10.9. Comparison of ablative and non-ablative lasers.

Source: https://external-content.duckduckgo.com/iu/?u=https%3A%2F%2Fwww.allwhitelaser.com%2Fwp-content%2Fuploads%2F2023%2F06%2Fblog-thumbnail5-06-scaled.jpg&f=1&nofb=1&ipt=04356327400ab4443af8dc4984c579c023b724d18cee4436c3daaccf4a8d30f1.

Test Your Knowledge

1. What are the main types of lasers commonly used in dermatology, and how do their wavelengths determine their clinical applications?
2. How do laser treatments achieve targeted tissue effects through principles such as selective photothermolysis?

10.3. Benefits of Skin Resurfacing and Laser Treatments

Learning Outcome

1. Discuss the Improvement in Skin Texture and Tone
2. Explain Reduction of Fine Lines and Wrinkles
3. Focus on Treatment of Acne Scars and Pigmentation Issues

Laser and skin resurfacing treatments are becoming promising devices that provide a great advantage in dermatological practice to patients who want to enhance the look and feel of their skin. The key advantage of these procedures is that they are able to address a range of skin issues, from acne scarring, fine lines, and photoaging, to mention a few. For instance, a dual-wavelength laser machine has been proven to be useful in the healing of atrophic acne scars of the face, with skin texture improvements and considerable reduction of scars being observed after therapy (Amoruso et al., 2023). The patients experience minimal downtime with five to six days on average as their recovery period, thus allowing them to return to their normal routine immediately. This dual potential to enhance cosmetic outcomes with less recovery disturbances renders laser therapy the best choice for individuals who want to rejuvenate their skin. Another benefit of laser therapy and skin resurfacing is that they can be used to treat an array of skin ailments, including actinic keratoses (AKs) and other premalignant lesions. With the high rate of occurrence of AKs in aging populations, especially among those with intensive sun exposure, these treatments provide intensive modalities to repair skin health and prevent possible progression into squamous cell carcinoma. Various treatment methods, including topical treatments, photodynamic treatment, and laser resurfacing, provide practitioners with the ability to customize the treatment to suit specific patient needs and types of lesions. The ability to cure focal lesions and broad facial areas emphasizes the efficacy of field-directed therapies, particularly in facilitating global treatment of sun-damaged skin and enhancing global skin integrity (Ferara et al., 2024). Moreover, the psychosocial and social benefits of laser therapy and skin resurfacing cannot be overlooked. Improved skin health can mean greater self-esteem and confidence, particularly for those patients who have endured long-term skin issues such as scars or irregularities in skin pigmentation. As these treatments become more widely available and are subject to greater popular scrutiny, patients become increasingly aware of the safety and effectiveness of laser technologies. With a constant high rate of patient satisfaction documented following such procedures, many individuals experience both physical and psychological relief from cutaneous illness. Thus, the psychological relevance of successful skin treatment emphasizes the critical role that progress in dermatological treatments assumes, transforming not just the appearance of skin but also overall well-being in many (Amoruso et al., 2023; Ferara et al., 2024).

10.3.1. Improvement in Skin Texture and Tone

The enhancement of skin texture and color is a major objective among many skin resurfacing and laser treatments. These are applied using newer technologies, such as fractional photothermolysis (FP), to deliver precise outcomes in skin renewal. FP specifically targets the dermal layers and does not affect the surrounding tissues, leading to collagen synthesis stimulation and cellular turnover. In one experiment among Korean patients with wrinkles on the face, physicians noticed varying degrees of improvement following a number of treatment sessions, illustrating the efficacy of FP in enhancing the appearance of the skin. Surprisingly, 12% of patients achieved excellent results, while 40% improved notably, demonstrating the ability of

FP to perfect not only cosmetic attributes like tone and texture but also to restore the radiance of aged skin (Chan et al., 2009). In contrast to fractional approaches, ablative and non-ablative laser combination offers a synergistic remodeling modality for texture and tonality improvement. The combined treatment modality utilizes the unique features of both ablative and non-ablative lasers to deliver an optimal aesthetic outcome with less patient downtime. Sequential application, supported by histologic examination, reveals that skin responds favorably to bidirectional energy pulses of dual-wavelength lasers. The augmented lesion coverage with heat increases texture improvement in skin, alongside stimulating the remodeling of collagen and giving improved skin tone as a whole (Bennardo et al., 2022).

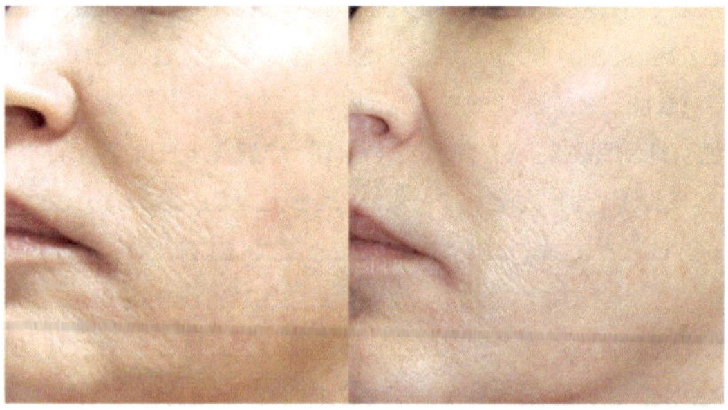

Figure 10.10. Improvement in skin texture and tone.

Source: https://external-content.duckduckgo.com/iu/?u=http%3A%2F%2Fdermasweep.com%2Fwp-content%2Fuploads%2F2014%2F12%2FDermaSweep_Before_and_After_Tone-Texture_2-e1424543995182.jpg&f=1&nofb=1&ipt=1d650a90cedfb504374d7cfed8ca28836dcc36d6af1b54f3a5c92ef77d51e6d2.

The discovery focuses on the importance of new techniques for enhancing curative responses. Moreover, pursuit of better skin texture and tone through such laser treatments is not merely cosmetic but also crucial in restoring patient confidence and psychological health. Improved skin health can have a significant effect on patients' self-esteem and social contacts because smoother and more even skin is typically connected with considerations of health and attractiveness. The patients' positive comments reported in research studies highlight the psychological advantages that ensue from improvements in skin texture and appearance. Therefore, as laser technologies improve, the dual priority of aesthetic results as well as psychological impact serves to explain the increasing popularity of skin resurfacing treatments among different patient groups (Chan et al., 2009; Bennardo et al., 2022) (Figure 10.10).

10.3.2. Reduction of Fine Lines and Wrinkles

The quest for more youthful-looking skin generally involves fine lines and wrinkles reduction, a universal issue encountered when getting older. Skin resurfacing and lasers have also been effective therapies for the condition, providing noticeable respite in the texture and appearance of patients' skin. Traditional technologies such as chemical peels and microdermabrasion opened the door to newer and more advanced systems employed nowadays. These new therapies take advantage of the ability of light and heat to induce collagen synthesis and yield tighter, smoother skin. The success of these therapies emphasizes the significant role played by technological innovation within dermatology in anti-aging techniques. Perhaps the most important development in this field is the launch of non-ablative fractional photothermolysis, which was FDA-approved in 2003. This revolutionary treatment touches only a proportion of the skin and leaves up to 95% of the surrounding tissue undisturbed, stimulating rapid healing and minimizing recovery time. The synergy of the twin benefits of stimulating skin rejuvenation without enhancing the risk of complications is elevating this treatment to greater popularity among the practitioners as well as the patients. Additionally, the arrival of ablative fractional photothermolysis further enhances the treatment efficacy by using lasers, i.e., erbium yttrium aluminum garnet (Er:YAG) and carbon dioxide, to treat a variety of skin imperfections, such as fine lines and wrinkles, effectively. The utility of laser treatments goes beyond mere aesthetic enhancement; it also encompasses a safety profile consistent with today's healthcare models. It was demonstrated that a combination of deep ablation and thermal stimulation would significantly improve the elasticity and texture of the skin, which are vital to the alleviation of wrinkles and fine lines. With more than one layer of skin being addressed, these technologies promote a more complete process of skin resurfacing, and this leads to longer-lasting results. As such, patients can now gain not just superficial improvements but also deeper structural rejuvenation, thus fulfilling their desire for a younger appearance. With the ongoing evolution of aesthetic dermatology, the relentless refinement of laser technology promises ever greater efficacy and safety, ensuring the war against fine lines and wrinkles an honorable niche at the frontier of cosmetic science (Cannarozzo et al., 2014; Allemann & Kaufman, 2018) (Figure 10.11).

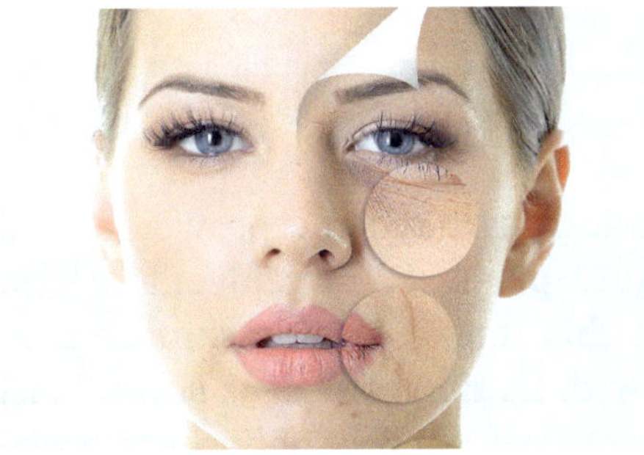

Figure 10.11. Reduction of fine lines and wrinkles.

Source: https://external-content.duckduckgo.com/iu/?u=https%3A%2F%2Fapexmedicalspa.com%2Fwp-content%2Fuploads%2Ffine-lines-and-wrinkle-reduction.jpg&f=1&nofb=1&ipt=6ea0d6d5dfc4e677c25f93e9bbccec190267e5276ef4621f82387667bd303e40.

10.3.3. Treatment of Acne Scars and Pigmentation Issues

The search for effective treatments for acne scars and pigmentation remains a topical matter in dermatology, particularly through the medium of skin resurfacing and laser treatments. These treatments have evolved a long way, presenting clinicians and patients with several options based on skin type and condition. Amongst such therapies, fractional laser therapy is a promising one for melasma treatment as it has the ability to penetrate superficial and deeper levels of skin, allowing remodeling of the collagen that leads to smoother skin and diminished pigmentation. Furthermore, the selectivity of laser therapies allows targeted interventions that have the ability to reduce injury to surrounding tissues, thereby hastening recovery and lessening downtime. Through addressing a number of issues simultaneously, such as atrophic scars and dyschromia, these treatments are a multifaceted approach to improving the appearance and functioning of the skin in a general manner. In the realm of treating skin hyperpigmentation, laser machines have been extremely effective. They are composed of ablative lasers and non-ablative lasers, each of which is utilized for particular purposes based on the depth and character of pigmentation targeted. Ablative lasers, including CO_2 and Er:YAG, peel off layers of pigmented skin, thus destroying the pigmented lesions while helping in the formation of new skin. Non-ablative lasers, however, target the deeper dermis and stimulate the production of collagen without damaging the surface of the skin and are thus perfect for patients who opt for less invasive treatment with shorter recovery times. Treatment protocols consist of a combination of modalities, including topical treatments and chemical peels, to enhance overall results and limit recurrence of hyperpigmentation, according to current dermatologic literature (Halim et al., 2016). Non-surgical interventions have gained prominence as an alternative to traditional surgery, providing patients with acne scarring and pigmentation another treatment option. Such processes are generally accompanied by little pain and short recovery periods, and individuals can resume their normal lives within a matter of minutes. Some of these methods, such as intense pulsed light (IPL) therapy and chemical peels, can significantly reduce the appearance of scars and pigmentation by stimulating cellular turnover, in addition to exfoliating. Although some minor side effects, such as swelling and erythema, may occur, these are reversible and spontaneously resolve, establishing the safety profile of such therapies (Timraz et al., 2025). The increased popularity of non-invasive treatments reflects a broader trend towards obtaining clearer, healthier-looking skin using effective but less invasive methods, highlighting their role in modern dermatological practice (Figure 10.12).

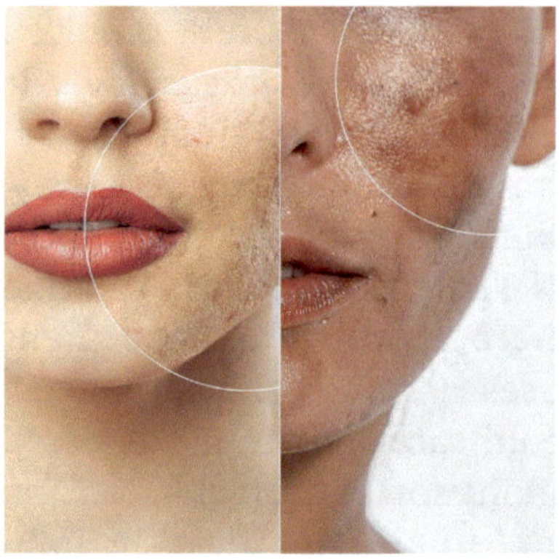

Figure 10.12. Treatment of acne scars and pigmentation issues.

Source: https://external-content.duckduckgo.com/iu/?u=https%3A%2F%2Fcdn05.zipify.com%2FKGwRCf3wCrnWNE05P_WrrNCccDs%3D%2Ffit-in%2F2048x0%2F9e03779a3e794a4f977c3334d46f04b8%2Fgold-cosmetics-pigmentation-vs-acne-scars_blog-image-5.jpeg&f=1&nofb=1&ipt=9069c7512fc9e39b0797984af7aa71df80a501dad23715db48ef2435126cae51.

Test Your Knowledge

1. How do skin resurfacing procedures help improve overall skin texture and tone?
2. What mechanisms make resurfacing treatments effective in reducing fine lines and wrinkles?
3. In what ways can skin resurfacing and laser therapies help treat acne scars and pigmentation disorders?

10.4. Risks and Side Effects

Learning Outcome

1. Explain the Common Side Effects of Laser Treatments
2. Focus on Potential Complications and Long-Term Effects
3. Discuss the Importance of Professional Consultation

The innovation of skin resurfacing and laser treatments has transformed cosmetic dermatology through the provision of diverse techniques purposed at rejuvenating the skin. Despite this, the quest for skin enhancement comes with its downsides, as several risks and side effects are inherent with these procedures. Some of the most common concerns are hyperpigmentation and dyspigmentation of the skin, which can be experienced after laser treatments, particularly among those with dark skin pigmentation. These are conditions that can be caused by inflammatory reactions to the lasers' heat, causing an unnatural proliferation of melanin production. Furthermore, lesions cannot react uniformly to treatment; whereas some react significantly, others may even re-emerge, complicating laser treatment outcomes (Halim et al., 2016). Practitioners should alert patients about such potential sequelae to enable realistic expectations and allow for informed decisions about their skin health. Apart from hyperpigmentation, patients also complain of frequent side effects such as chronic erythema, edema, and acneiform eruptions following treatment. Traditional ablative lasers, even though successful, have classically been said to induce more side effects compared to their nonablative counterparts. This leads to not only a greater risk to the patient but also an extended recovery period, resulting in potential emotional trauma and extended durations of disturbances in normal functions (Barikbin et al., 2011). The psychological impact of having to endure these side effects cannot be overemphasized, since patients are not pleased with their appearance during the course of recovery. Providers must adopt a thorough pre-treatment assessment, keeping in mind the individual patient factors, to minimize the occurrence of poor outcomes and establish an enhanced overall experience. Despite better technology with lasers, things remain complex when it comes to risks and side effects. Nonablative fractional resurfacing was promoted as able to decrease complications without sacrificing efficacy; although it must be noted that even this new method does not remove risk entirely. Complications exist in the form of slight irritation or temporary redness, which, while more generally less pronounced, still are a departure from the ideal of flawless skin (Barikbin et al., 2011). On top of this, inadequate technique or inadequate post-treatment care can highlight and exacerbate these conditions, which strongly underscores the need for well-trained practitioners familiar with the nuances of each modality. Thus, a general familiarity with the benefits and drawbacks of skin resurfacing treatments is key to building patient confidence and to fostering the safe practice of cosmetic dermatology.

10.4.1. Common Side Effects of Laser Treatments

Laser treatments are gaining popularity within dermatology due to their versatility in resurfacing the skin; however, they are not without side effects. Among the most common short-term reactions are erythema, or redness, most frequently resulting from the heat effect of the lasers on the skin. This reaction most typically resolves from a few hours to several days, depending on the intensity and depth of the treatment. Other common side effects include swelling and tenderness at the site of treatment, which may be accompanied by symptoms similar to a mild sunburn. While these initial side effects are usually temporary, they highlight the importance of proper pre- and post-procedure care, which can have a significant impact on recovery and outcome. The clinicians should be mindful of the common effects because a good process can reduce patient anxiety and increase overall satisfaction with the result of the treatment (Madnani et al., 2022). Apart from the short-term effects, there are also side effects that appear over the long term for treatments with lasers, which may be more worrying. A very common risk is the appearance of post-inflammatory hyperpigmentation (PIH), especially in patients with darker skin types. This occurs when the skin produces too much melanin in response to injury and may lead to darker patches appearing at the point of treatment. On occasion, loss of pigment or hypopigmentation can also occur, which is upsetting for patients who are attempting to improve the appearance of their skin. A greater appreciation of these risks is required, particularly in the context of field cancerization, when there are pre-existing lesions that can complicate the healing and outcome of the treatment. The complexities of these side effects reinforce the importance of close patient selection and management strategies according to individual needs and risk profiles (Anliker et al., 2014). In the management of these side effects, the role of individualized patient care cannot be overemphasized. Proper assessment of a patient's skin type, history, and cosmetic goals is necessary before the start of laser treatments. Pre-treatment counselling could make patients aware of realistic expectations and potential risks involved in the procedure. Finally, treatment regimens after the procedure, like the use of sunscreen and avoidance of sun exposure, are an important factor in the prevention of side effects like changes in pigmentation. Clinicians aware of these complications can enable their patients' recovery and optimize their treatment outcomes. Furthermore, continuous education of patients and professionals, as well as shifting expectations and realities of laser treatments, continues to be required for achieving the desired outcome without unnecessary side effects (Madnani et al., 2022) (Figure 10.13).

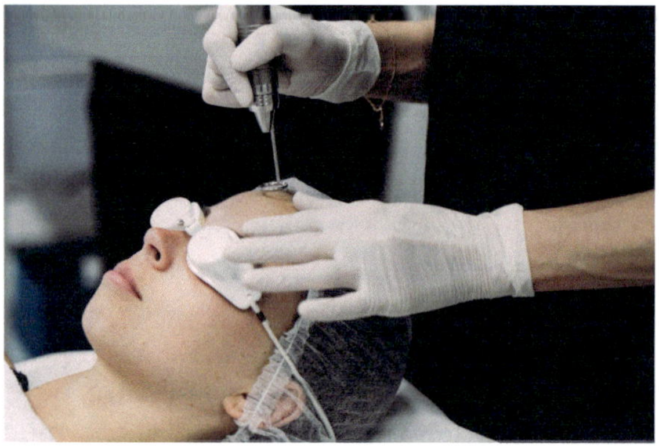

Figure 10.13. Common side effects of laser treatments.

Source: https://external-content.duckduckgo.com/iu/?u=https%3A%2F%2Fsoutherncosmetics.com.au%2Fwp-content%2Fuploads%2F2017%2F05%2FLaser-Skin-Resurfacing.jpg&f=1&nofb=1&ipt=2ffffe2a16565a97921159512ab56452ebc27f89c769b005856a627e52eab2e6.

10.4.2. Potential Complications and Long-Term Effects

Skin resurfacing and laser procedures are becoming increasingly common procedures to cosmetically improve the texture and look of the skin. But related complications and long-term effects of such procedures have to be considered carefully. Immediate complications of erythema, edema, and pain are common problems that typically resolve within weeks. Severe complications such as scarring, infection, and alteration in pigmentation also occur. In fact, post-inflammatory hyperpigmentation is particularly of concern, especially in patients with darker skin tones, since their skin responds erratically to the resurfacing procedures. Development of non-ablative fractional photothermolysis, addressing issues of the skin in a more conservative manner, was a development aimed at minimizing such risks without compromising effects (Allemann & Kaufman, 2018). Thus, it is critical to understand the minute differences in individual skin reactions to the procedures to achieve effective patient results. Resurfacing of the skin and laser treatments have long-term consequences, relying mostly on the type of procedure and on individual skin reactions. Ineffective post-procedure skin care can raise the danger of developing complications like long-standing erythema or abnormal pigmentation patterns. In particular, those with a history of hyperpigmentation may experience heightened symptoms as a result of the inflammatory response generated by resurfacing procedures. Accordingly, many dermatologists recommend continued protection of the skin, including the application of sunscreen daily, in order to minimize long-term negative effects and shield treated areas from the sun's UV rays. The introduction of ablative fractional photothermolysis maximized treatment options with degrees of resurfacing controlled for different skin concerns while trying to minimize complications. Post-follow-up procedures are also capable of being crucial in managing adverse reactions, further supporting the necessity of a tailored post-treatment plan to achieve optimum results (Halim et al., 2016). In addition to the immediate complications, long-term effects of skin resurfacing and laser treatments can include psychological effects on patients. The expectation of rapid recovery of skin status might be one cause of dissatisfaction due to divergence from pre-procedure expectations. Furthermore, prolonged erythema or unsatisfactory aesthetic outcomes might be one cause of psychological distress, and this requires physicians to have good communication with patients. Themcomplexities of healing the skin and individual variation should be addressed to set realistic expectations. Thus, dermatologists should provide candid counseling that outlines potential risks and the need to adhere to post-treatment guidelines. This multi-disciplinary strategy not only deals with physical outcomes but also deals with the psychological well-being of patients undergoing these transformative cosmetic treatments, hence adopting a whole-person perspective to skin health and appearance (Allemann & Kaufman, 2018).

10.4.3. Importance of Professional Consultation

The valuc of professional consultation regarding skin resurfacing and laser treatment cannot be overstated. As these methods have become more popular, informed consultations are necessary to ensure both efficacy and safety of the treatments. A trained consultation allows practitioners to evaluate a patient's skin type, medical history, and specific aesthetic wishes and adjust recommendations accordingly to address individual needs. Such a personalized approach significantly eliminates risks of unwanted reactions or poor results. As highlighted by recent studies, the aesthetic treatment setting is ever-evolving, and thus it becomes mandatory for both the patient and practitioner to engage in thorough discussions of expectations and choices (Bowler, 2009). In aesthetic treatments, emerging technology makes for a quintessentially complex setting in the sense of treatment options. The discovery of new procedures necessitates both practitioners and patients being updated on the latest advancements. Specialist consultations are essential learning tools, teaching clients about new technology and how this impacts treatment outcomes. Furthermore, systematic evaluation during the consultations can identify potential contraindications or complications that may arise, guiding patients to safer and more effective treatments (Ambrosio, 2018). Therefore, sparing time for such consultations establishes a mutual relationship between clients and practitioners, eventually yielding trust and satisfaction. Professional consultations are also important in closing the existing skills gap common in the beauty and medical industries.

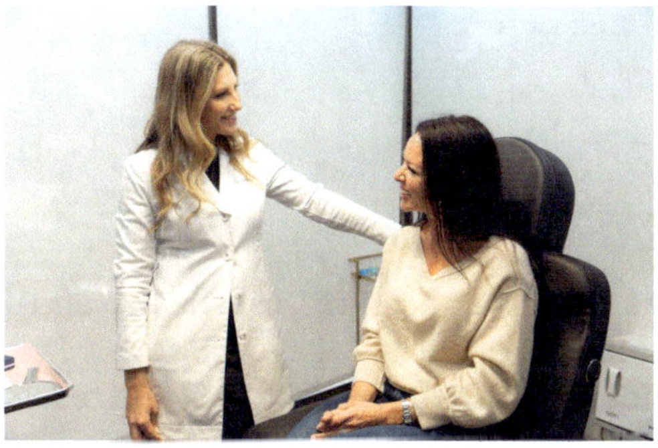

Figure 10.14. The significance of professional consultation.

Source: https://external-content.duckduckgo.com/iu/?u=https%3A%2F%2Fwww.houstonplasticsurgery.pro%2Fwp-content%2Fuploads%2F2023%2F01%2FHeights-Plastic-Surgery-Filler-0955.jpg&f=1&nofb=1&ipt=84cb3222eeca00f08b783c6993023c623a398e636868675922e4a7e97bebb70e.

As pointed out by the need for standard education of aesthetics, consultation helps in identifying areas where practitioners would require more training (Ambrosio, 2018). As there is now a wider variety of aesthetic treatments, practitioners are being encouraged to become more competent in high-end aesthetic treatments. Such sharing not only enhances the skill level of practitioners but also provides clients with a better level of awareness in terms of the therapies they are choosing. Hence, professional consultation is not only a concern of initial treatment planning but also encourages a spirit of continuous learning and enhancement to the advantage of both practitioners and clients in the rapidly evolving environment of skin resurfacing and laser treatments (Figure 10.14).

Test Your Knowledge

1. What are the most common side effects associated with laser skin treatments, and how long do they typically last?
2. What potential complications or long-term effects can occur after laser procedures if not performed properly or without proper aftercare?

10.5. Pre-Treatment Considerations

Learning Outcome

1. Discuss Skin Assessment and Consultation
2. Preparing the Skin for Treatment
3. Focus on Setting Realistic Expectations

Before undertaking skin resurfacing and laser treatments, there are several pre-treatment considerations that must be addressed in order to offer both safety and effectiveness. Long patient screenings are essential, such as medical history, skin type, and previous experiences with treatments. Practitioners will need to assess the overall health of the patient's skin and assess any contraindications. Skin conditions, medications, and evidence of any previous adverse reactions to treatments similar in nature must be carefully noted. Patient education regarding what to expect during and after treatment is also critical; this involves discussing potential side effects such as redness, swelling, or peeling. Having realistic expectations plays a significant part in patient satisfaction and lowers the chance of post-procedure frustration or anxiety. In addition, selecting the appropriate protocol of treatment is key to receiving optimal outcomes. For instance, lasers come with varying wavelengths and mechanisms that tend to address specific skin issues. A personalized approach that considers the individualizing characteristics of each individual's skin is needed. These conditions, such as actinic keratosis (AK), must be thought about just as carefully, particularly in regard to their association with chronic ultraviolet radiation exposure, which complicates treatment. As current clinical guidelines attest, providers must carefully weigh the severity of the lesions and adjust management accordingly. Individual risks, and an individualized treatment plan, targeting them enhances the possibility of favorable results without compromising patient safety when receiving skin resurfacing treatments (Anliker et al., 2014). The regulatory framework further plays a role in the decision-making process concerning skin resurfacing and laser treatments. Aspiring practitioners must understand the legal issues surrounding cosmetic lasers, including the lack of exhaustive regulations governing their use. As highlighted in past discussions of the laser sector, issues of safety must be of paramount concern, particularly concerning the training and qualification of the practitioners performing these procedures. Proper regulation can balance the very risks of the operation of these very powerful appliances. In addition, pre-treatment protocols must include rigorous informed consent processes, which do not simply recommend but actively engage patients in shared decision-making. By incorporating these regulatory considerations into the pre-treatment process, practitioners are able to bridge the gap between successful treatment outcomes and patient safety (Youngerwood, 2012).

10.5.1. Skin Assessment and Consultation

Successful skin consultation and assessment are required for creating a successful treatment plan for skin resurfacing and laser therapy patients. Through the consultation, practitioners must carefully inspect the patient's skin type, condition, and particular concerns. Such an assessment not only involves physical examination but also detailed interviews about the patient's medical history, lifestyle patterns, and previous treatments (Doorn et al., 2017). This thorough examination makes it possible for dermatologists to tailor intervention so that the chosen resurfacing technique can be made to enhance the patient's individual biological characteristics of the skin. Besides, the answer to the patients' concerns and expectations during consultation results in a trusting relationship required to achieve maximum patient compliance and satisfaction. Hence, successful skin assessment forms the foundation of an individualized approach and eliminates the possibility of adverse outcomes and optimization of follow-up laser treatment efficacy. Then, following assessment, the consultation should also include addressing possible side effects as well as analgesia. Patients are most concerned about pain associated with laser procedures and therefore, emphasize the significance of open discussion regarding such concerns. From current literature, it can be seen that local anesthetics, i.e., lidocaine/prilocaine cream, can induce remarkable pain relief when it comes to laser procedures, so they are included as obligatory pre-treatment protocols (Doorn et al., 2017). Incorporating such anesthetic measures into treatment plans allows practitioners to ensure patient comfort, which will eventually translate into increased treatment acceptance and satisfaction. An understanding of the possibilities of pain control allows practitioners to warn patients adequately, minimizing anxiety and allowing a less stressful experience.

Thus, success with laser treatments depends not only on technical competence but also on adequate measures of pain control dealt with at consultation. Lastly, post-treatment treatment and realistic expectations regarding outcomes need to be addressed during the consultation. Patients tend to expect rapid and dramatic results following laser therapy, but must be instructed that the process of healing is unpredictable based on patient reaction and the specific method utilized. Aftercare education, including guarding and hydration of the skin, allows patients to become an active participant in their own recovery following treatment (Barikbin et al., 2011). In addition, clinicians should impress upon patients that although nonablative fractional laser treatments can yield significant advantages with fewer side effects, their outcomes may not be fully realized for some time. Proper communication in the consultation can effectively align expectations, promoting patient participation and compliance with post-procedure measures. Therefore, a successful consultation not only readies the patients for treatment but also establishes the patients' expectations towards evidence-based outcomes, ultimately optimizing the outcome of the skin resurfacing treatment (Figure 10.15).

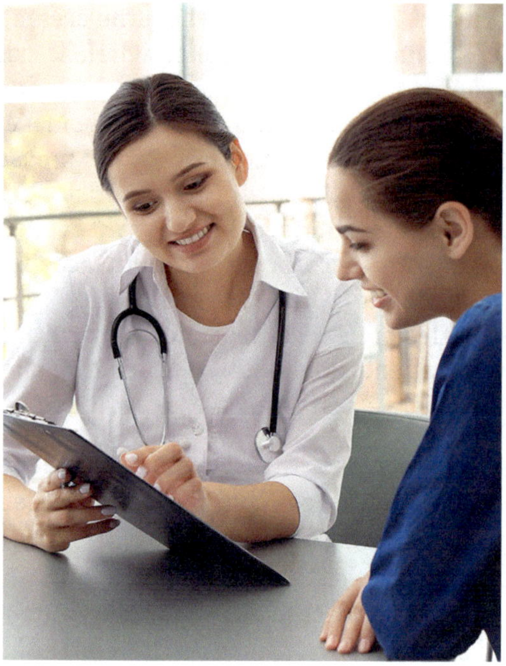

Figure 10.15. Skin assessment and consultation.

Source: https://external-content.duckduckgo.com/iu/?u=https%3A%2F%2Fwww.facetofacemedical.com.au%2Fwp-content%2Fuploads%2F2021%2F12%2Fskin-assessment-and-consultation-613x806.jpg&f=1&nofb=1&ipt=3ecc50dc406449e7aca92f5ee9548ec8406bc293f5b112293a5a0c1ed15e6d57.

10.5.2. Preparing the Skin for Treatment

Proper skin preparation prior to resurfacing of the skin and laser therapy is critical in achieving optimal outcomes as well as minimizing post-procedure complications. Preparatory treatments typically involve a cleansing process that removes excess oils, dirt, and cosmetics from the surface of the skin, allowing active ingredients in treatments to better penetrate deeper within the skin. In addition, skin hydration needs to be ensured, as hydrated skin is stronger and better placed to heal following invasive procedures. Use of serums with antioxidants, such as Vitamin C, can also enhance the skin's health by removing free radicals and giving an even pigmentation, thus making it a more favorable platform for subsequent treatments. Without such a foundation preparation, patients are left with suboptimal outcomes and prolonged recovery periods that compromise the overall efficacy of the skin resurfacing procedure. In addition to good cleansing and hydration, there is a requirement to assess the skin's individual needs in order to individually guide the treatment protocol. Patients with atrophic acne scarring, for instance, can significantly gain from a pre-treatment regimen aimed at maximizing dermal matrix health and integrity. Strategies can entail the application of topical retinoids to promote cell turnover, hence exfoliation and regeneration of the skin. As has been explained in the literature, a multimodal treatment is often necessary to sufficiently correct complex skin problems, such as acne scars, by preparing the skin to receive procedures like chemical peels or laser modalities (Yug et al., 2011). The importance of treatment personalized to the skin cannot be overstressed, as having knowledge about the nature of skin in each patient allows practitioners to customize treatment protocols more effectively and achieve more satisfying outcomes for patients. Finally, patient education plays a very crucial role in skin preparation for resurfacing and laser treatment. Patients need to be well educated about the possible side effects of these treatments and adherence to pre-treatment requirements. For example, avoidance of exposure to the sun, which can raise the risk of complications after treatment, is crucial. Secondly, knowledge of the molecular responses induced by fractionated nonablative laser resurfacing facilitates patient compliance with prep procedures designed to precondition dermal layers to respond favorably to treatment (Alster et al., 2010). Creating open lines of communication and issuing precise instructions on what patients can expect regarding the timeline for change in their skin and healing helps to manage their expectations and create a more rewarding treatment experience. Preparation, therefore, is not an isolated step but an extensive process that maximizes the overall effectiveness of skin resurfacing treatments.

10.5.3. Setting Realistic Expectations

In skin resurfacing and laser treatments, realistic expectations are most crucial for treatment success and patient satisfaction. A majority of patients undergoing these procedures do so on the basis of anticipating picture-perfect skin without understanding the complexities involved. The variable and unpredictable nature of healing of the skin renders the results extremely variable from individual to individual. As was noted in clinical experience, management of expectation is critical; patients must be instructed by clinicians what realistically can be achieved with both invasive and noninvasive therapies. Through the understanding that none of the therapies can guarantee a perfect outcome, the patient can have a better sense of what outcomes and limitations are achievable with skin resurfacing procedures. This realistic expectations platform not only decreases the likelihood of disappointment but also enhances patient-clinician communication during the course of treatment, ultimately leading to more satisfying outcomes on the whole (Chan et al., 2017). Further still, an individual's own skin type, condition, and overall health all play a strong role in determining how successful skin resurfacing and laser procedures can be. These factors necessitate an individualized treatment plan, wherein clinicians evaluate each patient's specific needs and desired outcomes. This broad evaluation includes inspection of the patient's medical history, skin concerns, and cosmetic goals, allowing for an informed treatment plan taking into account both expected benefits and risks. The understanding that treatment is not universal in every patient is the motivation for tailoring interventions to suit individual circumstances. Also, ongoing dialogue between clinician and patient is crucial; as the progress of treatment is achieved, adjustments can be made to fit patients' evolving expectations and outcomes. This back-and-forth process is the foundation for maintaining satisfaction and realistic expectations among patients, which contributes towards making them emotionally well in their aesthetic pursuit (Boulle et al., 2010). Finally, realistic expectations cannot be overlooked psychologically. The majority of patients go into skin resurfacing and laser treatment with preconceived notions from idealized photographs in the media and advertising. These idealized assumptions result in unwarranted expectations and discontentment following therapy. It is therefore important to inform patients that patience and gradual improvement in the skin are of utmost significance for guaranteeing positivity in the healing process. Physicians need to emphasize that progress will be possible, but not immediately and possibly through ongoing therapy to achieve the best effects. By establishing a perception that these therapies are not stand-alone procedures but one aspect of a complete aesthetic strategy, patients are better able to embrace the gradual alteration available in the skin. This emphasis on realistic expectations, qualitative as well as temporal, can be a significant consideration in offering long-term happiness and well-being to those patients who are being treated with these new dermatologic therapies (Boulle et al., 2010).

Test Your Knowledge

1. What key factors should be evaluated during a skin assessment and consultation before choosing a resurfacing or laser treatment?
2. How should patients prepare their skin prior to treatment to minimize risks and enhance outcomes?

10.6. Post-Treatment Care

Learning Outcome

1. Discuss the Immediate Aftercare Instructions
2. Focus on Long-term Skincare Regimen
3. Explain Monitoring for Adverse Reactions

Post-treatment care in laser treatments and skin resurfacing cannot be overemphasized, as it dictates healing outcomes and overall patient satisfaction. During the initial recovery phase, the patients typically experience varying degrees of redness, swelling, and pain in the treated areas. To offset such effects, practitioners typically recommend specific post-procedure care protocols, for example, careful cleaning and use of prescribed creams for healing. Maintaining a clean and humid environment can significantly enhance the skins healing and regeneration processes. Also, compliance with post-treatment instructions and guidelines will help prevent complications like infection or scarring that can impair the cosmetic results achieved from laser treatments. In turn, adherence to post-treatment is necessary to ensure that patients achieve their best recovery and satisfaction with skin resurfacing procedures. Also, sun protection is an integral part of post-treatment treatment that needs immediate attention following skin resurfacing or laser treatments to prevent trauma to recovering skin. Patients are usually advised to avoid direct sun and use broad-spectrum sunscreen strictly, since treated skin is particularly sensitive to ultraviolet. Curiously, exposure to intense sunlight has the potential to produce hyperpigmentation, undermining the very outcome that the treatment has been intended to achieve. Consequently, dermatologists usually stress the use of protective apparel and shade in sunny times until full healing is achieved. Education on the potential dangers of UV exposure in addition to the appropriate application of sun protection measures is a part of the post-treatment regimen. Hence, creating such sun-safe habits not only safeguards the skin but also enhances the longevity of the treatment results. Furthermore, follow-up communication with the healthcare team becomes important during the post-treatment period in order to address any issues or complications arising. Follow-up visits are scheduled for patients, where practitioners can observe healing patterns and make interventions early on in case any issues are noted. This forward-thinking process allows practitioners to alter care habits, like recommending supplemental treatment or adapting skin care plans. The significance of this interaction is underlined by the complexity of skin healing and the variability of individual responses to treatment. Ultimately, the goal of full post-treatment care is to promote optimal healing, allow optimal aesthetic outcomes, and have patients supported with the recovery process (Branney et al., 2011; Youngerwood, 2012) (Figure 10.16).

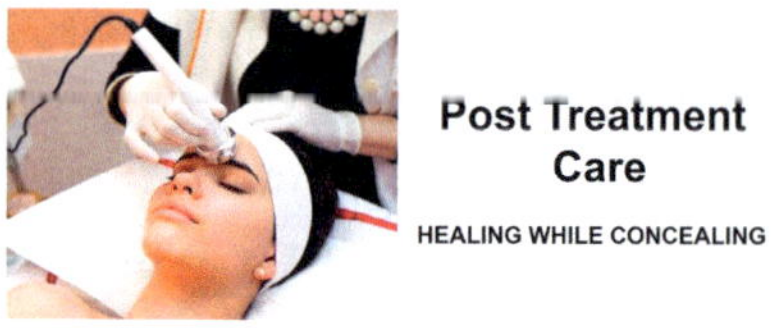

Figure 10.16. The significance of post-treatment care.

Source: https://www.inclinic.com.au/image/cache/catalog/Blog/Post%20Treatment%20Care%20Banner-1140x379.jpg.

10.6.1. Immediate Aftercare Instructions

Following skin resurfacing and laser procedures, instant aftercare instruction is crucial for optimal healing and outcomes. Patients are generally directed to keep the treated region clean and moisturized, preventing infection and promoting healing of the skin. Gentle cleansing with a bland, non-irritating soap is generally recommended, being careful not to scrub or apply harsh exfoliants. One must also apply an appropriate post-procedure cream or moisturizer as instructed by the clinician. These initial measures enable hydration and create the optimal setting for regeneration of the skin. Lacking proper aftercare, the patient may develop delayed redness, swelling, or even jeopardize the aesthetic outcome that they are seeking through such advanced modalities. Thus, the need for compliance with post-treatment regimens assumes greater significance. Sun protection is an integral component of the immediate post-skin resurfacing aftercare. The skin, after having been exposed to the process of resurfacing, is highly sensitive and at greater risk for hyperpigmentation if it is exposed to ultraviolet (UV) light. Doctors often recommend the use of a broad-spectrum sunscreen with SPF 30 or higher in order to minimize such a risk. Moreover, patients are typically not recommended direct sun exposure, with protective attire or avoiding shade outside. This protection is most crucial in the early recovery phase as the new, healed skin is still vulnerable. According to compromise presented in various clinical guidelines, behavior of sun protection has notable effects on the overall efficacy of laser treatments and can avoid re-appearance of improvement in texture and tone of the skin (Gauglitz et al., 2021). Also, patients should be aware of potential side effects and signs of complications that can arise after the treatment. The immediate post-treatment care involves monitoring the skin for any unusual reaction, such as swelling, redness, or infection, like pus or a foul smell. Under such circumstances, early consultation with the doctor who performed the treatment is the first order of business to attend to the issue. In addition, instructions may include precautions against strenuous exercise and perspiration for an interval of time, allowing the skin to heal with minimum stress. Including these detailed immediate aftercare instructions can bring about significant enhancements in outcomes from treatment and patient satisfaction and underscores education at this critical stage of healing (Giroux et al., 2019).

10.6.2. Long-term Skincare Regimen

A solid long-term skincare regimen is paramount in maximizing the results of skin resurfacing and laser treatments. These state-of-the-art treatments, as effective as they are in refining the skin, also require proper post-treatment care in order to maintain effects and prevent complications. The reepithelization time following laser treatments typically takes 8–42 days, whereby patients are typically advised to maintain their regular skincare routine using active elements such as antioxidants and retinoids. Surprisingly, over 76% of dermatology experts advise doing so, citing its value in stimulating skin regeneration and health following treatment, as quoted in the findings of a recent study (Al-Niaimi et al., 2025). Moreover, personalized skincare regimens enhance treatment outcomes, particularly in patients with variable Fitzpatrick skin types, whose reaction to resurfacing may be varied. Further, the incorporation of adjunct treatments into a complete skincare program maximizes the outcome yielded by laser therapy. As also indicated by over 81% of the dermatologists surveyed, incorporation of adjunct therapies, i.e., neuromodulators and Intense Pulsed Light Therapy, can aid in the global improvement of the outcome of skin resurfacing. The adjunctive treatments are particularly beneficial in addressing particular skin concerns, e.g., laxity or uneven tone, providing an improved treatment modality for skin well-being (Al-Niaimi et al., 2025). This holistic methodology not only takes care of short-term beauty requirements but also contributes to long-term skin well-being and resilience, hypothesizing the interaction among laser treatments and daily skincare as synergistic, prolongation of effects, and minimizing potential side effects. Lastly, the role of education and training within the domain of skincare cannot be emphasized enough. Because the art of somatology is now also encompassing a broader focus, that of beauty and consequences on health, professional continuing education is necessary. The professionals in this field, including dermatologists, somatologists, and skincare experts, must stay up to date with the best practices and newest trends if they are to be able to deliver the best results for patients undergoing laser treatment. A report highlighted the necessity of continuous training and updated curricula to stay current with industry developments and develop stronger referral networks among medical practitioners and skincare specialists. Not only do these proactive steps enhance the efficacy of long-term skin regimens, but they also sustain the importance of coordinated care to achieve long-term skin health results.

10.6.3. Monitoring for Adverse Reactions

In the area of laser therapy and skin resurfacing, monitoring for side effects is a vital aspect of ensuring the safety of the patient while also allowing for desired outcomes. Laser treatments, although largely successful in treating most dermatologic syndromes, have risks intrinsic to them that need close follow-up and monitoring. Physicians must vigilantly monitor both the immediate and delayed reactions, i.e., erythema and edema, as well as occasionally more severe events such as scarring or post-inflammatory hyperpigmentation. Developing a systematic process for monitoring these side effects not only increases patient satisfaction but also enables the identification of trends that may indicate bigger issues in treatment processes, as found in existing literature for the regulatory framework in laser use in cosmetics (Youngerwood, 2012). Patient education forms the core of preventive monitoring for adverse reactions to skin resurfacing. Engaging patients in dialogue regarding the potential side effects before treatment informs them of their individual risk profiles and allows them to recognize early complications. If patients are aware of what to look out for during the recovery period, they are more likely to report abnormal symptoms in a timely fashion, allowing for prompt medical intervention. The process emphasizes the importance of patient outcomes and experience being recorded and utilized to accumulate a database of evidence to further develop treatment processes. There is evidence presented in recent studies that well-educated patients have fewer long-term adverse effects since they are likely to adhere to recommended aftercare processes and inform health practitioners of any fearful symptoms in due time (Cuomo et al., 2024). Finally, clinical follow-up should be stressed as much as possible in monitoring for adverse reactions from laser treatment. Regular post-treatment consultations allow medical professionals to observe the healing process and readily address any complications that may occur. These follow-ups not only allow practitioners to measure the efficacy of treatments, but also the quality of patient satisfaction and overall quality of life improvement. These assessments are important in bridging the gap between clinical effectiveness and patient care. By offering a forum where feedback is given and addressed, practitioners can modify their techniques and protocols, thus enhancing outcomes and safety in laser treatment and skin resurfacing procedures, underscored as imperative by the rising debates over regulation in this increasingly dynamic industry (Youngerwood, 2012).

Test Your Knowledge

1. What immediate aftercare steps should patients follow to promote healing and reduce irritation after skin resurfacing or laser treatment?
2. How can a long-term skincare regimen support and maintain the results of resurfacing procedures?

SUMMARY

We are able to identify that fractional ablative and non-ablative laser technology are both viable options for improvement in the appearance of skin, with particular application in the treatment of acne scars. Research has indicated that while fractional CO_2 lasers have slightly more efficacy, erbium-doped glass non-ablative laser provides a strong alternative due to their lower discomfort and quicker recovery rates. In general, patient satisfaction with the two treatments would be a measure of efficacy and safety of the two, suggesting a two-way option for the candidates seeking skin rejuvenation therapy. The heterogeneity in the efficacy of the therapy further emphasizes the importance of customized treatment in clinical practice, such that the patient's expectation is met with the appropriate treatment (Elsaie et al., 2017). Moreover, non-invasive treatment technologies have significantly revolutionized dermatology practices, with various forms emerging that are patient safety and satisfaction-focused. Chemical peeling, Intense Pulse Light (IPL), and radiofrequency treatments all join laser treatments, offering diverse options depending on individual patient needs. A claimed 40% rise in the use of minimally invasive techniques since 2021 further reiterates the growing trend towards less onerous procedures in the realms of recovery and complication rates for traditional plastic surgery procedures. The shift not only reflects changing patient tastes but also toward the efficacy of modern aesthetic treatments that utilize new technology and methodologies (Timraz et al., 2025). Briefly, the landscape of laser resurfacing and treatments is one of tremendous advances in patient results as well as technique. Fractional ablative and non-ablative laser comparisons enhance our knowledge base of their respective roles in the treatment of skin imperfections, and the development of non-invasive procedures provides practitioners with additional modalities to more effectively treat patients. Lastly, ongoing research and innovations in these fields are required in order to advance methods, improve patient safety, and increase overall satisfaction, in the end making it simpler for patients to make more informed decisions about skin rejuvenation procedures. Ongoing studies will be pivotal in continuing to evaluate outcomes and patient acceptance, contributing further to dermatological aesthetic innovation (Elsaie et al., 2017; Timraz et al., 2025).

In recent years, laser and skin resurfacing treatments have become very popular as highly efficient solutions for skin problems and improving the overall appearance of the skin. Using these cutting-edge technologies, the minimally invasive and non-invasive treatments leverage the advantages of these techniques to revitalize the skin, decrease the visibility of imperfections, and stimulate collagen formation. In light of recent advances, cosmetic procedures such as laser therapy and intense pulsed light treatment enhance the cosmetic value of the skin while at the same time playing a therapeutic function in conditions such as actinic keratosis (AK). The latter, symbolized by prolonged ultraviolet radiation exposure, calls for comprehensive treatment that addresses discrete lesions as well as global damage to the skin, which is characteristic of affected areas (Anliker et al., 2014). In addition, the use of non-ionizing radiation (NIR) technology in cosmetic treatment attests to the wide array of advantages such treatment has to offer. These modalities include laser technologies, LED therapy, and electromagnetic field treatments that serve different aesthetic objectives, such as skin remodeling, body reshaping, and scar reduction. Of particular interest, though early research on these technologies has centered on their effectiveness, consideration should also be given to potential side effects that occur. It is reported that minor reactions such as swelling and erythema may be encountered by the patients, but there is always a risk of severe effects such as burns or pigmentary changes, particularly in vulnerable populations (International Commission on Non-Ionizing Radiation Protection, 2020). Thus, practitioners must weigh the risk-benefit ratio before prescribing such treatments. Clinicians must stay abreast of the constantly changing landscape of guidelines and best practices in treating skin resurfacing and laser therapy. The Working Group of the Swiss Registry of Actinic Keratosis Treatment (REAKT) releases helpful clinical practice guidelines that assist healthcare clinicians with making informed decisions about the treatment of AK and related skin damage commonly described as field cancerization. These recommendations stress a patient-specific treatment approach, taking into account patient-specific factors, individual risk estimation, and preventive measures. Clearly, an evidence-based and multidisciplinary treatment approach is needed in order to obtain the best long-term results for patients undergoing laser treatments and skin resurfacing (Anliker et al., 2014). Finally, ongoing research and surveillance by the regulating bodies will be the determining factor in assuring the safety and effectiveness of these increasingly popular cosmetic treatments.

KEY TERMS FROM THIS CHAPTER

- Ablative Laser
- Fractional Resurfacing
- Er:YAG Laser
- Fluence
- Wavelength
- Dermal Remodeling
- Photothermolysis
- Microdermabrasion
- Non-Ablative Laser
- CO_2 Laser
- Laser Parameters
- Pulse Duration
- Epidermal Ablation
- Collagen Stimulation
- Chemical Peels
- Radiofrequency Resurfacing

CRITICAL THINKING QUESTIONS

1. **The primary goal of skin resurfacing procedures is to:**
   a. Increase skin oil production
   b. Improve texture and reduce wrinkles
   c. Reduce bone prominence
   d. Lighten hair color
2. **Ablative lasers work by:**
   a. Stimulating melanocytes
   b. Vaporizing water in epidermal and dermal tissues
   c. Increasing collagen thickness only
   d. Shrinking sebaceous glands
3. **Which laser is considered an ablative resurfacing laser?**
   a. Nd:YAG 1064 nm
   b. CO_2 laser 10,600 nm
   c. Pulsed dye laser
   d. Alexandrite laser
4. **Er:YAG laser is preferred over CO_2 laser for:**
   a. Deep dermal resurfacing
   b. Lower risk of thermal damage
   c. Tattoo removal
   d. Hair removal
5. **The principle behind laser therapy known as "selective photothermolysis" refers to:**
   a. Destroying all skin layers
   b. Targeting specific chromophores using light energy
   c. Increasing sebum production
   d. Cooling the tissue before heating

Short Answer Questions

1. What is the primary goal of skin resurfacing procedures in facial cosmetic practice?
2. How do ablative lasers differ from non-ablative lasers in terms of tissue effects?
3. What is the principle of selective photothermolysis in laser treatments?
4. What skin conditions can be effectively treated with fractional laser technology?
5. How does chemical peeling differ from laser resurfacing in mechanism of action?

Answers to Critical Thinking Questions

1. (b) 2. (b) 3. (b) 4. (b) 5. (b)

REFERENCES

1. Ahn, Banzhaf, Bernstein, Brown, Calzavara-Pinton, Catalano, Gangatirkar, et al. (2016). *Quantitative monitoring of laser-treated engineered skin using optical coherence tomography*. https://core.ac.uk/download/79708971.pdf (accessed on 14th July 2025).
2. Timraz, J. H., Bakour, H. A., Samman, R. R., Alawi, K. M., Bava, F. S. M., Alkhdaidi, F. A., AlGhorab, M. A., Alabbassi, M. A., Thalib, H. I., Khan, S., Makki, F., & Alsolamy, A. (2025). Advancements in Non-Invasive Plastic Surgery Techniques: Evaluating Efficacy, Safety, Patient Outcomes and Potential Complications. *South Eastern European Journal of Public Health*, 4078–4099. https://doi.org/10.70135/seejph.vi.5983 (accessed on 14th July 2025).
3. Allemann, B., & Kaufman, J. (2018). *Fractional Photothermolysis—An Update*. https://core.ac.uk/download/159154189.pdf (accessed on 14th July 2025).
4. Al-Niaimi, F., Artzi, O., Beachkofsky, T. M., Biesman, et al. (2025). *Expert consensus on clinical recommendations for fractional ablative CO_2 laser, in facial skin rejuvenation treatment*. https://core.ac.uk/download/624140100.pdf (accessed on 14th July 2025).
5. Alster, Alster, Bak, Falanga, Goldberg, Karimipour, Karimipour, et al. (2010). *Molecular mechanisms of nonablative fractionated laser resurfacing*. http://deepblue.lib.umich.edu/bitstream/2027.42/79267/1/j.1365-2133.2010.09998.x.pdf (accessed on 14th July 2025).
6. Ambrosio, D. V. (2018). *Incidence and need of advanced aesthetic somatology in South Africa*. https://core.ac.uk/download/222968033.pdf (accessed on 14th July 2025).
7. Amoruso, G. F., Belletti, S., Bennardo, L., Fusco, I., Madeddu, F., Nistico, S. P., Provenzano, E. (2023). *An innovative dual-wavelength laser technique for atrophic acne scar management: A pilot study*. https://core.ac.uk/download/614035653.pdf (accessed on 14th July 2025).
8. Anliker, M., Boehncke, W. H., Brand, C., Braun, et al. (2014). *Swiss clinical practice guidelines on field cancerization of the skin*. https://core.ac.uk/download/77197804.pdf (accessed on 14th July 2025).
9. Arunachalam, M., Bassi, A., Bonan, P., Bruscino, et al. (2012). *Highlights of thirty-year experience of CO2 laser use at the Florence (Italy) Department of Dermatology*. https://core.ac.uk/download/pdf/8724335.pdf (accessed on 14th July 2025).
10. Baldin, G. C., & Liedtke, F. S. (2023). *Use of ablative fractional CO2 laser in facial rejuvenation: A prospective observational cohort study*. https://core.ac.uk/download/622811929.pdf (accessed on 14th July 2025).
11. Barikbin, B., Ghavam, S. A., Karimi, S., Moravvej, et al. (2011). *Nonablative Fractional Laser Resurfacing*. https://core.ac.uk/download/483636065.pdf (accessed on 14th July 2025).
12. Bennardo, L., Cannarozzo, G., Fusco, I., Magni, G., Nistico, S. P., Pieri, L., Rossi, F., et al. (2022). *Synergistic sequential emission of fractional 10.600 and 1540 nm lasers for skin resurfacing: An ex vivo histological evaluation*. https://core.ac.uk/download/592025060.pdf (accessed on 14th July 2025).
13. Boone, B., Creytens, D., De Schepper, S., Genouw, et al. (2018). *Laser-assisted photodynamic therapy for superficial basal cell carcinoma and Bowen's disease: A randomized intrapatient comparison between a continuous and a fractional ablative CO_2 laser mode*. https://core.ac.uk/download/157573232.pdf (accessed on 14th July 2025).

14. Bowler P. J. (2009). Impact on facial rejuvenation with dermatological preparations. *Clinical interventions in aging, 4*, 81–89. https://doi.org/10.2147/cia.s3524(accessed on 14th July 2025).

15. Branney, P., Eardley, I., & Witty, K. (2011). *Patients' Experiences of Penile Cancer*. https://core.ac.uk/download/29018642.pdf (accessed on 14th July 2025).

16. Cannarozzo, G., Chiricozzi, A., Morini, C., Nisticò, et al. (2014). *Deep pulse fractional CO_2 laser combined with a radiofrequency system: Results of a case series*. https://core.ac.uk/download/80267194.pdf (accessed on 14th July 2025).

17. Carniol, E. T., Carniol, P. J., & Hamilton, M. M. (2015). *Current Status of Fractional Laser Resurfacing*. https://core.ac.uk/download/46962931.pdf (accessed on 14th July 2025).

18. Chan, Chan, Collawn, Fisher, Geronemus, Hun Lee, Jih, et al. (2009). *Fractional laser photothermolysis for treatment of facial wrinkles in Asians*. https://core.ac.uk/download/pdf/8356817.pdf (accessed on 14th July 2025).

19. Chan, D., Ducic, Y., Jategaonkar, A., Kadakia, et al. (2017). *Scar Revision: Surgical and Nonsurgical Options*. https://core.ac.uk/download/160494272.pdf (accessed on 14th July 2025).

20. Cuomo, R., Han, J., Hou, S., Lv, et al. (2024). *Treatment of atrophic acne scarring with fractional microplasma radiofrequency: A multicentric experience*. https://core.ac.uk/download/618720889.pdf (accessed on 14th July 2025).

21. De Boulle, K., Fagien, S., Glogau, R., Sommer, et al. (2010). *Treating glabellar lines with botulinum toxin type A-hemagglutinin complex: A review of the science, the clinical data, and patient satisfaction*. https://core.ac.uk/download/pdf/8403709.pdf (accessed on 14th July 2025).

22. Madnani, N., Vedmurthy, M., Parthasarthi, A., Dhawan, S., Kandhari, R., Pillai, R., & Nischal, K. C. (2022). Expert opinion on pre and post procedure care in aesthetic dermatology. *International Journal of Research in Medical Sciences, 10*(4), 991–1000. https://doi.org/10.18203/2320-6012.ijrms20220999(accessed on 14th July 2025).

23. Doorn, M. B. A. van, Greveling, K., Prens, E. P., ten Bosch, et al. (2017). *Comparison of lidocaine/tetracaine cream and lidocaine/prilocaine cream for local anesthesia during laser treatment of acne keloidalis nuchae and tattoo removal: Results of two randomized controlled trials*. https://core.ac.uk/download/154410899.pdf (accessed on 14th July 2025).

24. Elsaie, M., Ibrahim, S. M., & Saudi, W. (2017). *Ablative fractional 10,600 nm carbon dioxide laser versus non-ablative fractional 1540 nm erbium-glass laser in Egyptian post-acne scar patients*. https://core.ac.uk/download/483636308.pdf (accessed on 14th July 2025).

25. Ferara, N., Franceschi, N., Šitum Čeprnja, Z., Šitum, et al. (2024). *Treatment of actinic keratoses and field cancerization – Croatian perspective*. https://core.ac.uk/download/620817167.pdf (accessed on 14th July 2025).

26. Gauglitz, G. G., Middelkoop, E., Mustoe, T. A., & Téot, et al. (2021). *Textbook on Scar Management*. https://core.ac.uk/download/478135440.pdf (accessed on 14th July 2025).

27. Giroux, P. A., Hersant, B., La Padula, S., Meningaud, J. P., Pizza, C., & SidAhmed-Mezi, M. (2019). *The outcomes assessment of the plasma blade technology in upper blepharoplasties: A prospective study on a series of 25 patients*. https://core.ac.uk/download/541661638.pdf (accessed on 14th July 2025).

28. Halim, A. S., & Yan, T. K. (2016). *Treatment modalities for hyperpigmented skin lesions: A brief overview*. https://core.ac.uk/download/132566787.pdf (accessed on 14th July 2025).

29. International Commission on Non-Ionizing Radiation Protection. (2020). *Intended human exposure to non-ionizing radiation for cosmetic purposes*. https://core.ac.uk/download/552405446.pdf (accessed on 14th July 2025).

30. Vosloo, M. (2025). *A framework to position the somatology profession in South Africa*. https://core.ac.uk/download/222966444.pdf (accessed on 14th July 2025).

31. Youngerwood, A. (2012). *From creams to lasers: Regulating the beauty industry in the new millennium*. https://core.ac.uk/download/28938988.pdf (accessed on 14th July 2025).

32. Yug, A., Chapas, A. M., Layton, A. M., Mendelson, B. C., Jacob, C. I., Collier, C. N., Hanke, C. W., et al. (2011). *Multimodal Management of Atrophic Acne Scarring in the Aging Face*. https://core.ac.uk/download/pdf/8656199.pdf (accessed on 14th July 2025).

PRINCIPLES OF FACIAL RECONSTRUCTION

11

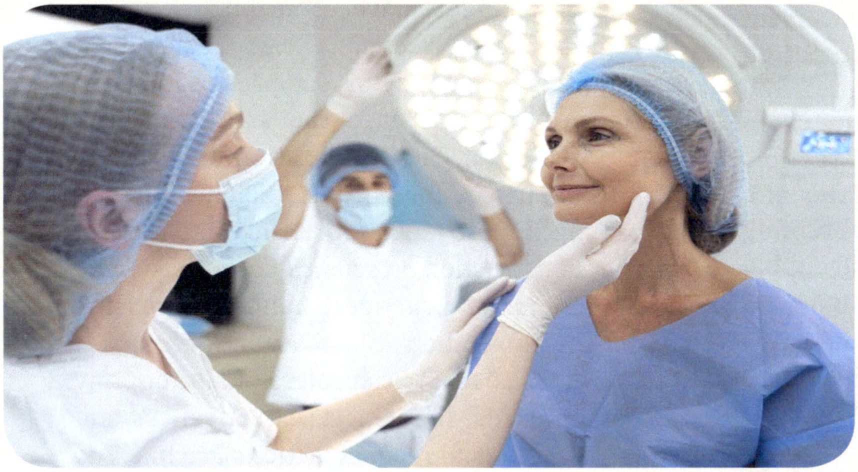

Introduction

Facial reconstruction is a critical area of study and practice with a collection of techniques to bring back the shape and function of the face following trauma, congenital defects, or medical conditions. Facial reconstruction has evolved significantly due to advances in surgical methods, technologies, and knowledge regarding facial anatomy. Because the face is the focal area of human identity and expression, not only does the reconstructive surgery correct the physical deformity, but it also restores the individual's psychological well-being. Facial reconstruction, furthermore, is founded on the holistic study of the anatomical structures, the integration of dynamics, and the individually tailored application of various reconstructive methods based on the patient's specific requirements. Among many challenges inherent in facial reconstruction, the treatment of irreversible facial paralysis is of great concern. It is characterized by the loss of mimetic muscle tone and function, delivering a serious social and psychological impact to patients. Restoration of facial motion and expression has been made possible by employing

LEARNING OBJECTIVES

After studying this chapter, you will be able to:

1. Discuss the science of facial reconstruction;
2. Describe the methods of facial reconstruction;
3. Highlight applications of facial reconstruction;
4. Know ethical considerations;
5. Deal with challenges in facial reconstruction;
6. Learn about future directions in facial reconstruction.

dynamic facial reanimation techniques, which are vital to interpersonal communication and self-image. While a vast amount of literature has been published regarding such new techniques, a thorough review of the methodologies and respective musculature for dynamic reanimation is absent. This lack warrants deeper investigation and documentation of the field of facial reconstruction for the aim of facilitating accurate and effective treatment processes in irreversible facial paralysis patients, as per the respective literature (Schutte et al., 2025). The advancement of three-dimensional (3D) reconstruction technology has completely transformed the practice of facial reconstruction with more accuracy and personalization in reconstruction. Techniques such as photometric stereo and shape-from-shading are pivotal to obtaining extremely accurate facial models capturing the uniqueness of patients. 3D reconstruction is not only aesthetically appealing but also has applications in biometrics, medicine, and even in cybersecurity. However, challenges to be overcome exist, including occlusion management and facial expression changes that can interfere with effective modeling. Despite these obstacles, ongoing research into real-time use and ethical considerations reflects the potential of 3D technology to transform facial reconstruction methods. Ultimately, integrating these advanced methods into proven reconstructive principles may pave the way for improved treatments and improved patient outcomes in facial rehabilitation (Suo, 2023).

Definition of Facial Reconstruction

Facial reconstruction is an interdisciplinary technique that merges science and art to restore the face of human beings using skeletal remains. Facial reconstruction is a crucial aspect of forensic science that is applied primarily to assist in the identification of unidentified deceased persons. The method employs anatomical data, forensic anthropology, and artistic skill to produce a three-dimensional representation of the face that can be instrumental in solving criminal cases or reacting to missing persons cases. By employing a working model created out of available anatomical landmarks, forensic artists can generate a reconstruction for efficient identification. This is necessary due to the criticism usually associated with forensic science, particularly those relying on artist interpretations, which can be rejected as being subjective.

Several models have come into existence to regulate facial reconstruction procedures, highlighting the need for set procedures and guidelines that increase the validity of the results achieved. The Organization of Scientific Area Committees for Forensic Science (OSAC) gives emphasis to basing forensic methods like facial reconstruction on science-based reasoning and established practices, hence addressing criticisms about the subjectivity in forensic art (Casey et al., 2018). With professionals adopting these standards, the general effectiveness and credibility of facial reconstructions are likely to improve, maintaining the discipline's position in the scientific community. Besides, the advancement of facial reconstruction has also been problematic for its status within forensic art and the requirement of strict training and ethics by practitioners. Representational issues within facial reconstructions suggest an area of fine line between artistic license and fact-based representation, raising questions about professional responsibility and the establishment of best practices. Ongoing criticism of the discipline functions as encouragement for continual research and development to establish its validity within forensic science (Wilkinson, 2025). Ongoing debate also highlights the importance of reaching a consensus regarding the definitions, methods, and standards upon which facial reconstruction is conducted. In consideration of such arguments, they revolve around facial reconstruction's potential to move from a controversial practice to an esteemed and legitimized forensic science, eventually confirming its worth in legal proceedings and public safety measures (Figure 11.1).

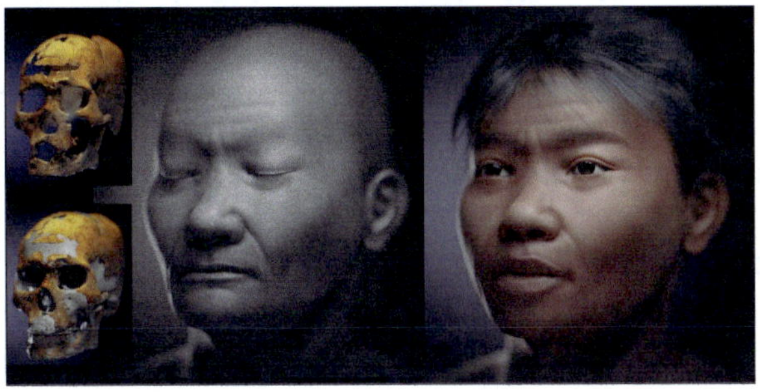

Figure 11.1. Facial reconstruction.

Source: https://external-content.duckduckgo.com/iu/?u=https%3A%2F%2Fgreekreporter.com%2Fwp-content%2Fuploads%2F2023%2F02%2Fthe-lifelike-face-of-zuzu-a-man-who-lived-9600-years-ago-credit-moacir-elias-santos-and-cicero-moraes.jpg&f=1&nofb=1&ipt=383e5d1817b0f3dc2854f7ec2461a3d091fb71938716afca5a260820ba42057e.

Historical Context and Significance

History has firmly rooted facial reconstruction in past practices and conceptions regarding human anatomy and identity. The origins of modern facial reconstruction trace back to early scientific endeavors when pioneers like Sir Francis Galton and Thomas Troward tried to account for the physical representation of human characteristics. This fascination with the human face not only laid the ground for reconstructive procedures but also illuminated the intersection of science, culture, and ethics. The significant historical conflicts, particularly in the times of United States positivist criminology, impacted the concept of identity and the application of scientific methods for analyzing individuals based on their physical characteristics. Thus, the history explains how cultural perspectives about appearance have evolved over time, reflecting broader cultural themes about justice, morality, and human nature (Burton, 2019). In the later evolution of facial reconstruction methods, the historic importance of forensic science breakthroughs cannot be exaggerated. The processes utilized in facial reconstruction in the late 20th and early 21st centuries, especially through the use of digital technologies, are a reflection of how innovation sat side by side with the eternal desire for accuracy in the representation of human likenesses. This shift can be discussed in the context of the ongoing debate regarding equal protection and the way marginalized communities are treated, as indicated by legal transformations questioning facial recognition and biometric technology.

Facial reconstruction is thus not simply a duplication of a scientific process but is also embedded with societal effects at a broader level, revealing how reconstruction methods can inadvertently result in stereotypes or social prejudices arising due to their historical background (Lau et al., 2017). Furthermore, facial reconstruction's importance extends beyond purely forensic application into social identity and representation. Group-wide understandings of identity, difference, and reconstructive technology's meaning in society have been shaped by the history of such practices. Anatomical correctness is paramount, yet the ethical value and conditions of facial reconstruction bring with them questions of authenticity and representation in a multicultural society. The way in which facial characteristics are read and reconstructed typically reflects the dominant prejudices and values of a time. This historical backdrop sheds light on the more profound ramifications of facial reconstruction, to the point of pursuing a critical examination of the influence of such procedures on the cultural and legal representation of identity, hence forming a contextual awareness of justice and representation in contemporary society (Burton, 2019Lau et al., 2017; Burton, 2019).

11.1. The Science of Facial Reconstruction

Learning Outcome

1. Discus the Anatomy of the Human Face
2. Explain Role of Forensic Science in Reconstruction
3. Focus on Techniques Used in Facial Reconstruction

Facial reconstruction is a science that surfs the wave of technology, anatomy, and art, and has a great example of how the three cooperate. The science can begin with the study of the skeletal part of the subject, which is a first-hand observation of the underlying bones that would guide the reconstructive process. Forensic anthropologists and artists utilize standard anatomical measurements to position features like the nose, eyes, and mouth with great accuracy. This attention to detail is a pointer to how important anatomical accuracy is, as misplaced features can result in unrealistic facial renderings. The application of imaging technology has also transformed this area, making it possible to achieve more accuracy when reconstructing facial features from bones. However, anatomical guidelines by themselves cannot properly mimic the nuances of individual facial characteristics, particularly soft tissue variations due to genetics and the environment. Incorporating technological innovations has increasingly become crucial in facial reconstruction. Three-dimensional modeling software, combined with digital imaging, has revolutionized the accuracy and efficiency of reconstructive techniques. Techniques such as 3D printing have emerged as potential tools in the creation of realistic physical models that can be used for crime investigation or education. These technologies enable specialists to produce more accurate facial representations from skull morphology, thus offering higher-quality reconstructions. With biometric facial recognition technology continually advancing, it is essential to understand how technology can be applied during facial reconstruction. The growing body of works in the literature emphasizes the need for cross-disciplinary research between computer science, legal studies, and forensic science to improve the accuracy and application of automated forensic facial comparison systems, especially since current automatic systems remain far from achieving acceptable quality for court admissibility, as noted in current writings on forensic identification systems (Ali et al., 2010).

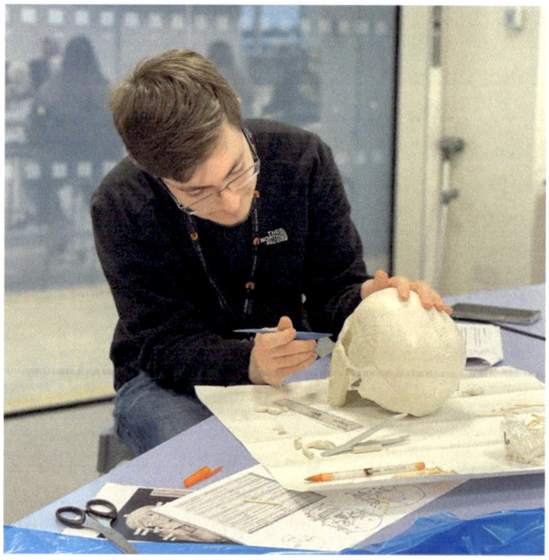

Figure 11.2. Science of facial reconstruction.

Source: https://external-content.duckduckgo.com/iu/?u=https%3A%2F%2Fwrexham.ac.uk%2Fmedia%2Fmarketing%2Fscience%2FFacial-Reconstruction.jpg&f=1&nofb=1&ipt=78d8bfaa71b45ccf6707ef1cf930c0f01d1cec8bdcd49b55368b4335c0295022.

One major consideration for evaluating the success of facial reconstruction is the realism with which such depictions can provide the appearance of an individual. Deep learning techniques, most especially in feature learning, have been revolutionary in providing facelifts to the capabilities of facial recognition systems and reconstructions. Compared to previous techniques that require massive amounts of data to learn, recent breakthroughs in transfer learning present new solutions for bridging data availability gaps. Through access to constraints in the target domain, researchers can make reconstructions more faithful by ensuring that aspects learned through more robust datasets can be appropriately transferred to more specific cases and therefore transcend the confines inherent in practitioners ' ability to handle in the forensic context (Ji et al., 2017). This approach not only improves the fidelity of facial reconstruction efforts but also lends further momentum to the growing use of technological innovation to improve results in forensic science, highlighting the need for ongoing research and interdisciplinarity (Figure 11.2).

11.1.1. Anatomy of the Human Face

Human face anatomy involves the intricate organization of structures that make up both functional and cosmetic characteristics. The human face consists mainly of the skull, which contains facial bones such as the maxilla, mandible, nasal bones, and zygomatic arches. These bones create the support upon which the overlying soft tissues lie, such as muscles responsible for facial expression, fat pads that add contour, and the dermal layers required for skin integrity. Understanding of this anatomic configuration is significant to reconstructive surgery because alterations in these support structures are of enormous potential to affect appearance and function. Considering that facial reconstruction typically works towards restoring the functional and aesthetic integrity of such areas, a sound understanding of the underlying anatomy becomes critical for successful outcomes in surgical procedures (Mohapatra et al., 2023). Besides the skeletal structure, facial vascular and neural structures are equally important in facial reconstruction. The face is well supplied with blood vessels and nerves that not only give nutrients to the tissues but also sensory functions and motor controls for expressions. Facial nerve and branches, for instance, innervate various muscles that facilitate facial expressions, while blood vessels supply adequate oxygenation and nutrients to these vital areas. The interplay between innervation, musculature, and facial vascularity is key to success in any reconstructive surgery. Interfering with the relationship between them leads to complications such as necrosis or impaired sensation.

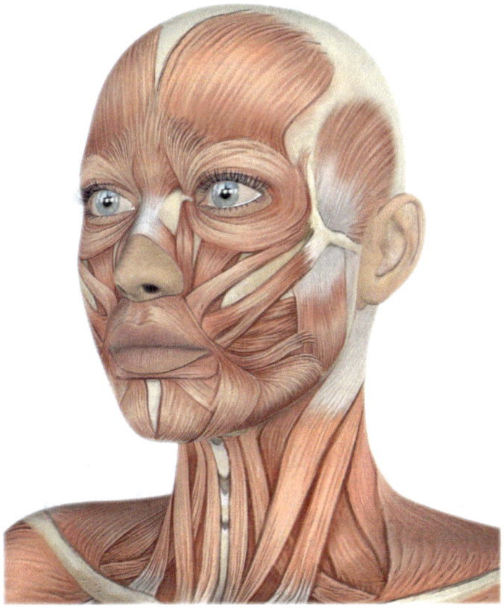

Figure 11.3. Anatomy of the human face.

Source: https://img.freepik.com/free-photo/3d-head-with-muscles_1048-4722.jpg?semt=ais_hybrid&w=740.

For this reason, reconstructive surgeons have to be highly knowledgeable about the vascular and neural relationships to enable them to optimize healing and preserve facial function (Burrows et al., 2011). Another important component of facial anatomy beneficial for reconstruction is the concept of aesthetic subunits, which are beneficial in facial restoration of appearance. The face is made up of recognizable regions that are beneficial in delineating the symmetry and proportion necessary in aesthetic achievement.

Surgeons like to use these subunits, such as the upper, middle, and lower thirds of the face, even specific areas such as the nose, cheeks, and chin, in an effort to plan interventions. It can be seen within many reconstructive methods, from flap techniques to skin grafts, which attempt to harmonize the reconstructed areas with the surrounding tissue. Alongside this, considering the role of evolutionary adaptation, for instance, the relationship between the shape of the face and functional need, will be more effective in reconstruction. Surgeons are able to provide results that can restore form along with function in facial reconstruction by correlating surgical habits with these anatomical and aesthetic needs (Mohapatra et al., 2023) (Figure 11.3).

11.1.2. Role of Forensic Science in Reconstruction

In forensic science, the reconstruction of facial features to accurately represent a key aspect in the identification of missing or unidentified persons when trauma or decomposition is extensive. Forensic facial reconstruction employs an application of scientific technique and artistic skill to create a likeness that can aid in the identification of witnesses or relatives. This process typically begins with a study of the skeletal remains, with the forensic anthropologists providing valuable information concerning the shape and size of the skull. The reconstruction is heavily dependent on empirical data regarding soft tissue thickness, which varies from individual to individual according to age, gender, and ethnicity, making the likeness as realistic as possible. Furthermore, advancements in digital technology have enhanced the creation of three-dimensional models that enhance facial reconstructions' precision and efficiency for forensic purposes. The integration of forensic science with new approaches has also helped establish more precise ways of facial soft tissue thickness measurement, a critical component of facial reconstruction. Previously, various procedures were not accurate, involving limited landmarks and employing outdated measuring procedures. New technologies have introduced contactless methods, including low-dose CT scanning and holographic data storage, which produce high-resolution tissue thickness maps in various populations. This evidence is underpinned by work emphasizing the necessity of such knowledge to create realistic reconstructions that play a central role in forensic identification. As this technological coming together continues, the field moves towards the creation of standardized guidelines that may enhance the collective reliability and acceptability of facial reconstructions in forensic cases, securing further the role of forensic science as a central element in identification processes. In addition, the interaction between technological progress and forensic methods becomes increasingly relevant in courtroom arguments regarding the admissibility of facial reconstruction evidence. While legal systems are having a hard time integrating advanced biometric technologies, there remains a critical focus on the need for multi-disciplinary research that intersects such innovation with traditional law. While automatic facial recognition technology has a lot of promise, concerns over its reliability and admissibility in court criteria still linger, as highlighted by controversies in forensic literature. Although the field works towards improving biometric techniques, forensic professionals must adhere to strict standards and guidelines during training, so that the application and interpretation of facial recognition technology are not only scientifically sound but also legally acceptable, closing the gap between forensic science and legal processes (Ali et al., 2010; Hering et al., 2018).

11.1.3. Techniques Used in Facial Reconstruction

Facial reconstruction techniques are now much more refined, using increasingly sophisticated techniques based on biological theory and computer science. A central technique is the use of anatomical landmarks as reference points upon which to project facial features onto a three-dimensional form. The landmarks, derived from anthropometric analysis, provide the basis for reconstructing facial shape and structure. Additionally, the integration of forensic facial identification techniques ensures improved reconstructions. Reconstructed images are typically compared with existing photographs through a manual validation procedure by forensic experts in order to ascertain accuracy. Although the process is traditionally manual, more recent innovations seek to automate the process, even as matters of court admissibility and system reliability continue to present challenges, highlighting the need for ongoing research to reconcile such techniques into legal frameworks (Ali et al., 2010). Another significant technique of facial reconstruction employs the assessment of micro-expressions, which can represent underlying emotions usually suppressed in facial displays. Recent research has established that such hidden expressions can be identified using sophisticated recognition algorithms. Considering the dynamics of facial muscles for momentary emotional expressions, specialists could potentially refine their reconstructions not only for physical characteristics but even for depth of emotion states. This approach uses sparse spectral and temporal patterns to concentrate on the most relevant facial motions while discarding redundant details. The effectiveness of this approach can be observed in improved performance metrics in automated identification systems for spontaneous subtle emotions, providing richness to the story constructed through facial reconstructions (Ngo et al., 2016). Finally, interdisciplinary approaches in facial reconstruction incorporate ideas that integrate various applied technologies within the field. The Bayesian strategy, for example, is of particular importance in statistical analysis of facial recognition systems, integrating prior experience with empirics to enhance the quality of inference. This strategy is beneficial in assessing the validity of facial reconstruction outcomes, particularly in forensic contexts where accuracy matters most. Researchers advocate for an interdisciplinary approach that not only optimizes reconstruction techniques but also tackles legal issues and social attitudes towards facial recognition technologies. Working on these areas is key to the future of facial reconstruction, ensuring that techniques are not only scientifically feasible but also ethically viable in actual practice (Ali et al., 2010) (Figure 11.4).

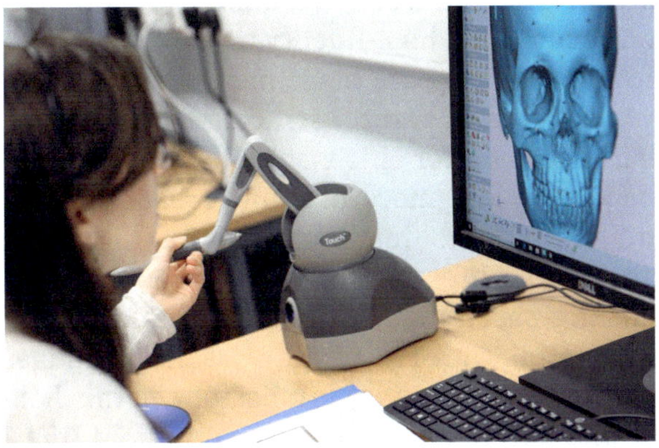

Figure 11.4. Facial reconstruction techniques.

Source: https://www.digitscotland.com/wp-content/uploads/2022/04/3D-FR.png.

Test Your Knowledge

1. Which key anatomical structures of the human face must be understood for accurate facial reconstruction?
2. How does forensic science contribute to identifying individuals through facial reconstruction methods?
3. What are the main techniques used in facial reconstruction, and how do they differ in approach and accuracy?

11.2. Methods of Facial Reconstruction

Learning Outcome

1. Focus on 2D Reconstruction Techniques
2. Explain 3D Modeling and Printing
3. Discuss the Traditional Sculpting Methods

Facial reconstruction has progressively made more use of the promise of deep learning, particularly in the case of 3D face reconstruction. This methodology represents a paradigm shift from typical methods that were largely dependent on labor-intensive input or rudimentary algorithms, often lacking the high degree of granularity required for precision. Current methodologies utilize convolutional neural networks (CNNs) to analyze and extrapolate data from two-dimensional images and reconstruct high-fidelity three-dimensional models. Not only are these methods increasing the quality level of reconstructed faces, but they also ensure better efficiency, allowing for faster processing and more uses in forensic science and animation. Current research highlights the promising progress caused by deep learning-based methods, which can detect fine information and create more realistic images, representing a significant milestone in this field. Despite the rapid progress in this field, there are still issues, particularly with occluded facial structures. Traditional techniques are ineffective when large facial regions are occluded, leading to incomplete or misleading reconstructions. As a way of overcoming this stumbling block, researchers have turned to GAN-inspired and bump mapping-like methods that normalize the facial topology and provide realistic details even though significant areas are occluded. This new approach maintains the integrity of the global shape and works on finer internal details necessary for realism. Furthermore, these approaches have been found to generalize extremely well over a broad spectrum of 3D reconstruction problems at the expense of the conventional methods that typically require occlusion removal manually. Emphasizing mid-level shape refinement techniques points towards a significant paradigm shift towards more computationally efficient facial modeling. Moreover, the empirical underpinning supporting the efficacy of such deep learning methods highlights their potential to transform facial reconstruction methods. Experiments on large scales performed in the context of general 3D face reconstruction tasks have validated the superior flexibility of such sophisticated models as opposed to traditional models. In providing various examples where these methods have outperformed general algorithms, researchers provide tangible evidence of their transvaluator power. The relevance of these advances is profound, for not only can they provide more accurate reconstructions, but also provide the door to revolutionary uses in virtual reality, computer games, and digital forensic analysis. Therefore, as the field develops, the integration of sophisticated algorithms promises to uncover new horizons in the art and science of facial reconstruction (Figure 11.5).

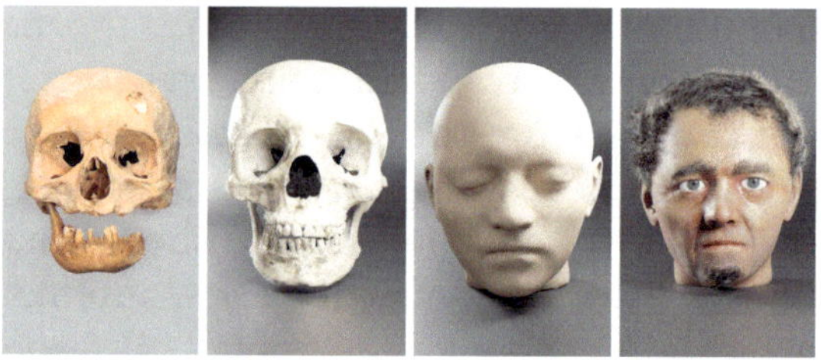

Figure 11.5. Methods of facial reconstruction.

Source: https://iscd.sorbonne-universite.fr/wp-content/uploads/2021/09/4head.png.

11.2.1. 2D Reconstruction Techniques

In facial reconstruction, 2D reconstruction techniques are supporting techniques that transform dimensional data to a visual form that can be read by humans. They are essential in applications ranging from historical artifact restoration to contemporary cosmetic surgery. Traditionally, 2D reconstruction relies on a suite of image processing techniques like edge detection and feature extraction that are applied in the detection and reconstruction of face structures from 2D images. Its efficiency is enhanced when used in combination with data-driven approaches that aggregate information from large collections of images or figures. The data-driven approaches enable one to derive geometric and structural relationships between different facial elements, thus enhancing the accuracy of reconstructions and general quality of visualization in facial analysis (Huang et al., 2015). Further, the use of 2D reconstruction techniques in pre-surgical planning has revolutionized plastic surgery, particularly facial aesthetics. Plastic surgeons now increasingly rely on computer software capable of warping 2D photos or 3D scans to offer simulations of potential post-operative appearances. The pre-emptive step results in improved decision-making regarding surgical outcomes. Using a holistic database of the best facial features, surgeons can quantitatively compare the patient's face to ideal standards. The method not only targets improvements in certain features but also in overall balance and proportion of the facial structure (Bottino et al., 2008). Consequently, through data aggregation and advanced imaging, facial reconstruction experts can make significant improvements in the aesthetic appeal and functional rehabilitation of facial structures. In addition, an increase in artificial intelligence and machine learning has the potential to bring further strengths to 2D reconstruction techniques. By subjecting large sets of facial images to deep learning technologies for processing, such systems can automatically identify patterns and correlations that exceed human sensory limits. Using such technologies, it is possible to significantly enhance the accuracy of reconstructions, including nuanced modeling and customized aesthetic guidance. Future research in the field will aim to combine computational techniques with human aesthetic experience, developing more sophisticated reconstruction techniques that balance subjective definitions of beauty against objective biological standards. Ongoing innovation in such tools speaks to the merit in integrating new methodologies into the foundations of facial reconstruction (Huang et al., 2015) (Figure 11.6).

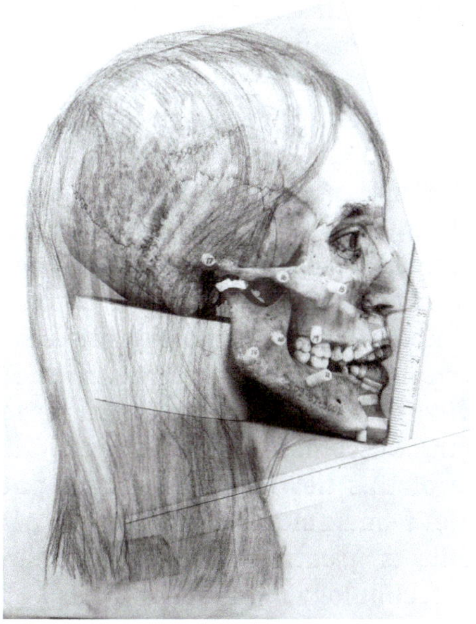

Figure 11.6. 2D reconstruction techniques.

Source: https://billinghamforensicimages.weebly.com/uploads/1/0/4/2/10427857/3106188_orig.jpg.

11.2.2. 3D Modeling and Printing

The advent of 3D modeling and printing has dramatically altered the facial reconstruction landscape with greater precision and customized strategies in surgical care. Traditional methods were typically faced with the limitations of universal methods and implants not accounting for individual patient anatomies. With the use of high-resolution 3D imaging technology, surgeons are able to create accurate virtual models of a patient's facial anatomy. This computer modeling is an accurate assessment of deformities or defects, hence a firmer foundation for planning the surgery. This advancement is important as it not only improves the fit and functioning of implants but also plays an important role in aesthetic outcomes, yielding more harmonious facial reconstruction. A crucial aspect of the application of 3D printing in facial reconstruction is its capability to produce tailored implants with custom shapes to suit every patient. An advanced software platform facilitates pre-operative planning of miniplates with an exact shape to match the patient's bone structure. According to studies quoted, the software enables surgeons to place various models of implants virtually within the patient's 3D anatomy, as well as to provide room for the complexity of facial bone defects. With the ability to manipulate the orientation and placement of the implants, the technology reduces intra-operative material realignments, therefore improving the time required for surgeries and improving outcomes among patients. Through the use of this new technology, the potential to achieve maximum stabilization of bone fragments is greatly improved, stressing the place of technology in modern surgical practice (Chen et al., 2017). The act of printing itself brings about major efficiencies, with surgeons able to speedily create the requirement for osteosynthesis material specific to a range of anatomical issues. Such capability has cost-saving and time-saving implications, both of which are important factors in surgical planning. The resulting models can be printed out as an STL file format, which is compatible with the multi-purpose 3D printing technologies that are increasingly prevalent and affordable. It is possible to save operating room time by using 3D printed implants or bending devices, meaning that patients will recover faster. In the broader context of facial reconstruction principles, the intersection of 3D modeling and printing not only enhances surgery but also opens up avenues for patient-specific healthcare solutions, ultimately enhancing quality of care and patient satisfaction (Chen et al., 2017) (Figure 11.7).

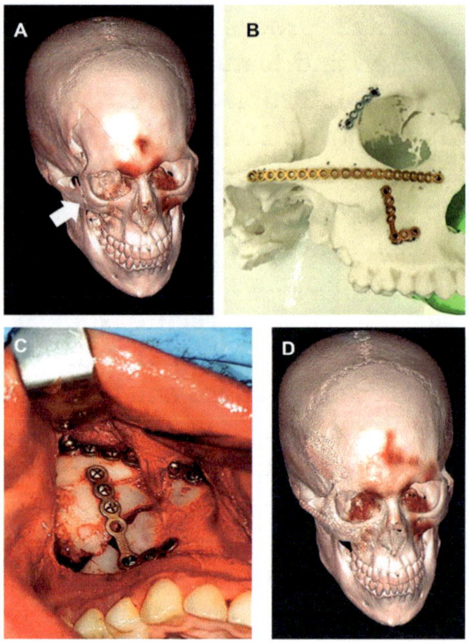

Figure 11.7. 3D modeling and printing of facial reconstruction

Source: https://www.researchgate.net/publication/360173268/figure/fig5/AS:11431281210649614@1702064686427/3D-design-and-printing-for-midface-reconstruction-Volumetric-representation-of-a.tif.

11.2.3. Traditional Sculpting Methods

The application of ancient sculpting methodologies has been a fundamental process in facial reconstruction, particularly in the creation of facial prosthesis. The methods are typically manual manipulation of materials, either wax or silicone, to replicate facial characteristics for individuals with injury or deformity. The delicacy of this work demands high levels of skill, artistry, and knowledge of anatomy as accuracy is critical in producing realistic and usable results. Artisans use their facial structure and proportion knowledge to create replicas that are like life, employing tools that support fine details. These traditional methods, though labor-intensive, have proven to be effective in creating personalized prostheses that match the unique characteristics of every patient's face, thereby enhancing the cosmetic and psychological health of the reconstructing patient. The effectiveness of traditional sculpting procedures in reconstructive facial reconstruction has been compared with more contemporary technology, including computer-aided design (CAD) and three-dimensional morphable models (3DMM). Comparative analysis of the different methods showed that 3DMMs were more repeatable and consistent in construction, but the traditional methods should not be discounted as they are hands-on and easily malleable with the sculptor's ideas (Jablonski et al., 2024). The hands-on process allows for adjustments that may not be achievable through digital methods, offering a personal touch that can be the difference between beautiful faces. So while new techniques are emerging, there remains relevance in traditional sculpting methods for a broad spectrum of clinical challenges, particularly in challenging cases where flawless detail matters. As advanced as facial reconstruction software has evolved, classical sculpting methods remain applicable and valid due to their rich history and fundamental principles that guide current practice. These methods, which focus on the fine details of facial features, rely on an in-depth understanding of human anatomy and artistic skillfulness required to replicate it exactly. Complications arising from varying levels of tissue laxity and patient-specific anatomical differences highlight the necessity for an individualized strategy in sculpting (Gi-Hong et al., 2024). As clinicians deal with such challenges, harmonizing the old methods with modern innovations can contribute to both aesthetics and functional outcomes of facial prostheses. Ultimately, the enduring validity of conventional sculpting practices is their continued application, which attests to the importance of maintaining these fundamental practices amidst advancing technology in facial reconstruction.

Test Your Knowledge

1. How do 2D facial reconstruction techniques use photographs or skeletal measurements to approximate a person's appearance?
2. What advantages does 3D modeling and printing offer over traditional reconstruction methods in terms of accuracy and visualization?

11.3. Applications of Facial Reconstruction

Learning Outcome

1. Discuss the Forensic Investigations
2. Explain the Medical Applications in Reconstructive Surgery
3. Describe the Historical and Archaeological Reconstructions

The diverse applications of facial reconstruction prove its valuable contribution to a wide range of fields, most notably forensic science and archaeology. In forensic contexts, facial reconstruction is employed primarily to support the identification of unidentified remains, particularly in cases where skeletal remains are involved. By reconstructing surface appearance from bones, facial reconstruction enables forensic artists to create realistic images that support the identification process. This is complemented by technological development in the shape of computer-based reconstruction techniques that maximize precision and speed in facial reconstructions. Despite the potential of such technologies, concerns exist regarding the integration of automatic facial recognition technology into the law, pointing toward the necessity for large-scale interdisciplinary research drawing on forensic practice and technological development in facial reconstruction (Ali et al., 2010). Facial reconstruction in archaeology is an important aspect when learning about populations and cultures in the past. Through close anatomical study of bones, scientists can reconstruct the faces of ancient individuals and thereby enhance our understanding of ancient societies. This method not only facilitates understanding demographic features and health conditions of such groups but also aids educational initiatives in museums, where such reconstructions can potentially render people visually connected to the past. Low-cost measures, as evident in recent studies, demonstrate that great facial analysis can be achieved without heavy technological investment, therefore making these applications feasible for scientists and teachers (Payne, 2013). This democratization of technique in facial reconstruction also has the potential to bridge resource disparities among various archaeological groups. In addition, advances in techniques of facial reconstruction have had significant implications in medicine, most notably in reconstructive surgery and prosthesis design. Accurate facial reconstructions can help surgeons pre-operatively plan surgery that restores a patient's aesthetic and functional potential following trauma or birth defects. High-end 3D imaging and modeling software allow personalized prosthetics that most accurately fit the patient's unique anatomical shape. With their confluence of artistic talent and medical knowledge, clinicians can greatly enhance patient satisfaction and results. Generally, applications of facial reconstruction extend beyond visualization for its own purposes; they are actually advancing interdisciplinary evolution in forensic science, historical studies, and medicine, emphasizing the need to continuously enhance the principles that underlie these fields (Figure 11.8).

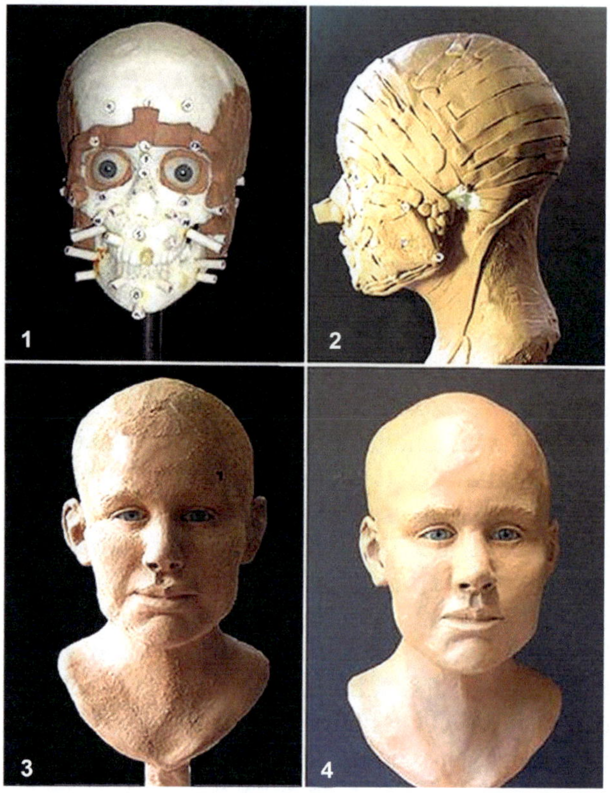

Figure 11.8. Multifaceted applications of facial reconstruction.

Source: https://static.wixstatic.com/media/683256_dfe559acff7344aca8dba0c7f23db65d~mv2.jpg/v1/fill/w_510,h_670,al_c,lg_1,q_80/683256_dfe559acff7344aca8dba0c7f23db65d~mv2.jpg.

11.3.1. Forensic Investigations

Forensic investigations are a key component of criminal justice through the application of an array of scientific techniques to analyze evidence and identify individuals who have participated in a crime. One of the most important aspects of these investigations is facial reconstruction, which is usually a tool that needs to be employed when other identification procedures, fingerprinting or DNA analysis, are ruled out because human remains are in a form that does not allow for such applications. Facial reconstruction from skeletal remains provides investigators with a visual image of a face, and this is utilized to create recognition and potentially result in victim identification. These portrayals have evolved over the years, evolving with technological progress and societal changes in regard to portraying dead individuals, and thus the ethical implications of these processes are a vital aspect in modern forensic practice, as outlined in the background history provided by literature on post-mortem facial portrayal and the social implications of such portrayals (Achenbach et al., 2014). Facial reconstruction reliability finally rests in the proper use of human anatomy-related biological principles. The ability to successfully carry out these reconstructions relies considerably on measuring facial soft tissue thickness, a pivotal factor that will offer precision in the portrayal of a person's features. Historically, a variety of methods have been employed to establish these measurements, but many were derived from limited data sets and subjective processes, and these might have influenced the accuracy of the results. Progress in recent years, such as the development of low-dose CT and holographic data measurement techniques, has transformed forensic science with promise for more precise and non-invasive ways of generating detailed facial soft tissue layer maps (Hering et al., 2018). This turn of events emphasizes the importance of combining technological developments within forensic methods for greater assurance of the reliability of facial reconstruction. Furthermore, the intersection of facial reconstruction and forensic science raises particular ethical issues that must be dealt with sensitivity. The implications of creating reconstructions are more than mere identification; they are associated with deeper public issues regarding dignity and respect for the dead. It is valued that the portrayal of human remains will often provoke intense emotional responses on the part of family members and the broader public, and thus careful consideration regarding how those images are produced and circulated is essential to respectful forensic practice. As facial reconstruction methods become more technological, researchers and practitioners are faced with establishing the balance between the requirements of creating successful identifications and having to be sensitive and respectful to the lives expressed through these reconstructions. The literature explaining the ethical considerations of facial reconstruction takes precedence, as debated in current arguments concerning the roles of forensic practitioners (Achenbach et al., 2014).

11.3.2. Medical Applications in Reconstructive Surgery

In reconstructive surgery, the integration of medical applications has opened up new avenues for facial aesthetics and the restoration of function. A noteworthy improvement is the use of three-dimensional (3D) printing technology in creating personalized molds for auricular reconstruction. Through the utilization of an empty, porous structure mirroring the anatomical character of the human ear, surgeons can place successful grafts consisting of diced cartilage mixed with platelet-rich plasma (PRP). This pioneering approach has yielded encouraging results, showing great fidelity to the auricle's natural shape and with the best viability of chondrocytes upon implantation. The implications of such approaches extend beyond cosmetic purposes; they are a step towards individualized surgical intervention that enhances patient results for facial reconstruction, successfully bridging technology with the traditional art of surgery (Chen et al., 2019). Another major aspect of medical application in reconstructive surgery is the exploration of tissue engineering and regenerative medicine. In the wake of the changing picture of autologous reconstructive options, the field has recognized the need to minimize donor-site morbidity. Advances in microsurgery and imaging modalities have provided bases for the development of engineered tissues that have the potential to replace or complement deficient structures.

Plastic surgeons are becoming more involved in the multidisciplinary discussion driving the innovation of biomanufacturing and clinical translation of tissue-engineered constructs. Even though this technological revolution promises to transform reconstructive results, issues such as determining the best cell sources and long-term safety of these constructs are still significant hurdles to be addressed (Abbott et al., 2017). The future of reconstructive surgery relies on integrating various medical and scientific specialties. The integration of these specialties is essential for overcoming current challenges in employing tissue engineering solutions efficiently. As accumulating evidence directs its current focus towards personalized approaches to surgery, the future becomes clearer to engineer customized grafts and scaffolds. But translating tissue-engineered solutions into practice involves a realistic appreciation of the time scale in bringing the basic sciences to clinical applications, typically decades (Abbott et al., 2017). In search of a revolution in facial reconstruction science, the stakeholders need to monitor the ongoing evolution of techniques and technology that have the potential to redefine the facial reconstruction procedures (Abbott et al., 2017) (Figure 11.9).

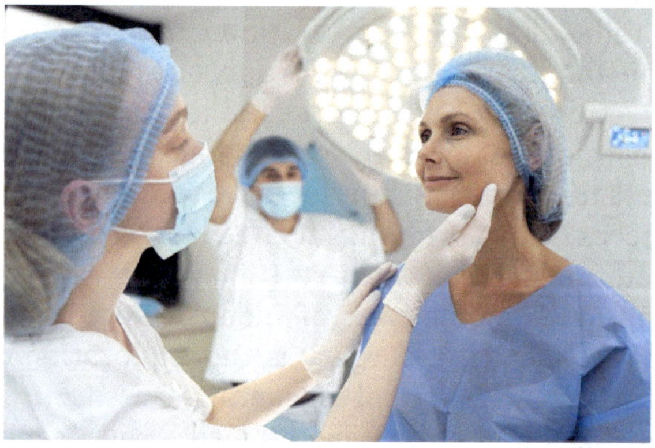

Figure 11.9. Medical applications in reconstructive surgery.

Source: https://florencehealthcare.international/wp-content/uploads/2024/03/Plastic-and-Reconstructive-Surgery-Center.jpeg.

11.3.3. Historical and Archaeological Reconstructions

In historical and archaeological reconstructions, craniofacial reconstruction (CFR) methods have revolutionized visualization and understanding of individuals in the past. The techniques allow researchers to reconstruct faces based on appearance using soft tissue depth mapping onto skeletons, providing valuable information regarding cultural, social, and biological contexts of the people in the past. For instance, applying computerized tomography to mummies, recent studies have been able to reconstruct a 17th-century Korean individual's face. This is not merely a technical exercise of applying CFR but one involving archaeological testimony of personal adornment, coiffure, and clothing, which results in a plausible portrait that secures both the appearance and essence of the moment and deepens our engagement with the stories of history (Lee et al., 2014). In addition, the intrinsic challenges of accurately reconstructing hairstyles, a very important aspect of facial reconstruction, have made it interesting to delve into new digital approaches. The traditional methods do not succeed due to a lack of sufficient available visual information and over-reliance on artistic impression. This deficiency has led to digital hair production techniques that claim to offer more accuracy and flexibility in approximating hairstyles. Referring to specific examples, such as the case of George Dixon, the last commander of the HL Hunley submarine, researchers have initiated a methodological process beginning with data gathering and concluding with the sophisticated integration of digitally simulated hair into facial models. The recursive reconstruction process enhances the realism and authenticity of reconstructions to facilitate the potential of having several various stylistic versions based on archaeologically obtained findings and historical evidence (Emerson, 2023). Synergy between technological advancement and archaeological data not only fosters the growth of facial reconstruction as an area of study but also interdisciplinary interaction. Through the integration of archaeological data and current graphic modeling techniques, scientists can construct holistic reconstructions that map the intricate aspects of historical identities. Such overlap of methodology assists in demystifying the intricacies of reconstructing historical figures, including hairstyle and facial structure changes that appropriately reflect their socio-cultural setting. Lastly, such detailed reconstructions are of immense educational significance, enabling one to understand the historical accounts better and triggering broader debate across identity, culture, and the human condition throughout history (Emerson, 2023Lee et al., 2014; Emerson, 2023) (Figure 11.10).

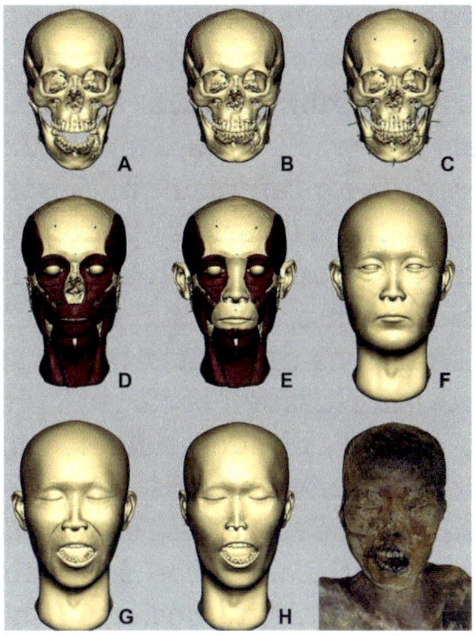

Figure 11.10. Historical and archaeological reconstructions.

Source: https://ars.els-cdn.com/content/image/1-s2.0-S0305440314002003-gr2.jpg.

Test Your Knowledge

1. How is facial reconstruction used in forensic investigations to aid in identifying unknown individuals?
2. How do historical and archaeological facial reconstructions help researchers understand past populations or significant historical figures?

11.4. Ethical Considerations

Learning Outcome

1. Discuss the Consent and Privacy Issues
2. Explain the Cultural Sensitivity in Reconstruction
3. Focus on Implications of Misrepresentation

Ethical issues are a cornerstone both for patient and practitioner in the case of facial reconstruction. The intrinsic difficulties of reconstructive surgery call for unambiguous ethical frameworks for decision-making, particularly in managing patient expectations and requirements. Patient discussion concerning patient wishes for aesthetics must take notice of fine psychological impacts because face reconstruction directly influences altering a person's perception of self, as well as their social life. Moreover, the practitioner must balance the ethical requirements of beneficence, acting in the patient's best interest, against principles of autonomy and informed consent. This balance is crucial, as informed patients will more actively engage in realistic outcome discussion, which will yield a more acceptable therapeutic process and highlight the importance of detailed preoperative counseling. Another key factor in the ethical concerns of facial reconstruction is the management of patient expectations. As surgical techniques and technologies improve, the line between realistic expectations and idealistic hopes becomes blurred. Therapists are ethical professionals who educate patients about the limits of reconstructive surgery, particularly regarding natural appearance and functional restoration. Failure to articulate these limits persuasively can result in dissatisfaction and emotional suffering post-procedure. Furthermore, consideration of resource allocation of reconstructive surgery must also be given. In situations where healthcare resources are limited, prioritization of surgical procedures based on ethical considerations is paramount to advancing equity and ensuring all persons have access to care regardless of socioeconomic status. Finally, ethical concerns extend beyond direct patient contact to societal and cultural considerations on a larger level. This is especially true in multicultural populations where cultural expectations about beauty and facial appearance are quite different. Ethically, providers will have to negotiate these cultural axes with great care so as not to impose a homogenous definition of beauty that will not connect with all patients. Additionally, the application of imagination, as underscored in ethical decision-making literature, points to a vulnerability to new ideas that will revolutionize conventional presumptions in facial reconstruction. Drawing on both creativity and imagination can provide a more embracing practice that is responsive to diverse identities while fortifying rehabilitation techniques for patients (Mar et al., 2008; Angelopoulou et al., 2016). An ethical approach to facial reconstruction thus encompasses the individual, society, and community in a holistic practice that is dignified and equitable and emphasizes the well-being of all parties.

11.4.1. Consent and Privacy Issues

It is important to steer clear of consent and privacy concerns in facial reconstruction, especially in relation to the ethical questions surrounding personal information in modern society. The greater accessibility of online platforms has made individuals' biometric data more accessible but vulnerable to misuse. When applying ethical thinking to facial reconstruction, one needs to confront the reality that data from web social networks can include a wealth of personal information of individuals and therefore consents become complex. Researchers must be confident that they are conducting ethically sound data collection and management, understanding the full non-anonymity of network data to potentially jeopardize individual privacy. Failure to navigate these nuances can lead to crossing the boundaries of ethical norms, eventually invading an individual's right to informed consent within the larger psychological and legal context of their facial identity (Betts et al., 2017). In addition, the responsibility of keeping informed consent is even more tenuous when facial reconstruction subjects are adolescents. The psychological impact of facial surgery can be far-reaching, particularly in the context of motivations derived from cultural pressure regarding physical appearance. Informed consent cannot be a procedural formula; it must involve close attention to a patient's mental condition, body image, and family dynamics. Relevant counseling sessions should be implemented to provide understanding and capacity for decision-making, with the minors' best interests at heart. An organized process such as this can prevent exploitation and manipulation so that a more ethical environment is provided within cosmetic surgery procedures. Lastly, any procedure must be measured against patients' psychological and physical well-being to ensure that consent is indeed real and informed (Luca et al., 2018). These debates underscore the imperative to create comprehensive ethical frameworks addressing consent and privacy issues regarding facial reconstruction procedures. The evolving character of technology and its interaction with human identity demand ongoing examination of ethical practice. Ethical principles need to adapt as they address increased sophistication in data handling and personal consent, particularly where personal identifiers would offer a means of unwarranted revelation of sensitive information. The debate concerning the ethical considerations of reconstruction treatments should be inclusive of stakeholders such as practitioners, patients, ethicists, and lawyers. A multidisciplinary approach will enable practitioners to sail through the issues in ethics with ease and hence maintain the integrity of the consent process alongside ensuring patient privacy of patients undergoing facial reconstruction therapy (Betts et al., 2017; Luca et al., 2018).

11.4.2. Cultural Sensitivity in Reconstruction

Facial reconstruction and cultural sensitivity are the key to ensuring that historical individuals are portrayed correctly and respectfully. Facial approximation procedures are likely to rely on a combination of art and scientific technology, and therefore, it is critical that cultural contexts be recognized and integrated into reconstructive procedures. For instance, in reconstructing historic personalities, scientists must gather not only morphological data but cultural data regarding hairstyle, attire, and norms of society during the period when the individual lived. This approach is synchronized with the notion that reconstructive practice cannot solely be founded upon aesthetic interests; it must move through the intricate dynamics between culture, history, and identity, so that the end product is not just scientifically true but also culturally resonant (Emerson, 2023). That sensitivity not only brings richness to the precision of the reconstruction but also brings better insight into the role of the individual within their historical and cultural setting. Inclusion of cultural sensitivity in facial reconstruction also necessitates a multi-disciplinary process that includes historians, archaeologists, and representatives of the descendant community. That multi-disciplinary process can bring the authenticity and applicability of the reconstruction to a higher level. Engaging with different groups who could have genealogical or cultural linkages to the reconstructed individual creates a better understanding of how such a person would have perceived his/her identity. This work belongs to the overall recognition that history isn't a single tale but a web of viewpoints that must be noted and corroborated (Fellmann Widmann, 2017). By forming connections with communities that are invested in the subject, researchers are able to assure that the reconstructions will not inadvertently perpetuate stereotypes or distort cultural heritage, thus allowing a more representative and diverse portrayal of historical figures. The inclusion of cultural sensitivity in facial reconstruction ultimately comes to underscore the broader ethical implications of reconstructive practice. When technologies of facial approximation advance, so too must the responsibility to honor the identity that is being rebuilt. Scholars need to balance the impact their research has on living communities today and on the legacy of the deceased. .11).

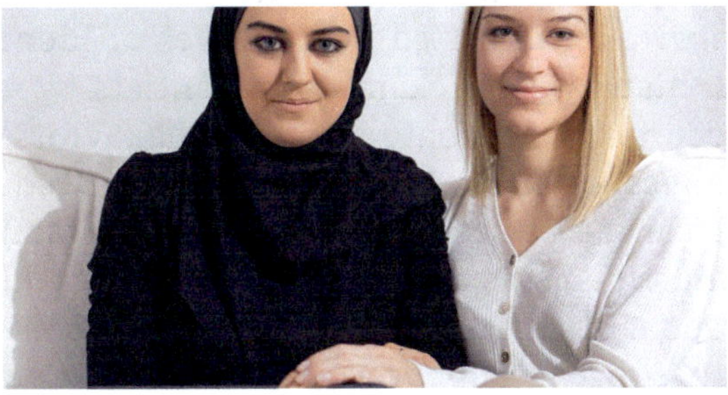

Figure 11.11. Cultural sensitivity in facial reconstruction.

Source: https://thecenterforgrowth.com/assets/uploads/images/_1200x630_crop_center-center_82_none/cultural-sensitivity.jpg?mtime=1703376541.

This responsibility also involves an understanding of the specific cultural features that make an individual unique, as these facets are at the heart of their historical significance. By prioritizing cultural sensitivity, facial reconstruction not only brings back the past but also initiates a dialogue about cultural representation, identity, and respect. This dialogue can bridge the gap between the past and the present by establishing a two-way dialogue of comprehension, which can be utilized to upgrade the narrative of people whose lives have been lost or misremembered for centuries (Emerson, 2023) (Figure 11

11.4.3. Implications of Misrepresentation

Scientific integrity is not only threatened by misrepresentation in facial reconstruction, but it also has important implications for society. Accuracy in reconstructive procedures is important in representing individuals with respect, particularly if reconstructions are being utilized in legal proceedings or for cultural heritage studies. When reconstructions are based on false assumptions or anthropomorphic readings, as the process of anthropomorphization indicates, then it results in providing distorted perspectives of identity and history. For example, scientists would inaccurately attribute complex behaviors to biological entities such as neurons, a procedure that can be equated to the misrepresentation of individuals in facial reconstruction, where personal attributes are removed from context in an effort to support a broader narrative of action and identity, ultimately depreciating the unique human experience in scientific and social contexts (Nizami, 2017). The ramifications of misrepresentation extend further into ethical concerns, particularly against marginalized populations whose race or ethnicity may be oversimplified or misrepresented in faulty facial reconstructions. Such determinations can contribute to reflecting and reinforcing existing stereotypes and result in negative societal consequences. If facial reconstructions stray from reality, they can also potentially reinforce system-level bias and misconceptions about race, gender, and culture. This creates a necessary tension within the field, whereby the scientific need for exact imitations has to contend with the moral imperative to represent the complex, multifaceted identities of people realistically. Repeat misrepresentation within these processes can potentially fuel broader social biases, undermining efforts to engender understanding and acceptance between demographically distinct populations (Gooya, 2020). In addition, misrepresentation during facial reconstruction has profound implications for the individuals undergoing reconstruction, particularly in cases involving remains of historical or archaeological significance. Misrepresentation can confuse public understanding or lead to the misallocation of cultural significance, thereby influencing how history is recorded and taught. These reconstructions have a tendency to become integrated into popular memory and identity for groups; as such, not depicting people as well as possible can erase their stories or distort their legacies. As the consequences of misrepresentation within academia are further established, the procedure of facial reconstruction will have to move towards a more robust methodology that demands ethical responsibilities and community engagement. Determining that representation is accurate and respectful will not only enhance the integrity of facial reconstruction procedures but also enable communities to reclaim and narrate their own stories (Nizami, 2017).

Test Your Knowledge

1. What consent and privacy issues must be addressed when performing facial reconstruction, especially in forensic or medical contexts?
2. Why is cultural sensitivity important in facial reconstruction, particularly when recreating features of historical or indigenous populations?

11.5. Challenges in Facial Reconstruction

Learning Outcome

1. Discuss the Limitations of Available Data
2. Explain the Variability in Human Features
3. Focus on Technological Constraints

Facial reconstruction is a field with a high number of sophisticated challenges that may result in failed practices. Facial anatomy complexity is one of the primary obstacles in this field. The face consists of a web of complex structures, such as bones, soft tissues, and nerves, each with a vital role in both form and function. In reconstructive surgery, the surgeons have to work within these sensitive interactions to re-establish not just the appearance but also the functional integrity of the face. This is made more complex by the differences from one individual to another, making template-based methods inadequate. Technological innovations in data-driven methods are beginning to bypass these challenges, allowing more intricate investigation of geometric and structural interrelations between 3D forms. Application of such techniques, however, requires comprehensive training and familiarity to ensure accuracy in model and reconstruction (Huang et al., 2015). Apart from anatomical complexity, another problem with facial reconstruction is the handling of soft tissue injury and scarring. Soft tissue injury can significantly influence the cosmetic result of reconstructive operations, resulting in scarring, skin necrosis, and loss of tissue. Successful reconstruction is highly dependent on the accurate evaluation and management of these injuries, which may range from being mild and superficial to being severe and deep. An evaluation of oral and maxillofacial injury at Muhimbili National Hospital unearths the incidence of laceration and bruising requiring immediate medical care and planned reconstruction (Kileo, 2012). A comprehensive understanding of healing mechanisms, scar behavior, and how best to choose the optimal surgical techniques to prevent long-term sequelae to appearance and function is required in soft tissue trauma management. Furthermore, psychological factors significantly influence the overall success of facial reconstruction. A majority of patients experience a broad spectrum of emotional distress, anxiety, and dissatisfaction with appearance following traumatic injury. Psychological ruin can interfere with recovery from surgery and might cause the patient to become resistant to pursuing further procedures. Unsatisfactory cosmetic outcomes can result in dissatisfaction independent of technically satisfactory surgery. Therefore, the inclusion of psychological support and counseling in the reconstruction process is essential. By addressing the emotional needs of patients in conjunction with their physical reconstruction, healthcare workers are able to enhance the overall success of facial reconstruction as well as promote an inner feeling of well-being that is not dependent on physical characteristics, leading ultimately to improved patient outcomes (Figure 11.12).

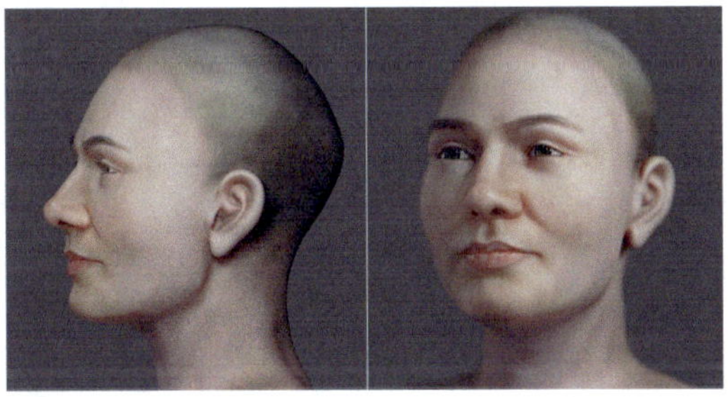

Figure 11.12. Facial reconstruction in-colour with eyes.

Source: https://www.researchgate.net/publication/377075677/figure/fig11/AS:11431281215451547@1704254115514/Facial-reconstruction-in-colour-with-eyes-opened.jpg.

11.5.1. Limitations of Available Data

Facial reconstruction, as much as it is a vital element of forensic anthropology and science, is immensely troubled by data constraints. Reconstruction relies solely on the psychological and anatomical profiles gathered from a small number of digital databases. Representation inconsistencies of individual features in the databases are typical and lead construction to make faulty inferences about a subject's features. As is outlined, reliance on general models can obscure important variation within populations and create the potential loss of specificity required for successful reconstructions. Accordingly, a consideration of the variability and limitations of data sets is a key consideration in developing the methods and ensuring that they are representative of the diversity that occurs in human facial anatomy. Moreover, technological constraints of data collection remain to fuel the shortcomings in facial reconstruction. For instance, imaging technology has improved significantly, yet most of the existing databases are not revised to reflect the newest findings that add to anthropological knowledge. As noted in emergent technology discussions, the evolution of the field is not only reliant upon developments in capture methods but also upon the incorporation of this information into holistic platforms that can allow for a richer familiarity with facial features. As a result, without continued updates and additions to available data sets, the field may stagnate, restricting the use of facial reconstruction methods in forensic and archaeological applications. During the era of sudden digital transformation, the importance of privacy concerns over data accumulation cannot be overstated. Increased use of digital representations and avatars in environments such as the metaverse raises questions about ethical standards in managing data. Likenesses of users can be duplicated and utilized without explicit consent, further speeding up the map of available data for facial reconstruction. The line between innovation and ethics is fine; emerging technologies must be focused on transformation and efficiency, but must also incorporate robust privacy measures to form trust in their consumers. This dynamic between the potential for data-driven innovation and ethical concerns highlights the imperative need for an infrastructure of encourages the use of data responsibly in the discipline of facial reconstruction to ensure that scientific progress does not come at the expense of the inherent rights of the individuals involved.

11.5.2. Variability in Human Features

Human facial variation is at the heart of understanding principles of facial reconstruction, reliant on the accurate representation of solitary features. Human variation in traits is a broad spectrum of factors, such as genetic, environmental, and developmental factors. The unique interaction of these factors in each individual is responsible for typical facial features that must be interpreted when reconstructing facial appearances from skeletal remains or forensic evidence. Research underscores the importance of manual facial comparison methodology, as forensic examiners subject this variation carefully in an effort to make correct identifications (Ali et al., 2010). While methodologies used today consider the general trends in forensic identification, these are significantly enhanced with the incorporation of a full understanding of human variation across populations. Thus, recognition of variability comes into play while determining the nuances of facial reconstruction as each individual is shaped by a unique combination of heredity and life experiences. In facial reconstruction, precise modeling of the facial structure is critical, particularly in forensic analysis. Variability is a major challenge in the reconstruction process, demanding advanced techniques that are also accommodating differences in shape, size, and proportions among different ethnic groups and individual genetic patterns. As research continues, data-driven techniques are increasingly define how geometric and structural issues presented by variability in human facial traits are understood. These methods aggregate data from huge databases of human faces and allow for the detection of patterns and correlations that enhance single reconstructions (Huang et al., 2015). In embracing this data-driven methodology, researchers can enhance the accuracy of facial reconstructions while also conquering the inherent difficulties brought about by the variability of human facial appearances.

The result is a more unified and science-oriented approach to understanding the diversity of human appearance, essential for forensic application as well as anthropological inquiry. Implications of human variability extend beyond theoretical discussion into practical application in the fields of forensic science, anthropology, and even artificial intelligence. With facial recognition technology more in demand than ever, the need to understand this variability becomes increasingly urgent. Recent research emphasizes that the majority of recent biometric technologies do not properly take into account the complexities of human facial variability, and this can lead to errors and potential misidentifications. Resolution of such problems is best approached using interdisciplinary approaches by combining technological innovation with human factors. One significant area of ongoing research is in developing models that can learn from large datasets to accommodate the changing facial characteristics present in different groups (Huang et al., 2015). These advances come after the basic necessity for a complex sense of variability across human traits, ultimately to enable more effective facial reconstruction techniques and better facial recognition technology accuracy across varied scenarios (Figure 11.13).

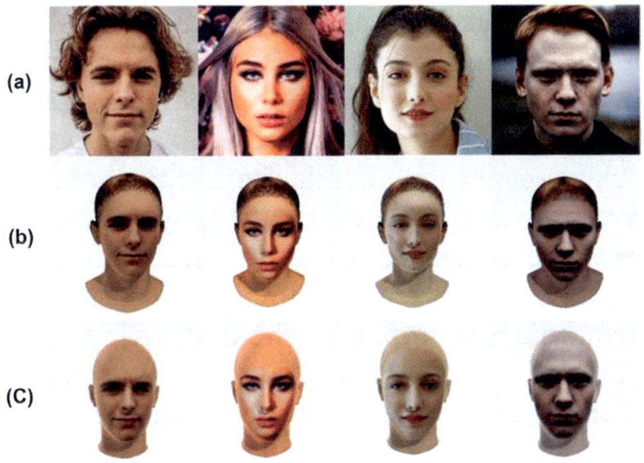

Figure 11.13. Human facial variability.

Source: https://media.springernature.com/lw685/springer-static/image/art%3A10.1007%2Fs11042-024-19583-0/MediaObjects/11042_2024_19583_Fig11_HTML.png.

11.5.3. Technological Constraints

Technological limitations of the methods developed in facial reconstruction come with unprecedented magnitude that ultimately governs their efficiency and reliability. A significant limitation arises from the intrinsic difficulties in accurately modeling the human body, which needs to be respected in reconstructing facial structures. Traditional methods have the tendency to base themselves upon accurate anatomical landmarks, not considering individual variation, thereby forming an inability to develop exactly personalized reconstructions. Against such challenges, data-driven techniques have emerged, as they combine data from multiple sets of shapes to enhance the analysis of individual facial structures. Through the application of such techniques, researchers can overcome various biases of conventional techniques to generate more accurate reconstructions that are informed by a broader knowledge of geometric relations in facial anatomy (Huang et al., 2015). Technological development has also been held back by the access and precision of image technology used in facial reconstruction. While methods like photogrammetry and 3D scanning have become more readily available and easier to use, these too are hampered by limitations such as resolution boundaries and the potential for capturing fine detail, particularly on complex areas like the nose or the eyes. These limitations can likely lead to significant variations in reconstructed models, thus affecting their usability for application in clinical settings or forensic examination. In addition, emerging technologies also face the challenge of imposing extensive data processing requirements, which normally require significant amounts of computation. The creation of synchrotron X-ray sources and related equipment has enabled the investigation of interfacial structures, meaning that such developments in the field of imaging could be of immense significance when it comes to addressing these weaknesses in facial reconstruction (Ahn et al., 2020). Further, the computational techniques applied in facial reconstruction are typically constrained by the software and algorithms available for researchers to use. While contemporary technology makes possible the analysis and processing of facial features in new realms, there remains a reliance on pre-established parameters that may be less than perfectly suited for any specific reconstruction. These restraints can hinder the creation of adaptive models, which otherwise might accommodate the unique quality of individual cases. Though researchers are still researching the joining of machine learning techniques, there's a chance to get past such limitations by developing self-learning algorithms that learn to improve based on new information and become more precise with time. Ultimately, the breaking of the technological barrier in facial reconstruction is essential to further enhancing the overall efficiency of reconstruction procedures and making them universally accepted in medicine, law enforcement, and historical reconstruction (Figure 11.14).

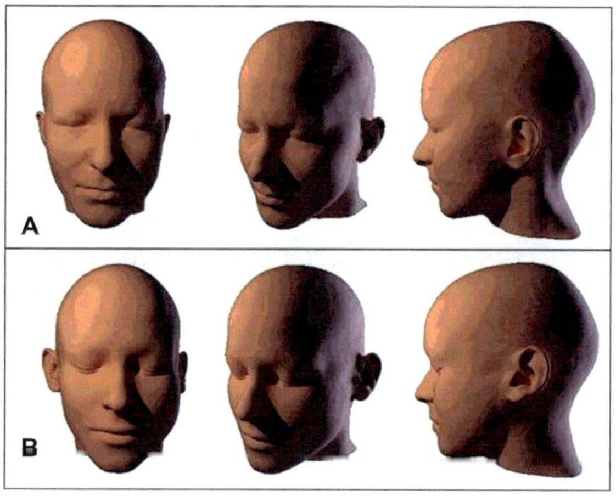

Figure 11.14. Evolution of facial reconstruction technological constraints that ultimately shape their effectiveness and reliability.

Source: https://www.tandfonline.com/cms/asset/9b330eef-fbbd-421b-8302-35cd708fa6cd/tfsr_a_1469185_f0016_c.jpg.

Test Your Knowledge

1. How do limitations in available skeletal or soft-tissue data affect the accuracy of facial reconstruction results?
2. Why does natural variability in human facial features make reconstruction challenging, even with detailed anatomical knowledge?

11.6. Future Directions in Facial Reconstruction

Learning Outcome

1. Explain Advances in Technology and Software
2. Focus on Integration of Artificial Intelligence (AI)
3. Discuss Potential for Virtual Reality (VR) Applications

Advances in computer hardware are poised to transform facial reconstruction, particularly through the synthesis of sophisticated hair modeling and simulation methodologies. Traditional approaches fall short of recreating realistic hairstyles because archaeologists do not have hard evidence and because artistic interpretation is extremely subjective. The research, with a focus on computer-generated hair, as in the reconstruction of George Dixon on the HL Hunley submarine, offers a glimpse into the capability of a more realistic and dynamic process. This multi-phase method uses archaeological data, 3D modeling through computed tomography, and current computer graphics to simulate hair's physicality in a realistic way. Improvements in this field not only hold out for more accuracy in the facial reconstructions but also for more research into the aesthetic range in variations depicting historical accuracy, and both technical and artists' interpretative problems are thus addressed at once (Emerson, 2023). Another field with potential for new developments in facial reconstruction involves the application of facial recognition technologies. With the expanding adoption of facial recognition technologies across various industries, from security to healthcare, the rising need for integrating these technologies with effective defenses against face spoofing attacks cannot be ignored. Recent studies indicate the need to develop more sophisticated detection approaches, which translate into raising descriptors as well as classifiers. This analysis's findings can be applied to guide future development of facial reconstruction techniques with real-time recognition potential that can be integrated, which would not only be more accurate but also safer for forensic use. These advances make necessary interdisciplinary studies between facial reconstruction specialists and computer scientists to ensure that these technologies become more advanced to meet contemporary challenges as well as improve the reliability of reconstructed images (Oliveira et al., 2018). Finally, the ethical aspect of facial reconstruction is gaining momentum with advancing technology. The ability to reproduce a person's image provokes fundamental questions about consent, privacy, and the potential for its misapplication, particularly in forensic applications. Whereas facial reconstruction as an increasing and less challenging prospect develops with technological advancements, ethical frameworks must develop alongside to address these matters. Future research must not only prioritize technical accuracy but also engage stakeholders like communities, attorneys, and ethicists in developing comprehensive guidelines to govern the use of reconstructed images. An integrative framework will ensure that facial reconstruction practices are consistent with ethical standards while tapping into cutting-edge techniques, hence encouraging public confidence in applications of this critical field (Emerson, 2023Oliveira et al., 2018; Emerson, 2023).

11.6.1. Advances in Technology and Software

New technology and computer software have revolutionized the appearance of facial reconstruction, allowing for improved accuracy and efficiency in planning and conducting surgery. An example is high-resolution real-time three-dimensional (3-D) shape measurement technology that uses digital micromirror devices (DMD) to achieve simultaneous 3-D shape acquisition and reconstruction at a 30 Hz rate.

This capability not only enhances the precision of facial modeling but also ensures surgeons can also visualize anatomical structures in real time, ensuring enhanced educational outcomes and surgery decision-making. The integration of such advanced measurement techniques is evidence of the significant role technology plays in demystifying the axioms of facial reconstruction, taking the discipline towards more individualized and effective interventions for particular patient requirements (Bell et al., 2014). Artificial intelligence (AI) and computer-assisted planning software are also poised to be critical elements in optimizing facial reconstruction surgery. These technologies enable surgeons to utilize virtual surgical planning according to the individual anatomy of each patient. AI can also be used to predict surgical results, thereby enhancing the preoperative preparation process. Furthermore, 3-D printing technology is facilitating the ability to design customized surgical templates and bioprinted prosthetics, changing reconstructions to be done in a more sophisticated manner. As the software itself becomes more sophisticated, it can potentially provide even more sophisticated tools that simplify workflows and reduce the likelihood of surgery-related complications. The rising application of these technologies is a sign of an intriguing turn towards a data-driven approach to facial reconstruction that enhances surgical efficacy as well as patient safety (Alfertshofer et al., 2023). With progress still being made within the field, there are still concerns about applying and standardizing these technologies. While fibula free flap procedures have seen tremendous advances in their application to facial deformities, the addition of new technologies is still a field that remains untapped. Improved donor site morbidity and adequate blood supply are two of the primary motives for research on new applications of technology for the field. Moreover, there exists an imperative for extensive studies that analyze the interface of 3-D modeling, virtual planning, and real-time monitoring systems in postoperative care. These are imperative needs because they can lead to better clinical results while promoting a shared knowledge base that will facilitate future developments in the concepts of facial reconstruction (Alfertshofer et al., 2023).

11.6.2. Integration of Artificial Intelligence (AI)

AI use in facial reconstruction is a significant breakthrough in digital imaging technologies and forensic science. The scientists utilize AI's pattern recognition and data analysis abilities to significantly enhance the speed and accuracy of reconstructing facial features from bones or other inconclusive sources. AI algorithms facilitate easier matching of facial structures to biological profiles, leading to enhanced identifications. This technology is of profound importance, particularly in criminal investigations where timely and accurate identifications can make or break a case. Moreover, the flexibility of AI systems in working with various datasets makes them efficient in modeling facial features of any nature, capable of adapting to any ethnic population and age group, thus promoting inclusivity in forensic applications. Apart from traditional methods, AI-backed processes such as computational ghost imaging have transformed 3D facial reconstruction's visual and interpretative processes. As elaborated in recent studies, the new approach utilizes single-pixel sensors at many positions to collect 2D images under various illumination directions to make it possible for the analysis of surface gradients reconstruction of a 3D model. This technology, furthermore, not only enhances resolution and detail of face reconstructions, but it accomplishes this at a fraction of the expense of more conventional multi-camera systems. With more effective accessibility to high-end imaging technology made possible through AI, opportunities exist to use it to a higher degree in consumer markets as well as specific forensic settings, satisfying a high-priority requirement for high-fidelity reconstructions in both contexts (Bowman et al., 2013). In addition, AI integration implies the technological development of collaborative technologies that impact the communication of non-verbal facial expressions in facial reconstructions. As described in research surrounding Mixed Reality systems, AI can make an insightful interpretation of facial expressions and social relations within the reconstructive process. Through marrying immersive projection technology with telepresence technology, AI provides for collaborative environments in which cohorts are capable of working and exploring facial reconstruction scenarios in real-time, both facilitating learning as well as real-world applications. This technological model allows for an enhanced context within which to explore not only the structural components of face reconstruction, but the implicit emotional and communicative elements that are a part of human interaction. With the advancement of AI technology, so will the role of AI in facial reconstruction, crossing disciplinary boundaries and informing new approaches (Campion et al., 2017).

11.6.3. Potential for Virtual Reality (VR) Applications

Research on VR applications to facial reconstruction offers great promise, particularly in preoperative planning and simulation of surgery. Surgeons can visualize and interactively manipulate facial anatomy with computer-generated 3D models prior to complex procedures being carried out. Pre-planning helps in the correct positioning of osteosynthesis material, as implemented with recent advances like computer-aided position planning of miniplates for facial bone defects. Surgeons can customize the virtual models to the individual anatomical features of patients, ultimately resulting in greater accuracy during surgery and a reduction in time spent adapting in the operating room. With the potential for the creation of prototypes of implants or individual bending tools using 3D printing, the use of VR in surgical preparation has the potential to dramatically change the way facial reconstructive surgery is performed (Chen et al., 2017). Besides, VR can be employed to enhance collaboration among surgical teams where high-quality communication is of utmost significance. Using the mixed reality systems, teams engage in discussions in common spaces that mimic the operating room, thus improving the non-verbal understanding of facial expressions and spatial position. The systems facilitate an immersive approach that heightens teamwork dynamics, critical in the proper execution of complex facial reconstruction procedures. For instance, the combination of telepresence technology and immersive screens has been promising in facilitating interaction beyond geographical locations. Besides making it possible for experts to address strategy, it has also facilitated real-time evaluation of surgical methods so that preoperative planning can be more inclusive and elaborate (Campion et al., 2017). Lastly, the application of VR technology in combining facial reconstruction concepts will revolutionize education and clinical practice. Training future surgeons with simulations based on reality confronts them with experiential learning in a safe situation. These virtual simulations are able to simulate various situations, thus subjecting learners to the unpredictability of actual surgeries. Thus, VR is not only a tool for planning surgery but also a learning tool that facilitates a better understanding of facial anatomy and surgical procedures. As VR technology evolves, so do applications, opening up the potential for dramatic improvement in both surgical results and surgical education in facial reconstruction. The marriage of medicine and technology portends a revolutionary future in which precision and collaboration can improve surgical art and aesthetics (Campion et al., 2017) (Figure 11.15).

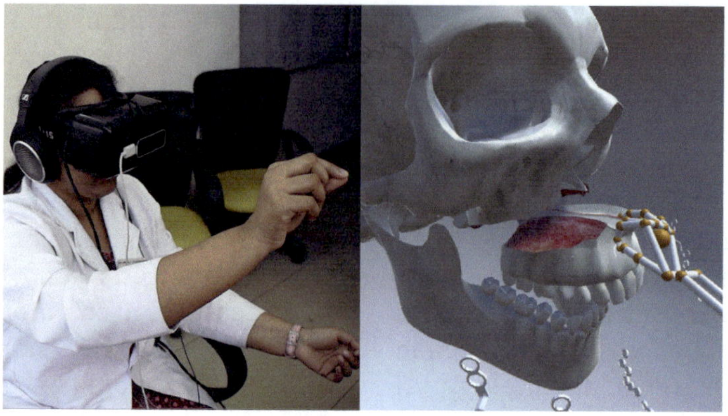

Figure 11.15. Exploration of virtual reality (VR) applications.

Source: https://www.joms.org/cms/10.1016/j.joms.2017.10.002/asset/c6867d56-5e69-498b-8d23-6e9c9024fd91/main.assets/gr2_lrg.jpg.

Test Your Knowledge

1. How might artificial intelligence (AI) improve accuracy and predictive capabilities in facial reconstruction models?
2. What potential applications could virtual reality (VR) offer in visualizing and refining facial reconstructions for forensic or medical use?

SUMMARY

Facial reconstruction principles involve a multi-disciplinary approach integrating art, science, and forensic use. Integration of heterogeneous technologies, like biometric face recognition, enhances the accuracy and reliability of reconstructive outcomes. The inability of automatic systems to cope with the demands of forensic facial identification reinforces the gap between technology and law, thus necessitating the need to continue research to bridge it. The inter-disciplinary collaboration identified in the literature reflects the need for ways of enhancing reconstruction techniques, along with satisfying court admissibility, a key factor when testimonies must be consistent with the degree of rigor of forensic demands. It is noted in Ali et al. (2010) that existing frameworks must adjust to function in accordance with judicial needs, with an emphasis placed on facial reconstruction as an integral aspect of both criminology and identity rehabilitation. Furthermore, statistics gathered from research studies of maxillofacial injuries show the urgent repercussions injury has on the process of facial reconstruction. For instance, research shows that road traffic accidents are a prevalent cause of the same and pose grave issues related to public safety and socio-economic determinants of the accidents. Comprehensive knowledge of why facial injuries occur is essential to optimize prevention and treatment practice. As illustrated in Kileo (2012), enhanced comprehension of population trends in the context of facial trauma can inform public health policy and enable more effective training of medical personnel engaged in facial reconstruction. This nexus of evidence and practice serves to solidify the foundation upon which effective reconstructive interventions are based. Finally, as we incorporate the guidelines that direct the reconstruction of the face, the importance of continued discourse in scholarly and professional circles cannot be overstated. The debate should include progress in surgical technique, the incorporation of technology, and the ongoing review of ethical matters surrounding facial identity. The complexities involved in facial reconstruction necessitate commitment to both refining procedural methods and understanding the broader implications for people and society. The agenda for future research must be interdisciplinary, with studies that analyze the evolving environment of facial reconstruction technology and its applicability for both forensic science and plastic surgery procedures. Through the collaboration of disciplines, there can emerge a clearer context for facial reconstruction, ultimately leading to better and more humane results for victims of trauma or disfigurement.

The discipline of facial reconstruction is also related to various complicated principles that guide its practice, particularly in clinical and surgical practice. One of the key concerns is achieving anatomical accuracy in rebuilding facial structures that have been damaged due to trauma, congenital malformations, or disease. The reconstruction of a face with success demands broad knowledge of craniofacial anatomy, coupled with the application of new methods involving the use of advances in technology. Surgeons today are employing computer-aided design systems that allow for precise planning of operations that maximize patient outcomes. The suggested software systems, for instance, the one in Chen et al. (2017), make it easy to select standard implant models that adapt to the exact contours of every patient's bones, significantly reducing intra-operative procedures and material readjustments. In addition to technology integration, the utilization of data-driven methods marks the root of facial reconstruction. From the utilization of large datasets by tapping into them, such methods reveal geometric, structural, and semantic connections that are inherent in 3D shapes and contribute heavily to facial reconstruction procedures. The move from the traditional methods, most often constrained by hard-coded rules, marks more sophisticated data-driven analysis, improving the modeling, editing, and visualization of facial structure. As noted by Huang et al. (2015), these techniques improve facial feature classification, segmentation, and matching to support more natural-looking reconstructions that adhere closely to the aesthetic and functional characteristics of the human face. This not only helps in producing accurate reconstructions but also provides a foundation for future facial reconstruction breakthroughs. Lastly, the protocols that guide facial reconstruction are based on collaboration among clinical practice and technological development. Continued research and advancements in surgical technique as well as analytical analysis techniques are required to strive for optimal restoration outcomes. The integration of bespoke techniques, e.g., personalized implant model design in Chen et al. (2017), highlights how surgery can be refined through precision and patient-specific planning. With analytical intelligence gained from data-driven practices outlined in Huang et al. (2015), the art of facial reconstruction stands at the threshold of transformative advancement. Not only does the future hold promise for more aesthetically beautiful reconstructions, but it also maximizes the function restoration of facial units, the true determinant of general quality of life.

KEY TERMS FROM THIS CHAPTER

- Reconstructive Ladder
- Wound Bed Preparation
- Regional Flaps
- Skin Grafting
- Tissue Matching
- Vascular Supply
- Scar Camouflage
- Bone Reconstruction
- Tissue Viability
- Local Flaps
- Free Tissue Transfer
- Aesthetic Subunits
- Functional Restoration
- Donor Site Morbidity
- Facial Nerve Preservation
- Soft Tissue Coverage

CRITICAL THINKING QUESTIONS

1. **The primary goal of facial reconstruction is to:**
   a. Reduce scars only
   b. Restore form and function
   c. Increase skin thickness
   d. Tighten facial muscles
2. **The "reconstructive ladder" refers to:**
   a. Steps of fracture management
   b. A hierarchy of reconstructive options from simple to complex
   c. Sequence of anesthesia techniques
   d. Sequence of cosmetic procedures
3. **Which of the following is the simplest option on the reconstructive ladder?**
   a.. Free flap transfer
   b. Skin graft
   c. Local flap
   d. Primary closure
4. **Local flaps are preferred because they:**
   a. Require no anesthesia
   b. Match color and texture best
   c. Require microsurgery
   d. Do not scar
5. **The aesthetic subunit principle is MOST relevant in reconstruction of the:**
   a. Ear only
   b. Nose
   c. Neck
   d. Scalp

Short Answer Questions

1. What is the main goal of facial reconstruction following trauma or tumor excision?
2. Explain the reconstructive ladder and its importance in planning facial reconstruction.
3. What factors determine the choice between local flaps, regional flaps, and free tissue transfer in facial reconstruction?
4. What role does vascular supply play in flap selection for facial reconstruction?
5. What are the key considerations when planning reconstruction in highly visible areas such as the nose or lip?

Answers to Critical Thinking Questions

1. (b) 2. (b) 3. (d) 4. (b) 5. (b)

REFERENCES

1. Abbott, Anderson, Asano, Atala, Baiguera, Barnes, Berry, et al. (2017). *Tissue-engineered solutions in plastic and reconstructive surgery: Principles and practice.* https://core.ac.uk/download/78862846.pdf (accessed on 14th July 2025).
2. Achenbach, Aitken, Algemeen, America's Most Wanted, Aries, Arnow, Barron, et al. (2014). *A review of the changing culture and social context relating to forensic facial depiction of the dead.* https://core.ac.uk/download/42477688.pdf (accessed on 14th July 2025).
3. Ahn, C., Disa, A., & Walker, F. (2020). *High-resolution crystal truncation rod scattering: Application to ultrathin layers and buried interfaces.*
4. Alfertshofer, M., Baecher, H., Hoch, C. C., Kauke-Navarro, et al. (2023). *From bench to bedside – current clinical and translational challenges in fibula free flap reconstruction.* https://core.ac.uk/download/590331043.pdf (accessed on 14th July 2025).
5. Ali, T., Spreeuwers, L., & Veldhuis, R. (2010). *Forensic Face Recognition: A Survey.* https://core.ac.uk/download/pdf/11478879.pdf (accessed on 14th July 2025).
6. Angelopoulou, M. V., Artopoulou, I. I., Emmanouil, D., Maroulakos, et al. (2016). *Removable partial dentures vs overdentures in children with ectodermal dysplasia: Two case reports.* https://core.ac.uk/download/213075195.pdf (accessed on 14th July 2025).
7. Bell, T., & Zhang, S. (2014). *Toward superfast three-dimensional optical metrology with digital micromirror device platforms.* https://core.ac.uk/download/38936128.pdf (accessed on 14th July 2025).
8. Betts, L. R., Binder, J. F., Buglass, S. L., Underwood, et al. (2017). *Online Social Network Data as Sociometric Markers.* https://core.ac.uk/download/46563167.pdf (accessed on 14th July 2025).
9. Bottino, A. G., Laurentini, A., & Rosano, L. (2008). *A new computer-aided technique for planning the aesthetic outcome of plastic surgery.* https://core.ac.uk/download/pdf/11398829.pdf (accessed on 14th July 2025).
10. Bowman, A., Bowman, R., Edgar, M. P., Padgett, et al. (2013). *3D Computational Ghost Imaging.* http://arxiv.org/abs/1301.1595 (accessed on 14th July 2025).
11. Burity, J., Fonte, I. B. da, & Melo, P. B. de (2014). *Radiological Society of North America (RSNA) 3D printing special interest group (SIG): Guidelines for medical 3D printing and appropriateness for clinical scenarios.* https://core.ac.uk/download/212867900.pdf (accessed on 14th July 2025).
12. Burrows, K., Muldoon, A., & Sylvester, A. (2011). New models and insights into primate evolutionary morphology. *Anatomy Research International, 2011.* https://www.semanticscholar.org/paper/3657881e687d71af517b1a6028ea462c3dfb71ab (accessed on 14th July 2025).
13. Burton, C. S. (2019). *Republican monsters: The cultural construction of American positivist criminology, 1767–1920.* https://core.ac.uk/download/287621833.pdf (accessed on 14th July 2025).
14. Campion, S. P., Fairchild, A. J., Fernando, T. P., Garcia Jimenez, et al. (2017). *A mixed reality telepresence system for collaborative space operation.* https://core.ac.uk/download/42590329.pdf (accessed on 14th July 2025).

15. Casey, E., Gladyshev, P., Jaquet-Chiffelle, D. O., Pollitt, et al. (2018). *A framework for harmonizing forensic science practices and digital/multimedia evidence.* https://core.ac.uk/download/151212923.pdf (accessed on 14th July 2025).
16. Chen, J., Chen, Y., He, B., Li, et al. (2019). *Auricle Shaping Using 3D Printing and Autologous Diced Cartilage.* https://core.ac.uk/download/323068973.pdf (accessed on 14th July 2025).
17. Chen, X., Egger, J., Gall, M., Reinbacher, et al. (2017). *Computer-aided position planning of miniplates to treat facial bone defects.* http://arxiv.org/abs/1708.05711 (accessed on 14th July 2025).
18. Di Luca, N. M., Marinelli, E., Napoletano, S., Vergallo, et al. (2018). *Ethics and/or aesthetics? Reflections on cosmetic surgery for adolescents.* https://core.ac.uk/download/188823836.pdf (accessed on 14th July 2025).
19. Dwivedi, Y. K., Hughes, L., Baabdullah, A. M., Ribeiro-Navarrete, S., Giannakis, M., Al-Debei, M. M., Dennehy, D., et al. (2022). Metaverse beyond the hype: Multidisciplinary perspectives on emerging challenges, opportunities, and agenda for research, practice and policy. *International Journal of Information Management, 66*, 102542–102542. https://doi.org/10.1016/j.ijinfomgt.2022.102542 (accessed on 14th July 2025).
20. Emerson, Robert, "Digital Hair Creation for Archaeological Facial Approximation: George Dixon, the Last Captain of the Hl Hunley" (2023). *All Theses*. 4105. https://open.clemson.edu/all_theses/4105 (accessed on 14th July 2025).
21. Fellmann, F., & Redolfi Widmann, E. (2017). *Aspects of sex differences: Social intelligence vs. creative intelligence.* https://core.ac.uk/download/141469975.pdf (accessed on 14th July 2025).
22. Gooya, N. C. (2020). *The contemporary porn debate – Perceptions of sexual health of porn actors, the 2013 HIV crisis, and recognizing the complexities of the porn industry.* https://core.ac.uk/download/322983186.pdf (accessed on 14th July 2025).
23. Hering, P., Hirsch, S., & Prieels, F. (2018). *Holographic topometry for a dense visualization of soft tissue for facial reconstruction.* https://core.ac.uk/download/159145958.pdf (accessed on 14th July 2025).
24. Hong, G. W., Hu, H., Park, S. Y., Wan, J., & Yi, K. H. (2024). What are the factors that enable thread lifting to last longer? *Cosmetics, 11*, 42–42. https://doi.org/10.3390/cosmetics11020042 (accessed on 14th July 2025).
25. Huang, Q., Kalogerakis, E., Kim, V. G., Xu, et al. (2015). *Data-Driven Shape Analysis and Processing.* http://arxiv.org/abs/1502.06686 (accessed on 14th July 2025).
26. Jablonski, R. Y., Malhotra, T., Shaw, D. S., Coward, T., Shuweihdi, F., Bojke, C., Pavitt, S., et al. (2024). Comparison of trueness and repeatability of facial prosthesis design using a 3D morphable model approach, traditional computer-aided design methods, and conventional manual sculpting techniques. *Journal of Prosthetic Dentistry*. https://doi.org/10.1016/j.prosdent.2024.03.006 (accessed on 14th July 2025).
27. Ji, Q., & Wu, Y. (2017). *Constrained Deep Transfer Feature Learning and Its Applications.* http://arxiv.org/abs/1709.08128 (accessed on 14th July 2025).
28. Kileo, B. F. (2012). *The pattern of oral and maxillofacial injuries among patients attending Muhimbili National Hospital, Dar es Salaam, Tanzania.* https://core.ac.uk/download/pdf/11307821.pdf (accessed on 14th July 2025).

29. Lau, H., & Li, H. (2017). *American Equal Protection and Global Convergence*. https://core.ac.uk/download/144232668.pdf (accessed on 14th July 2025).

30. Lee, W. J., Shin, D. H., Song, M. K., Wilkinson, et al. (2014). *The archaeological contribution of forensic craniofacial reconstruction to a portrait drawing of a Korean historical figure*. https://core.ac.uk/download/74237934.pdf (accessed on 14th July 2025).

31. Mar, M. D. (2008). *Creativity and Imagination in the Practice of Philosophy*. https://core.ac.uk/download/131179506.pdf (accessed on 14th July 2025).

32. Mohapatra, D., Friji, M. T., DineshKumar, S., Chittoria, R. K., Pathan, I., & Koliath, S. (2023). Reconstruction of defects following excision of basal cell carcinoma of face: A subunit-based algorithm. *Journal of Cutaneous and Aesthetic Surgery*, *16*, 1–13. https://www.semanticscholar.org/paper/131c1df2a30d473c3041c6126b961ef96c2a9aca (accessed on 14th July 2025).

33. Ngo, A. C. L., Phan, R. C. W., & See, J. (2016). *Sparsity in dynamics of spontaneous subtle emotions: Analysis & application*. http://arxiv.org/abs/1601.04805 (accessed on 14th July 2025).

34. Nizami, L. (2017). *I, Neuron: The Neuron as the Collective*. https://core.ac.uk/download/186332026.pdf (accessed on 14th July 2025).

35. Oliveira, L., Pamplona, M., Papa, J., Souza, et al. (2018). *How Far Did We Get in Face Spoofing Detection?* http://arxiv.org/abs/1710.09868 (accessed on 14th July 2025).

36. Payne, Michael G., "The Reliability Of Facial Soft Tissue Landmarks With Photogrammetry" (2013). Master's Theses (2009 -). Paper 198. http://epublications.marquette.edu/theses_open/198(accessed on 14th July 2025).

37. Schutte, H., Maat, R., Muradin, M., & Rosenberg, A. J. W. P. (2025). Technique and muscle preferences for dynamic facial reanimation in irreversible facial paralysis—A literature review. *Craniomaxillofacial Trauma & Reconstruction*, *18*. https://www.semanticscholar.org/paper/82a799c35d57ae8120d8d37ed9bb28eb47b5847a (accessed on 14th July 2025).

38. Suo, X. (2023). Overview of 3D human face reconstruction techniques and a novel approach. In *2023 Congress in Computer Science, Computer Engineering, & Applied Computing (CSCE)*. https://www.semanticscholar.org/paper/997583949e0f35a40ea8a4c108ffcff0041bfabe (accessed on 14th July 2025).

39. Wang, Y., Su, Z., Zhang, N., Xing, R., Liu, D., Luan, T. H., & Shen, X. (2022). A survey on metaverse: Fundamentals, security, and privacy. *IEEE Communications Surveys & Tutorials*, *25*, 319–352. https://doi.org/10.1109/comst.2022.3202047 (accessed on 14th July 2025).

40. Wilkinson, C. (2025). *A Review of Forensic Art*. https://core.ac.uk/download/42477686.pdf (accessed on 14th July 2025).

TRAUMA RECONSTRUCTION IN FACIAL COSMETIC

12

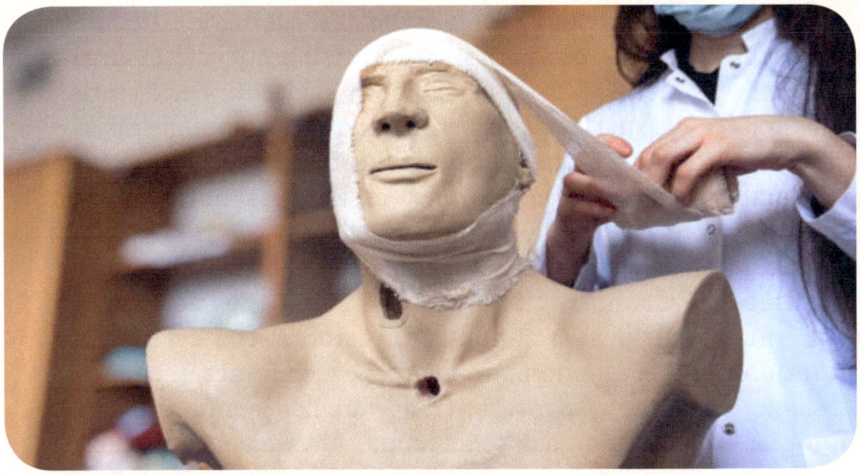

LEARNING OBJECTIVES

After studying this chapter, you will be able to:

1. Discuss facial trauma types;
2. Describe the psychological impact of facial trauma;
3. Highlight surgical methods of facial reconstruction;
4. Describe the cosmetic procedure contribution to reconstruction;
5. Understand a multidisciplinary treatment approach;
6. Know ethical issues in facial reconstruction.

Introduction

The discipline of trauma reconstruction in the field of facial cosmetic surgery has gained significant interest owing to the increasing number of cases of facial trauma, either from accidents or violence or surgery. Facial structures are very important in both aesthetic and functional demands; efforts to reconstruct such structures to their pre-trauma state are prioritized. The face's reconstruction complexities are not just physical reconstruction of bone and tissue, but also the psychological effects of trauma. The most optimal reconstructive outcomes are capable of improving patients' self-esteem and quality of life, thereby highlighting the need for developments and innovations in surgical techniques and materials during the process of trauma management. Autologous grafting has been the gold standard in these situations for many years, providing good cosmetic outcomes at low risk of rejection from foreign substances (Abbott et al., 2003). The more demand there is for improved reconstructive techniques, the greater the quest for alternative techniques and materials. Though autologous bone grafting possesses numerous benefits, such as optimal biocompatibility and mechanical durability, its potential drawbacks, such as donor-site morbidity and protracted operation time, led to the development of alloplastic materials. These attempts to prevent the attendant complications of acquiring bone from the donor site while offering sufficient structural support and ultimately leading to increased patient recovery times. Clinical studies have yielded promising results regarding the use of synthetic bone substitutes and their ability to complement or even replace autologous grafts in certain instances (Neovius, 2016). Therefore, understanding the risks and benefits of traditional and new reconstruction techniques is paramount to achieving optimal surgical outcomes and lowering the rate of complications. Also, the integration of surgical and technical developments into trauma reconstruction processes is proof of the evolving nature of the field. The incorporation of minimally invasive surgical processes along with high-tech image-making technologies has allowed the surgery process to make more precise and effective restorations. Other seminal research in bioactive materials includes the bone morphogenetic proteins (BMPs) in enhancing bone repair and regeneration, but caution should be exercised in the variable reported success rates and complications with the use of such therapy. Further, comprehension of the multifaceted complexities of facial trauma involves an individualized consideration of each patient's unique circumstance, taking into account the type of injury, psychological issues, and long-term expectation for function. This multidisciplinary approach emphasizes the necessity of research and extensive training in trauma reconstruction (Abbott et al., 2003; Neovius, 2016).

Definition of Trauma Reconstruction

Trauma reconstruction is a multidisciplinary approach attempting to restore form and function to the facial form following traumatic injuries. This subject of study is not only critical for treating physical deformity but also for the alleviation of the psychological effects of facial trauma. The reconstructive process entails careful examination of the condition of the patient, as well as an appreciation of the cause of injury, for instance, vehicular accident, falling, or assault. Effective trauma reconstruction entails interdisciplinary cooperation between surgeons, orthodontists, and other healthcare workers as they strive to achieve the best aesthetic outcome while ensuring the underlying structural integrity of the facial bony skeleton. The nature of such cases often demands a combination of surgical techniques, like bone graft and soft tissue repositioning, to address both short-term and long-term needs at the same time. One of the most important features of trauma reconstruction is implementing advanced surgical techniques to restore facial aesthetics and function. Among those techniques, the facial artery perforator (FAP) flap has been attracting attention due to its unique advantages. Based on reports, this new technique has the potential to transform a normally two-stage procedure into a more efficient one-stage operation, therefore reducing the time and risks associated with surgery. FAP flaps are favored since they can provide better aesthetic results, especially for those patients seeking trauma reconstruction. Extensive use is, however, constrained by the need for extensive knowledge of the requisite anatomical features, which form the basis of successful application. Through cadaveric dissections, vast data regarding the facial artery, its perforating branches, and their diameter have been gathered, with better consistency of FAP flaps in reconstructive surgery on various parts of the face (Fogg et al., 2010). The psychological aspects of facial trauma cannot be ruled out, as they also hold equal value to the physical aspect. Trauma reconstruction not only aims at reversing the form of a patient but also restoring self-worth and rehabilitating them to re-integrate them into society. Patients typically experience shame or embarrassment resulting from external deformities that lead to social isolation or emotional distress. The multidisciplinary aspect of trauma reconstruction emphasizes the coordination of care that includes emotional and psychological care in addition to surgical control. Comprehensive treatment regimens must also consider the application of adjunctive treatments, such as counseling or support groups, which are also able to supplement the healing process. Prioritizing both physical and psychological recovery is what makes trauma reconstruction such a crucial stepping stone towards achieving the quality of life in patients who have endured facial injuries (Bosio et al., 2008) (Figure 12.1).

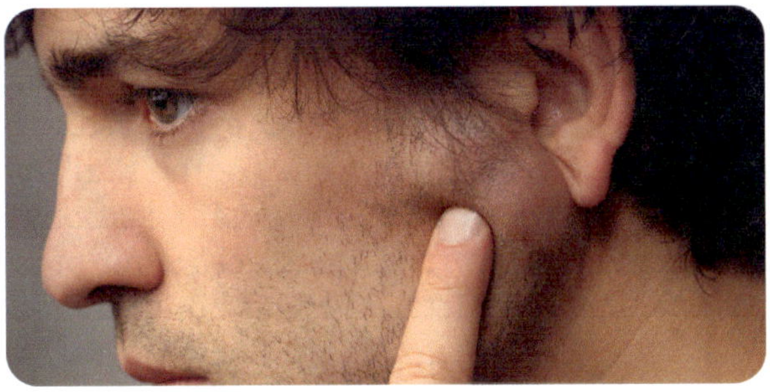

Figure 12.1. Trauma reconstruction.

Source: https://external-content.duckduckgo.com/iu/?u=https%3A%2F%2Fswosa.com%2Fwp-content%2Fuploads%2F2024%2F06%2FSWOSA_Procedures_Facial-Trauma-1024x512.png&f=1&nofb=1&ipt=e2abe8f4acbd96208c2452e8cc5e1722a10508118bdc347e84953073e717fa61.

Facial Aesthetics In Psychological Rehabilitation

The function of facial aesthetics in psychological rehabilitation cannot be overstated, especially in trauma reconstruction. In patients who have experienced disfiguring conditions or injuries, rebuilding of facial appearance generally leads to increased levels of self-esteem and self-confidence. It has been researched that an aesthetically pleasing face significantly contributes to how people see us, and thus affects interpersonal relationships as well as social interactions. In addition to cosmetic changes, a successful outcome in terms of facial aesthetics following trauma can also be a driver of emotional recovery. Patients are often said to feel psychologically more well when they perceive a return to a more familiar self, connecting physical presentation with mental health recovery on a direct level. This connection between beauty and emotional hardiness emphasizes the need for holistic methods that maximize facial aesthetics as fundamental aspects of psychological recovery. In craniofacial reconstruction, advancements in surgical techniques and technology have greatly improved the outcomes of aesthetic repair. The use of new devices, such as ultrasound-guided osteotomes, has enabled surgeons to perform fine procedures in the craniofacial region more accurately. For all this, studies have evidenced that such advanced devices lead to more quality micromorphological outcomes in bone healing, i.e., a smoother healing process for patients who are reconstructing (Anesi et al., 2014). These advancements are necessary since they improve not only the cosmetic results but also the psychological status of individuals. By reducing recovery time and complications, such strategies allow for an early return to regular life, thereby eliminating worry and providing confidence to patients who undergo traumatic facial injury. In addition, the exploration of tissue engineering and stem cell therapy also provides promising pathways for facial aesthetic enhancement and psychological healing. Recent studies indicate that stem cell therapy can regenerate damaged craniofacial tissue more effectively than existing methods (Hughes & Song, 2016). New technology aligns therapeutic goals and esthetic goals with a common emphasis on the structure and function of the face throughout the healing process. The integration of scientific findings with craniofacial surgery not only optimizes physical rehabilitation but also addresses the psychological implications of trauma. With patients finding new hope and identity from such cutting-edge treatments, psychological resilience is also increased. The convergence of cosmetic enhancement with medical technology ultimately underscores the reality that creation of facial aesthetics constitutes a key component in the overall rehabilitation of traumatized patients (Figure 12.2).

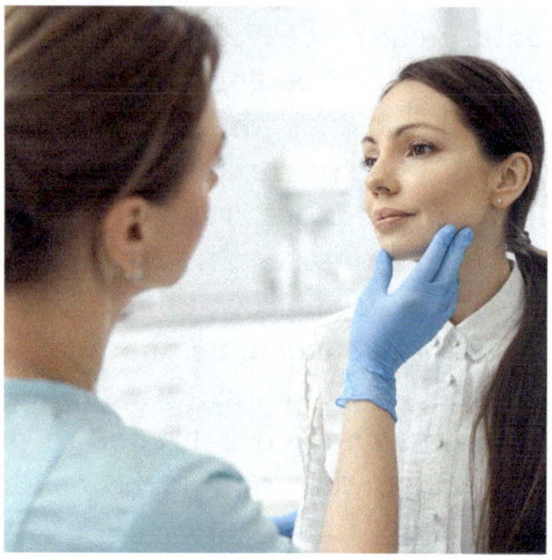

Figure 12.2. Importance of facial aesthetics in psychological recovery.

Source: https://external-content.duckduckgo.com/iu/?u=https%3A%2F%2Fthedentalsurgeries.co.uk%2Fwp-content%2Fuploads%2F2023%2F08%2Ffacial-aesthetics-consultation-1024x1024.jpeg&f=1&nofb=1&ipt=a9c2630f6869873a72c1b477add4378aeb0778b5db7bf51331462480354f0960.

12.1. Types of Facial Trauma

Learning Outcome

1. Discuss the Common Causes of Facial Injuries
2. Explain Classification of Facial Trauma
3. Impact of Trauma on Facial Structure

Facial trauma is a very critical area of investigation in the domain of trauma reconstruction due to its involvement with various types of trauma that have different implications on function and aesthetics. Facial trauma can occur in a variety of common forms, namely, soft tissue trauma, fracture, and laceration, each of which presents unique challenges during reconstruction. Soft tissue injury most commonly creates defects that compromise both protective and aesthetic roles of facial structures, necessitating advanced reconstruction techniques for optimal recovery. One such example is when trauma results in extensive lacerations that not only disrupt the skin but also involve underlying muscle and vascular components, which affect both cosmetic and functional outcomes, e.g., speech and swallowing. Understanding of the individual mechanisms and implications of such trauma is significant in the development of effective reconstructive methods, particularly in the restoration of facial integrity and patient confidence. Fractures are also a broad category of facial trauma involving bones of the skull and mandible, which would lead to complications if not attended to early and effectively. Some of the most commonly fractured facial bones include the nasal bones, zygomatic arch, and maxilla. All types of fractures require proper realignment and stabilization, which is typically done via surgery. Methods of reconstruction employed can make use of plates, screws, or grafts to restore harmony in the architecture and maintain functionality intact. Delayed intervention can exacerbate complications such as malocclusion or asymmetry, thus making later reconstruction more difficult. This timing value is also stressed by research that shows delayed intervention is expressed in greater aesthetic failures and increased patient morbidity, which necessitates that surgical procedures for facial fractures be timely and effective. When it comes to facial reconstructive modalities, the significance of newer surgical modalities cannot be overstated, particularly when facial injuries are very severe (Bodiwala et al., 2025). Newer surgical techniques, such as the pedicled forehead flap, have become indispensable tools in the quest for form and function restoration, particularly in challenging cases where standard methods are not effective. For example, the pedicled forehead flap has pertinent advantages regarding vascular assistance to enable the reconstruction of large traumatic soft tissue deficits. It has been shown to provide not just cosmetic rehabilitation but also functional recovery, as evidenced by the gain in improved oral competence and facial symmetry post-surgery. These methods emphasize how crucial it is for surgeons to have a clear knowledge of the nature of facial trauma, as clearly explicated in recent studies, revealing that personalized approaches concerning the nature of injury exhibit the best outcomes in trauma reconstruction in facial cosmetic conditions (Yu et al., 2022) (Figure 12.3).

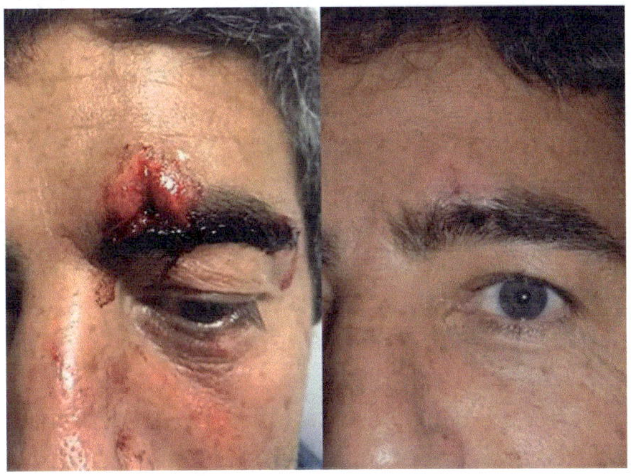

Figure 12.3. Facial trauma.

Source: https://www.darrensmithmd.com/wp-content/uploads/2023/08/facial-trauma-ba-2.webp.

12.1.1. Common Causes of Facial Injuries

Facial trauma is more common, and it most frequently results from different accidents and traumatic injuries. Car accidents are among the most common causes, whereby crashes result in high impact forces leading to fractures of the facial bones or damage to the soft tissues. Facial trauma from car crashes constitutes a high percentage of emergency department presentations and typically mandates complex surgical treatment, as witnessed in a review of trauma data. The degree of the injury can be highly variable, ranging from lacerations of soft tissue to fractures involving the mandible or maxilla. In treating these injuries, it is critical to understand the mechanisms of injury as they directly affect the reconstruction techniques used in trauma surgery. Understanding these allows surgeons to plan successful reconstruction in order to restore function and aesthetic appearance in patients with such traumas. Interpersonal violence, such as physical assaults and cases of domestic violence, is also a significant cause of facial injuries. Statistics indicate that facial trauma due to brawls or domestic disputes is very high, particularly among certain populations. Injuries of this nature are most commonly reported as midface fractures, zygomatic bone fractures, and lacerations. Management of such injuries often entails unique challenges as patients not only require physical therapy but also psychological counseling due to the nature of their trauma. Furthermore, facial nerve and vascular exposure during surgeries requires cautious attention to avoid long-term consequences of aesthetic and functional deficits. Therefore, classification of various etiologies of facial trauma introduces the topics of prevention and management with emphasis on particular strategies in reconstructive trauma. Injuries secondary to sports are a frequent cause of facial trauma seen in patients of all ages. Contact sports such as football, hockey, and boxing have a high incidence of facial injuries, mainly due to direct blows, falls, or impact against another participant. They most commonly present as fractures of the nasal and zygomatic bones and soft tissue damage in the patterns of contusions and lacerations. Protective equipment, such as helmets and face masks, plays an important role in reducing the number and degree of injuries. Rates are still high with precautions, emphasizing the need for continued research and development in preventive techniques and surgery. As trauma reconstruction emerges, advanced imaging modalities and minimally invasive surgical approaches must be included to enhance recovery outcomes in athletes with facial injuries due to sporting activities (Figure 12.4).

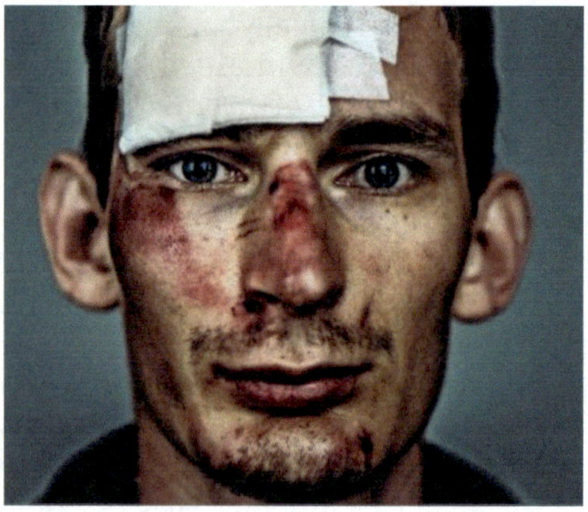

Figure 12.4. Facial injuries.

Source: https://external-content.duckduckgo.com/iu/?u=https%3A%2F%2Fhpasolicitors.com%2Fwp-content%2Fuploads%2Felementor%2Fthumbs%2FFace-Injury-Claims-r0agjx97hbzl4y5mzi3yr0z6s29s2emlymrirc940s.jpg&f=1&nofb=1&ipt=d1525ea2115a227695fcb5f8623e492020b521257da5146f4cb6fa09b0853bda.

12.1.2. Classification of Facial Trauma

Facial trauma must be classified in order to guide treatment plans in trauma reconstruction. Facial trauma can in general be classified into soft tissue and hard tissue trauma, both with varying implications for reconstruction surgery. Soft tissue damage typically involves laceration, abrasion, and contusion that represents a continuum of injury to the skin, muscles, and underlying structures. It is classically divided into depth and distribution, with special emphasis on preserving function and aesthetic outcome. Conversely, hard tissue injuries entail fractures of facial bones such as the maxilla, mandible, and zygomatic arch that can potentially significantly impact function and aesthetics. Proper classification helps in determining the most appropriate reconstructive approach depending on the severity and extent of the injuries, thus ensuring better patient outcomes for reconstructive procedures. In the area of facial trauma, a broad-based classification system attempts to address the variability of numerous injury patterns found in the clinical environment. Tuli et al.'s suggested broad-based system distinguishes facial fractures as either high-energy or low-energy forms and offers insights regarding mechanisms of trauma based on impact forces. This differentiation is crucial for reconstructive surgeons when scheduling operations, as high-energy trauma causes more extensive damage that may require advanced techniques and materials for reconstruction (Desai et al., 2020). Second, understanding the location and pattern of mandibular and maxillary fractures, which are most common in facial trauma, allows for a more tailored treatment strategy whereby not only structural reconstruction but also aesthetic restoration of the patient's face can be addressed by surgeons. Such subtle classification allows surgeons to optimize surgical procedures effectively. The growing application of technological advancements, such as three-dimensional (3D) printing, is reshaping facial trauma classification and reconstruction. While traditional classifications are significantly reliant on clinical examination and imaging, 3D models from Digital Imaging and Communications in Medicine (DICOM) data are ultimately more accurate in preoperative planning and education. Through the production of three-dimensional models of intricate fractures, reconstructive surgeons can comprehend facial anatomy and spatial relationships more clearly in a trauma environment. Not only does this new modality improve the precision of surgical procedures, but it is also beneficial for patient counseling and visualization of anticipated results. As proposed in recent literature, there is some expectation that use of 3D-printed models will grow in reconstructive procedures, particularly cementing further the association between innovative technologies and maximized classification in the management of facial trauma (Mitsouras et al., 2015).

12.1.3. Impact of Trauma on Facial Structure

Trauma radically transforms facial structures, both in terms of appearance as well as functional integrity. Facial trauma can be brought about by a variety of reasons like road accidents, falls, and violent confrontations. The traumatic injury is prone to cause fractures, cuts, and displacements of the bone as well as soft tissue. These alterations can provide overt deformities as well as impaired functions, such as chewing, speech, and breathing. Also, the psychological impact of facial trauma is prominent, with patients showing reduced self-esteem and withdrawal from society. Hence, learning about the different methods by which trauma affects facial contours is necessary to incorporate clinical interventions and psychological therapy as part of the reconstruction process. Reconstruction of facial trauma encompasses numerous surgical techniques and cutting-edge technology to recapture both the contour and function. One of the notable advancements in this field is the use of piezosurgery, which offers a more precise method for osteotomies compared to traditional instruments. Studies have established that techniques like Piezosurgery Medical® result in more precise incisions without injuring surrounding tissues such as the dura mater and nervous tissue. The reduced trauma to the surrounding tissues promotes better healing and reossification of the injured bone surfaces, addressing not just the short-term cosmetic problems but also long-term sustainability of the bone and associated tissues (Anesi et al., 2014). The improvements point to the necessity of selecting proper surgical methods that are crafted based on the unique character of the trauma, as well as the desired outcomes of the reconstruction. Secondly, the integration of 3D body-surface scanning technology has revolutionized the planning and assessment stages. Advanced imaging modalities such as these facilitate the accurate visualization and measurement of a patient's facial anatomy, which remains critical for the creation of individualized treatment plans. The accurate information provided by 3D scanning aids surgeons' predictions and designs prosthetics or grafts required for effective reconstruction (Figure 12.5).

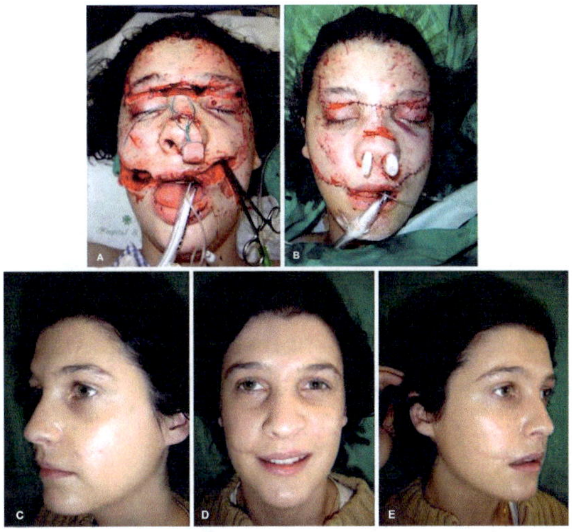

Figure 12.5. Trauma on the facial structure.

Source: https://media.springernature.com/lw685/springer-static/image/chp%3A10.1007%2F978-3-642-38482-0_133-2/MediaObjects/272888_0_En_133-2_Fig2_HTML.jpg.

Test Your Knowledge

1. What are the most common causes of facial injuries, and how do these mechanisms typically affect different facial regions?
2. How is facial trauma classified, and what criteria are used to distinguish between soft-tissue and skeletal injuries?

12.2. Psychological Effects of Facial Trauma

Learning Outcome

1. Discuss the Emotional and Mental Health Implications
2. Explain Social Stigma and Its Effects on Recovery
3. Focus on Role of Self-image in Psychological Healing

The psychological consequences of facial trauma are profound and intricate, typically leading to extreme emotional pain that impacts individuals' quality of life. Facial traumas, when they occur, not only jeopardize physical appearances but also challenge personal identity and social relationships. Patients may experience a range of psychological reactions, including anxiety, depression, and post-traumatic stress disorder (PTSD), as they cope with altered self-concept and social perceptions. Research indicates that the seriousness of facial injury correlates with the seriousness of psychological symptomatology observed, illustrating an intricate relationship between physical and psychological well-being. The unique form of each individual's experience calls for a personalized approach to trauma reconstruction, where the overriding priority lies in psychological support as well as physical rehabilitation. The psychological trauma has to be treated in the patient with facial trauma so that complete recovery can be facilitated. Cosmetic reconstructive surgery can play a pivotal role in facilitating this process, both restoring the physical damage and healing emotionally as well. As discussed, utilization of autologous bone grafting in facial reconstruction has distinctive advantages, including improved aesthetic outcomes that are able to significantly boost a patient's self-esteem and psychological rehabilitation (Abbott et al., 2003). Successful surgery can lead to enhanced social contact and reduced social isolation, thus allowing individuals to restore their sense of identity. However, the psychological recovery cannot be left out because the patients can still go on struggling to get used to the new appearance and cope with social interactions after the surgery. Additionally, advances in surgical techniques, for example, utilization of Piezosurgery® for surgical osteotomies, have been shown to have potential positive outcomes for both physical and psychological recovery (Anesi et al., 2014). Maintenance of the surrounding tissues during surgery with meticulousness minimizes complications and improves cosmetic results, which can minimize recovery-related anxiety. By improving not just the structural support for facial structures but also the psychosocial aspect of healing, such technologies can result in better overall outcomes for patients. Ultimately, there is a need for an effective global approach that addresses both physical and psychological consequences of facial trauma in trauma reconstruction, giving the person assistance in their healing process and reintegration into society (Figure 12.6).

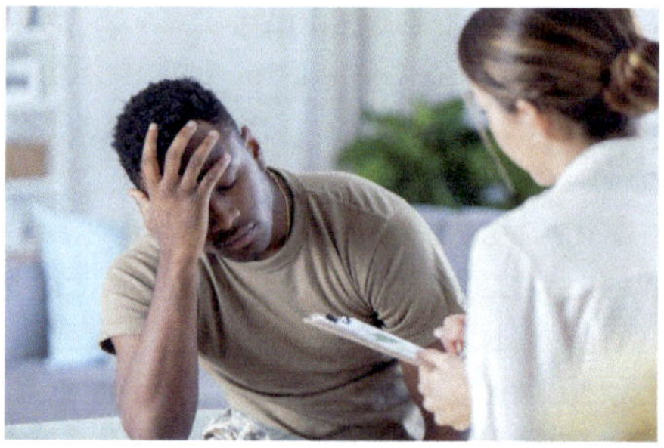

Figure 12.6. Psychological effects of facial trauma.

Source: https://www.sanantoniobehavioral.com/wp-content/uploads/2021/12/psychological-trauma.jpg.

12.2.1. Emotional and Mental Health Implications

Facial cosmetic surgery, particularly in trauma reconstruction, has emotional and mental health implications which are myriad and extensive. Patients undergoing such procedures often wish for changes that not only aim to restore the physical but also to heal the psychological. Research has established that patients who undergo reconstructive surgeries such as rhinoplasty are likely to experience extensive alterations in mental health status, particularly with regard to depression. In a trial of 200 rhinoplasty patients, there was a great decline in depression scores at six months after the operation (p=0.032) (Bazgir et al., 2023). The finding illustrates how cosmetic surgery can enhance emotional well-being by addressing feelings of inadequacy or social embarrassment that could be caused by facial disfigurements or injuries. But it is also critical to look at the psychological factors why and how these procedures are done so that maladaptive body views do not result from them. In addition, all emotional outcomes are not positive. The interplay between early life and body image can be a deciding factor in whether cosmetic procedures work for an individual's mental health. Surgery patients with a history of childhood trauma and neglect may have deep-seated body shame-related issues, which thus manifest as body dysmorphic disorder after surgery. Body dysmorphic disorder is characterized by obsessive concerns regarding perceived flaws and persistent dissatisfaction regardless of surgery (Constantian, 2022). If the patients carry unresolved psychological trauma related to their concept of self, then the expectation that cosmetic surgery will be an overall increase in mental health may remain unfulfilled. Thus, resolution of the psychological concerns on which a patient's motivation for surgery lies is of special significance for trauma reconstruction in the field of facial cosmetic surgery. In general, the emotional and psychological impacts of facial cosmetic surgery trauma reconstruction must be tackled with complex insight. Although evidence has shown that these procedures can lead to improvement in mental well-being, it is also important to note that the psychological factors and individual histories play significant roles in such cases. A careful assessment concerning patients' pre-surgery mental health may potentially identify at-risk individuals for ill effects, for instance, anxiety or body dysmorphic disorder. By including psychological counseling and guidance in the cosmetic surgical intervention, clinicians are better able to make certain that the benefits of trauma reconstruction transition from physical changes to facilitate long-term emotional recovery (Figure 12.7).

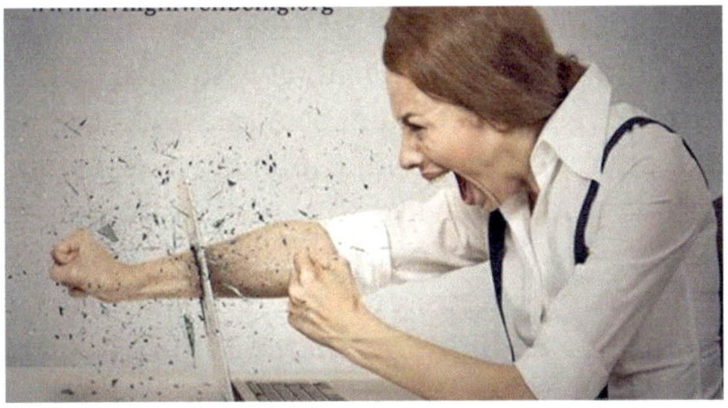

Figure 12.7. Emotional and mental health implications of facial cosmetic procedures.

Source: https://www.livinginwellbeing.org/wp-content/uploads/2019/05/Emotional-Mental-Health-Problems-1200x675.jpg.

12.2.2. Social Stigma and Its Effects on Recovery

The process of healing from facial trauma is normally tainted by the pervasive social stigma that accompanies altered appearances. Victims of extreme facial injuries are often confronted with current social attitudes that characterize them as different or unfortunate. Stigma does this to cut one off and make them feel inferior, and over time, this impedes emotional healing. Research demonstrates that the psychosocial effects of facial disfigurements have a tendency to surpass the bodily injuries, extending to affect self-esteem and interpersonal relations. The stigma is also bolstered by the cultural emphasis on aesthetics and beauty, which tends to enhance the psychological disturbance in recovering patients. Identification of these dynamics is important, given the fact that the social world has a profound impact on one's ability to metabolize trauma and react positively to rehabilitative efforts. The effects of social stigma are multifaceted and function differently across different demographic populations. Individuals recuperating from facial trauma, be it due to accidents or medical procedures, may be subjected to gendered nuances in the practice and perception of stigma. For example, women may experience more judgment over their looks and the beauty standards of society. Men may experience stigmas related to challenging their sense of masculinity and being strong. Both populations have to navigate complex social environments that can either reinforce healing or disrupt healing. Because of this, supportive networks are needed that take into consideration the individual needs of each population. These types of networks can promote dialogue and sharing of experience, thereby reducing the stigmatizing segregation of recovery paths. In cosmetic reconstruction, addressing social stigma is not only demanded for cosmetic improvement but also for general recuperation. The innovation of prosthetic design and production, for instance, custom-made artificial eyes, is a demonstration of collaboration of technological advancement and social acceptance in recuperation. Despite these advances, studies indicate that there is still limited knowledge of the psychosocial impacts of wearing appearance-transforming devices, such as artificial eyes, which can perpetuate stigma (Chinnery et al., 2016). At the same time, what cisgender and transgender patients go through in the performance of cosmetic surgeries is found to be parallel as far as motivation and postoperative satisfaction are concerned, but accentuates differential access to support systems along gender status (Windsor, 2011). This means a demand for certain therapeutic techniques with stigmatization of altered aesthetics in mind for purposes of encouraging broader understanding and acceptance within society.

12.2.3. Role of Self-image in Psychological Healing

The relationship between self-image and psychological healing is of profound significance, specifically in facial cosmetic surgery of trauma reconstruction. Self-concept, one's own definition of one's own physical appearance and one's overall worth, is a deciding factor in the direction of mental health outcomes. In cosmetic facial patients, the desire to improve is typically linked with a past history of traumatic incidents in which their self-concept has been negatively impacted. This interaction suggests that individuals who perceive a disparity between the inner being and outward appearances may suffer from low self-esteem as well as social anxiety. Thus, treating these elements through surgery is not only able to alter an individual's outer appearance but also invoke powerful psychological healing. The psychological effects of bodily deformity or perceived ugliness can manifest in the form of social anxiety, depression, and a severe effect on inter-relations. The majority of individuals who experience trauma, particularly where the facial aesthetics are altered or disfigured, do have self-view concerns that affect their mental health. Recovery towards redefinition of one's self-perception involves a sensitive therapy process where people can modify their pre- and postoperative selves. To reiterate, incorporating psychological care into the cosmetic surgical process cannot be overstressed. These treatments benefit patients not only through the physical changes but also through the emotional effects that accompany them, so that a very holistic approach to reconstruction of trauma in facial cosmetic surgery is possible. Furthermore, self-image extends beyond the individual and into interpersonal relationships and social interaction. Following reconstructive surgery, patients may have higher self-esteem, which translates into more positive social interactions and relief from feelings of disconnection and isolation that the surgery client may have experienced before surgery. Research indicates that a positive change in self-image can lead to tangible benefits in a person's overall quality of life, such as healthier relationships and an increased social support network. Furthermore, successful outcomes from reconstructive surgery can confirm a patient's identity and agency, restoring their resilience to previous traumas. It is where the role of self-image not just facilitates psychological healing but develops a new sense of self, enabling individuals to regain control over their lives following trauma (Anesi et al., 2014; Cheung et al., 2014) (Figure 12.8).

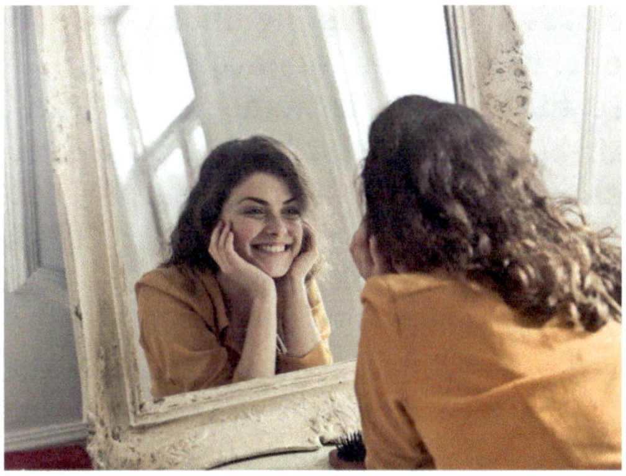

Figure 12.8. Role of self-image in psychological healing.

Source: https://cdn2.psychologytoday.com/assets/styles/manual_crop_4_3_1200x900/public/teaser_image/blog_entry/2024-11/pexels-olly-774866.jpg?itok=jiIeR7Fe.

Test Your Knowledge

1. What emotional and mental health challenges are commonly experienced by individuals following facial trauma?
2. How can social stigma related to visible facial injuries affect a patient's confidence and overall recovery process?

12.3. Surgical Techniques in Facial Reconstruction

Learning Outcome

1. Give an Overview of Surgical Options Available
2. Discuss the Innovations in Surgical Technology
3. Explain Importance of Personalized Treatment Plans

Accuracy of surgical technique is the essence of facial cosmetic surgery for the restoration of form and function, as well as aesthetic form, in the process of trauma reconstruction. The multidisciplinary nature of facial plastic surgery, which involves composite techniques from otolaryngology, oral maxillofacial surgery, dermatology, ophthalmology, and plastic surgery, provides a complete approach to the management of traumatic injury. Reconstructive surgery often entails the use of new flap techniques, which aim to restore the integrity of the cutaneous and promote healing with minimal scarring. These techniques are continually evolving since they are governed by advances in surgical skills and adjunctive technologies, necessitating surgeons to remain updated on existing practice of facial reconstruction to enhance patient results (Chuang et al., 2016). Among the many surgical techniques, the bicoronal flap technique has emerged as a so-called catch-all procedure when dealing with troublesome facial and skull fractures. Popularized by Tessier, the technique offers wide exposure to the field while preserving all the essential neurovascular structures intact, thus significantly reducing postoperative morbidity. Bicoronal incision is where the incision is made within the area of hair-bearing skin, which not only gives the necessary exposure to the site of surgery but also optimizes the cosmetic outcome upon recovery. Each case of the application of this technique has underscored its versatility, in that it may be tailored to suit different pathological conditions within the frontal region (Balachandar et al., 2012). The benefits of this flap operation extend beyond enhancing aesthetic looks; it provides potential for functional reconstruction that is critical in reconstructive trauma. Beyond traditional flap techniques, the integration of minimally invasive procedures is transforming the component of facial reconstruction surgery. Techniques such as injectables and lasers have gained popularity to the extent that they provide surgeons with the ability to enhance facial aesthetics with fewer traumatic maneuvers. These methods can correct texture defects, soft tissue deficiency, and aging alterations that can occur after trauma.

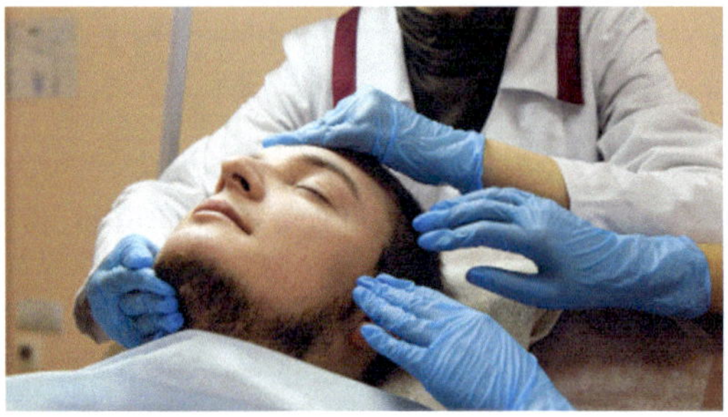

Figure 12.9. Surgical techniques in facial reconstruction.

Source: https://www.medstarhealth.org/-/media/project/mho/medstar/services/h1_doctor-examining-paitents-face.jpg?h=410&iar=0&w=730&hash=7108613E91018EEFFD7F7F490816C63D.

The incorporation of these non-surgical adjuncts into practice complements surgery, allowing for a more extensive solution to facial reconstruction. Surgeons are thus encouraged to integrate highly innovative surgical techniques with innovative cosmetic procedures in order to attain optimal recovery and patient satisfaction when patients need trauma reconstruction in facial cosmetics (Chuang et al., 2016) (Figure 12.9).

12.3.1. Overview of Surgical Options Available

For trauma reconstruction within facial cosmetic purposes, surgical options vary significantly based on the severity and nature of injuries incurred. One of the more significant techniques employs autologous bone grafts, which are harvested from the patient's own body to facilitate the reconstruction of facial shape and function. This technique is particularly suited to the repair of craniomaxillofacial fractures, as it ensures biological compatibility and low risk of rejection. However, there are consequences, as harvesting these grafts runs the risk of additional surgical sites and complications. With the aim to enhance the results of surgery, the application of emerging technologies such as 3D printing has emerged as a viable option, allowing for the fabrication of personalized implants and surgical guides to fit the unique anatomical features of the patient's face, resulting in improved function and aesthetics. Along with 3D printing and bone grafting, other surgical techniques have also been established to address the different needs of patients undergoing facial reconstruction. As an example, soft tissue grafting is used to restore volume and shape, especially in the area of trauma. This can involve the transfer of skin, muscle, or fat from the rest of the body, tailored to fit the defect resulting from injury. The success of the procedure relies largely on the meticulous planning of the surgical site and the source of donor tissues. Besides, technology in microsurgical techniques has also enhanced the precision of soft tissue reconstruction to the extent that the complex anastomosis of veins and arteries, and also nerves, can be achieved with good perfusion and function of the transplanted tissue. The evolving techniques make it possible for a better quality of life for patients through the enhancement of both form and function. The application of technology and emerging techniques in trauma reconstruction recognizes the need for a multidisciplinary approach between surgical teams. Craniofacial, plastic, and reconstructive surgeons also often work with specialists from other fields to offer comprehensive care of facial trauma. Teamwork is crucial, especially when treating complex trauma that can involve bones, soft tissue, and ocular tissues. For instance, in cases like anterior staphyloma, where complicated ocular deformities resulting from trauma develop, surgery and prosthetic rehabilitation afterward have been successful, as shown in comparative studies (Yadav et al., 2025). Besides, the use of 3D-printed devices has been effective in producing patient-specific results, which contribute to facial symmetry and functional capacity restoration (Oley et al., 2024). These novel techniques reflect the ongoing evolution of surgical methods observed in trauma reconstruction of facial cosmetic surgery, ending in enhanced patient outcomes and experience (Figure 12.10).

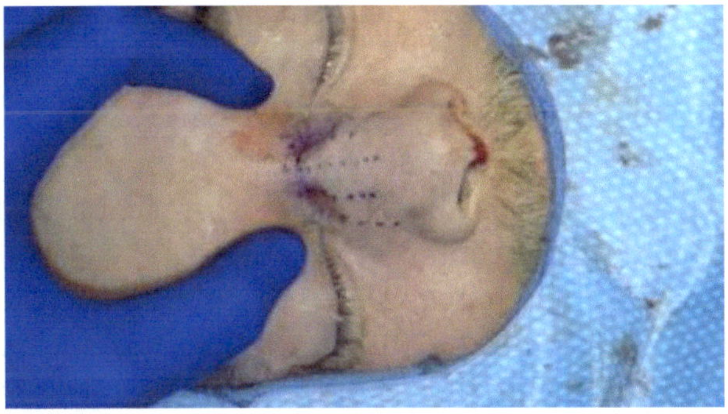

Figure 12.10. Surgical options for trauma reconstruction.

Source: https://cfvod.kaltura.com/p/1315631/sp/131563100/thumbnail/entry_id/1_x80jwhen/version/100011/height/197/width/350.

12.3.2. Innovations in Surgical Technology

The recent technological advancements in surgical technology have significantly changed the dynamics of trauma reconstruction in facial cosmetics. Developments such as minimally invasive surgery, computer-assisted surgical planning, and newer imaging technologies have vastly improved surgical outcomes and recovery of the patient. One of them is the development of ultrasonic osteotomes that have replaced traditional cutting technologies in craniofacial surgeries. These devices make precise cuts with minimal trauma to the encompassing tissue, promoting better healing and less intraoperative complications. As a result, the application of such technologies not only ensures optimal aesthetic results but also enhances functional restoration of facial morphology. This convergence of innovation serves to put the central role of technology into focus to revolutionize the standard practice of reconstructive surgery to offer new hope for patients with facial trauma and deformities (Chuang et al., 2016). Developments in 3D printing technology have also changed preoperative planning and intraoperative control for facial cosmetic reconstruction. Surgeons can now create patient-specific facial anatomy models to allow precise surgical plans individualized to specific needs. These models are capable of being used to develop custom-designed implants, reducing the risk of biocompatibility complications and allowing for greater ease of integration with the surrounding tissues. Coupled with virtual reality environments for simulating operations, accuracy in trauma reconstruction has never been greater. These customized methods not only enhance the surgeon's capability for predicting complications but also improve the patient's experience through enhanced translucence of the surgical process. To this end, these innovations introduce a paradigm shift in solving facial cosmetic procedures, leading to improved patient outcomes and satisfaction (Anesi et al., 2014). Aside from the surgical devices themselves, the use of artificial intelligence and digital technology in patient management and postoperative care also contributed to advancements in the field. Predictive analytics using patient data analysis can ensure better selection of surgical procedures and interventions after surgery, resulting in a more tailored approach to recovery. The use of augmented reality is on the agenda to assist surgeons in actual surgery, providing immediate feedback and visualizations of critical anatomical structures. The application of digital technology in the surgical workflow is not a plus but is becoming pivotal to the achievement of trauma reconstruction excellence. Constant research into the newest technological advances is an allegiance to refine surgical methods, ultimately resulting in decreased complications, faster recovery times, and better overall patient results in facial cosmetic surgery (Chuang et al., 2016) (Figure 12.11).

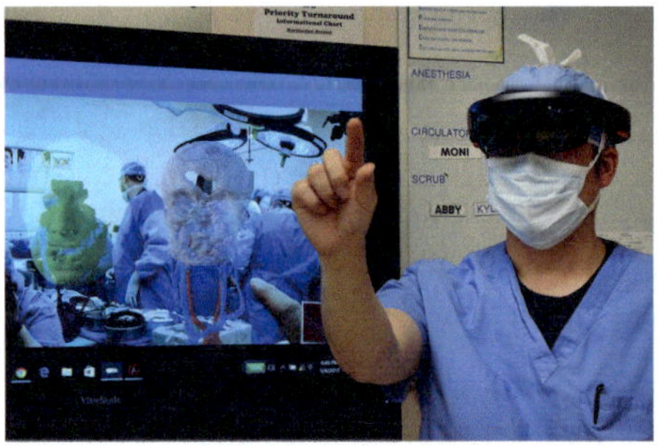

Figure 12.11. Innovations in surgical technology.

Source: https://medical-technology.nridigital.com/medical-technology/medical_technology_yb20/how_is_technology_transforming_facial_reconstruction_surgery/788339/Researcher_using_Halo_Lens.960_0_1.jpg.

12.3.3. Importance of Personalized Treatment Plans

Personalized treatment planning and its execution are of the highest priority in the practice of trauma reconstruction in cosmetic facial surgery. Every patient possesses a one-of-a-kind set of anatomical features, medical background, and aesthetic aspirations that must be carefully planned for in order to achieve optimal results.

Personalized approaches allow for customized intervention that not only addresses the physical component of the trauma but also the psychological needs of the patient. This personalized care improves patient satisfaction and creates the illusion of control, thereby facilitating a better healing process. It has been established through research that the psychological status of patients who are about to undergo reconstructive procedures can also have a tangible effect on their recovery, and therefore, the treatment plan should not only be physically responsive to the patients' needs but also psychologically. Technological advancements, such as the application of precision surgical equipment and the use of artificial intelligence, have further emphasized the need for such customized plans. As an example, technologies such as ultrasonic osteotomes have shown benefits over traditional osteotomes when used to prevent damage to surrounding tissues and enhance bone healing results. These advancements allow surgeons to choose methods most appropriate to the specific requirements of the trauma being treated, ensuring high levels of precision and efficiency in reconstructive surgery. The ability to individualize operative procedures both to the anatomy of the patients as well as the nature of the trauma puts personalized treatment protocols in the very center of modern facial cosmetic surgery. The inclusion of technology such as AI can automate this process further, ultimately leading to better surgical planning and treatment of patients (Aguayo et al., 2024). Moreover, the incorporation of data-driven insights within individual treatment plans can significantly increase the predictability of surgery outcomes. Advanced imaging techniques and analysis help create deep profiles of patients, leading to improved decision-making. They can also outline realistic cosmetic expectations in harmony with the patient's lifestyle and wants, which can directly impact postoperative satisfaction. Personalization even extends to the postoperative recovery, where customized rehabilitation programs can enable functional recovery and emotional well-being. Therefore, not only is it helpful, it is a critical practice of reconstructive facial cosmetic surgery for trauma that acknowledges the diverse realities and fantasies of patients, ultimately leading to improved care and outcomes (Anesi et al., 2014) (Figure 12.12).

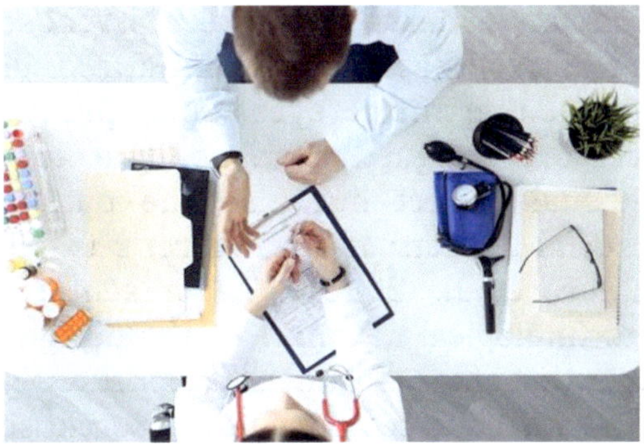

Figure 12.12. Importance of personalized treatment plans.

Source: https://www.indiapharmaoutlook.com/uploaded_images/newstransfer/r6e2Captureujiklo.JPG.

Test Your Knowledge

1. How have recent innovations in surgical technology improved precision and outcomes in facial reconstruction procedures?
2. Why is developing a personalized treatment plan essential for achieving optimal functional and aesthetic results in facial reconstruction?

12.4. Role of Cosmetic Procedures in Reconstruction

Learning Outcome

1. Discuss the Integration of Cosmetic Techniques in Trauma Recovery
2. Explain Non-Surgical Options for Facial Enhancement
3. Focus on Patient Satisfaction and Quality of Life Improvements

The use of cosmetic surgery in reconstruction is a crucial element in enhancing the welfare of patients suffering from facial trauma. Psychological and emotional effects of the trauma are extremely debilitating, leading to significant psychosocial disabilities. For instance, facial deformities caused by trauma can significantly alter one's image and interpersonal functioning, and thus reconstruction is not merely a physical restoration issue but also a mental health emergency. By applying new cosmetic surgery techniques, surgeons attempt to reestablish not only the structure but also the aesthetic appearance of the face. These procedures typically utilize new technology and techniques, where the accuracy and success of surgical operations are further enhanced. This is best observed through the implementation of ultrasonic osteotomes, which provide unique advantages compared to traditional tools through minimizing damage to the surrounding tissue, thereby promoting better healing outcomes (Anesi et al., 2014). Apart from that, cosmetic procedures used in reconstruction are not just surgical interventions; they tend to be a multidisciplinary intervention involving psychological counseling and aesthetic treatments. Patients exposed to ocular trauma, for instance, face severe psychosocial impediments that can be minimized using customized artificial eyes. Such prosthetic devices are designed to rehabilitate not just the visual aspect but also the emotional and social aspects of the wearer's existence (Chinnery et al., 2016). The present report and technological advances in the design and construction of these artificial prosthetics signify the heightened acceptance of the psychosocial aspects that accompany facial trauma. As such, the integration of cosmetic aspects in reconstructive surgery has a considerable role to play in ensuring patient satisfaction and quality of life by meeting both the functional and aesthetic needs of the patient. Finally, the role of cosmetic surgery in reconstruction points to the importance of considering the needs and wishes of individual patients during recovery. Individualization of the reconstructive processes ensures physical restoration is compatible with the psychological as well as social desires of the patient. Physicians are becoming more patient-focused, engaging individuals in discussions about their expectations and goals.

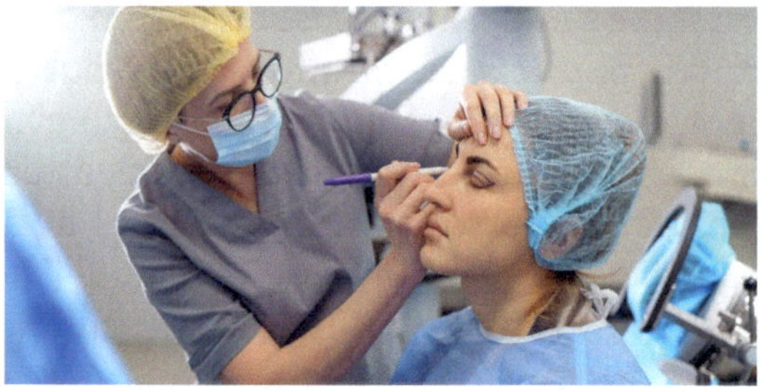

Figure 12.13. Cosmetic procedures.

Source: https://cachevalleyent.com/storage/2023/10/Reconstructive-Surgery-by-Cache-Valley-ENT-in-Logan-UT-scaled-2560x1280.jpeg.

This cooperative process enhances patients' feelings of agency and empowerment, which contribute to improved psychological outcomes after surgery. With the progress of cosmetic surgeries, not only do they have the potential to enhance physical looks, but they also allow emotional recovery, thereby changing the trajectory of recovery from trauma. Thus, the combination of cosmetic procedures with reconstructive surgery clearly evinces a sense of the subtle interaction between physical rehabilitation and psychosocial restoration (Figure 12.13).

12.4.1. Integration of Cosmetic Techniques in Trauma Recovery

Combining cosmetic methods with trauma recovery has emerged as an essential component in facial reconstruction, with important benefits on both aesthetic results and functional performance. As patients recover from traumatic facial injuries, focus shifts more and more to restoring physical appearance and psychological well-being. This dual strategy is important because the external consequences of trauma are capable of seriously degrading self-esteem and social interactions. Through the application of cosmetic techniques that prioritize careful tissue handling and aesthetic enhancement, caregivers can reduce scarring and maximize overall facial symmetry. These treatments are usually supplemented by technological advances that enable proper surgical techniques, thereby optimizing recovery avenues for patients with facial trauma, finally bridging the gap between medical necessity and esthetic demand, evident in today's research on craniofacial surgery (Neovius, 2016). The application of advanced surgical techniques, including ultrasonic osteotomes, has totally revolutionized the practice in the treatment of facial trauma. In contrast with traditional methods that can injure surrounding tissues, the innovative devices not only enhance bone cut precision but also preserve essential soft tissue morphology. Research indicates that piezosurgical procedures not only achieve improved micromorphology of osteotomized surfaces but also facilitate better healing and reossification (Anesi et al., 2014). This is particularly advantageous in trauma healing, where aesthetics and integrity of bone are simultaneous objectives. These developments highlight the importance of integrating cosmetic principles during trauma surgery, equipping surgeons with the tools to achieve optimal functional and aesthetic results, ultimately enhancing patients' quality of life following injury and rebuilding their bodies and also their resilience. Moreover, a full system of trauma rehabilitation entails multidisciplinary teamwork between surgeons, psychologists, and rehabilitation professionals. Such an association not only assures to focus on the physical aspects of recovery through advanced cosmetic treatments but also underscores the necessity of mental health treatment for trauma victims. Because facial trauma can profoundly affect self-concept, psychological ramifications need to be addressed for complete recovery. By integrating cosmetic with psychosocial treatments, treatment planning can be tailored to individual patient needs to create an environment conducive to healing and personal growth. Lastly, the synthesis of cosmetic surgery with trauma recovery is an innovative paradigm shift in facial reconstruction, demonstrating how aesthetic artistry in cosmetic surgery can smoothly complement medical treatments to provide greater degrees of patient satisfaction and improved general outcomes in trauma treatment (Ancsi et al., 2014; Neovius, 2016).

12.4.2. Non-Surgical Options for Facial Enhancement

In contemporary facial cosmetic surgery, enhancement without surgery is a dominant trend, particularly with trauma reconstruction. The procedures allow patients to achieve their desired appearance without exposing themselves to the risks and recovery times associated with invasive interventions. One of the most popular non-surgical procedures is dermal fillers, which can easily restore the cheeks and lips, among other features, to make the face appear young. Besides, neuromodulators like Botox are often employed to minimize the appearance of wrinkles by paralyzing specific facial muscles for a temporary period of time. The rapid result and relative simplicity of these procedures render them attractive for individuals desiring quick changes after facial injury, allowing for more prompt return to social functioning and regular activity, as well as to aesthetic considerations. Another fundamental feature of non-surgical facial enhancement involves the role of advanced skin treatments. Chemical peels and laser resurfacing, along with other treatments, have the potential to dramatically improve skin texture, tone, and overall appearance. These procedures induce collagen production and are employed to manage many of the sequelae of trauma, such as scarring or dyspigmentation. In cases of facial trauma, these treatments offer a non-invasive alternative to restoring skin integrity and thereby maximizing facial form. Furthermore, their tailoring to the individual requirements and skin types proves their adaptability and renders them a consideration in trauma reconstruction cases worth exploring. Non-surgical treatment can be tailored, raising its effectiveness and providing a more holistic means of facial recreation. While celebrating all these triumphs, though, it should be remembered that there are limitations and complications to non-surgical facial augmentation techniques. Though normally safe, procedures such as fillers and Botox can produce side effects such as swelling, bruising, or allergic reactions. Moreover, since favorable outcomes usually depend on the practitioner's skill set and level of experience, extensive consultations and examinations prior to treatment are required. As highlighted in more current studies, incorporating new technologies into planning and conducting non-surgical procedures can diminish some of these risks as well as improve outcomes (Xu et al., 2022). This is particularly important in reconstructive cases where precision is of utmost importance. With growth in the field, ongoing study and development will undoubtedly shape the new face of non-surgical facial enhancement (Figure 12.14).

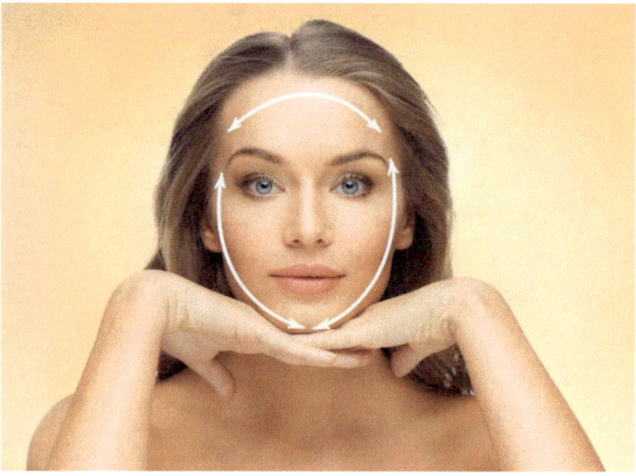

Figure 12.14. Non-surgical options for facial enhancement.

Source: https://drkaranshetty.com/wp-content/uploads/2024/04/non-surgical-facelift-glasgow-e1712837681310-1024x752.jpg.

12.4.3. Patient Satisfaction and Quality of Life Improvements

The complementarity of patient satisfaction and quality of life improvement for cosmetic facial surgery in the reconstruction of trauma is increasingly valued in reconstructive surgery. Correction of aesthetic as well as functional defects is required for enhanced overall patient care, with successful outcomes significantly affecting psychological function and social rehabilitation. Various surgical techniques, such as utilizing cutting-edge ultrasonic osteotomes, have been developed to enhance surgical precision and minimize postoperative complications. These advancements not only optimize the structural stability of the reconstructed facial framework but also facilitate a better healing process, ultimately leading to enhanced patient satisfaction. Studies that examine the micro-morphologies and roughness values of osteotomized surfaces, as published in Anesi et al. (2014), are just one of the ways technological advancement in operating tools is tantamount to improved patient outcomes, lending credence to the fact that innovation in surgery improves quality of life. Furthermore, understanding patient experience is important when evaluating the effectiveness of trauma reconstruction treatments. The focus shifted from merely achieving surgical success to incorporating patient-reported outcomes. For instance, autologous fat grafting studies in the eyelid have focused on the improvement rate overall among recipients of such procedures, and this has revealed that most of the patients indicate significant improvement not just in terms of looks but also in emotional and social areas of life. The systematic review outlined in Bannani et al. (2016) elaborates on the relationship between reconstructive surgeries and enhanced patient satisfaction, underscored by the crucial role of subjective experience in determining the success of surgery. Improved patient experience, testified to in the form of minimal complication rates and satisfactory aesthetic results, necessarily extends to enhanced quality of life, thus patient satisfaction being a fundamental aspect of reconstructive surgery. The repercussions of these findings extend beyond the patient to shape the overall healthcare practice. As patient satisfaction increasingly becomes a metric for successful outcomes with trauma reconstruction, healthcare providers are increasingly tasked with tailoring interventions to the individual. This patient-centered approach facilitates communication between the patient and the surgeon that fosters trust and goal-driven treatment. The insights obtained from recent advances, for example, as reported in Anesi et al. (2014) and Bannani et al. (2016), not only shape clinical practice but also further enhance surgical procedure and protocol improvement. Lastly, as these technologies are applied to work in the context of improved patient experiences, the face of medicine will experience an enormous paradigm shift towards prioritizing patient satisfaction as a driving force of quality-of-life improvements in facial cosmetic trauma reconstruction (Figure 12.15).

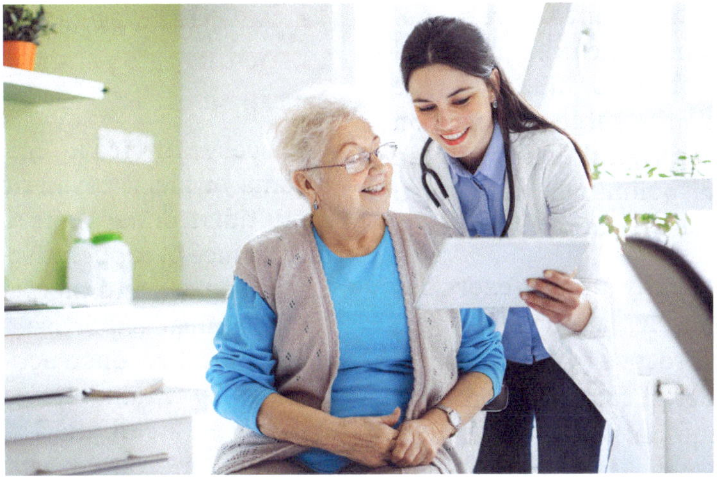

Figure 12.15. Patient satisfaction and quality.

Source: https://external-content.duckduckgo.com/iu/?u=https%3A%2F%2Fwww.performancehealthus.com%2Fhubfs%2Fimproving%2520patient%2520satisfaction.png&f=1&nofb=1&ipt=d7323a349af5ab66debc1ae5dbfb239ded792fd4fce622ba6867a732b08e5d96.

Test Your Knowledge

1. How are cosmetic techniques integrated into facial trauma recovery to improve both function and appearance?
2. What non-surgical options are available for facial enhancement during or after reconstructive treatment?
3. How do cosmetic procedures contribute to patient satisfaction and overall quality of life following facial reconstruction?

12.5. Multidisciplinary Approach to Treatment

Learning Outcome

1. Explain Collaboration Between Surgeons, Psychologists, and Therapists
2. Discuss Importance of a Holistic Treatment Plan
3. Identify Case Studies Demonstrating Successful Multidisciplinary Outcomes

The complexity involved in trauma reconstruction for facial cosmetics necessitates a multidisciplinary approach to treatment through the application of respective specialists' expertise. Facial trauma patients require orthodontists, prosthodontists, and oral and maxillofacial surgeons to collaborate closely to produce optimal outcomes. Initial stages often involve surgical reconstruction, during which maxillofacial and oral surgeons manage fractures and soft tissue injury. Orthodontic therapy may be required after surgery to correct misalignments, both through trauma and surgical methods. This cooperation guarantees that function and esthetic outcomes are optimized together, treating both the jaw's structural stability and the patient's appearance. This broad-based care ultimately enhances patient satisfaction and emotional health, reflecting the importance of a team-based approach in efficiently addressing the complex aspects of facial trauma. In addition, the incorporation of other medical professionals, including physical therapists and psychologists, adds to the overall treatment. While the surgeons focus on reconstructing the face, physical therapists can aid in rehabilitation, dispelling any functional limitation that can hinder the patient's recovery.

The therapists typically utilize exercises that strengthen facial muscles, allowing for both functional and cosmetic recovery. Alternatively, the psychological impact of facial trauma may be enormous, which requires intervention from mental health professionals. It is also critical to treat the psychological aspects of recovery, such as body image and self-esteem, because patients may become anxious, depressed, or withdrawn. The development of a cohesive treatment plan incorporating these various disciplines not only improves physical well-being but also assists in the emotional recovery process, critical to successful recovery. In the specific instance of facial trauma, management of complications such as open gingival embrasures also demonstrates the necessity of a multidisciplinary approach.

The fact that such cosmetic complications, typically the aftermath of periodontal disease or surgical intervention, will arise only serves to highlight the importance of involving the services of orthodontists and periodontists in treatment. Management of the aesthetic ramifications of such conditions can significantly enhance patient results and satisfaction. As noted by research, there are multiple means of treating open gingival embrasures, but it is the cooperation of the interdisciplinary team that usually yields the most successful results (Bosio et al., 2008). Thus, incorporating multiple specialties ensures that not just the surgical defects, but also the esthetic components are carefully addressed, fulfilling the holistic demands of trauma reconstruction patients.

12.5.1. Collaboration Between Surgeons, Psychologists, and Therapists

The very intricate task of reconstructing trauma in facial cosmetic surgery necessitates a multidisciplinary approach, emphasizing the importance of cooperative work among surgeons, psychologists, and therapists. Surgeons provide the technical expertise necessary to perform the physical reconstruction of facial structures affected by trauma. However, the psychological impact of facial disfigurement tends to be profound, more than just physical appearance, affecting individuals' self-esteem, interpersonal relationships, and mental health. This beautiful dance of physical and emotional recovery calls for the integration of psychologists who can assess and treat the psychological well-being of patients. With an integration of surgical techniques and psychological treatment, teams can offer patients complete care, leading to improved outcomes and building resilience to adversity. The alliance extends beyond the operating theatre and into rehabilitation and psychological preparation. Psychologists are engaged in prepping patients for reality surgery and potential results, reducing anxiety and emotional barriers to recovery. Speech and occupational therapy-trained therapists intervene further by addressing the functional and rehabilitative aspects of recovery. Patients' physiological and psychological demands are, in this manner, coordinated, making it possible to treat trauma reconstruction as an overall phenomenon. Such multidisciplinary interaction is paramount in minimizing the risk of post-operative complications as patients are mentally prepared to cope with the changes that surgery creates. The work of these professionals ultimately leads to improved patients' quality of life during recovery. The newer trend towards trauma reconstruction highlights the importance of building strong networks between facial transplantation and reconstruction professionals, as reported in the face allotransplantation literature (Coiante et al., 2022). A network of surgeons, psychologists, and therapists enables the sharing of information, strategies, and best practices that work to enhance patient care and outcomes. By creating a synergy of professionals, cross-disciplinary education has the potential to bring forth novel approaches and therapies to match each patient's needs. Also, ethical considerations that stem from such sophisticated procedures demand integrated debates among these experts. Patient choice, rejection management, and long-term follow-up are best managed by honest communication and collaboration to maintain the ethical standards of treatment while advancing the specialty of facial cosmetic surgery trauma reconstruction (Cimasi et al., 2011). By such an approach of collaboration, the procedure is legitimized, and a support system is made stronger on a holistic level for the patient during their recovery processes.

12.5.2. Importance of a Holistic Treatment Plan

In reconstructive trauma in facial cosmetic surgery, the role of a holistic treatment plan becomes even more evident. A holistic approach not only deals with the physical aspects of the procedure but also deals with the emotional and psychological well-being of the patient. With the disfiguring impact facial injury and reconstruction can have on a patient's self-esteem, a comprehensive approach must be employed to effectively recover. This involves a detailed work-up that incorporates medical history, psychological evaluations, and the patient's wants, facilitating more individualized surgical planning that addresses particular concerns. Such a holistic approach is most frequently linked with enhanced patient satisfaction and improved results, which underscore the requirement that surgeons anticipate more than mere technical skill when redefining facial structures. Moreover, through an overall treatment plan, the medical team can design a facilitating environment that answers the multifaceted challenges inherent in trauma reconstruction for patients. The coordination between surgeons, mental health specialists, and rehabilitation specialists is crucial in the process of ensuring that all recovery facets of a patient are properly addressed. The multidisciplinary care not only ensures optimum surgical results but also provides emotional healing and coping skills to tackle psychological effects. Evidence has shown that when patients feel supported emotionally during recovery, they will be more likely to take additional rehabilitative measures and adhere to post-operative instructions, thus working towards even better long-term results in facial appearance and self-esteem (Anesi et al., 2014). It is also important to observe the strange interplay of medical care and emotional support within the overall treatment plan, particularly in cases such as the O'Donnabhain case, which shows how competing ideas of medical necessity can affect patient treatment (Pratt, 2016). In patients who are reconstructing facial trauma, cosmetic benefit is usually entangled with psychological well-being. The experts should be aware of the psychological impact of surgical outcomes and social stigmatization. Thus, by the incorporation of elements such as counseling, peer counseling, and patient education into treatment protocols, surgeons can enhance the healing process so that people can recover not only their physical appearances but also self-confidence. Consequently, physical and psychological care as well constitute a vital component of an integrated treatment plan for trauma reconstruction.

12.5.3. Case Studies Demonstrating Successful Multidisciplinary Outcomes

Integration of various medical specialties has been found crucial in providing effective outcomes for trauma reconstruction, particularly in cosmetic surgery of the face. Recent case studies depict how a multidisciplinary approach enhances recovery and patient satisfaction. For instance, collaborative works between oral and maxillofacial surgeons, plastic surgeons, and rehabilitation specialists assure functional and esthetic reconstruction of facial trauma. Not only do these collaborative works make surgery more effective, but they also maximize postoperative care to an optimum extent, resulting in a reduction of complication rates and improved overall patient satisfaction. The effectiveness of such an approach is evidenced by a report indicating the necessity of integrating multiple expertise to achieve the best surgical outcomes in complicated facial reconstructions. Finally, a synergistic team setting encourages innovative solutions, as evidenced by perfect multidisciplinary outcomes in trauma reconstruction. Extraprimordial attention to innovative surgical approaches, such as Piezosurgery® use for osteotomies, underscores the innovation achieved by working in multidisciplinary teams. Comparative research on the micromorphologies and roughness values of bone surfaces after osteotomies has shown that ultrasound-assisted osteotomes have definite advantages over conventional practice. The use of Piezosurgery® allows selective cutting of mineralized tissue with preservation of the surrounding soft tissues, a key to maximizing healing and minimizing complications in craniofacial surgery. This technological application is an example of how surgical innovation and collaboration can bring superior outcomes in structural and functional rehabilitation. These findings point to the continuous evolution of techniques mixed with interdisciplinarity controversy to enable surgeons to further establish practices on empirical evidence. Therefore, the application of such modern techniques reflects the viability of successful multidisciplinary practice in facial trauma reconstruction. The inquiry into bone substitutes in craniofacial reconstruction further substantiates the benefit of multidisciplinary management. Conventional methods often involve the use of autologous bone to avoid donor-site morbidity, but studies indicate growing interest in artificial bone substitutes as a means of addressing this problem (Neovius, 2016). For instance, current studies on the comparison of the healing potential of next-generation materials, such as BMP-2 in hydrogel, reveal promising results that are equivalent to conventional autograft results. These analyses highlight the central role of coordination between material scientists and surgeons to streamline treatment modality. Such evolving practices not only aim to eliminate donor site complications but also enhance the efficacy of bone healing. The cross-fertilization of knowledge among disciplines is thus a vision-oriented effort towards achieving fruitful results in the realm of trauma reconstruction, heading towards optimum patient care and surgery success.

Test Your Knowledge

1. How does collaboration between surgeons, psychologists, and rehabilitation therapists enhance outcomes for patients undergoing facial reconstruction?
2. Why is a holistic treatment plan essential for addressing both the physical and psychological needs of patients recovering from facial trauma?

12.6. Ethical Considerations in Facial Reconstruction

Learning Outcome

1. Discuss the Informed Consent and Patient Autonomy
2. Explain Balancing Aesthetic Desires with Medical Needs
3. Focus on Addressing Disparities in Access to Care

The ethical issues of facial reconstruction, particularly after trauma, serve to underscore the nuance of patient autonomy and consent. Because reconstructive surgery of the face tends to be extensive in terms of altering the patient's appearance, it is very important that practitioners engage patients in lengthy preoperative discussions. These discussions must not only address the medical aspect of the procedure but also the emotional and psychological consequences that may arise due to cosmetic change. Ethical practice demands that patients are properly informed and that they provide consent freely, without coercion, so that they know about the probable outcome and risks of the procedure. Moreover, respecting a patient's wish where trauma has already resulted in emotional distress is paramount to establishing trust and feelings of control in the reconstructive process. Another basic ethical issue is the allocation of resources and access to facial reconstruction services. Notably, the disparities of access to healthcare can significantly decide who benefits from ideal advanced reconstructive treatments. Ethical issues necessitate that professionals critically examine the socio-economic determinants of quality of care received and patient care. The professionals must engage in the struggle to provide equal access to these life-critical reconstructive services, particularly among patients who are less affluent and therefore would be least able to pay for these services. The approach is consistent with the general healthcare equity framework that each patient, irrespective of socio-economic standing, ought to be provided with sufficient care. Thus, efforts to narrow these disparities can significantly improve aggregate patient outcomes and adherence to ethical standards in the medical profession. Finally, integrating leading-edge technologies into facial reconstruction comes with ethical concerns about the ramifications of such technologies. Although techniques like free tissue transfer and advanced imaging significantly enhance surgical precision and patient results, they also pose challenges. Informed consent questions arise when patients have to make decisions about new technology that has not been widely tried. The ethical burden on surgeons is to be up to date on the most current studies and to freely discuss the potential benefits and limitations of new procedures. Additionally, the evolving nature of reconstructive surgery requires ongoing debate in medicine in terms of best practices, ethics, and the patient-centered care mandate, which underlies the argument for sustaining clinical excellence while ensuring patients undergoing trauma reconstruction come first (Turner et al., 2021; Morales et al., 2023).

12.6.1. Informed Consent and Patient Autonomy

In trauma reconstruction for cosmetic facial surgery, informed consent is a paramount principle in maintaining patient autonomy. This ethical principle enables patients to make decisions about their medical care, so they are better informed about the risks, benefits, and options of their treatment regimen. The complexities of facial reconstructive surgery mandate extensive consultations between the surgeon and the patient, establishing an environment in which the patients are able to express their fears and expectations. The nuances of informed consent involve not just a detailed understanding of the procedures themselves, but also an understanding of the psychological impact of trauma and body changes. This ensures that patients are engaged in shared decision-making, which is essential in maintaining their autonomy and enhancing their satisfaction after surgery. Furthermore, the cosmetic surgery environment is also influenced by varied legal settings that decide how paramount informed consent is. The growing evaluated nature of cosmetic treatments has provoked debate on the medical professional's ethical role to prioritize patient understanding. Regulations and legislation are quite diverse throughout jurisdictions, which mirrors the evolving understanding of consent throughout the surgical fields. Comparative research highlights that it is crucial for medical professionals to be well educated about local and international practices, as Levon & Valančienė (2021) stress. This is a sign that there is a need to create a standard model of informed consent that responds to best practices and in the long term, allows patients to take charge of their health decisions while safeguarding their rights. The history of surgical practices also provides an impetus for upholding the importance of informed consent and patient autonomy, especially where treatments before were not disclosed. For instance, routine recommendation of sex reassignment surgery for intersex infants is ethically questionable in terms of consent because the majority of parents were persuaded to enroll for radical procedures without being fully aware of everything they stood to risk. This cautionary tale, quoted in Beh et al. (2000), necessitates a paradigm shift from the response to patient autonomy employed in modern medicine, particularly in trauma reconstruction. By putting informed consent first, healthcare professionals can establish trust and a culture of respect for patient autonomy, opening the way for ethical practice in healthcare in line with evolving conceptions of autonomy in medical advancement.

12.6.2. Balancing Aesthetic Desires with Medical Needs

There is a special challenge in the field of trauma reconstruction in facial cosmetic surgery in balancing aesthetic desires and medical needs. Reconstructive patients typically possess intense emotional and psychological motivations behind their interest in appearance, resulting from trauma. A desire for beauty can at times conceal underlying medical factors, and there can be conflict where the medical need is overshadowed by a desire to attain standards of beauty. The ramifications of this conflict are far-reaching; not only do they complicate surgical planning and patient consultation, but they also raise ethical concerns regarding the prioritization of aesthetic want over authentic medical need.

By closely examining these dynamics, practitioners are able to determine a framework that respects patients' aesthetic wants while keeping clinical imperatives as the priority for treatment planning. The globalized beauty of cosmetic surgery is a cultural trend whereby aesthetic interventions are becoming normalized, imposing societal pressures to maintain the need for cosmetic upgrades. In such an environment, the reasons for elective surgeries, even in the context of trauma, can be shaped by wider social constructs such as economic means and cultural ideals of beauty. As highlighted by studies, historical and sociopolitical backgrounds hold significant relevance for patient expectations, notably in developing nations where Western beauty perception is likely to affect personal aspiration (Riggs et al., 2012). The combined presence of the aforementioned factors makes the healthcare decision-making process challenging for healthcare providers, as they must balance patients' sociocultural demands with their medical needs. Reconstructive surgeons are thus confronted with ethical dilemmas, with a clear understanding of the social constructs that define what desires in a patient are, to provide holistic, ethical treatment. The problem of differentiating between medical and cosmetic motivations for surgical use also implies that there must be an apprehensive process of patient assessment and surgical planning. Research indicates that the majority of patients request treatments with both dental and cosmetic problems in mind, often driven by psychosocial reasons not always easily identifiable to practitioners (Broers, 2025). This highlights the importance of strict screening processes with mental health in view, and post-surgery long-term satisfaction in mind. Surgeons must establish an environment that fosters open communication about expectations, in which patients are fully informed of risks associated with any surgery. By highlighting ethical principles such as nonmaleficence and patient autonomy, clinicians can establish a work environment for teamwork whereby aesthetic desires are openly discussed without compromising medical integrity. Therefore, achieving an optimal equilibrium between cosmetic desires and medical needs is based on an integrated understanding of patients' motivations, hence enhancing outcomes and patient satisfaction.

12.6.3. Addressing Disparities in Access to Care

The accessibility of healthcare, particularly trauma reconstruction for facial cosmetic surgery, is highly disproportionate. Socioeconomic standing, geographical location, and systematic inequalities are significant determinants of an individual's access to necessary surgery. Patients from disadvantaged groups often face obstacles that not only hinder their access to timely treatment but also influence the quality of treatment they attain. As an example, those in rural communities might have limited specialized services available, which would require a lot of travel to access, thus discouraging patients from seeking proper treatment. Besides, inequalities also often stem from weak insurance coverage, which can significantly affect patients' decisions regarding whether or not to access reconstructive surgeries, thus limiting their potential for successful treatment of trauma. This dynamic of interdependence perfectly illustrates the actual need to reform policies to eliminate these inequalities and ensure equal access for everybody. Another aspect of complexity in achieving access imbalances is identity intersectionality, i.e., gender, race, and socioeconomic status, which overlaps with the existing healthcare disparities. Transgender individuals, for instance, have specificity of experiencing difficulties in accessing reconstructive services that might not be clearly understood by the health professionals. Evidence shows that the majority of practitioners are given minimal extensive training on the specific requirements of transgender patients, thus leading to misperceptions and suboptimal treatment choices. In addition, gender-affirming operations, normally inseparable from reconstructive and cosmetic procedures, are less likely to be taken care of by insurance programs, creating additional barriers in terms of access. Patient reluctance to seek healthcare for fear of discrimination or stigmatization denies them the opportunity to address trauma on time. Addressing the disparities requires a multi-disciplinary approach that is sensitive and responsive to differences in patient identity and experiences within the healthcare system. To reduce inequalities in access to trauma reconstruction care, advanced measures need to be taken that prioritize patient-centered strategies. Policymakers and healthcare professionals need to make committed efforts toward broad educational endeavors that heighten awareness of the singular needs of various populations, including gender-diverse populations. This is imperative in creating an environment that is helpful in delivering quality care and healing. In addition, leveraging technology to offer remote consultation services can potentially transcend spatial differences in access. Having community-based programs that offer financial assistance or sliding scales for the underinsured can enhance equity of healthcare access as well. Further, longitudinal studies are essential to an understanding of how these differences impact patient outcomes over the longer term and emphasize the importance of targeted interventions. Such attempts not only presage greater direct access to care but also promote a more sensitive healthcare system to the diverse needs of patients navigating through trauma reconstruction in facial cosmetic surgery.

Test Your Knowledge

1. Why is informed consent essential in facial reconstruction, and how does it support patient autonomy during treatment planning?
2. How should clinicians balance a patient's aesthetic desires with their medical and functional needs when determining treatment options?

SUMMARY

The complexities of trauma reconstruction in facial cosmetics attest to a rich interaction between cutting-edge surgical technology and patient-centered outcomes. With the advent of new tools such as ultrasound-guided osteotomes, the potential for improving surgical precision and restricting trauma to surrounding tissues has increased. Literature has revealed considerable differences in osteotomized bone surfaces using outdated versus newer techniques, suggesting that technologies such as Piezosurgery might aid in promoting more favorable patterns of postoperative healing and reducing donor-site morbidity. The development of such surgical tools plays an important role in the greater objective of attaining not only aesthetic improvement but functional reconstruction as well, thus validating the motivation for continued research and innovation in facial trauma surgeries (Anesi et al., 2014). In addition, growing interest in artificial bone substitutes is a turning point in the art of facial reconstruction. Historically, the autologous bone grafting has been considered the gold standard, but donor-site morbidity limitations and complications make it essential to search for alternative solutions. Results from research emphasize the necessity of assessing risks and complications following craniofacial surgeries, thereby simplifying surgical protocols for enhancing patient safety. The relative comparison between grafting techniques, e.g., the effectiveness of BMP-2 in hydrogel systems, illustrates the complex interplay between innovation and resilience in bone healing progress. These results bring the field closer to the implementation of safer and more efficient biomaterials for reconstructive surgery (Neovius, 2016). Finally, the future of trauma reconstruction in facial cosmetic surgery lies at a crossroads, with emerging evidence still defining best practices and surgical methodologies. With continuing evolution, the focus must be put on minimizing sequelae like diplopia and sensory impairment, which have a profound impact on patients' quality of life after trauma. Advanced surgical techniques and minimal-access modalities promise to minimize complications while still achieving aesthetic and functional outcomes. However, keeping the synergism of sound clinical studies and patient participation active is critical to advancing treatment protocols to a level of comprehensiveness. Ultimately, it is by holding to a vision of innovation and patient-centricity that the topic of study in facial trauma reconstruction is actually able to advance, making outcomes effective as well as enduring over the long term (Neovius, 2016).

A balanced overview of trauma reconstruction in aesthetic facial surgery illustrates several important aspects of surgical methods and their implications for patient outcomes. Among the primary issues has been technology in surgical instruments, specifically the advent of ultrasonically activated devices, such as Piezosurgery®, that revolutionized the practice of osteotomy. Studies highlight the disparity in micromorphology and roughness of bone surfaces attainable by standard methods compared to modern ultrasonic osteotomes. The latest technology facilitates the selective removal of mineralized tissues with the maintenance of the integrity of surrounding soft tissues, which is especially important for optimal recovery and healing in facial reconstruction. The evaluation of such tools reflects high potential to improve cranio-facial surgery outcomes, as is the demand for cosmetic reconstruction and functional rehabilitation of facial beauty from trauma patients (Anesi et al., 2014). Rhinoplasty remains at the core of trauma reconstruction as it addresses aesthetic and functional grievances that have their origin in facial trauma. The book Contemporary Rhinoplasty provides a clear insight into the complexities of orbital reconstruction surgery, discussing various points such as nasal beauty, and how to plan for the operation. This source highlights the importance of identifying the interaction between the surgery techniques and patient-specific anatomical differences, particularly in cases where skeletal abnormalities caused by trauma are a factor. In particular, correcting deformities like saddle nose deformity requires not only technical competence but also an intuitive understanding of morbidities underlying them, which can be sleep breathing disorders or cleft diseases. Adequate consideration of these factors during the surgical process guarantees enhanced results and patient satisfaction in trauma reconstruction (Kalaskar et al., 2016). With evolving experience in cosmetic reconstruction of the face, the incorporation of new methods and a deeper understanding of anatomical issues is critical. There is an obligation for surgeons to remain current with the latest happenings in surgical technology and technique, such as the efficacy of various osteotomes and the value of individualized rhinoplasty. Ongoing research into the impact of different surgical techniques on healing processes even more underscores the necessity for critical review and adaptation within the practice of surgery. This commitment to continued education ultimately ensures enhanced patient outcomes, validates the relevance of trauma reconstruction, and determines its role within the restoration of both form and function in facial trauma patients. With these technologies, clinicians can make a significant difference in the trajectory of healing from trauma by incorporating goals of cosmetic repair with the required aspects of patient rehabilitation and care.

KEY TERMS FROM THIS CHAPTER

- Facial Fractures
- Zygomaticomaxillary Complex (ZMC)
- Maxillofacial Trauma
- Avulsion Injuries
- Open Reduction and Internal Fixation (ORIF)
- Titanium Plates and Screws
- Orbital Floor Repair
- Mandibular Fracture Fixation
- Soft Tissue Laceration Repair
- Contusion Management
- Rigid Fixation
- Bone Grafting

CRITICAL THINKING QUESTIONS

1. **The main goal of facial trauma reconstruction is to:**
   a. Reduce wrinkles
   b. Restore anatomy, function, and aesthetics
   c. Improve facial pigmentation
   d. Increase skin thickness
2. **The first priority in managing facial trauma is:**
   a. Aesthetic evaluation
   b. Airway assessment and stabilization
   c. Scar revision
   d. Bone grafting
3. **The "golden period" for primary closure of facial lacerations is usually within:**
   a. 6–8 hours
   b. 24 hours
   c. 48 hours
   d. 72 hours
4. **Which bone is most commonly fractured in facial trauma?**
   a. Nasal bone
   b. Frontal bone
   c. Zygoma
   d. Mandible
5. **Blowout fractures typically involve which structure?**
   a. Nasal septum
   b. Orbital floor
   c. Zygomatic arch
   d. Mandibular symphysis

Short Answer Questions

1. What are the primary goals of facial trauma reconstruction?
2. How does the concept of "functional and aesthetic subunits" influence facial reconstruction planning?
3. What imaging modality is most commonly used to evaluate facial fractures and why?
4. What is the role of rigid fixation in facial fracture reconstruction?
5. How does soft tissue swelling affect surgical timing in trauma reconstruction?

Answers to Critical Thinking Questions

1. (b) 2. (b) 3. (a) 4. (a) 5. (b)

REFERENCES

1. Abbott, Amstutz, Arden, Arnaud, Arnaud, Asano, Axhausen, et al. (2003). *Bone autografting of the calvaria and craniofacial skeleton: Historical background, surgical results in a series of 15 patients, and review of the literature.* https://core.ac.uk/download/pdf/53848962.pdf (accessed on 14th July 2025).
2. Aguayo, S., García-Huidobro, R., Villena, F., Véliz, et al. (2024). *Generative artificial intelligence in dentistry: Current approaches and future challenges.* http://arxiv.org/abs/2407.17532 (accessed on 14th July 2025).
3. PRELIMINARY FINDINGS OF A POTENZIATED PIEZOSURGERGICAL DEVICE AT THE RABBIT SKULL / Anesi, A;Palumbo, C; Ferretti, M; Salvatori, R; Cavani F, .; Chiarini, L. - (2014). ((Intervento presentato al convegno 22° Congressof European Association for Cranio-Maxillofacial Surgery (EACMFS) tenutosi a Praga (Repubblica Ceca) nel 23-26September 2014(accessed on 14th July 2025).
4. Anger, J. T., Case, L. K., Baranowski, A., Berger, A., Craft, R. M., Damitz, L. A., Gabriel, R. A., et al. (2024). Pain mechanisms in the transgender individual: A review. *Frontiers in Pain Research, 5.* https://doi.org/10.3389/fpain.2024.1241015 (accessed on 14th July 2025).
5. Balachandar, L., & Thiagarajan, B. (2012). *Versatility of bicoronal flap approach in head and neck surgeries.* https://core.ac.uk/download/pdf/9634063.pdf (accessed on 14th July 2025).
6. Bannani, S., Bertheuil, N., Boureaux, E., Carloni, et al. (2016). *Eyelid fat grafting: Indications, operative technique and complications; a systematic review.*
7. Chuang, J., Barnes, C., & Wong, B. J. F. (2016). Overview of Facial Plastic Surgery and Current Developments. *Surgery journal (New York, N.Y.), 2*(1), e17–e28. https://doi.org/10.1055/s-0036-1572360 (accessed on 14th July 2025).
8. Bazgir, N., Fazli, M., Gachkar, L., Ghazizadeh Hashemi, et al. (2023). *Comparison of depression and anxiety levels before and after rhinoplasty: A longitudinal study.* https://core.ac.uk/download/643598101.pdf (accessed on 14th July 2025).
9. Beh, H. G., & Diamond, M. (2000). *An emerging ethical and medical dilemma: Should physicians perform sex assignment surgery on infants with ambiguous genitalia?* https://core.ac.uk/download/32299494.pdf (accessed on 14th July 2025).
10. Beneti, I. M., Rezende, L. S., & Sena Sobrinho, M. A. de. (2023). *Access to the upper third of the face: A literary review of indications, techniques, and intercurrences.* https://core.ac.uk/download/622811946.pdf (accessed on 14th July 2025).
11. Bodiwala, N., Bhola, N. D., Gupta, C. S., & Anukula, H. S. (2025). Single-staged islanded forehead flap for cheek defect in recurrent buccal mucosa cancer: A case report. *Journal of Clinical and Diagnostic Research.* https://www.semanticscholar.org/paper/f7a004a2d47c79169392b6345cfe58ed1b40559b (accessed on 14th July 2025).
12. Bosio, J. A., Furquim, B. D'Aurea, Maruo, H., Pascotto, et al. (2008). *The dilemma of the open gingival embrasure between maxillary central incisors.* https://core.ac.uk/download/213084039.pdf (accessed on 14th July 2025).
13. Broers, D. L. M. (2025). *Is the customer king?: Ethical and psychological considerations regarding tooth removal.* https://core.ac.uk/download/655140725.pdf (accessed on 14th July 2025).

14. Cheung, L. K., Ho, M. Y. S., Luk, W. K., McGrath, et al. (2014). *Psychosocial and quality of life outcomes of prosthetic auricular rehabilitation with CAD/CAM technology*. https://core.ac.uk/download/38046618.pdf (accessed on 14th July 2025).
15. Chinnery, H., Dyer, B., Noroozi, S., Thompson, et al. (2016). *Scoping review of the development of artificial eyes throughout the years*. https://core.ac.uk/download/163076643.pdf (accessed on 14th July 2025).
16. Cimasi, R. J. (2011). *Adviser's Guide to Health Care: Volume 2, Professional Practices*. https://core.ac.uk/download/335347929.pdf (accessed on 14th July 2025).
17. Coiante, E., D'Andrea, F., Hersant, B., La Padula, S., Longo, B., Meningaud, J. P., Pensato, R., et al. (2022). *Face transplant: Indications, outcomes, and ethical issues—Where do we stand?* https://core.ac.uk/download/636949002.pdf (accessed on 14th July 2025).
18. Constantian, M. B. (2022). *Childhood Abuse, Body Shame, and Addictive Plastic Surgery*. https://core.ac.uk/download/520261637.pdf (accessed on 14th July 2025).
19. Dean, J. H., Hoch, C. C., Wollenberg, B., Navidzadeh, J., Maheta, B., Mandava, A., Knoedler, S., et al. (2025). Advancements in bioengineered and autologous skin grafting techniques for skin reconstruction: A comprehensive review. *Frontiers in Bioengineering and Biotechnology, 12*. https://doi.org/10.3389/fbioe.2024.1461328 (accessed on 14th July 2025).
20. Desai, S. C., & Seth, R. (2020). Shifting paradigms in head and neck reconstructive surgery during the COVID-19 crisis. *Facial Plastic Surgery & Aesthetic Medicine, 22*, 152–154. https://doi.org/10.1089/fpsam.2020.0186 (accessed on 14th July 2025).
21. Fogg, Q., Ng, Z. Y., & Shoaib, T. (2010). *Where to Find Facial Artery Perforators: A Reference Point*. https://core.ac.uk/download/10521.pdf (accessed on 14th July 2025).
22. Hughes, D., & Song, B. (2016). Dental and Nondental Stem Cell Based Regeneration of the Craniofacial Region: A Tissue Based Approach. *Stem cells international, 2016*, 8307195. https://doi.org/10.1155/2016/8307195 (accessed on 14th July 2025).
23. Kothandaraman, S., Nair, V. B., & Narasiman, S. (2013). *'Old Foley's in a new bottle' – Use of Foley's catheter in anterior maxillary wall fractures*. https://core.ac.uk/download/pdf/9634091.pdf (accessed on 14th July 2025).
24. Levon, J., & Valančienė, D. (2021). *Ar pasaulinės kosmetinės chirurgijos teisinės problemos aplenkia Lietuvą?* https://core.ac.uk/download/479942901.pdf (accessed on 14th July 2025).
25. Mitsouras, D., Liacouras, P., Imanzadeh, A., Giannopoulos, A. A., Cai, T., Kumamaru, K. K., George, E., et al. (2015). Medical 3D printing for the radiologist. *Radiographics, 35*, 1965–1988. https://doi.org/10.1148/rg.2015140320 (accessed on 14th July 2025).
26. Deepak M. Kalaskar, Peter E. Butler, Shadi Ghali. (2016). *Textbook of Plastic and Reconstructive Surgery*. ISBN: 978-1-910634-37-0 (Hbk.) https://core.ac.uk/download/79526588.pdf
27. (accessed on 14th July 2025).
28. Neovius, E. (2016). *Development of Surgical Techniques in Craniofacial Reconstruction*. https://core.ac.uk/download/70344167.pdf (accessed on 14th July 2025).
29. Oley, M. H., Oley, M., Sukarno, V., & Faruk, M. (2024). Advances in three-dimensional printing for craniomaxillofacial trauma reconstruction: A systematic review. *The Journal of Craniofacial Surgery, 35*, 1926–1933. https://www.semanticscholar.org/paper/21a3e3ce98ec2c77b146be237e9136f3c4ae035a (accessed on 14th July 2025).

30. Pratt, K. (2016). *The tax definition of medical care: A critique of the startling IRS arguments in O'Donnabhain v. Commissioner*. https://core.ac.uk/download/232700370.pdf (accessed on 14th July 2025).

31. Riggs, L. E. (2012). *The Globalization of Cosmetic Surgery: Examining BRIC and Beyond*. https://core.ac.uk/download/216977885.pdf (accessed on 14th July 2025).

32. Turner, B., Collin, J., & Fernandes, R. (2021). Soft tissue reconstruction of the maxillofacial region. *Oral and Maxillofacial Surgery for the Clinician*. https://www.semanticscholar.org/paper/7fa97a061fae0906be70c91e2a8c23ee0518c768 (accessed on 14th July 2025).

33. Vega Morales, A. Q., Lara Pérez, M. A., & Ruiz Reyes, D. P. (2023). Advancements in plastic surgery and facial reconstruction: A comprehensive review of surgical techniques and outcomes. *International Journal of Medical Science and Clinical Research Studies*. https://www.semanticscholar.org/paper/971665dbda7c1828e2089ce662d4c434d4fb8f13 (accessed on 14th July 2025).

34. Windsor, E. J. (2011). *Regulating healthy gender: Surgical body modification among transgender and cisgender consumers*. https://core.ac.uk/download/71423075.pdf (accessed on 14th July 2025).

35. Xu, Y., Zhang, F., Zhai, W., Cheng, S., Li, J., & Wang, Y. (2022). *Unraveling of advances in 3D-printed polymer-based bone scaffolds. Polymers, 14*, 566–566. https://doi.org/10.3390/polym14030566 (accessed on 14th July 2025).

36. Yadav, N. K., Singhal, S., Sadaphale, S. V., & Srivastava, A. K. (2025). Cosmetic reconstruction of post-traumatic anterior staphyloma by customized ocular prosthesis. *International Journal of Research and Scientific Innovation*. https://www.semanticscholar.org/paper/078ba885b3e5eada4add5f573b1d7bb73cf7d8c4 (accessed on 14th July 2025).

37. Yu, A., Ference, E., Ge, M., Su, P., Smith, S., Moayer, R., Levin, K. M., et al. (2022). Facial plastic and reconstructive surgery poster presentations. Otolaryngology–*Head and Neck Surgery, 167*, P182–P192. https://www.semanticscholar.org/paper/e467d5d0d3f13c11f7cf2c4402802ca47316c419 (accessed on 14th July 2025).

38. Zhou, G., Jiang, H., Yin, Z., Liu, Y., Zhang, Q., Zhang, C., Pan, B., et al. (2018). In vitro regeneration of patient-specific ear-shaped cartilage and its first clinical application for auricular reconstruction. *EBioMedicine, 28*, 287–302. https://doi.org/10.1016/j.ebiom.2018.01.011 (accessed on 14th July 2025).

CONGENITAL AND DEVELOPMENTAL DEFORMITIES IN FACIAL COSMETIC

13

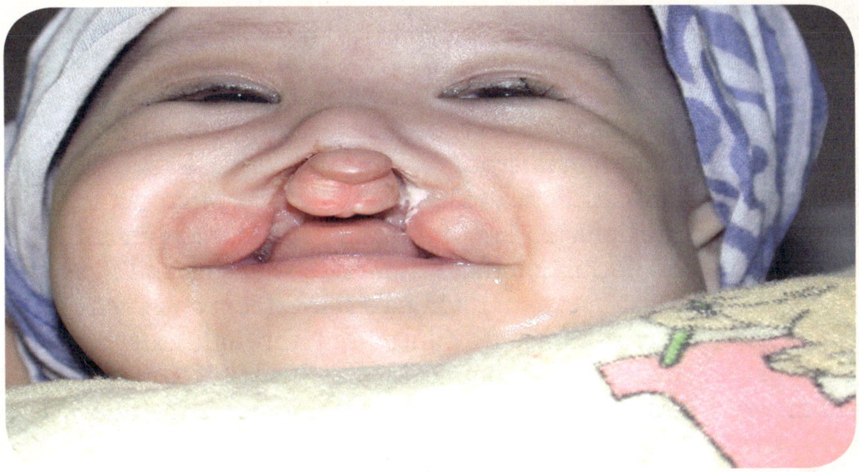

LEARNING OBJECTIVES

After studying this chapter, you will be able to:

1. Discuss the type of congenital deformities;
2. Describe the type of developmental deformities;
3. Assess causes of the congenital deformities;
4. Understand the psychological impact of facial deformities;
5. Highlight treatment of facial deformities;
6. Know advancements in facial aesthetic procedures.

Introduction

The facial aesthetics are an interdisciplinary combination of biological, aesthetic, and psychological problems, particularly when we talk about congenital and developmental deformities. These are likely to occur during childhood and can potentially have a significant impact on a person's quality of life. Such studies address not just the morphological aspect of facial shape but also the social and emotional impact of such conditions on patients. Advances in surgical techniques, including orthognathic surgery, have led to improved patient outcomes, modifying the concept of aesthetic beauty and function. A complete understanding of these deformities calls for an examination of the genetic histories, fetal influences, and neonatal developments responsible for their occurrence, ultimately informing treatment methodologies as well as prevention in craniofacial deformities, thus breaking up the normal development (Zammit et al., 2023). Wherever facial deformities intersect with neurodevelopmental processes, it is a critical field of research to explore. Evidence suggests that stomatognathic abnormalities are either a cause or a consequence of neurological illnesses. Because facial growth is intricately interwoven with neural inputs, it is important to know how such correlates with facial growth, especially in diagnosing and managing congenital defects. The presence of the "brain-oral axis" highlights the intricate intertwining of neurological and facial beauty, necessitating multidisciplinary management of such conditions. An understanding of the crosstalk between the nervous system and facial deformities can reveal the processes of congenital anomaly formation, thus shaping therapy intervention and enhancing the quality of care (Wu et al., 2023). Lastly, evaluation of congenital and developmental deformities of facial aesthetics is a multi-faceted task of careful assessment of physical as well as psychological conditions. Practitioners must seek out comprehensive treatment protocols that address not only structural abnormalities but also the psychosocial ramifications that these impose on patients. The growing number of studies warrants intervention measures that are supplementary to surgical procedures, psychological treatment, and patient education at an initial stage. As technology improves and multidisciplinary approaches evolve, the aim is to encourage better patient outcomes for patients suffering from such complex deformities. Achieving harmony in both form and function remains an inherent goal in the domain of facial aesthetics, and this ensures that afflicted patients can lead productive lives irrespective of their status (Zammit et al., 2023).

Definition of Congenital and Developmental Deformities

Congenital and developmental deformities represent a significant area of study within medical and aesthetic disciplines, particularly regarding facial aesthetics. Congenital deformities are structural growth developmental anomalies that arise during fetal development and growth, which are usually caused by genetic defects, environmental exposure, or both. The deformities can manifest in many forms, such as but not limited to cleft palate, cleft lip, and auricular deformity in the form of microtia. On the other hand, developmental deformities are often brought about by an interruption in typical postnatal patterns of growth due to nutrition, disease, or trauma. The differentiation between the two categories is significant to health professionals, as this influences intervention choices and strategies in surgical reconstruction, rehabilitation, and psychological counseling of individuals who possess such conditions. In studying the specific form of facial deformities, scholars observed that certain conditions, including microtia, significantly alter functional and aesthetic attributes of the face. Microtia, or the deformation of the outer ear, is a congenital malformation that can threaten hearing abilities and affect an individual's self-esteem and social interactions. As illustrated through existing research, the complexity of auricular deformities transcends outward physical appearance; they also impact psychological well-being as well as social growth in children. This multifaceted impact is a persuasive argument in favor of an interdisciplinary approach to considering the etiology and implications of such deformities. Understanding how the developmental origin and formation of such deformities take place is valuable in designing effective clinical methods specifically tailored to restore form and function in patients presenting with such conditions (Lin et al., 2024). The advancement of medical technology has also enhanced our ability to diagnose and assess congenital and developmental deformities better. For instance, novel imaging technologies and automated measuring algorithms, the focus of recent research, provide for a precise evaluation of facial structures that allows for customized treatment plans to be devised. These new technologies are significant in standardizing methods of assessment, hence improving clinical outcomes for auricular malformation patients. Moreover, the use of objective measuring devices provides for uniform tracking of treatment performance over time, thereby culminating in improved patient confidence and satisfaction. With heightened awareness of congenital and developmental deformities, medical practitioners are better positioned to advocate for the needs of the affected individuals, putting restoration of function and aesthetic enhancement at the top throughout the treatment continuum (Lin et al., 2024) (Figure 13.1).

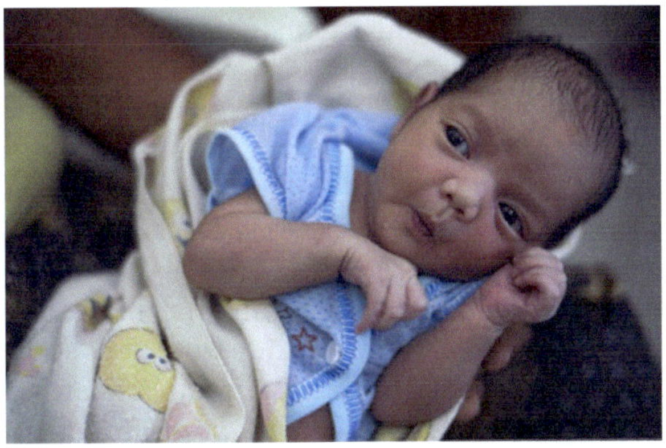

Figure 13.1. Congenital and developmental deformities.

Source: https://cdn.who.int/media/images/default-source/mca/maternal-nb/un0304684.tmb-479v.jpg?sfvrsn=d91cee2_3%20479w.

Importance of Facial Aesthetics in Social Interactions

Facial beauty is of utmost significance in social encounters, as facial beauty determines the way people see one another and are treated. The human face is a principal vehicle of emotion and attachment expression; therefore, positive facial beauty has the ability to shape social experiences greatly. Individuals who have congenital and developmental disfigurements, such as hemifacial microsomia (HFM), tend to struggle with peer relationships because their typical facial appearance is disrupted. Research confirms that HFM children tend to struggle to form social relationships and are extremely susceptible to peer rejection, which will have adverse effects on their self-esteem and mental health. These issues underscore the paramount importance of not only the medical management of facial deformities' physical conditions but also their psychosocial effects, as espoused in research connecting the face's appearance and social acceptability and developmental traits (Pniak et al., 2024). Moreover, facial aesthetics' impacts continue into peer relations during adolescence and adulthood. Teenagers with congenital facial abnormalities are likely to be more socially isolated and may face challenges in establishing romantic relationships, as they are perceived to be lacking aesthetically. Social challenges in such instances are most likely accompanied by internalized stigma that causes individuals to avoid social engagements altogether. The impact of such isolation is extremely profound; it might hamper emotional and cognitive development, resulting in widespread educational and career inequalities in later life. As observed in follow-up studies on psychosocial adaptation among individuals with facial deformities, the interventions that optimize physical appearance and confidence can be decisive in cushioning against such adverse effects and overall quality of life (Lone et al., 2023). The pressure for facial beauty during interactions is also increased by cultural and societal expectations that strongly favor symmetry and beauty. In the majority of social interactions, individuals with conventionally attractive facial structures are assessed as more competent, honest, and likable. This halo effect leads to unfair treatment in all aspects of life, including employment opportunities and social standing. Thus, individuals carrying facial congenital malformations can resist preconceptions and stereotypes that reduce their social standing. Understanding these dynamics is central to developing comprehensive support programs aimed at fostering acceptance and accommodation for individuals with abnormal facial aesthetics. Awareness, education, and empathy-driven programs can be central in shifting attitudes in society and supporting social interactions for individuals affected by congenital and developmental facial abnormalities, ultimately leading to a more accommodating society (Lone et al., 2023) (Figure 13.2).

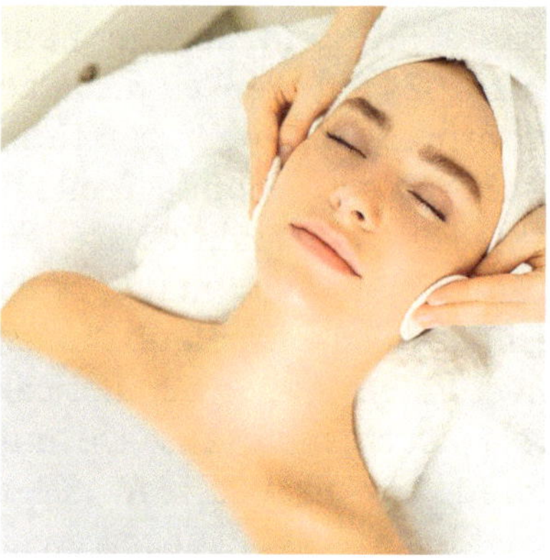

Figure 13.2. Facial aesthetics in social interactions.

Source: https://www.bellissimaclinic.com/wp-content/uploads/2023/05/facial-aesthetics-blog.jpg.

13.1. Types of Congenital Deformities

Learning Outcome

1. Discuss Cleft Lip and Palate
2. Explain the Craniosynostosis
3. Focus the Hemifacial Microsomia (HFM)

Congenital deformities occur in varied forms and have a strong impact on facial appearance, presenting individualistic difficulties in diagnosis, treatment, and psychosocial acceptance. The most common types are craniofacial microsomia and cleft lip and palate. Craniofacial microsomia occurs as a result of underdevelopment of the mandible and ear, resulting in asymmetry as well as functional disability, especially speech and mastication. By comparison, cleft lip and palate are due to a failure of facial structures to fuse early in development, usually resulting in conspicuous aesthetic discrepancies and feeding and speech problems. A perspective on these specific deformities is necessary to establish effective intervention protocols that maximize both functional and aesthetic results in affected patients. A second crucial category of congenital deformities involves the more complex syndromic presentations, like Treacher Collins syndrome and Pierre Robin sequence. Treacher Collins syndrome can be associated with a combination of facial dysmorphisms, e.g., underdeveloped jaw and cheekbones, that lead to impaired facial symmetry and hearing deficit. Conversely, the Pierre Robin sequence is primarily defined by a triad of anomalies: a decreased jaw size, cleft palate, and tongue displacement, which will occlude the airway. Both conditions have significant influences on the developmental trajectory and social experience of the affected, as facial appearance is a central ingredient in both social interaction and self-concept. These syndromic congenital anomalies need a multi-disciplinary treatment plan to optimize treatment protocols based on both the external and functional aspects of facial appearance (Rutger ter Horst et al., 2021). Congenital anomalies also happen on the basis of genetic and environmental factors, like hemifacial microsomia, where the face is underdeveloped on one side, affecting overall symmetry and aesthetic balance. The presentation and severity of the condition can widely differ from one individual to the next, emphasizing the importance of individualized treatment approaches. Treatment approaches tend to involve surgical corrections to restore symmetry to the face and enhance functional abilities, as well as psychological counseling to manage the emotional impact of having a visible difference. Hence, a comprehensive treatment plan is required, keeping in view not only the physical rectification but also the psychosocial well-being of patients, thereby facilitating a holistic approach to care in the domain of congenital and developmental deformities of facial aesthetics (Rutger ter Horst et al., 2021) (Figure 13.3).

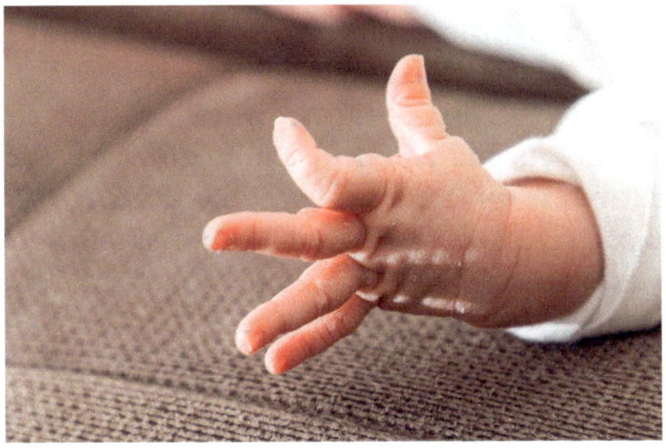

Figure 13.3. Congenital deformities manifest.

Source: https://www.spirehand.com.sg/wp-content/uploads/2024/04/spire-blog-congenital-hand-scaled.jpeg.

13.1.1. Cleft Lip and Palate

The impact of cleft lip and palate extends much further than mere physical characteristics, affecting numerous aspects of a child's life and health. The birth defects happen in fetal formation during early pregnancy when tissues employed to form the lip and palate fail to fuse together. Prevalence of cleft lip and palate also varies geographically, from 1 in 500 to 1 in 2,500 live births, reflecting a significant health concern that necessitates all-embracing intervention strategies. The nuances of these deformities tend to give rise to a complex set of functional deficits, such as feeding disorders and speech pathology, and psychological and social implications, yet further complicate the life of the affected person. This heterogeneity of cleft lip and palate highlights the need for multidisciplinary treatment and care, which introduces the significance of addressing the physical and psychological needs of patients. Multidisciplinary care coordination is the key to the care of cleft lip and palate since it maximizes treatment outcomes and facilitates overall rehabilitation. These children are typically cared for by an interdisciplinary team of professionals, including surgeons, orthodontists, speech therapists, and psychologists, to address the broad variety of issues presented by the deformity. Available literature suggests that integrated management with a tiered system is extremely useful, allowing for increased functional potential and restorative esthetics. For instance, Eshiev et al. (2025) emphasize the necessity of interdisciplinary collaboration on an everyday basis, one that is not only necessary in surgical operations but also in constant observation and treatment throughout childhood.

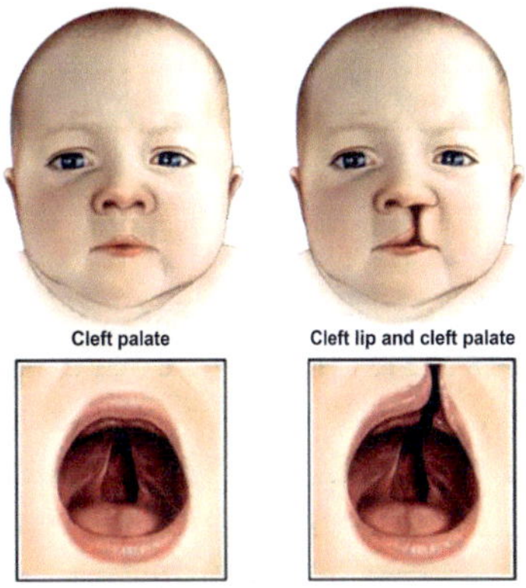

Figure 13.4. Cleft lip and palate.

Source: https://www.mayoclinic.org/-/media/kcms/gbs/patient-consumer/images/2013/08/26/10/45/ds00738_ds00998_im02607_fl7_cleft_palatethu_jpg.png.

This active interprofessional collaboration guarantees the development of a practice arena in which healthcare professionals can work collaboratively toward solving the physical and psychosocial problems involved in treating children for cleft lip and palate. Apart from the direct issue resulted by cleft lip and palate, patients also bear a higher risk for dental abnormalities, such as Molar-Incisor Hypomineralization (MIH), complicating orthodontic treatment and oral health overall (Pérez Sánchez et al., 2022). Such dental anomalies bring about high burdens, affecting the psychosocial outcomes of children in dealing with their own circumstances. Effective and prompt dental care becomes inevitable, not just for the reason that untreated dental conditions exacerbate underlying functional deficits but also because they are likely to induce compromised social acceptance and self-confidence. It is thus necessary that the healthcare practitioners apply methods with the priority of employing holistic treatment approaches involving dental rehabilitation with other modalities to optimize facial aesthetics, function, and quality of life in these patients. By adopting a comprehensive approach to treatment and rehabilitation, the medical community can improve the life course of the victims of cleft lip and palate (Figure 13.4).

13.1.2. Craniosynostosis

Craniosynostosis is a severe congenital abnormality resulting from the premature closure of an individual or more cranial sutures. This abnormal fusion restricts skull expansion and can lead to elevated intracranial pressure and potential developmental delays, ultimately influencing overall facial appearance. The illness most frequently occurs in multiple forms, the most common of which is single-suture craniosynostosis. For instance, sagittal synostosis results in a short, narrow head form, while coronal synostosis results in asymmetrical skull features. These deformities not only may jeopardize the cosmetic shape of the skull but also facial architecture, with significant social implications for the manner in which an individual is perceived. As such, craniosynostosis necessitates careful evaluation and multi-modal therapy to prevent aesthetic as well as functional morbidity. Craniosynostosis is typically diagnosed in infancy with the aid of imaging modalities such as X-rays or CT scans for assessment of suture involvement. Prompt diagnosis is crucial, as it will dictate the treatment plan aimed at the remodeling of skull shape and alleviation of intracranial pressure. Surgical intervention remains the modality of choice, with the surgery planned to allow the skull to grow and develop in a normal fashion. Prompt treatment is associated with improved neurological function and cosmetic results. Additionally, thorough care will sometimes go beyond surgery, including continued observation and possible orthodontic work as the child matures. As indicated in companion research, treatment for such cranial deformities can radically improve quality of life and psychosocial adjustment, especially among children as they continue to cope with social interactions. The psychosocial nature of craniosynostosis is important and too often underemphasized in clinical reports. Kids with typical cranial morphologies may be stigmatized or bullied, in turn influencing their social relationships and self-perception. These issues must be approached from a multidisciplinary point of view, not only from medical and surgical treatment but also from psychological intervention. Family counseling and education play an important role in developing patients' and families' resilience. For instance, the importance of psychosocial intervention coupled with physical therapy has been highlighted in order to achieve the best possible developmental results. Research shows that by integrating these factors into care, clinicians can significantly improve the quality of life in affected individuals, ultimately leading to increased overall function and form, combining both therapeutic and aesthetic results (Figure 13.5).

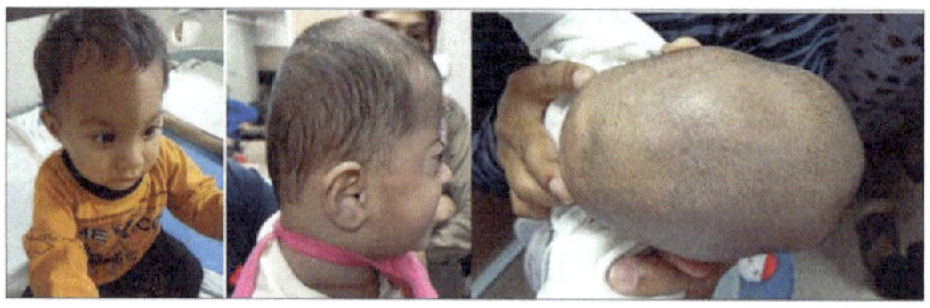

Figure 13.5. Craniosynostosis.

Source: https://www.researchgate.net/publication/363687463/figure/fig1/AS:11431281085248531@1663688286727/Abnormally-shaped-head-as-a-presentation-of-craniosynostosis-in-a-child-of.ppm.

13.1.3. Hemifacial Microsomia (HFM)

HFM is a significant congenital craniofacial deformity, with clinical presentations that can dramatically impact an individual's aesthetic and functional features. Second only to cleft lip and palate as the most frequent congenital facial deformity, HFM is characterized by a vast spectrum of facial asymmetry, typically including the mandible, maxilla, and associated soft tissue. The heterogeneity of presentation creates complex challenges like underdevelopment of the jaw, malformations of the ear, and potential hearing impairment. In addition to the physical status, the psychosocial impact of having HFM can significantly contribute to the patient's self-concept, communication, and interpersonal relationships. Facilitating early intervention and appropriate management strategies reduces such problems, which proves that there is a need for a multidisciplinary team in the delivery of care, including operative interventions as well as psychosocial intervention. The impact of HFM extends even into the area of neurodevelopment and education, particularly for the affected children. Studies indicate that HFM patients are at a higher risk of verbal, non-verbal, and educational problems, particularly if accompanied by other anomalies such as microtia and mandibular hypoplasia. These challenges can hinder skills that are crucial to social interaction and mental development, and cause feelings of isolation or peer rejection to persist. Although some children get by in the beginning, research states that as they progress with their education, they experience declining outcomes later. This also emphasizes the need for early assessment and targeted interventions that enhance social and language skills, eventually improving the quality of life of patients with HFM (Pniak et al., 2024). Recent advances in surgical techniques have promising potential in the treatment of HFM, and more importantly, the use of virtual surgical planning (VSP) and 3D-printed surgical assistants, which have been used to great benefit in reconstructive procedures. Through the application of modern technology, surgeons are able to accurately plan and execute surgical procedures that rectify deformity, in addition to obtaining the most optimal aesthetic outcomes. Combined application of 3D-printed titanium mesh and iliac cancellous bone grafts, for instance, has been found to significantly improve facial function and symmetry. The precision that these tools provide not only enhances the efficacy of surgery but also decreases the rate of complications and postoperative bone resorption. As additional research continues to illuminate the benefits of such new techniques, the possibility for improved surgical results in patients with HFM grows, ultimately leading to a more favorable prognostic profile in congenital facial anomalies (Zhao et al., 2023) (Figure 13.6).

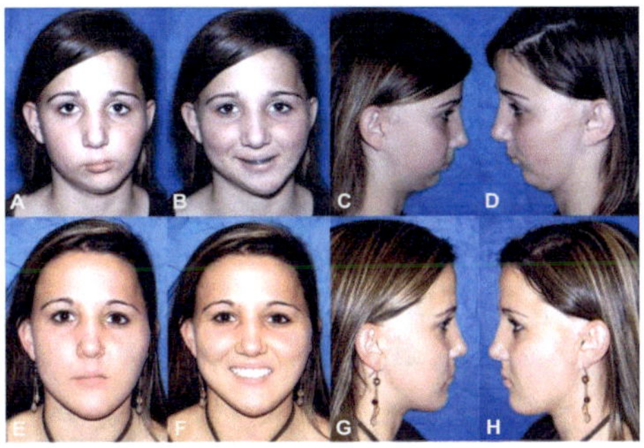

Figure 13.6. Hemifacial microsomia (HFM).

Source: https://drlarrywolford.com/wp-content/uploads/2015/01/Screenshot-2015-02-14-12.14.48.png.

Test Your Knowledge

1. What developmental abnormalities lead to cleft lip and palate, and how do these conditions affect feeding and speech?
2. How does craniosynostosis occur, and what impact does premature fusion of cranial sutures have on skull and brain development?

13.2. Types of Developmental Deformities

Learning Outcome

1. Discuss the Facial Asymmetry
2. Explain Acquired Deformities Due to Trauma
3. Focus Deformities Resulting from Medical Conditions

Developmental facial deformities are grouped in facial aesthetics as a broad range of conditions that may be caused by genetic, environmental, or multifactorial etiologies. Of these, craniosynostosis, or deformity through premature closure of one or more of the cranial sutures, has profound effects on the development of the face. Irregular head shapes often ensue from this deformity, and facial structure position and symmetry can be compromised. In some cases, surgery is required to prevent elevated intracranial pressure and permit normal craniofacial growth. The significance of treatment and diagnosis at an early stage is rendered evident by the possibility of more favorable aesthetic and functional outcomes, illustrating the relationship of developmental processes and beauty of the face within the broader framework of congenital deformity. Another extremely prevalent category of developmental anomalies is cleft lip and palate, which results from an incomplete closure of the lip and/or palate during embryogenesis. Incidence of this syndrome varies across the globe but is among the primary indications for surgical repair in children. Along with the main cosmetic defect, cleft lip and palate will have major impacts on the acquisition of speech, oral health of the dentition, and psychosocial adaptation. Medical specialists have a penchant for adopting an interdisciplinary strategy, combining surgical correction with orthodontic treatment and speech therapy in order to address the numerous challenges posed by these deformities. This integrated mindset is dedicated to the intricate relationship between congenital conditions and the resulting effect on facial morphology, and the importance of patient-specific interventions to achieve functional and esthetic goals. More complex developmental deformities, such as those requiring advanced surgical techniques, have been enhanced by recent advances in technology. One prime example of a useful improvement to craniofacial surgery is the introduction of ultrasound-guided osteotomes, such as Piezosurgery®. Comparing research on traditional osteotomes with the new devices has shown advantages in terms of micromorphological precision and preservation of surrounding tissues, which can enhance healing outcomes (Anesi et al., 2014). Additionally, new treatments utilizing stem cells hold promising directions for regenerating specific craniofacial structures, providing solutions for what may not best heal with conventional surgical intervention (Hughes & Song, 2016). With the continued advancement of scientific research in the field, it is clear that the nature of developmental facial appearance deformities is complex, thus necessitating continued study of new remedies and methods for improving patient outcomes (Figure 13.7).

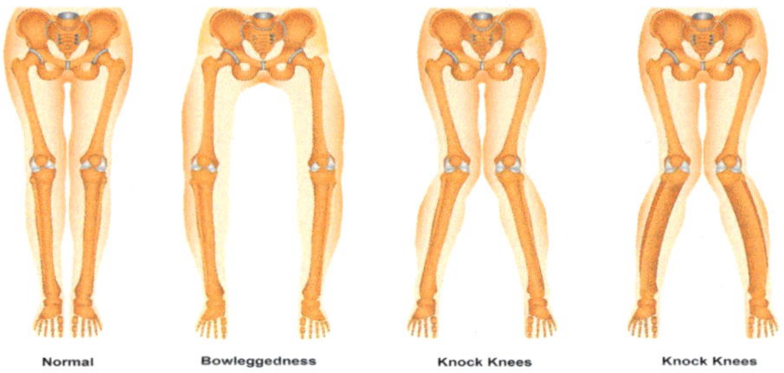

Figure 13.7. Types of developmental deformities.

Source: https://external-content.duckduckgo.com/iu/?u=https%3A%2F%2F1.bp.blogspot.com%2F-L97YYXcp5qA%2FXcCK1_EYsGI%2FAAAAAAABtz8%2F-a3whpQ_oV8EGT8bClZILJ60fL1SuqWSQCLcBGAsYHQ%2Fs1600%2FDevelopment%252Bof%252BAngular%252BDeformities.jpg&f=1&nofb=1&ipt=57e9a35a2d56658834412bb8fb783e71468808cff84e9b844a07f0e77d636de6.

13.2.1. Facial Asymmetry

Facial asymmetry is very prevalent in facial aesthetics, particularly as it relates to how congenital and developmental deformities look on individuals. As described as a non-symmetrical appearance between the two sides of the face, asymmetry can be brought about by some different factors, including genetic influences and environmental pressures on developmental critical periods. In the case of patients with congenital deformities such as microtia, facial asymmetry may bear severe consequences not only on their outward appearance but also on their psychological condition, typically presenting as self-esteem and social integration issues. Uncovering the etiology of facial asymmetry is essential in formulating specific therapeutic interventions, either through surgery or other means of enhancing facial symmetry and beauty. In the examination of specific conditions that lead to facial asymmetry, auricular deformities like microtia come to mind. Microtia is characterized by the underdevelopment of the outer ear and typically also by asymmetry of both the auricle and the facial complex closely related to it. Current research highlights the necessity for a precise measurement technique in the assessment of such deformities, as conventional techniques may not detect minor asymmetries, which potentially can affect the outcome of treatment. New technologies, such as a newly developed computerized 3D surface-based measurement of the auricle, offer higher accuracy in auricular feature and bilateral asymmetry measurement. This new technology is likely to be able to better optimize facial deformity patient diagnostic and treatment algorithms, such as those responsible for high levels of asymmetry, with the ultimate aim of improved aesthetic results and higher psychological benefit (Lin et al., 2024). Apart from surgical repairs, the psychological impacts of facial asymmetry should not be taken lightly. Individuals who have visible asymmetries, either congenital or acquired, are subject to societal bias, which can cause tremendous influences on their mental health as well as their general well-being. It has been shown through research that beauty is highly correlated with facial symmetry, thus placing more burdens on individuals with asymmetrical facial anatomy. Awareness of these psychological effects encourages a more sympathetic and integrated treatment approach that confronts not only the physical realignment of asymmetries but also the social and emotional ramifications of living with these conditions. By integrating psychological support with aesthetic procedures, medical experts can prescribe a more complete treatment program to patients with facial asymmetry, encouraging better body image and acceptance among patients (Lin et al., 2024) (Figure 13.8).

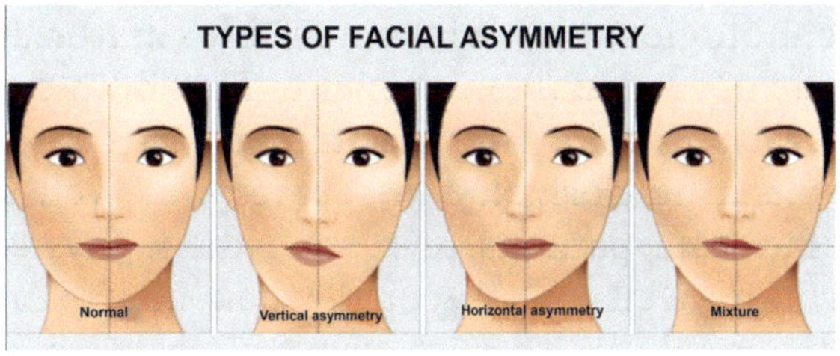

Figure 13.8. Facial asymmetry.

Source: https://external-content.duckduckgo.com/iu/?u=https%3A%2F%2Fgotobeauty.com%2Fwp-content%2Fuploads%2F2024%2F01%2FTYPES-OF-FACIAL-ASYMMETRY-1024x576.png&f=1&nofb=1&ipt=62b957f72b3f1d3b3d184b415ca0c9fd192030d0c09876f08b459a5db959fff4.

13.2.2. Acquired Deformities Due to Trauma

Trauma-caused deformities are a key issue of the field of facial aesthetics, distinguishing them from developmental or congenital deformities. These resulting conditions are a result of a variety of injuries, including accidents, athletic accidents, or brutal attacks, that can alter facial bone and soft tissue structural integrity. Trauma tends to have profound effects, as not only do they alter one's looks but also the psychological health of the patient. Patients can suffer chronic emotional distress resulting from disfigurement, which decreases quality of life. It is essential to understand the consequences of such deformities in the development of therapeutic interventions aimed at correcting both function and esthetics. It is frequent that the treatment of acquired facial deformities is carried out by a multidisciplinary team. Maxillofacial reconstruction surgeries are crucial in the correction of the underlying bony structure and esthetic contour of the face. Evolutionary facial jaw surgery techniques, which seek to repair structural deformities caused by trauma, have been introduced to achieve maximum patient benefit (Ugli, 2024). These treatments can involve the use of advanced imaging technologies and biocompatible materials to achieve maximum benefit. Rehabilitation operations following treatment are critical in ensuring normalcy in recovery, as well as to facilitate patients to restore their physical form, as well as self-belief when interacting with people. With such comprehensive care, the aftermath of trauma-related deformities can be effectively addressed. Furthermore, rehabilitation in patients with facial acquired deformities is a complex process that is generally not possible surgically. Prosthetic is also widely used to address aesthetic and functional deficits, particularly in children and adolescents who are victims of such injury at formative stages (Wojtyńska et al., 2024). Such prosthetics are not only used to cover the deformities but also to enable the normal facial movement during social interaction. With the treating clinicians interacting with these patients, it becomes necessary to assess their individualized needs and formulate a personalized care regimen involving both surgical and prosthetic components. This move emphasizes the importance of integral treatment models that take into account the multidimensional impact of acquired deformities on individuals who are in pursuit of aesthetic balance in facial appearance.

13.2.3. Deformities Resulting from Medical Conditions

The intersection of congenital disease and facial aesthetics is a complicated issue, particularly as it involves the treatment of deformities due to medical conditions. Congenital conditions such as cleft lip and palate are significant concerns due to their pervasive impact on both aesthetics and functionality. These disfigurements may disrupt essential activities such as feeding and speech and need intricate, multidisciplinary treatment. The psychosocial impact of the visibility of disfigurements may disrupt social interaction and self-esteem, further making the experience of affected individuals more complicated. As with studies among patient populations with heterogeneity, benefits from cooperative work among surgeons, orthodontists, and speech pathologists underscore the necessity for an integrated rehabilitation care strategy beyond the correction of aesthetics (Eshiev et al., 2025). In addition to birth conditions, acquired facial deformities due to illnesses such as trauma or surgery also significantly impact facial appearances. For instance, the results of injuries that manifest as craniofacial trauma can result in extreme asymmetry and malformation. The conditions reflected in such instances normally demand advanced reconstructive processes specifically designed to correct both the function and the aesthetics. Moreover, facial asymmetry, resulting from an array of medical conditions—such as developmental disorders—should be thoroughly analyzed in order to determine the etiology of the conditions. Understanding of the underlying causes can facilitate proper surgical planning and management, ultimately improving aesthetic outcomes. As research emphasizes, convergence of novel imaging technologies in diagnosis as well as surgical planning is crucial to providing optimal facial balance and patients' quality of life (Boymuradov et al., 2025). The role of interdisciplinary integration cannot be overemphasized in the treatment of deformities resulting from medical conditions.

Effective management of conditions like cleft palate and lip involves a lifelong effort from an interdisciplinary team of skilled health professionals, bringing together both physical and psychological components of treatment. Corrective surgery is usually staged, and ongoing reevaluation and intervention are required as the patient grows. Furthermore, participation of mental health professionals may help address the psychological burden of having visible defects and enhance the general therapeutic process. A treatment plan that is methodical in scope and incorporates not only operative correction, but also psychological guidance and rehabilitative therapy, realizes massive benefits both aesthetically and in terms of patients' overall well-being. Such a holistic model is crucial to instill resilience and foster an optimistic self-image among patients with congenital and developmental deformities (Eshiev et al., 2025).

Test Your Knowledge

1. What developmental abnormalities lead to cleft lip and palate, and how do these conditions affect feeding and speech?
2. How does craniosynostosis occur, and what impact does premature fusion of cranial sutures have on skull and brain development?

13.3. Causes of Congenital Deformities

Learning Outcome

1. Discuss the Genetic Factors
2. Explain the Environmental Influences
3. Focus on Maternal Health During Pregnancy

Congenital deformity pathogenesis is multifactorial and includes genetic, environmental, and epigenetic factors contributing to the adverse impact on fetal development. The majority of cases are caused by genetic defects in the forms of chromosomal and single-gene disorders. For instance, trisomy 21 disorders like Down syndrome are characterized by several physical deformities and predominantly facial structures. In addition, environmental influences, such as teratogenic agents, ranging from drugs to infectious diseases, have major roles to play in fetal morphology during periods that are critical for gestation. Maternal alcohol or drug exposure has been found to be a causative agent of facial deformities and therefore contributes importantly to the induction of disorders such as fetal alcohol syndrome. Therefore, an understanding of both environmental stimuli and genetic susceptibility is paramount in the development of the multifaceted processes of congenital deformities. In addition to environmental and hereditary causes, maternal health or nutrition also play a key role in the prevention of congenital disabilities. Deficiencies in some critical nutrients early in pregnancy have been found to increase vulnerability to neural tube defects and other birth defects. Pregnancy-associated maternal conditions like obesity and diabetes are additional threats, not only causing potentially fatal pregnancy-related complications but also increasing the chances of congenital facial abnormalities in offspring. As more research pours in, what becomes apparent is that the integration of a multidisciplinary strategy of maternal care can assist in reducing risk for congenital malformation. By promoting maximum prenatal health and filling in defects, doctors can improve outcomes and eventually reduce the prevalence of congenital deformities.

Advances in medical technology and genetic counseling have opened up new avenues for education about and possibly avoiding the dangers of congenital deformities. For example, the application of orthognathic surgery has evolved significantly, so that treatment of facial deformities resulting from congenital conditions is more successful.

Midface and mandible osteotomies are routinely done now, and the aesthetic and functional outcome is improved. Additionally, as craniofacial deformities (CFDs) as a science are continually changing, corrective procedures based on regenerative medicine and tissue engineering are of immense potential to correct severe deformities. However, congenital deformities still remain a challenge in the form of complex anatomical structures and individualized management. Consequently, ongoing research is an integral part of fine-tuning treatment modalities and enhancing patient outcomes within facial aesthetics, ultimately improving quality of life among congenital patients (Tahmasebi et al., 2023; Zammit et al., 2023) (Figure 13.9).

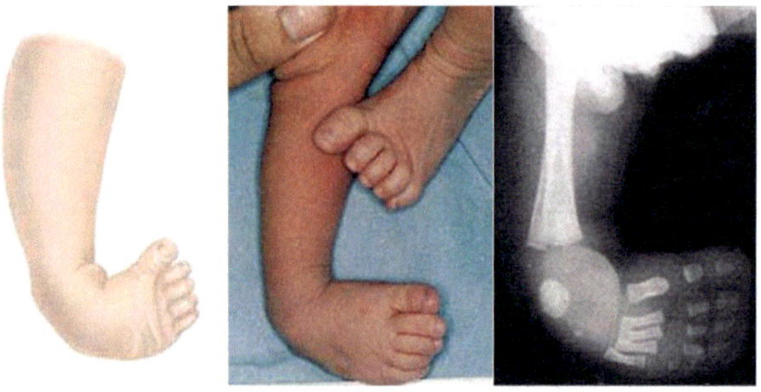

Figure 13.9. Causes of congenital deformities.

Source: https://external-content.duckduckgo.com/iu/?u=https%3A%2F%2Farchive.cdc.gov%2Fwww_cdc_gov%2Fncbddd%2Fbirthdefects%2Fsurveillancemanual%2Fphoto-atlas%2Fmuscu_html_files%2FCongenital-deformities-of-feet.jpg&f=1&nofb=1&ipt=963b6b0fbdcba7b2d99e63f1f664504c98c205a57ae886d08dac6b9a1986f979.

13.3.1. Genetic Factors

Genetic contributions towards the cause of congenital and developmental facial deformities are extensive and multifaceted. Genetic predispositions can lead to various craniofacial anomalies, which manifest through complex interactions among a number of genes. Studies have indicated that certain genetic diseases are directly related to abnormal facial patterns, i.e., cleft lip and palate, caused not only due to environmental reasons but also by the hereditary contributions of the genes. With continuous progress in genomic studies, determining the specific genetic markers and their role in craniofacial morphogenesis becomes increasingly important. With the identification of these genetic factors, clinicians are better able to assess risks, provide early interventions, and plan personalized treatment for patients who are facing such congenital challenges, thus optimizing clinical as well as aesthetic results in facial reconstruction. Exceeding isolated congenital deformities, the influence of genetic factors is present across a vast spectrum of facial aesthetic conditions that manifest themselves during the course of an individual's lifetime. For example, facial structures can be asymmetrical because they have both genetic and environmental influences. Facial directional asymmetry (DA) research indicates that genetic predispositions toward certain face shapes will work with the influence of aging to create unique developmental trajectories between populations. Three-dimensional measurements of DA over different ages are used in research to demonstrate how genes are involved in morphological change over time. In reviewing these findings, it is apparent that ongoing studies of genetic influences may shed light on the maintenance of facial beauty and the repair of a hereditary etiology of deformity, and ultimately the overall quality of life in such cases. Finally, neurodevelopmental genetics plays a part in the expression of facial beauty as the very interactive relation between nervous and stomatognathic systems. Genetic abnormalities may interfere with the highly complex processes of craniofacial development, causing congenital disorders that require in-depth clinical treatment. Recent research has highlighted the significance of the "brain-oral axis" in elucidating these connections, with a view to underlining that deviations from normal neural development can have downstream effects on facial features and overall aesthetic result. Diseases such as periodontitis were discovered in conjunction with neurodegenerative diseases, shedding light on the bidirectional interaction of the nervous and facial systems. As progress is made in science, it becomes increasingly important to combine genetic and neurological knowledge, fostering an interdisciplinary approach to treating congenital facial abnormalities and improving patient care in aesthetic and reconstructive surgery (Harnádková et al., 2023; Wu et al., 2023).

13.3.2. Environmental Influences

Environmental conditions are of utmost significance in the development and congenital deformities, particularly facial appearance. Various environmental factors, including maternal health, teratogenic effects, and nutrient deficiencies, have been shown to influence fetal development in a significant way. Malnutrition in pregnant women, for instance, has been shown to affect the craniofacial structures, leading to asymmetry and other types of deformities. The environmental role ranges from chemical exposure to psychosocial stressors known to influence fetal health. Therefore, it is paramount to comprehend these influences so that populations at risk can be identified and preventive interventions can be instated that can counteract adverse developmental impacts. Advances in imaging techniques have facilitated better comprehension and diagnosis of facial asymmetry and environmental deformities. As emphasized by recent research, discrimination between true and false facial asymmetries is important in formulating effective treatment plans. Diagnostic methods such as 3D CBCT scanning, cephalometry, and facial photometry enhance the clinician's ability to identify structural defects resulting from environmental causes (Boymuradov et al., 2025). Further, these assessments facilitate the correct preoperative evaluation so that the intervention provided is done in accordance with the precise needs of the patient, taking into consideration both aesthetic and functional deformities. The multifactorial nature of congenital and developmental deformities makes treatment a process that demands a holistic approach where genetic predispositions are balanced against environmental factors. Even though genetics might initiate the tendency towards the formation of facial deformities, environmental conditions are more likely to be the provocateurs of expression. For instance, environmental exposure in utero to pollutants or behavioral factors like smoking may worsen genetic susceptibilities to conditions such as facial asymmetry or cleft lip and palate (Boymuradov et al., 2025). Understanding these intersections is important for designing successful intervention strategies that treat both the genetic and environmental aspects, which in turn contributes to better treatment outcomes and enhancing the general quality of life of patients. With continued research continuing to reveal more and more of these factors, it highlights the importance of integrated healthcare policies which incorporate genetic counseling as well as environmental health literacy.

13.3.3. Maternal Health During Pregnancy

Pregnancy maternal health is a significant determinant of fetal as well as maternal outcomes, particularly regarding congenital and developmental defects. The intricate interrelationship among maternal diet, mental health, and environmental exposures plays a significant role in determining the trajectory of fetal health. Maternal nutrition plays a critical role in fetal development because dietary deficiency can make infants susceptible to congenital malformations, including orofacial clefts. For example, research has established that supplementation with folic acid can reduce the occurrence of neural tube defects, which highlights the importance of maternal food factors. The psychological well-being of the mother also cannot be overlooked since high levels of stress and anxiety during pregnancy have been proven to produce negative outcomes for the fetus, making pregnancy even more complicated during this period of maternal development. The challenges to neonate mothers with congenital abnormalities, such as cleft lip and palate, extend beyond the body's health. Such aberrations in anatomy are often complicated by a need for a multimodal care continuum, ranging from surgical intervention to a sophisticated feeding regimen. In cleft lip and palate, for instance, the issues of breastfeeding are compounded by the infant's characteristic anatomical deficits. Their management requires a multidisciplinary approach with surgical reconstruction and psychological treatment of mothers. Mothers must cope with the psychological aftermath of caring for a child with a congenital deformity. Stress and emotional status in mothers are two significant variables that not only affect lactation success but also the overall developmental outcome for the child. Therefore, emotional support and resources specific to these mothers can have a valuable impact on their capacity to care for their infants effectively. Furthermore, the prevalence of cleft lip and palate differs amongst populations, posing individual challenges based on genetic and environmental components. Insight into the epidemiology of these congenital anomalies can inform public health efforts towards enhancing maternal health practices and outcomes. For example, evidence shows that in Asian communities, clefting is more common than in African communities, which highlights the relevance of culturally sensitive healthcare provisions. The multifactorial etiology of these deformities implies that genetic vulnerabilities as well as maternal health behaviors during pregnancy, including smoking and alcohol consumption, play a major role in their occurrence. Controlling these risk factors by strengthening maternal health education and steering interventions can introduce more effective prevention strategies in congenital anomalies, thus guaranteeing optimum facial aesthetics as well as overall wellness of the affected person (Figure 13.10).

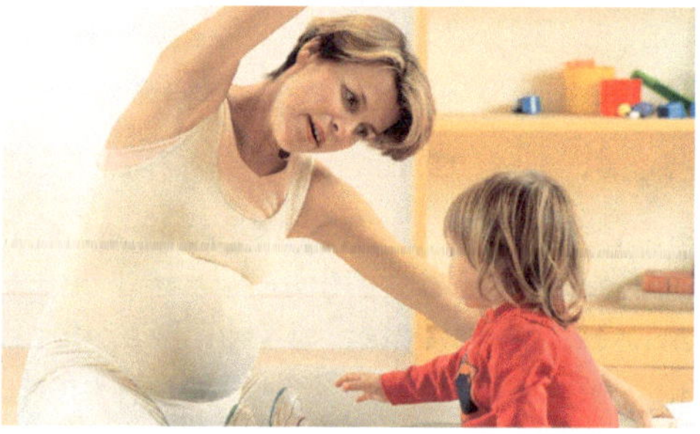

Figure 13.10. Maternal health during pregnancy influences a child's autism.

Source: https://external-content.duckduckgo.com/iu/?u=https%3A%2F%2Fsurvivethenews.com%2Fwp-content%2Fuploads%2F2025%2F03%2FHow-maternal-health-during-pregnancy-influences-a-childs-autism-risk.jpg&f=1&nofb=1&ipt=08feedd083146c2228509090a7ea26a8c19ce82abe3e4b1775af54dcf68268f5.

Test Your Knowledge

1. How do genetic mutations or inherited traits contribute to the development of congenital facial deformities?
2. What environmental factors during pregnancy may increase the risk of congenital deformities in a developing fetus?

13.4. Psychological Impact of Facial Deformities

Learning Outcome

1. Discuss the Self-esteem and Body Image Issues
2. Explain Social Stigma and Discrimination
3. Focus on Mental Health Implications

The psychological impact of facial deformities is quite wide-reaching beyond considerations of aesthetics alone, affecting the individual's self-esteem and relationships with others considerably. Congenital and developmental facial deformity patients usually express high levels of social distress and distress relating to their appearance. Research has demonstrated that individuals with craniofacial deformities experience higher levels of psychological distress than the general population, pointing to the fact that exterior stimuli of their look can lead to interior tension with their self-concept and identity. Negatively affecting mental health are depression, social withdrawal, and anxiety, which can significantly reduce quality of life. Emergence of addressing these psychological considerations underscores the need for interdisciplinarity that encompasses psychological counseling along with medical interventions for facial deformities, a primary determinant in healthcare providers crafting treatment protocols commensurate to patient needs (Bessell et al., 2015). Furthermore, the implications of facial deformity on other facets of life, including social inclusion, communication, and employment opportunities, cannot be ignored. As individuals with visible difference will struggle with negative stereotypes or prejudice, they are likely to face barriers that constrain full inclusion in many social contexts. Studies establish that such barriers lead to loneliness and a diminished sense of community, which further complicates mental illness. For instance, difficulties with chewing and speaking can generate feelings of inadequacy and anxiety, amplifying the impact their facial look has on social interactions. Incredibly, rehabilitative intervention, although beneficial, may still not restore people's self-esteem and quality of life to a position where they can be equated with nondisfigured counterparts. Along this line, it is crucial to pursue rehabilitation with a holistic perspective of the psychological dimension of facial beauty (Palmeiro et al., 2013). Last but not least, the issue of support systems is a significant one in mitigating psychological distress caused by facial deformity. Supportive comments from parents, peers, and health professionals can foster individuals' sense of self-concept and resilience in coping with adversity in society. Counseling and support groups may serve as a useful means of promoting acceptance and coping strategies, enabling one to cope with the intricacies associated with appearance in an improved manner. By building accepting environments that are centered on acceptance and understanding, the stigmatization of facial deformities can be reduced.

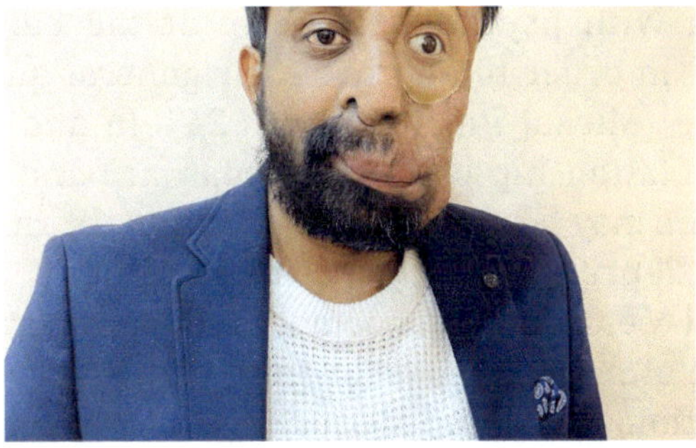

Figure 13.11. Psychological impact of facial deformities.

Source: https://www.camraredisease.org/wp-content/uploads/2023/08/image_50368513-1080x675.jpg.

Consequently, alongside the treatment of the physical aspect, the provision for the emotional and psychological aspects of the individual can significantly aid their general well-being and social incorporation, an essential process towards empathetic practice in facial aesthetics (Bessell et al., 2015) (Figure 13.11).

13.4.1. Self-esteem and Body Image Issues

Facial aesthetic deformities, whether developmental or congenital, have a significant impact on body image issues and low self-esteem. The overwhelming majority of individuals with conditions such as hemifacial microsomia experience the adverse views of their appearance and subsequently suffer from low self-esteem. Facial deformity has the greatest psychological impact at adolescence—a tender time marked by enhanced sensitivity to social acceptance and body image. As the research shows, hemifacial microsomia children have social integration problems and the risk of rejection by their peers, which aggravates their self-esteem issues. These issues are strongly entangled with their facial features, where perceived cosmetic abnormalities influence their interpersonal relationships and mental health results, which makes it critical to provide them with psychological help at the earliest stage in order to improve their general quality of life (Michał Pniak et al., 2024). In addition, the relationship between appearance and self-esteem may be seen in the higher rates of anxiety and depression in patients with congenital facial deformity. Abnormal facial appearance most often leads to feelings of inadequacy and isolation, which impede social relationships and reinforce negative self-concepts. In adolescents and young adults, these consequent impacts cause social avoidance or unwillingness to engage in relationships, perpetuating the cycle of low self-esteem. Moreover, individuals internalize cultural ideals of beauty, become unhappy with their own looks and distressed about their state. Resolution of such psychological and emotional problems is pivotal in developing self-acceptance and resilience in targeted groups, emphasizing the need for integrated treatment responses that involve psychological well-being (Pniak et al., 2024). As part of effective interventions, recognition of the part played by healthcare professionals in managing issues related to self-esteem and body image is important. Clinicians are also required to have attention not only to the physical treatments but also to the psychosocial consequences that accompany facial congenital deformities. The therapy may include working on open conversations about one's image, providing access to counseling interventions, and applying education as a strategy of achieving de-stigmatization by society. Studies have shown that patients suffering from conditions such as hemifacial microsomia, when provided with proper psychosocial support, show improved emotional functioning and an increased sense of belongingness among peers. Moreover, active intervention in the form of programs such as community awareness and outreach aids in creating a positive attitude towards diversity in facial aesthetics, in the end aiding affected individuals to enhance their body image and self-esteem in the long run (Pniak et al., 2024) (Figure 13.12).

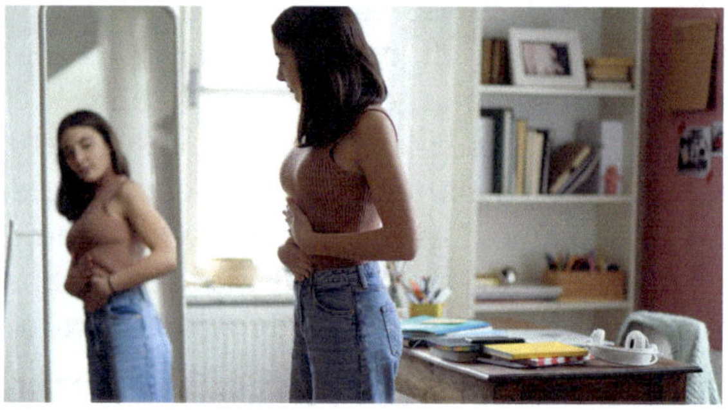

Figure 13.12. Self-esteem and body image issues.

Source: https://www.servicesforeducation.co.uk/wp-content/uploads/2024/07/Body-Image-and-Self-Esteem-1400x775.png.

13.4.2. Social Stigma and Discrimination

The social stigma that accompanies congenital and developmental deformities, particularly those affecting the beauty of the face, has drastic effects on the person's psychological and social well-being. Victims of deformity endure discrimination that gets to define their lifestyle and relationships. Social exclusion exists in the form of offensive statements, social rejection, and overall negative generalization. All these external forces tend to create the overwhelming emotional pain with resulting low self-esteem and mental illness. Drawing from research on oral reconstructive surgery, bullying and social experiences of loneliness persist to influence people before undergoing surgery, further underlining the urgent need for addressing these social perceptions of physical appearance (Sablada & Amparado, 2020). Not only do such stigmatizations undermine a person's feeling of belonging, but these stigmatizations also form a vicious cycle of discrimination that can deter individuals from accessing necessary medical or psychological care. Physical appearance discrimination is widespread in multi-ethnic social settings, including schools, the workplace, and healthcare facilities. Where those with facial disfigurements are discriminated against, their opportunities for social mobility, professional development, and access to basic services are compromised. A review of literature on cleft lip and/or palate individuals reveals that while the overall impact of these disorders on psychological adaptation was found to be low, the multigene nature of social experiences indicates significant barriers in terms of acceptance and satisfaction with appearance (Stock & Feragen, 2016). This dissonance between self and societal expectations generally increases feelings of isolation. Eradicating these inequalities requires an understanding of the stigma that exists and deliberate steps to bring inclusivity, thereby providing a space where individuals are valued for what they are able to do rather than being attacked based on their physical appearance. Steps towards avoiding social stigma and discrimination against individuals with congenital and developmental deformities require a holistic approach that includes education, advocacy, and community action. By raising awareness of the psychological impacts of experiencing such, society can demolish prevalent stereotypes surrounding physical appearance. Inclusivity and empathy programs can significantly improve the lives of people with facial deformities. Support groups and peer workshops, for instance, can allow individuals to voice their experiences, develop resilience, and overcome loneliness. In addition, medical personnel and teachers need to be educated on identifying and confronting biases in their settings, developing a more supportive environment for patients and students. Encouraging empathy and understanding can play a critical role in shifting societal attitudes and ensuring that individuals with congenital and developmental deformities are given the respect and support they need (Figure 13.13).

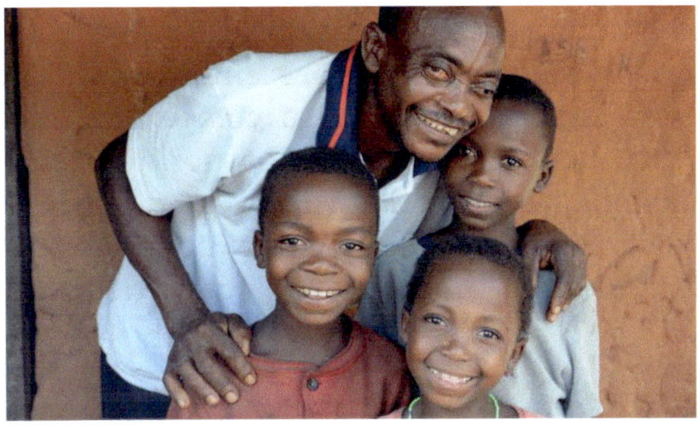

Figure 13.13. Social stigma and discrimination.

Source: https://www.infontd.org/sites/default/files/styles/crop_freeform/public/2020-05/CBM-Onchocerciasis-0011.JPG?h=34e69bba&itok=jOS2gSx1.

13.4.3. Mental Health Implications

The psychological effect on congenitally or developmentally deformed individuals who have facial aesthetic deformities is profound and intricate. Research shows that patients with craniofacial anomalies have heightened issues concerning their appearance, leading to high social anxiety and a diminished quality of life.

For instance, such patients have been found to register higher negative psychological impacts in terms of their appearance compared to patients presenting without deformities. Specifically, interventions using the Psychological Impact of Dental Aesthetic Questionnaire (PIDAQ) and the Derriford Appearance Scale (DAS) identify that patients with craniofacial abnormalities experience much more distress over their looks, which may prompt avoidance of social interaction and fear of others' reactions (Bessell et al., 2015). Hence, the psychological impact from it does not just manifest at the subjective level of well-being but also in the general capacity to engage in normal social rituals. Also adding to the intricacies of handling mental health among this population is the long-term nature of the issues they have. Individuals with congenital deformities also tend to have issues with chewing, speech, and social integration, all impacting their quality of life (QoL) vitally. The oral presentation of such deformities tends to be so complicated that it requires extensive rehabilitation to restore function and aesthetics. However, studies have shown that even with interventions like oral rehabilitation, patients with conditions like cleft lip and palate (CLP) continue to have impaired masticatory function and lower QoL scores than healthy controls. Therefore, the inability of rehabilitation efforts to completely achieve both functional and psychosocial needs underscores the importance of interdisciplinary-based care; integrating psychological support with physical treatments (Palmeiro et al., 2013). Generally, the psychological aspects of congenital and developmental deformities must be addressed with a comprehensive approach that values and addresses the emotional needs of the afflicted. Effective interventions should aim not just to correct physical appearance, but also to promote emotional ease through counseling and outreach. By self-acceptance and the strengthening of coping mechanisms, mental health treatment can improve social integration and quality of life among such people. It is critical to have such an integrated approach, for it realizes that the journey towards accepting one's appearance is as significant as the medical or surgical intervention that has already been done. The psychological climate for the cases of facial deformity, therefore, can be favorably altered, initiating enhanced overall results.

Test Your Knowledge

1. How do facial deformities influence self-esteem and body image, especially during childhood and adolescence?
2. In what ways can social stigma and discrimination affect the emotional well-being and social development of individuals with facial deformities?

13.5. Treatment Options for Facial Deformities

Learning Outcome

1. Discuss the Surgical Interventions
2. Focus on Orthodontic Treatments
3. Explain Psychological Support and Counseling

Treatment of facial deformities is case-specific and multidisciplinary in nature. Certain of the surgical options, such as orthognathic surgery, have also emerged as vital instruments in orthodontic correction of mismatched jaws and overall facial aesthetics. This type of surgery allows for the accurate realignment of facial bones to both restore functional deficits and address aesthetic concerns. Advances in technology, including computer planning and patient-specific fixation, have significantly enhanced the outcome of these operations. Surgeons are now better able to plan complex osteotomies with better predictability of outcome. Apart from this, the operations are also able to cure obstructive sleep apnea in a manner that makes the treatment doubly beneficial for patients who have both cosmetic and functional problems with their facial structures (Zammit et al., 2023). Apart from surgery, orthodontic treatments form part and parcel of facial deformity treatment, particularly in malocclusion. Malocclusion can interfere with one's oral function and also the aesthetic appearance, and identification and treatment of malocclusion have become extremely important in contemporary dentistry. Malocclusions were acknowledged by the World Health Organization as a main oral disorder that occurs with a high prevalence rate among the community. Interference at an early stage during the primary dentition period is capable of preventing the development of severe malocclusion into adulthood. The various malocclusion classifications, particularly the Angles classification system, enable understanding of unique dental alignment deviation forms to help orthodontists select the best treatment modalities based on specific cases (Lone et al., 2023). Lastly, non-surgical methods such as facial fillers and orthodontic appliances are becoming increasingly used to minimize or correct minor facial deformities and improve aesthetic results without surgery. For those patients who are not surgical candidates or wish less intrusive options, aligners and braces provide excellent improvement in facial form and function. Facial fillers are also an extremely viable option for volume and contour restoration of birth-defected areas. These treatments can enhance facial looks by providing rapid results with minimal downtime, which is appealing to those who appreciate rapid and effective treatments. With the development of facial aesthetics, possessing a general understanding of the variety of treatment modalities provides patients with the capacity to make informed choices regarding their treatment (Zammit et al., 2023) (Figure 13.14).

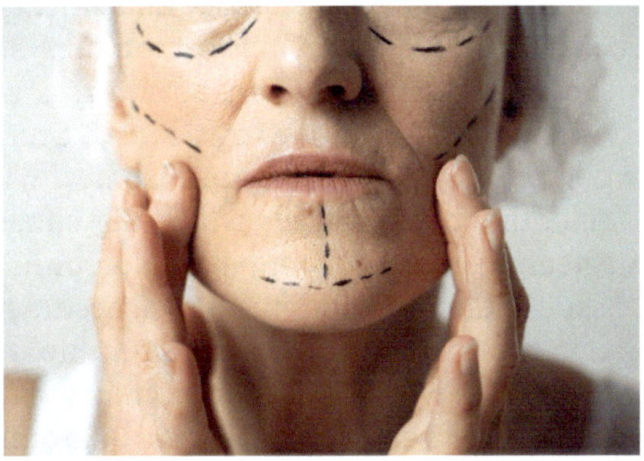

Figure 13.14. Treatment options for facial deformities.

Source: https://reconfaceindia.in/wp-content/uploads/elementor/thumbs/Post-trauma-facial-deformities-qf6ws1lmuvx33nip0n7m7qjv3gpywk5af1b92wtw5c.png.

13.5.1. Surgical Interventions

Surgical procedures play a pivotal role in the treatment of congenital and developmental facial aesthetic deformities, particularly for cases such as hemifacial microsomia (HFM). This is an asymmetric underdevelopment of first and second branchial arch components and is characterized by a variety of craniofacial anomalies that include mandibular hypoplasia, ear deformities, and other related structures. Surgical intervention generally requires a multidisciplinary approach to ensure holistic management and optimal aesthetic results. Several methods are utilized, including rib or fibular bone grafting, distraction osteogenesis, and orthognathic surgery, all of which collectively attempt to address functional and aesthetic deformities. The efficient synergism of such surgical techniques has far-reaching implications for improving not only the facial structural dimensions but also the psychosocial quality of life of the patients at a young age (Behnia et al., 2023). In addition to traditional surgical modalities, technological advancements have created sophisticated surgical instruments that further enhance the accuracy and efficacy of these interventions. Ultrasonic osteotomes, such as Piezosurgery, offer obvious advantages over conventional rotary or sawing devices. Studies have demonstrated that these ultrasonic devices yield smoother bone surfaces, which may enhance tissue healing and reduce injury to surrounding soft tissues during osteotomies. Such accuracy is crucial in the correction of complex craniofacial malformations, wherein collateral injury has to be avoided to preserve important anatomical structures. The comparative outcomes between ultrasonic and traditional osteotomes reveal a dramatic contrast in micromorphological features, again confirming the application of newer technology in operations to correct facial deformity (Anesi et al., 2014). The long-term benefits of surgical intervention in correcting congenital and developmental facial deformity extend beyond aesthetic purposes. Successful surgical outcomes can significantly enhance the psychosocial aspect of patients' lives, particularly at the time of adolescence, when perceptions of the peer group have an increasingly powerful influence. Procedures to correct jaw straightening or facial asymmetry have been found to enhance self-esteem and social function, producing a more positive self-concept. The integration of functional orthodontics along with surgical treatment, as validated by the findings of longitudinal follow-up in the instances of HFM, underscores the importance of a strictly planned treatment regimen that attempts to offer optimal facial esthetics and restoration of function. This multi-disciplinary strategy supports the imperative for ongoing research and communication among specialists to continue improving surgical techniques and overall patient care within the field of craniofacial surgery (Behnia et al., 2023) (Figure 13.15).

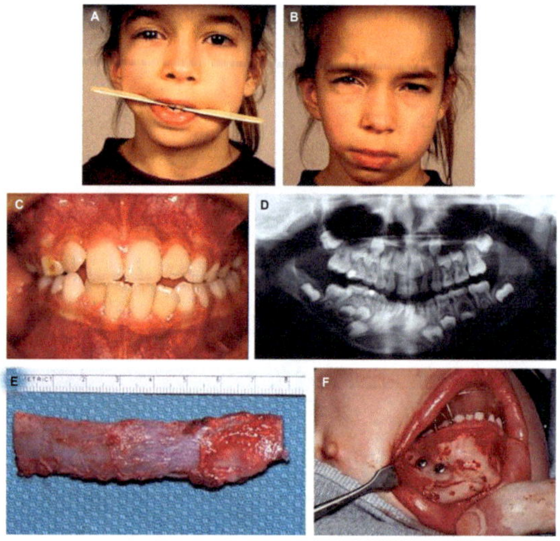

Figure 13.15. Surgical interventions play a pivotal role in addressing congenital and developmental deformities in facial aesthetics.

Source: https://ars.els-cdn.com/content/image/1-s2.0-S1042369907000386-gr7af.jpg.

13.5.2. Orthodontic Treatments

Orthodontics is a key component in the management of congenital and developmental facial aesthetic deformities. Orthodontic treatment has a tendency of aligning teeth, correcting issues with bites, and improving overall dental function, which can significantly improve a patient's facial appearance. With patients who have diseases such as Apert syndrome, which includes facial and dental abnormalities, orthodontics plays a crucial role. Early treatment using braces or other orthodontic devices can help in the proper alignment of the teeth and jaws, which in turn results in a more balanced facial esthetic profile. Since most of the congenital conditions can produce secondary functional impairment, orthodontic treatment not only has a purely aesthetic function but also corrects the underlying functional impairment and hence supports a better quality of life for the patients. With the progress in orthodontic treatments, integration of surgical treatments has become the standard, particularly if skeletal discrepancies exist. Orthognathic surgery is typically used in conjunction with orthodontic treatments to achieve optimum benefits. Improvements in surgical techniques in today's time, such as computer-aided planning and patient-specific fixation, have tailored the process in the correction of severe deformities (Zammit et al., 2023). This partnership between orthodontists and oral surgeons allows the face and oral structures to be treated more accurately and effectively, not only for their appearance, but also for the functional dynamics of the bite. Such comprehensive care is the focal point in multidisciplinary treatment plans for those with congenital deformities and strives to enhance aesthetic outcomes as well as oral health. Moreover, the psychosocial impact of orthodontic treatment cannot be overlooked, especially on individuals with obvious congenital or developmental deformities. Orthodontic therapy of dental and facial deformities exercises a significant influence on self-perception and social acceptance. Patients become less embarrassed and more confident following the treatment, which is evidence of the psychological significance of facial beauty (Kumari et al., 2023). By improving the symmetry and alignment of their smile, orthodontic treatments contribute to a satisfactory self-image, thereby maximizing the quality of life as a whole. To this end, healthcare providers are required to plan for treatment holistically, taking into consideration the emotional and psychological health of the patients along with the technical know-how of care in aesthetic dentistry (Figure 13.16).

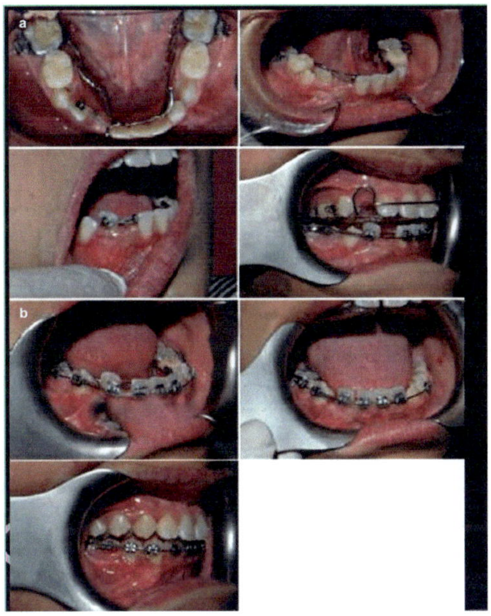

Figure 13.16. Orthodontic treatments.

Source: https://www.researchgate.net/profile/Biagio-Rapone/publication/320432128/figure/fig2/AS:580206029176833@1515343305438/a-Pictures-of-the-different-phases-of-the-orthodontic-treatment-b-Orthodontic.png.

13.5.3. Psychological Support and Counseling

Psychological guidance and support are of critical significance in the rehabilitation of congenital and developmental facial deformities in aesthetics, with direct impacts on emotional state as well as social integration. These individuals are often more anxious, self-conscious, and disabled in daily social contact, and hence they have a poorer quality of life. It entails the development of a therapeutic relationship between the patient and the mental health professional, in which the latter creates a comfortable environment where the patient can express their concerns and emotions. This kind of support is not only important in coping with the immediate emotional disturbance caused by their condition but also in preparing individuals to prepare for potential treatments or procedures that can alter the appearance of individuals, as the psychological impact can be as profound as the physical alterations inherent within these medical interventions. Counseling interventions specific to those with facial deformity should also take into account the special needs of this group. Cognitive-behavioral therapy (CBT) and other forms of therapy can successfully correct negative self-perception and distorted thinking about appearance. These therapeutic interventions assist patients in changing their perceptions and improving self-acceptance, thus building resilience against social stigma. In addition, support groups can prove to be priceless because they allow people to bond with their peers who are going through the same issues, fostering mutual healing. Sharing such group experiences not only offers emotional encouragement but also leads to the sharing of coping mechanisms and personal experiences, which ultimately strengthen people to deal with and overcome their fears concerning their facial looks, bolstering their mental strength. Further, the need for interprofessional teamwork among treatment professionals cannot be overemphasized when it comes to psychological care of patients with congenital and developmental deformities. Interprofessional collaboration ensures an integrated approach, involving plastic surgeons, mental health professionals, and genetic counselors to design an integrated plan of care. Interprofessional collaboration allows providers to address not only physical but also psychological issues, thus enhancing overall outcomes of treatment. As has been demonstrated in current literature, holistic management practices can lead to better patient outcomes and experiences, with the importance of shared decision-making in treatment highlighted. This inter-disciplinary strategy mirrors evidence regarding the complexity of most congenital conditions, highlighting the promise that integrated care networks hold to improve dramatically the quality of life for such individuals, allowing them to better navigate the complexity of their conditions with a lot more support and understanding, as in the management of neurofibromatosis type 1 (Bergqvist et al., 2020) and congenital heart disease (Pierpont et al., 2018).

Test Your Knowledge

1. What are the key surgical interventions used to correct common congenital facial deformities, and how do they improve function and appearance?
2. How do orthodontic treatments support facial deformity management, particularly in cases involving jaw or dental misalignment?

13.6. Advances in Facial Aesthetic Procedures

Learning Outcome

1. Discuss the Innovations in Surgical Techniques
2. Focus on Role of 3D Imaging and Modeling
3. Explain the Non-Surgical Aesthetic Enhancements

The field of facial aesthetics has experienced great advances that have widened the treatment options for patients with developmental and congenital deformities. Traditional practices, which were primarily surgical, have been revolutionized with the introduction of minimal access procedures that enhance safety and recovery. Emerging three-dimensional imaging and computer simulations have also become valuable in pre-surgical planning and patient education. These innovations provide professionals with a greater understanding of craniofacial anatomy, enabling them to provide customized treatment options better suited to individual patient needs. With fewer invasive and more precise surgeries, patients can expect improved functional and aesthetic results. More patient-centered treatment modalities for facial aesthetics place increased focus on improvements that assist in diminishing the psychological effect of congenital deformity, promoting overall quality of life for individuals so involved. Further, the development of non-surgical approaches to aesthetic enhancement has had a profound impact on the facial reconstruction and enhancement arena. Technologies such as fillers, neurotoxins, and other biocompatible agents in soft tissue augmentation provide some alternatives that can reduce the necessity for more invasive surgeries. For patients with congenital deformities, these technologies can correct the anomalies immediately, enhancing facial contours and symmetry without the extensive downtime associated with surgery. Also, the growing availability of Piezosurgery®, among other ultrasound-assisted osteotomes, adds the benefits of precision in osteotomies that provide smoother bone surfaces to heal and produce more acceptable aesthetics following surgical interventions (Anesi et al., 2014). With growing technological developments, the use of these non-surgical techniques not only transforms patterns of treatment but also opens a new frontier for the return of confidence in patients with congenital and developmental facial disorders. Cosmetic procedures' clinical practices have expanded due to a better understanding of the physiological and psychological details of congenital deformities. More advanced prosthetic therapies, including individually customized orthodontic appliances, address both functional and cosmetic problems maximally. These devices have a vital role in treatment regimens for patients with conditions such as cleft lip and palate, where rehabilitation is multifaceted and requires close consideration in terms of the optimal balance between form and function.

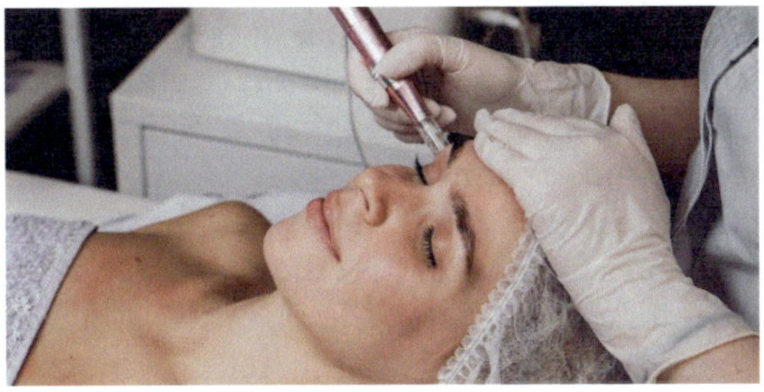

Figure 13.17. Facial aesthetics.

Source: https://iicad.org/wp-content/uploads/2024/01/IICAD-7.png.

Novel non-surgical treatment options, including novel orthodontic techniques, can now offer patients more comfortable and functional solutions for coping with extreme deformity and optimizing oral function (McNeil, 1951). As research ever more illuminates the correlation between aesthetic perfection and emotional well-being, it is increasingly evident that innovation in facial aesthetic surgery is paramount for transforming not just the physical topographies but also the psychosocial existence of individuals with congenital and developmental facial disfigurements (Figure 13.17).

13.6.1. Innovations in Surgical Techniques

Craniofacial surgery has witnessed significant new development as far as surgical techniques addressing congenital and developmental facial aesthetics deformities are concerned. Among the most promising of these is the use of stem cell therapy with tissue engineering. As highlighted in recent literature, this technique has immense potential for regrowing some craniofacial tissues but remains at its nascent stage of advancement in its clinical applications. The unique type of various stem cell sources makes personalized treatments for complicated facial deformity patients, hence promising improved surgical outcomes. While researchers seek to study the most appropriate cell sources, challenges that are unique to these new types of treatment need to be addressed to increase their efficacy and availability in clinics (Hughes & Song, 2016). The second essential innovation of surgical techniques is the application of ultrasonic osteotomes to enhance precision for osteotomies in craniofacial surgery. The traditional method of using turning or sawing tools will cause damage to the surrounding soft tissue, thus causing postoperative complications. However, studies have established that Piezosurgery, a technique assisted by ultrasound, not only preserves the integrity of adjacent tissues but also enhances bone healing and reossification. Micromorphological surface features of osteotomized surfaces mirror increased roughness values, which are crucial for effective healing and incorporation of graft materials. The minimally invasive surgery has monumental advantages, eventually leading to improved aesthetic and functional outcomes for individuals with craniofacial deformities (Anesi et al., 2014). With improving surgical techniques, integration of advanced imaging modalities and computer-aided design (CAD) has transformed preoperative planning as well as intraoperative navigation. Technological advances in 3D imaging make it possible to have personalized surgical strategies, and through this, surgeons are able to design patient-specific models that closely approximate the anatomical complexities of individual patients. Such precision guarantees that surgical procedures are customized to correct the specific deformities involved, as well as to maximize aesthetic outcome and functional abilities of reconstructions. Supported by intraoperative navigation devices, these developments facilitate accurate execution of surgical plans to the minimum possible extent, ensuring reduced opportunities for errors and overall patient safety. With growing popularity, these advances are likely to transform the quality of care for the correction of congenital and developmental facial anomalies (Anesi et al., 2014; Hughes & Song, 2016).

13.6.2. Role of 3D Imaging and Modeling

The intersection of three-dimensional (3D) imaging and modeling technology has revolutionized the field of reconstructive surgery for developmental and congenital facial aesthetic deformities. Advances in 3D imaging provide advanced visualization of craniofacial anatomy, which allow clinicians to examine deformities with unmatched precision. Such technological advances enable virtual surgical planning (VSP), which transforms cumbersome anatomical data into efficacious surgical plans. For instance, in the management of conditions such as hemifacial microsomia, 3D modeling enables planning of osteotomy lines and cutting guides that are tailored to the individual anatomical features of the patients. The technique enhances intraoperative precision and minimizes intraoperative complications, hence dramatically improving patient outcomes.

This innovation serves to underscore the basic significance of 3D imaging in transforming traditional surgical practices into more precise, streamlined procedures, ultimately resulting in enhanced success rates for reconstruction surgeries. In terms of orthognathic surgery, 3D imaging has facilitated unprecedented advances in the planning and execution of treatment. Surgeons can now execute precise osteotomies of the midface and mandible, aligning their surgical goals with an individually designed treatment plan. The precise combination of patient-specific fixation systems and advancing imaging technologies provides a rational approach to treating both functional and cosmetic issues in facial aesthetics. In the past two decades, this paradigm has seen enhancements in the fidelity of computer-assisted planning, making it simpler for surgeons to predict and avoid potential complications during surgery. These improvements have enabled improved integration of orthodontic treatments with surgical procedures, generating synergistic methods for treating congenital and acquired facial deformities (Zammit et al., 2023). This development strongly suggests growing prevalence and reliance on 3D imaging among the surgical community. As craniofacial surgery continues to advance, the significance of 3D imaging and modeling technology is bound to increase even more. The utility of such technologies is not just restricted to successful surgeries; they also enhance postoperative assessment and long-term follow-up of facial shape and function. In successful reconstructions, for instance, with 3D-printed surgical implants in hemifacial microsomia treatments, systematic evaluations show promising decreases in asymmetry parameters (Zhao et al., 2023). The use of digital software not only impacts the short-term results of surgeries but also contributes to ongoing learning and improvement in surgical procedures. As more use of 3D imaging techniques is seen, novel progress in the future may simplify surgical procedures, improve reconstructive procedures, and increase the standard of patient care in facial aesthetic surgery. Overall, the use of 3D imaging and modeling remains at the core of defining the future of craniofacial reconstructive surgery, particularly for complex congenital malformations.

13.6.3. Non-Surgical Aesthetic Enhancements

Non-surgical aesthetic enhancement has emerged as a flagship procedure in the facial aesthetic industry, particularly for individuals with congenital and developmental anomalies. Such enhancements, such as dermal fillers and neurotoxin injections, provide versatile solutions that can subtly remodel facial features without the dangers of surgical procedures. For those who have congenital asymmetries or facial development abnormalities, non-surgical interventions can be utilized to establish balance and aesthetic appeal. Procedures are favored because they are minimally invasive, recovery time is brief, and treatments can be individually designed to focus on particular facial issues. This adaptability not only empowers the patients but also promotes a more personalized modus operandi of aesthetic treatment in the scenario of congenital facial deformities. The increasing popularity of non-surgical augmentation of beauty evokes serious ethical concerns, particularly in children or congenital deformity cases. Although these interventions are effective in restoring self-esteem and enhancing quality of life, careful assessment must be conducted in order to determine the appropriateness of treatment and reality of treatment expectations. The practitioners must engage the patients in lengthy discussions of potential outcomes, risks, and limitations. Also, the fleeting nature of the majority of non-surgical enhancements necessitates repeated sessions, and this results in a continuous commitment, which could complicate the decision-making process by individuals with developmental disabilities. Healthcare providers then must walk the thin line between supporting self-betterment and making interventions match the psychosocial needs and maturity levels of the patients. Despite the efficacy of non-surgical measures, they should not be regarded as a substitute for complete surgical treatment for severe congenital and acquired facial deformities. For instance, conditions requiring extensive structural realignment, e.g., those being managed by orthognathic surgery, cannot rely on cosmetic enhancement alone to yield curative benefits. The overlap of non-surgical and surgical procedures indicates a growing pattern towards an amalgamation of the two in aesthetic medicine, both helping to complement each other. Both developments hold the potential for inter-disciplinary interaction, enhancing patient results and quality of life for sufferers of congenital conditions. As ongoing research and technological advancements continue, facial aesthetics will likely continue evolving, and non-surgical treatment will become a component of treatment modalities in harmony with the patient's individual profile and needs (Zammit et al., 2023; Ugli, 2024).

Test Your Knowledge

1. How have recent innovations in surgical techniques improved precision, safety, and outcomes in facial aesthetic procedures?
2. In what ways does 3D imaging and modeling enhance preoperative planning and patient communication in facial aesthetics?

SUMMARY

One can see in summarizing the complexity of congenital and developmental deformities in facial aesthetics that there must be a multi-dimensional approach to the successful treatment and rehabilitation. These deformities, such as cleft lip and palate, critically disrupt not only the facial beauty but also the functional aspect of speaking, breathing, and swallowing. By analyzing various case studies, the importance of interdisciplinary collaboration among the specialists, i.e., surgeons, orthodontists, speech therapists, and psychologists, is emphasized. Thus, successful treatment methods should be holistic to facilitate recovery of function and aesthetics equivalent to those of healthy children, thereby enhancing the quality of life in children so affected. Results from 1,415 children indicate that an integrated approach has a profound impact on outcomes of recovery, which is an indication that orderly methodological endeavor plays a pivotal role in addressing such multifaceted challenges (Eshiev et al., 2025). Also, facial symmetry issues are paramount to the art of maxillofacial surgery, most notably in the surgical correction of congenital deformities. Specifically, facial asymmetry requires careful diagnostic methodologies to formulate effective preoperative strategies. For 87 patients that were analyzed for skeletal malocclusions, of which 28 were asymmetries, advanced diagnostic tools such as 3D CBCT analysis and cephalometry were exceedingly useful. Such procedures not only allow for complete information regarding the deformities but also contribute to the precision of surgical restoration for restoring facial symmetry. Differentiation of authentic versus non-authentic asymmetries is crucial for the optimization of treatment planning. Addition of advanced imaging modalities, thus, has a direct impact on surgical procedures, affirming the need for individualized examination before intervention (Boymuradov et al., 2025). In essence, the landscape of treating congenital and developmental deformities in facial aesthetics is dynamically evolving, and this illustrates the necessity for consistent research and integration of varied disciplines. The profound impact of these deformities on an individual's functional and emotional well-being necessitates a concerted effort at treatment and rehabilitation. The future plans need to incorporate evolving technologies and methods in order to facilitate holistic care. These issues will not merely be alleviated with improved aesthetic and functional outcomes but also provide an environment where affected individuals can fulfill their full potential in social and personal domains. The integrated conclusions of studies from multiple fields corroborate the argument for systemic integration of treatment, yielding a path to enhance not just aesthetic appearance but also general quality of life for individuals afflicted by these complex disorders.

The study of congenital and developmental deformities in facial attractiveness reveals essential implications for physical and psychological well-being. Deformities can result from genetic, environmental, or combined causes and can lead to an array of disorders impacting craniofacial morphology. It is important to recognize the multifaceted character of such deformities, as they have the capacity not only to influence the facial structural qualities but also the functional capabilities such as speech and mastication. Visible deformities can be accompanied by stigma, leading to severe psychological torment, hence the importance of early diagnosis and treatment in children. A holistic strategy involving interdisciplinary collaboration by geneticists, psychologists, and maxillofacial surgeons is needed in an effort to address the intricate requirements of patients with such conditions both aesthetically and psychologically. Other types of maxillofacial injuries, which are often the outcomes of violence or accidents, are significant in explaining how facial deformity develops. There is a high correlation between social behaviors and the prevalence of such injuries, as evident from the pattern of incidence during events like the COVID-19 pandemic, when social distancing led to physically observable declines in such injuries (Canzi et al., 2023). Study of these injuries provides insight into the mechanical factors that shape facial morphology, in addition to the way surgical treatments may be used to restore form and function. Trauma-related deformity patients need advanced surgical techniques, continuous research, and new forms of therapy to achieve the best results and quality of life. Moreover, interdependency between neurological and developmental disorders complicates the facial aesthetic domain even further. The coordination between the stomatognathic system and the nervous system stresses gaining knowledge about congenital anomalies through the neural approach (Wu et al., 2023). Abnormalities in this complex interaction can result in severe craniofacial malformations, which can further exacerbate or cause neurological disorders. It illustrates the two-way effect of the two systems on health as well as form, suggesting that treatment approaches to the former should be made keeping these interdependencies in mind. Finally, the progression of clinical practice and research in the neurological complications of facial deformity will be very crucial in setting comprehensive care pathways for impacted patients, which consequently will yield improved aesthetic outcomes and psychological resilience.

KEY TERMS FROM THIS CHAPTER

- Cleft Lip
- Craniofacial Anomalies
- Micrognathia
- Craniosynostosis
- Midface Hypoplasia
- Multidisciplinary Management
- Cleft Palate
- Hemifacial Microsomia
- Macrognathia
- Syndromic Deformities
- Functional Impairment

CRITICAL THINKING QUESTIONS

1. **The most common congenital facial deformity requiring surgical correction is:**
   a. Craniosynostosis
   b. Cleft lip and palate
   c. Hemifacial microsomia
   d. Microtia
2. **The optimal age for primary cleft lip repair is usually:**
   a. At birth
   b. 2–3 months
   c. 1 year
   d. 5 years
3. **The "rule of 10s" for cleft lip repair includes all EXCEPT:**
   a. 10 weeks old
   b. 10 lbs weight
   c. Hemoglobin of 10 g/dL
   d. Oxygen saturation of 100%
4. **Hemifacial microsomia primarily affects which structure?**
   a. Orbit
   b. Maxilla
   c. Mandible
   d. Zygoma
5. **Goldenhar syndrome is a variant of:**
   a. Treacher Collins syndrome
   b. Hemifacial microsomia
   c. Cleft palate
   d. Pierre Robin sequence

Short Answer Questions

1. What are the common congenital deformities of the face that require cosmetic or reconstructive correction?
2. How does the concept of facial growth influence the timing of surgical intervention in congenital deformities?
3. What is the role of multidisciplinary care in managing congenital facial deformities?
4. What are the key principles for correcting craniofacial asymmetry?
5. How does hemifacial microsomia typically present clinically?
6. What types of grafts or implants are commonly used to correct congenital midface deficiencies?

Answers to Critical Thinking Questions

1. (b) 2. (b) 3. (d) 4. (c) 5. (b)

REFERENCES

1. Anesi, A., Cavani, F., Chiarini, L., Ferretti, et al. (2014). *Preliminary findings of a potenziated piezosurgical device at the rabbit skull.* https://core.ac.uk/download/80171725.pdf (accessed on 14th July 2025).

2. Behnia, H., Dehghani Soltani, A., Tehranchi, A., Zahedipour, et al. (2023). *Hemifacial Microsomia: A Mini-Review and Case Report.* https://core.ac.uk/download/588468504.pdf (accessed on 14th July 2025).

3. Bergqvist, C., Servy, A., Valeyrie-Allanore, L., Ferkal, S., Combemale, P., & Wolkenstein, P. (2020). Neurofibromatosis 1 French national guidelines based on an extensive literature review since 1966. *Orphanet Journal of Rare Diseases, 15.* https://doi.org/10.1186/s13023-020-1310-3 (accessed on 14th July 2025).

4. Bessell, A., Itthagarun, A., Marcusson, A., Thompson, A., Silva Da, A. P., McWilliams, B. J., Lorenzzaoni, D., et al. (2015). *Psychological impact of visible differences in patients with congenital craniofacial anomalies.* https://core.ac.uk/download/323891118.pdf (accessed on 14th July 2025).

5. Boymuradov, S. A., Yusupov, S. S., Rakhmanov, S. A., & Madraimova, K. (2025). The role of accurate diagnosis of the aesthetic parameters of the face in preoperative planning and successful surgical treatment for patients with asymmetric jaw deformities. *Frontline Medical Sciences and Pharmaceutical Journal.* https://www.semanticscholar.org/paper/cae33d20836eceafdb28638fab942820a03bfc73 (accessed on 14th July 2025).

6. Boymuradov, S. A., Yusupov, S. S., Rakhmanov, S. A., & Madraimova, K. (2025). The role of accurate diagnosis of the aesthetic parameters of the face in preoperative planning and successful surgical treatment for patients with asymmetric jaw deformities. *Frontline Medical Sciences and Pharmaceutical Journal*, *5*, 11–17. https://doi.org/10.37547/medical-fmspj-05-05-03 (accessed on 14th July 2025).

7. Boymuradov, S. A., Yusupov, S. S., Rakhmanov, S. A., & Madraimova, K. (2025). The role of accurate diagnosis of the aesthetic parameters of the face in preoperative planning and successful surgical treatment for patients with asymmetric jaw deformities. *International Journal of Medical Sciences and Clinical Research*, *5*, 29–36. https://doi.org/10.37547/ijmscr/volume05issue05-07 (accessed on 14th July 2025).

8. Canzi, G., Novelli, G., Mirabella, S., & Sozzi, D. (2023). The Comprehensive Facial Injury (CFI): A modern communication tool on maxillo-facial traumas characteristics. *Hellenic Archives of Oral and Maxillofacial Surgery, 24.* https://doi.org/10.54936/haoms242p74 (accessed on 14th July 2025).

9. Harnádková, K., Kočandrlová, K., Kožejová Jaklová, L., Dupej, J., & Velemínská, J. (2023). The effect of sex and age on facial shape directional asymmetry in adults: A 3D landmarks-based method study. *PLoS ONE, 18*, e0288702–e0288702. https://doi.org/10.1371/journal.pone.0288702 (accessed on 14th July 2025).

10. Hendrijantini, N., Dahlan, A., Husniya, J., Farha, M., Aziza, H., Rasheed, N., Joseph, S., et al. (2022). *Indonesian Journal of Prosthodontic, 3.* https://doi.org/10.46934/ijp.v3i2 (accessed on 14th July 2025).

11. Hughes, D., & Song, B. (2016). Dental and Nondental Stem Cell Based Regeneration of the Craniofacial Region: A Tissue Based Approach. *Stem cells international, 2016*, 8307195. https://doi.org/10.1155/2016/8307195(accessed on 14th July 2025).

12. Jar, A. A., Alotaibi, A. S., Alqahtani, H. A., Alshaqaqeq, G. A., Alandanoosi, H. I., Alsulami, S. R., Alosaimi, L. A., et al. (2023). Breastfeeding in children with cleft lip and palate and its effect on surgical outcomes. *International Journal of Community Medicine and Public Health, 10*, 4957–4961. https://doi.org/10.18203/2394-6040.ijcmph20233522 (accessed on 14th July 2025).

13. Katanaki, N., Makrygiannakis, M. A., & Kaklamanos, E. G. (2024). The prevalence of congenitally missing permanent teeth in a sample of orthodontic and non-orthodontic Caucasian patients. *Healthcare, 12*, 541–541. https://doi.org/10.3390/healthcare12050541 (accessed on 14th July 2025).

14. Kumari, K., Saleh, I., Taslim, S., Ahmad, S., Hussain, I., Munir, Z., Javed, T., et al. (2023). Unraveling the complexity of Apert syndrome: Genetics, clinical insights, and future frontiers. *Cureus*. https://doi.org/10.7759/cureus.47281 (accessed on 14th July 2025).

15. Lin, Y. (2024). *Objective analysis of anthropometric parameters of the auricle in health and disease*. https://core.ac.uk/download/631131682.pdf (accessed on 14th July 2025).

16. Lone, I. M., Zohud, O., Midlej, K., Awadi, O., Masarwa, S., Krohn, S., Kirschneck, C., et al. (2023). Narrating the genetic landscape of human class I occlusion: A perspective-infused review. *Journal of Personalized Medicine, 13*, 1465–1465. https://doi.org/10.3390/jpm13101465 (accessed on 14th July 2025).

17. McNeil, C. K. (1951). *Congenital malformation and acquired deformity of the oral and facial structure*. https://core.ac.uk/download/286712032.pdf (accessed on 14th July 2025).

18. Palmeiro, M. R. L. (2013). *Quality of life and masticatory ability of selected foods in cleft lip and palate subjects and maxillary denture wearers*. https://core.ac.uk/download/48139729.pdf (accessed on 14th July 2025).

19. Pérez Sánchez, C. F., Sierra Perilla, N., Inostroza, F., & Palomares, M. (2022). LATICFA abstracts. *The Journal of Craniofacial Surgery, 33*, 2276–2320. https://www.semanticscholar.org/paper/f0267c5d8c075cda6abe9b85fd5da8940b95efd7 (accessed on 14th July 2025).

20. Pierpont, M. E., Brueckner, M., Chung, W. K., Garg, V., Lacro, R. V., McGuire, A. L., Mital, S., et al. (2018). Genetic basis for congenital heart disease: Revisited: A scientific statement from the American Heart Association. *Circulation, 138*. https://doi.org/10.1161/cir.0000000000000606 (accessed on 14th July 2025).

21. Pniak, M., Miklis, P., Mawlichanów, M., Ciesielska, A., Sieradzka, A., Szerej, K., Czaplińska-Paszek, Z., et al. (2024). Understanding the educational and social difficulties in children with hemifacial microsomia – A literature review. *Quality in Sport, 36*, 56644–56644. https://doi.org/10.12775/qs.2024.36.56644 (accessed on 14th July 2025).

22. Renkema, R. W. (2020). European guideline craniofacial microsomia. *Journal of Craniofacial Surgery, 31*, 2385–2484. https://doi.org/10.1097/scs.0000000000006691 (accessed on 14th July 2025).

23. Sablada, J. R. P., & Amparado, M. A. P. (2020). *Living changed lives: Experiences of individuals after oral reconstructive surgery*. https://doi.org/10.31219/osf.io/xep6a (accessed on 14th July 2025).

24. Stock, N. M., & Feragen, K. B. (2016). Psychological adjustment to cleft lip and/or palate: A narrative review of the literature. *Psychology and Health*, *31*, 777–813. https://doi.org/10.1080/08870446.2016.1143944 (accessed on 14th July 2025).

25. Tahmasebi, E., Mohammadi, M., Alam, M., Abbasi, K., Gharibian Bajestani, S., Khanmohammad, R., Haseli, M., et al. (2023). The current regenerative medicine approaches of craniofacial diseases: A narrative review. *Frontiers in Cell and Developmental Biology*, *11*. https://doi.org/10.3389/fcell.2023.1112378 (accessed on 14th July 2025).

26. Ter Horst, R., van Weert, H., Loonen, T., Bergé, S., Vinayahalingam, S., Baan, F., Maal, T., et al. (2021). Three-dimensional virtual planning in mandibular advancement surgery: Soft tissue prediction based on deep learning. *Journal of Cranio-Maxillofacial Surgery*, *49*, 775–782. https://doi.org/10.1016/j.jcms.2021.04.001 (accessed on 14th July 2025).

27. Ugli, Y. B. D. (2024). Advancements in facial jaw surgery: Exploring surgical interventions and management of facial jaw diseases. *International Journal of Medical Sciences and Clinical Research*, *4*, 74–81. https://doi.org/10.37547/ijmscr/volume04issue02-11 (accessed on 14th July 2025).

28. Wojtyńska, E., Bączkowski, B., Cierech, M., & Mierzwińska-Nastalska, E. (2024). Assessment of children and "young" adult patients' quality of life after prosthetic treatment of disorders of the craniofacial region—A retrospective study. *Journal of Clinical Medicine*, *13*, 339–339. https://doi.org/10.3390/jcm13020339 (accessed on 14th July 2025).

29. Wu, Y., Lan, Y., Mao, J., Shen, J., Kang, T., & Xie, Z. (2023). The interaction between the nervous system and the stomatognathic system: From development to diseases. *International Journal of Oral Science*, *15*. https://doi.org/10.1038/s41368-023-00241-4 (accessed on 14th July 2025).

30. Zammit, D., Ettinger, R. E., Sanati-Mehrizy, P., & Susarla, S. M. (2023). Current trends in orthognathic surgery. *Medicina*, *59*, 2100–2100. https://doi.org/10.3390/medicina59122100 (accessed on 14th July 2025).

31. Zhao, Z., Bao, J., Shen, G., Cai, M., & Yu, H. (2023). Integrating virtual surgical planning and 3D-printed tools with iliac bone grafts for orbital and zygomatic reconstruction in hemifacial microsomia patients. *Journal of Clinical Medicine*, *12*, 7538–7538. https://doi.org/10.3390/jcm12247538 (accessed on 14th July 2025).

32. Zumba. C. N. E., Macas Caamaño, L. J., Cueva Flores, R. A., Sarmiento Ávila, S. A., Franco, P. F., Ayala, A., Lombeida Arias, J. J., et al. (2023). Cleft lip and palate, scoping review. *EPRA International Journal of Multidisciplinary Research (IJMR)*. https://doi.org/10.36713/epra14264 (accessed on 14th July 2025).

33. Eshiev, M., Khalmurzaev, D., Eshiev, N., Azimbaev, N., Taalaibekov, N., & Myrzasheva, N. (2025). A comprehensive approach to the treatment of patients with congenital defects and deformities of the maxillofacial area. *Bulletin of Science and Practice*. https://www.semanticscholar.org/paper/a7289489049c5bc9fb2f32a8327f2c2462834b7e (accessed on 14th July 2025).

ONCOLOGIC AND POST-TUMOR RECONSTRUCTION IN FACIAL COSMETIC

14

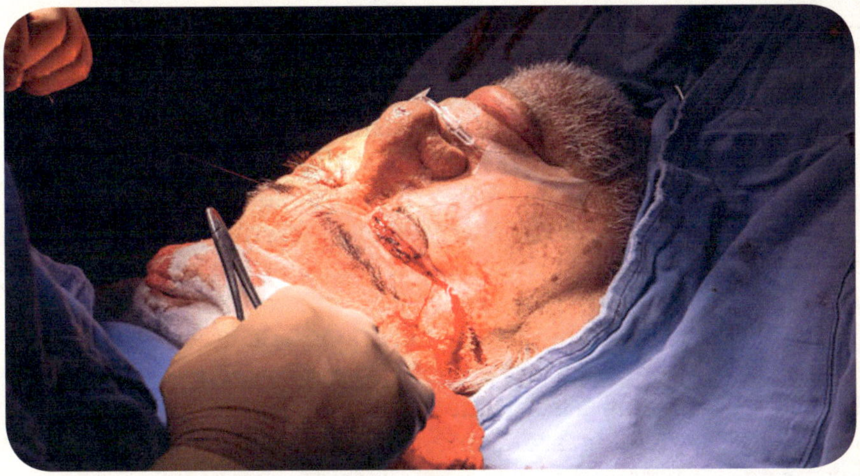

Introduction

The intricate interplay between oncologic surgery and subsequent cosmetic reconstruction has been a matter of considerable interest in the medical literature. In association with the evolution of facial cosmetic surgery, it increasingly recognizes the value of not only removing malignant tumors but also rehabilitating form and function post-surgery. Oncologic treatments have a great impact in changing facial structure and function, and therefore there has to be a holistic approach that transcends the primary operation. Therefore, measures of reconstruction must be pursued to reverse the physical and psychological impacts of such treatments. This dual focus on excision of cancer and cosmetic reconstruction underscores the importance of innovative surgical techniques that can optimize patient quality of life in the setting of oncologic surgery. To this end, there should be a clear understanding of the spectrum of reconstructive modalities. One of the watershed moments in post-tumor and oncologic reconstruction is the management of facial defects due to tumor excision, especially when defects

LEARNING OBJECTIVES

After studying this chapter, you will be able to:

1. Understand oncologic surgery;
2. Discuss reconstruction's role in facial cosmetic surgery;
3. Identify preoperative considerations;
4. Describe surgical techniques in reconstruction;
5. Identify postoperative care and recovery;
6. Understand ethical considerations in oncologic and reconstructive surgery.

compromise critical zones affecting function as much as aesthetics. The reconstructive surgeon must very carefully weigh the specific nuances of the tissue loss, the extent of resection, the facial site, and patient-specific anatomical subtleties. This comprehensive analysis of interest, since inadequate reconstruction can lead to psychosocial sequelae and compromised function. Techniques such as the use of pedicled perforator flaps have come under the spotlight based on their capacity to restore both volume and cutaneous integrity. Most importantly, an algorithm for partial breast reconstruction with these flaps demonstrated successful outcomes, serving as a model that can be used in facial reconstruction following tumor excision (Cillino et al., 2010). In addition, functioning impairment treatment, such as paralysis of the face resulting from oncologic therapy, is still within the realm of post-tumor cosmetic surgery. Facial nerve paralysis can significantly impair a patient's quality of life by interfering with their emotional expression, as well as with simple activities such as eating and speaking. Restorations that will restore facial movement need to incorporate a thorough assessment of nerve integrity and muscular function. Various types of surgeries, including nerve grafts and dynamic muscle transfers, can be employed to yield good results (Anderson et al., 2012). But the complexity of facial anatomy and nerve courses is a huge hindrance to achieving maximum functional recovery. Thus, it is necessary that there should be more research and surgical development in oncologic and post-tumor reconstruction to help patients by improving outcomes and enhancing their quality of life.

Definition of Oncologic Surgery

Oncologic surgery is a significant branch of surgical oncology that focuses on the resection of tumor, especially malignant tumors, which are harmful to health. The most critical aim of oncologic surgery is to ensure the removal of the cancer completely without sacrificing the surrounding healthy tissue to the extent possible. Not only is maintaining this delicate balance crucial for the success of the treatment, but it is done to preserve the functional integrity of the afflicted body part. The character of such an operation requires an operative multidisciplinary team in which radiologists, oncologists, and surgeons all work together to establish a correct surgical plan for each individual patient's condition. This teamwork is essential in determining the optimal timing and the extent of the surgical procedure, ultimately guiding prognosis, enabling postoperative recovery, and enhancing the overall results. Following tumor excision by surgery, post-tumor reconstruction is also a critical factor in the restoration of the shape and function of the involved anatomical structures. In facial aesthetic surgery, this is regarding the correction of oncologic surgical defects and attempting to permit the patient to regain their preoperative appearance or to obtain an improved aesthetic result. Free tissue transfer, local flaps, and fat grafting are a few of the refined techniques that are utilized in order to overcome these reconstructive challenges. Use of pedicled perforator flaps, such as in the reconstruction of breasts, also indicates advancement in the surgical technique of regaining volume and form after oncologic surgery (Cillino et al., 2010). These methods not only aim at eliminating the physical deformities in surgery but also help to reduce the psychological impact of cancer therapy-induced disfigurement. Further, the inclusion of new techniques such as fat grafting also introduces more potential for successful reconstruction in oncologic surgery. By means of transferring autologous adipose tissue to sites of deficiency, the surgeons can improve the contour deformities with the additional benefit of using the patient's tissue, thereby eradicating the foreign body complications (Vyas et al., 2016). This twofold benefit outlines the manner in which contemporary oncologic and reconstructive therapies are evolving with regard to both cosmetic and functional needs of patients. However, use of adipose-derived stem cells (ASCs) within fat grafting also raises oncological concerns regarding cancer microenvironments and possible tumorigenesis, and will continue to require more investigation to offer protection for patients and efficacy for reconstructive outcomes. Thus, the oncologic surgery definition goes beyond simple cancer removal, embracing restoration and rehabilitation as well, ultimately targeting the enhancement of the quality of life for post-treatment patients (Figure 14.1).

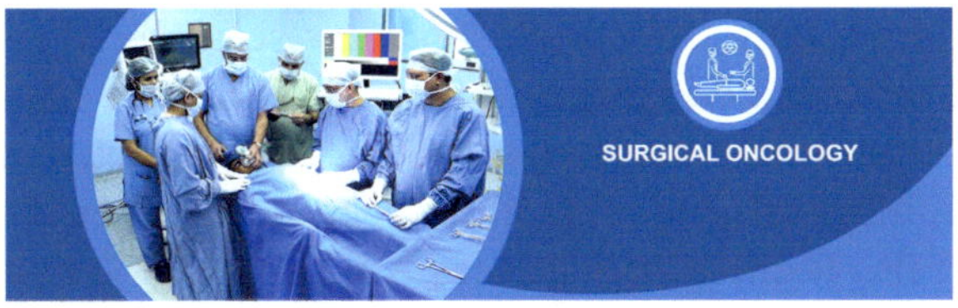

Figure 14.1. Oncologic surgery.

Source: https://external-content.duckduckgo.com/iu/?u=https%3A%2F%2Fwww.venkateshwarhospitals.com%2Fblog%2Fwp-content%2Fuploads%2F2019%2F04%2Fsurgical-oncology.jpg&f=1&nofb=1&ipt=0c7f13233510321641ccb59ff65dc731528d600152aa40d37b354d80017caa4e.

Role of Facial Cosmetic Surgery

Facıal cosmetic surgery plays a -affected facial structures. Post-surgical procedures, for example, maxillectomy, may lead to severe issues in the form of altered facial beauty and functional impairment in patients. Disfigurement has a psychological impact, leading to decreased self-esteem and withdrawal from society. To overcome such problems, effective post-tumor reconstruction is necessary, which facilitates not only physical construction but also psychological healing. Evidence indicates that through intensive cooperation among reconstructive surgeons and oncologists, results are likely to significantly improve both the cosmetic results and functional capacities of patients. Such collaboration fosters personalized prosthetic treatments to restore normalcy to speech, mastication, and social interaction, thus supporting the role of facial cosmetic surgery as an integrated component of worldwide cancer care (Fattah et al., 2012). Use of modern cosmetic surgical techniques also facilitates the other general aim of enhancing the life quality of cancer survivors. Reconstruction of tumors, particularly on the face, necessitates sophisticated techniques that provide natural appearances and appropriate restoration of function. Certain procedures by pedicled perforator flaps, for instance, have been used to recreate breast forms but have striking contrasts when translated to facial reconstruction (Cillino et al., 2010). Like breast tissue, facial structures need to be handled with great care so that both volume and shape are harmonized with surrounding tissue. With the use of these techniques, compromised structural form can be restored, enabling patients to re-enter their social milieu and feel normal. The psychological effects of successful restorative appearance cannot be underestimated, as patients report heightened confidence and improved mental well-being following such reconstructive therapy. Moreover, facial cosmetic surgery has more than just cosmetic consequences, penetrating into social and working life. In the majority of cases, appearance-based social biases may have negative effects on career opportunities as well as social relationships. Because cosmetic surgery enables individuals to represent themselves in a more conventionally approved manner, it can prevent discrimination or prejudice against individuals who are different physically. Recognition of this intersection between aesthetics and social dynamics highlights facial cosmetic surgery as a priority for individuals who are recovering from oncologic disease. Indeed, it provides them with the ability to more effectively manage social expectations, ultimately leading to reintegration and improved life satisfaction. Therefore, the role of facial cosmetic surgery is not one-dimensional but instead multi-dimensional and involves restoration of beauty, enhancement of function, and reintegration into society for oncologic and post-tumor reconstruction (Fattah et al., 2012) (Figure 14.2).

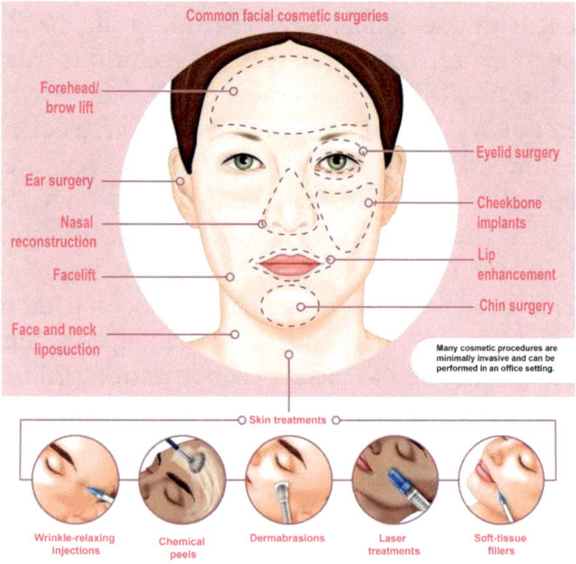

Figure 14.2. Facial cosmetic surgery.

Source: https://ekbybzt92zq.exactdn.com/wp-content/uploads/2021/12/facial_cosmetic surgery-662x1024-1.jpg?strip=all&lossy=1&ssl=1.

Overview of the Relationship Between Oncology and Reconstruction

That the evolving nature of facial cosmetic surgery, particularly tumor post-reconstruction, is highlighted by the intricate relationship between reconstruction and oncology is noteworthy. The oncologic procedures have a propensity to result in huge loss of tissue, particularly in cases of head and neck cancers, and thus necessitate innovative reconstructive techniques to enable both function and aesthetics. These procedures not only make the patients look more beautiful but also have a significant role to play in their psychological rehabilitation. Through the integration of reconstructive techniques with oncologic treatment, surgeons are able to offer a more complete approach to patients, emphasizing the necessity for multidisciplinary patterns of care for cancer survivors. The collaboration between these fields ensures that the functional and psychological outcomes of tumor resection are adequately accounted for, thereby improving the overall quality of life for treated individuals. Among the new areas of interest in oncologic and reconstructive surgery is the use of advanced technologies, such as ultrasonic osteotomes and lipotransfer techniques. Comparison of different instruments, including Piezosurgery®, reveals potential advantages in reducing tissue trauma during procedures. For example, micromorphology and roughness values comparisons between osteotomized bone surfaces indicate that ultrasound-assisted procedures can assist in maintaining significant structures intact while facilitating successful healing. These innovations not only facilitate better surgical outcomes but also improve understanding of bone regeneration and soft tissue integration in reconstructive surgery. The more researchers explore these new methods, the more their oncologic considerations deepen, enriching the armamentarium of surgery after tumor reconstruction. As with lipotransfer, concerns arise regarding the effects of interactions between lipoaspirates and tumor beds. While lipofilling has improved certain aspects of plastic surgery, foremost breast reconstruction, its cancer recurrence implications remain obscure. Research has shown that while the adipose-derived regenerative tissues have been found to promote healing and tissue repair, they may interact with latent cancer cells, raising an issue about the long-term safety of the procedure. Thus, extensive clinical studies are urgently required to clarify such interactions and secure the safety of lipotransfer in oncologic patients. It is only by an exhaustive amount of research that the oncology-reconstruction interface can be better described, with surgery advancements complementing the principles of cancer treatment and maximizing patient safety and efficacy of treatment results (Goldhirsch et al., 2011; Anesi et al., 2014).

14.1. Understanding Oncologic Surgery

Learning Outcome

1. Explain the Types of Cancers Affecting the Facial Region
2. Focus on Surgical Techniques Used in Oncologic Procedures
3. Discuss Goals of Oncologic Surgery in Facial Aesthetics

Oncologic surgery forms a critical intersection between reconstructive surgery and cancer treatment. The final intent of oncologic surgery is to excise tumors with minimal sacrifice of surrounding normal tissue, a norm especially important in facial structure surgery. The intricacy of oncologic surgery is amplified by the intricate anatomy of the face, where small error can result in aesthetic and functional compromise of significant magnitude. Surgeons also have to plan for the excision of the tumor with careful planning for the subsequent reconstructive procedure to avoid disfigurement. With advancing technology and technique, procedures such as ultrasonic osteotomes are now available, with the promise to minimize damage to the surrounding tissues while effectively facilitating the removal of cancerous cells (Anesi et al., 2014). The goal is to achieve maximum healing and functional preservation, which serves as the foundation for further aesthetic restoration with cosmetic techniques. In facial cosmetic surgery after oncologic surgery, the two pillars of reconstructive surgery are involved in the restoration of appearance and function. With oncologic lesion extirpation, most patients have physical difficulties and profound psychological sequelae resulting from changes in appearance. This necessitates a tailored method of reconstruction, such as through the application of advanced techniques, such as pedicled perforator flaps, which have been proven to effectively improve volume and revise skin envelope deformities after tumor excision. It has been proven that the flaps are capable of reconstructing breast volume and shape with minimal noticeability at the donor site (Cillino et al., 2010). This philosophy is then carried over to facial regions, where symmetry and the maintenance of natural contours take precedence; aesthetic issues are therefore harmoniously incorporated into the reconstructive design. Lastly, the importance of multidisciplinary team effort in cancer and reconstructive surgery cannot be stressed enough. Oncologists, surgeons, and cosmetic professionals must all work together to devise integrated treatment regimens involving the removal of the cancer as well as reconstruction afterward. This common model facilitates better-informed decision-making regarding when and how to integrate cosmetic procedures into oncologic surgery and therefore, enhance patient outcomes.

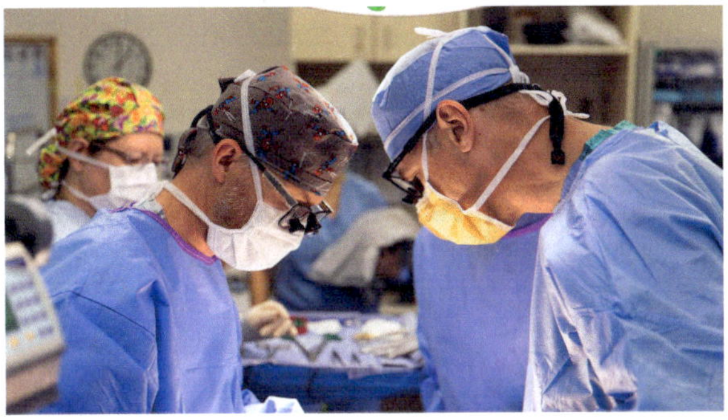

Figure 14.3. Oncologic surgery represents a critical intersection between cancer management and reconstructive techniques.

Source: https://www.childrenscolorado.org/globalassets/departments/surgical-oncology/2023-04-12-surgical-oncology_cost_roach_61_cropped.jpg?v=49ba92&width=1440&height=810&rxy=0.5,0.49.

Patient education and psychological counseling are also an integral part of care, as they address the emotional aftermath of cancer therapy. With the integration of a holistic model addressing both the technical and emotional aspects of surgery, the field of oncologic and post-tumor reconstruction itself expands, with the added emphasis on not only the extirpation of disease but also the reconstruction of patients' dignity and quality of life through successful cosmetic reconstruction (Figure 14.3).

14.1.1. Types of Cancers Affecting the Facial Region

Facial cancers are a diverse group of malignancies that mostly affect the skin, mucous membranes, and facial adnexal structures. Two of the most frequent types are basal cell carcinoma (BCC) and squamous cell carcinoma (SCC), often the consequence of prolonged exposure to ultraviolet (UV) radiation. BCC, while typically slow-growing and rarely metastasizing, can lead to extensive local tissue destruction if left untreated. On the other hand, SCC is at a higher risk of metastasis, particularly if it is on the lip or ear. In addition, melanoma, the more malignant skin cancer, develops from melanocytes in the epidermis and is notorious for the manner in which it rapidly spreads through the body. Awareness of these cancers is important in developing an effective oncologic treatment plan and later reconstructive plan in cosmetic facial surgery. Aside from skin cancers, oral cavity and salivary gland cancers also have a significant effect on the facial region. Oral squamous cell carcinoma (OSCC) arises from the mucosal lining of the oral cavity and is due to many risk factors, some of which include tobacco use and human papillomavirus (HPV) infection. OSCC commonly exhibits an aggressive nature and therefore most of the time needs wide resection surgically, which significantly damages the aesthetic as well as functional functions of the face. Salivary gland tumors, while uncommon, are also clinically formidable since their behavior is unpredictable and their histological subtypes may be extremely variable. These tumors may prove very difficult to operate on from a standpoint of intricate surgical techniques, and so the introduction of sophisticated postoperative reconstruction procedures must be utilized to optimize patient quality of life. Conquering these difficulties is an important step towards improving clinical outcomes in facial cosmetic surgery. Further, the intersection of oncologic treatment and post-tumor reconstruction testifies to the effectiveness of cooperative surgical approaches. Facially cancer therapy often requires an interdisciplinary group of oncologists, maxillofacial surgeons, and prosthodontists. More specifically, pre-prosthetic surgical conditioning in primary resections, i.e., maxillectomy, plays a pivotal role in the subsequent prosthetic rehabilitation process. Effective rehabilitative outcomes are much dependent on strategic planning and execution of reconstructive surgeries, rebuilding facial contours and function. With evidence provided by Fattah et al. (2012), incorporation of pre-prosthetic surgery with oncologic therapy optimizes patient rehabilitation, not only allowing for aesthetic recovery but also improving social interactions and quality of life. Therefore, optimal care encompassing both oncologic and reconstructive components is essential in addressing the implications of facial cancers (Figure 14.4).

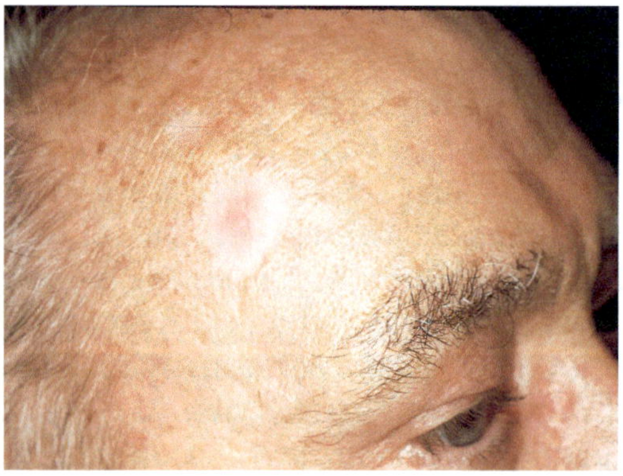

Figure 14.4. Cancers affecting the facial region.

Source: https://www.verywellhealth.com/thmb/z2UTB9_KBcE47gPA3R8Oe2PXzc0=/998x759/filters:no_upscale():max_bytes(150000):strip_icc()/basal-cell-carcinoma-4-scar-5304337d6b3e4b3b8c601fde7a0880f8.jpg.

14.1.2. Surgical Techniques Used in Oncologic Procedures

The trend in surgical oncologic procedures mainly utilizes advancements with the focus of efficiently removing the tumors while preserving functionality and aesthetics within the involved region. Techniques such as Mohs micrographic surgery are focal, especially in skin cancer treatment, and ensure complete removal of the tumor without causing excessive damage to the surrounding tumor tissue. This technique allows for real-time histological evaluation, eliminating the risk of recurrence to a large degree and allowing for more cosmetically pleasing results. Mohs surgery's precision specifically demands comprehensive knowledge of facial anatomy and demands reconstruction proficiency following excision. These principles further align with oncologic and post-tumoral reconstruction practices in stressing the preservation of the facial tissues' fine details as a way of achieving oncologic clearance. Another key area of concern for surgical techniques in oncologic treatments is the management of complications, in this case, in relation to facial nerve integrity. Surgical intervention for head and neck cancer can inadvertently cause facial paralysis of the nerves, providing unique challenges in post-operative rehabilitation and restoration of function. Such complications need to be addressed with individualized interventions, ranging from neurotization to facial reanimation procedures, to restore function as well as aesthetics. The complex anatomy of the facial nerve makes reconstruction difficult, but new and innovative methods keep appearing, allowing improved quality of life for patients post-treatment. As stated, extensive study and patient-specific treatment are most significant in developing effective management regimens in patients with nerve deficits following tumor removal (Anderson et al., 2012). Reconstructive interventions following oncologic surgeries are significant in modifying patient outcomes and enhancing psychological well-being. Pedicled perforator flaps are one of the effective methods employed in breast cancer surgery that enable the maintenance of breast volume following quadrantectomy. Thoraco-dorsal and intercostal perforator-based flaps were found to be effective in restoring the natural breast contour with fewer complications at the donor site. These not only reconstruct the physical contours of the breast, but also correct the emotional impact cancer patients must endure. As shown, all flap procedures in a study had total survival, giving proper restoration in size, shape, and volume without requiring extra corrective surgery of the opposite breast (Cillino et al., 2010). This shows the profound intersection between patient care and surgical progress in oncologic treatment (Figure 14.5).

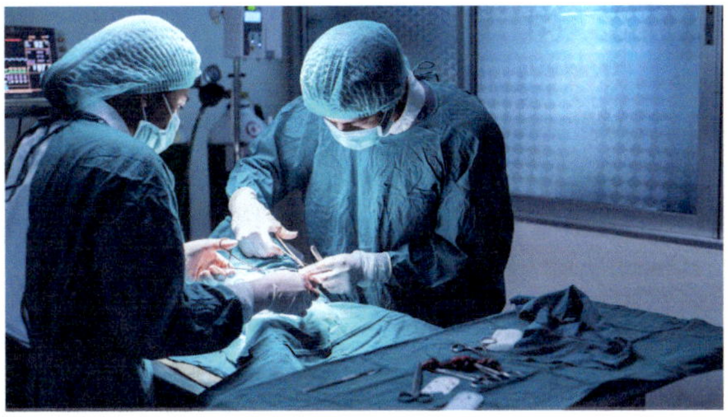

Figure 14.5. Surgical techniques used in oncologic procedures.

Source: https://www.krupamayihospitals.in/wp-content/uploads/2023/06/Onco-Surgery.jpg.

14.1.3. Goals of Oncologic Surgery in Facial Aesthetics

In oncologic surgery, particularly in facial beauty, one of the most critical aims is the complete eradication of malignant tumors without compromising the facial structure. Surgeons' target is not only successfully removing the malignant tissues but also preserving the functional and aesthetic components of the face. This dual focus is important as the face is at the core of individual identity and social interaction.

Patients often suggest that alterations in facial attractiveness carry considerable psychological implications, affecting self-esteem and eliciting emotional distress. Thus, a successful integration of oncologic and aesthetic concerns is paramount to achieving not only physical but also psychological well-being in patients who are treated for facial oncologic reconstruction. Aside from the removal of the tumor, another critical goal of oncologic surgery with facial esthetic consideration is the meticulous reconstruction of the surgical defect. Reconstruction plays a crucial role in restoring the functional capacity of the deficient area, such as speech, swallowing, and breathing. Techniques like locoregional flaps are frequently used in order to do so, as these allow surgeons to work with surrounding tissues in order to correct defects without excessive extraneous scarring and with optimal aesthetic results. Research suggests that certain types of flaps, such as infrahyoid and nasolabial types, provide good results for both medium-sized and smaller defects, which supports the concept that well-planned reconstruction has the power to greatly improve postoperative appearances (Accorona et al., 2024). By wise selection and application of reconstructive techniques, surgeons attempt to usher patients toward a symphonic equilibrium of healing and beauty. Furthermore, technological advancements and surgical techniques have had a revolutionary influence on oncologic surgery philosophy for facial aesthetics. The use of new practices such as preoperative planning of surgeries with Mixed Reality (MR) and navigation has been shown to enhance the success of procedures. MR technology provides improved visualization of anatomy, which may help surgeons to deliver more precise results, and also enhance patient communication on the outcome of their procedures (Kalaskar et al., 2016). Besides making surgery more accurate, these technological advances can also help in enhancing the aesthetic outcome. Thus, the goals of oncologic surgery increasingly are a combined policy that supports both cancer removal and, where feasible, restoration of facial form, with the ultimate aim to improve patients' quality of life after tumor excisions (Figure 14.6).

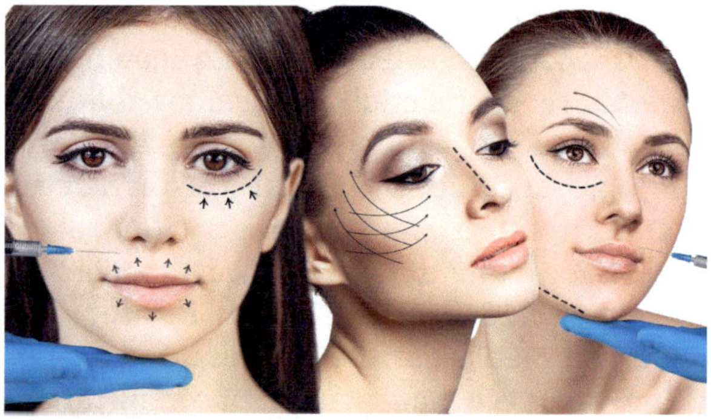

Figure 14.6. Goals of oncologic surgery in facial aesthetics.

Source: https://external-content.duckduckgo.com/iu/?u=https%3A%2F%2Fwww.boutiquedental23.com%2Fwp-content%2Fuploads%2F2022%2F10%2Fwhat-is-facial-aesthetics-1.jpg&f=1&nofb=1&ipt=3d30e27f00610de9a5f4e621d21adf8ddc11ce383a58a381fb2b20b0986969a3.

Test Your Knowledge

1. What types of cancers commonly affect the facial region, and how do their locations influence treatment planning?
2. What surgical techniques are used in oncologic procedures to remove tumors while preserving function and appearance?

14.2. The Role of Reconstruction in Facial Cosmetic Surgery

Learning Outcome

1. Definition and Purpose of Reconstructive Surgery
2. Discuss the Techniques Used in Facial Reconstruction
3. Explain Psychological Impact of Facial Reconstruction on Patients

The intricate relationship between reconstruction and facial cosmetic surgery is of utmost significance for the promotion of restoration of both functional and aesthetic outcomes in patients who have undergone oncologic surgery. In the facial reconstruction following tumor resection, the primary objective is the establishment of normal anatomy with the encouragement of preservation or enhancement of essential functions such as speech and swallowing. This multi-disciplinary procedure often includes cooperative activity between surgeons, prosthodontists, and other specialists to create individualized solutions tailored to unique needs. For instance, in maxillary defect reconstruction following maxillectomy, careful pre-prosthetic surgery planning plays a crucial role in the success of prosthetic rehabilitation. As pointed out by the study of Fattah et al. (2012), such preps would be able to enhance facial profile and overall aesthetic results, offering a foundation for successful rehabilitation and increased quality of life among patients suffering from cancer. Moreover, advancements in surgical tools and techniques likewise confirm the importance of innovation in facial reconstruction. Introduction of new technology, such as ultrasonic osteotomes, has revolutionized the field of bone manipulation for reconstructive surgery. Comparative studies on traditional rotating instruments and ultrasound-based systems illustrate natural differences in micromorphology and surface roughness of osteotomized bones and thus impact healing and functional restoration. Such technologies not only preserve soft tissue covering but also enhance osseointegration and health of the tissue and consequently deliver dramatically better outcomes for surgery. As highlighted in the work by Anesi et al. (2014), the application of such advanced devices in cranio-facial surgery is essential in achieving optimal results, particularly for oncology patients who require precise reconstruction after tumor excision. The psychological impact of facial cosmetic reconstruction after cancer treatment cannot be overstated. Facial disfigurements and alterations secondary to oncologic surgeries have a tendency to create severe emotional distress and social isolation among patients. By successfully restoring facial beauty through meticulous reconstruction, surgeons are able to mitigate these psychological challenges, facilitating enhanced social reintegration and self-concept. Furthermore, involving patients in the decision-making process for their reconstructive options provides a sense of control, facilitating wholesome mental health outcomes. Thus, the role of reconstruction in facial cosmetic surgery is more than corporeal, and it is an integral part of comprehensive cancer care intended to enhance quality of life as well as psychosocial well-being for survivors as they step into the bewildering realm of life after treatment (Figure 14.7).

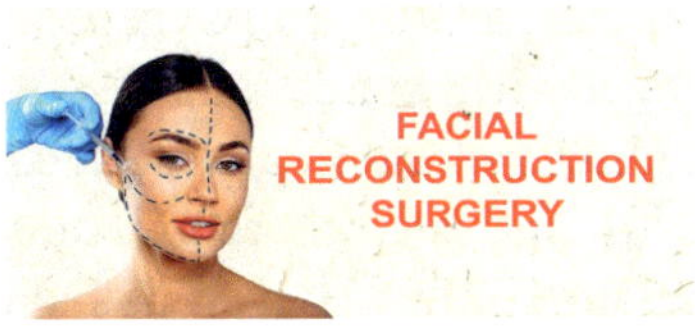

Figure 14.7. Role of reconstruction in facial cosmetic surgery.

Source: https://external-content.duckduckgo.com/iu/?u=https%3A%2F%2Famandeephospital.org%2Fwp-content%2Fuploads%2F2023%2F06%2FFacial-Reconstruction-Surgery.webp&f=1&nofb=1&ipt=83c386ff65aa8d01d146479063b17799f93538f2fa757da65fc6d0229d1e24f4.

14.2.1. Definition and Purpose of Reconstructive Surgery

Reconstructive surgery is a fundamental component of clinical treatment that entails the reconstruction of form and function following trauma, disease, or surgery. The term "reconstructive surgery" extends beyond the exclusive esthetic correction and comprises the rehabilitation of not only physical integrity but also psychological health of those patients who have experienced significant loss, particularly following oncological surgery. It frequently entails the rebuilding of complicated areas of anatomy in which malignancies have required massive excisions, for example, facial tumors. Reconstructive surgery, beyond cosmetic repair, is meant to allow for necessary physiological processes such as mastication, communication, and respiration, which can be impaired as a result of tumor resections or cancer therapy deformities. In particular, in the oncologic and post-tumoral reconstructive fields, the reconstructive surgery methodology is focused on enhancing the survivor's level of quality of life. The procedures may involve the use of a large variety of state-of-the-art methodologies, including flap techniques, which utilize the patient's own tissue to restore volume, shape, and function. The applicability of such procedures is best illustrated through breast reconstruction following lumpectomy, whereby incorporation of pedicled perforator flaps restores breast loveliness following cancerous tissue excision. The effectiveness of such procedures has been demonstrated in research to produce positive outcomes in functional as well as psychological reconstruction, substantiating the importance of reconstructive surgery in cancer management in its entirety (Cillino et al., 2010). Furthermore, improvements in surgical techniques, such as the development of ultrasonic osteotomes, illustrate the ongoing evolution of reconstructive surgery. These innovations have portrayed a noticeable improvement in the precision and outcomes of surgical interventions, minimizing destruction of adjacent tissues and refining recovery times. Understanding micromorphology and surface roughness of osteotomized bone surfaces has been beneficial, particularly in craniofacial reconstruction, where delicate facial bones require close attention. As reconstructive surgery advances and utilizes newer technologies, its purpose remains constant in rehabilitating function and form for the victims of cancer as well as the psychological impact of disfigurement and trauma (Anesi et al., 2014) (Figure 14.8).

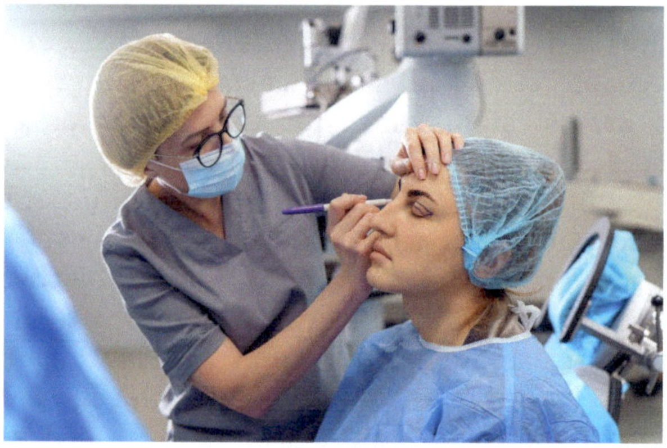

Figure 14.8. Purpose of reconstructive surgery.

Source: https://external-content.duckduckgo.com/iu/?u=https%3A%2F%2Fcachevalleyent.com%2Fstorage%2F2023%2F10%2FReconstructive-Surgery-by-Cache-Valley-ENT-in-Logan-UT-scaled.jpeg&f=1&nofb=1&ipt=2799cefeb77b86f258a57cf0c898ab54ff23c34f1626cfd74cfbd729e77d35d8.

14.2.2. Techniques Used in Facial Reconstruction

There are various surgical techniques used to attain facial function and aesthetics in oncologic and post-tumor reconstruction. Soft tissue reconstruction is generally performed through the usage of local flaps, such as the rotation or advancement flaps, which transfer tissue within the vicinity for the aim of covering defects with minimal disfigurement. Free tissue transfer techniques involving microvascular anastomosis have also become increasingly popular, with the possibility of transferring tissue from more distant sites. This technique not only facilitates the reconstruction of large defects but also facilitates the restoration of function, which is paramount to the overall quality of life in the patient. The nature of the technique varies significantly based on the size and location of the defect, the general well-being of the patient, and their desired aesthetic result; thus customized treatment planning is essential in achieving the most desirable outcome. Another significant feature of facial reconstruction is the management of facial paralysis of the facial nerve, a not uncommon complication of head and neck cancer surgery. The procedures employed to address this condition need to be tailored for each patient based on individual anatomy and functional requirements. For instance, reinnervation methods, where remaining segments of nerves are utilized to stimulate facial musculature, are able to offer more natural motion compared with static reconstructive methods. However, the intricacy of facial innervation often defies complete restoration, and surgeons find it necessary to combine neurotization with other surgeries, such as muscle transfers, to provide better function and cosmetic result. The subtle dance of anatomy and surgical potential demands close understanding of the pathway of the facial nerves and the patient's functional deficit (Anderson et al., 2012). Lastly, the incorporation of advanced technologies has transformed facial reconstruction methods in the recent past. Computational models and 3D printing have become useful resources when it comes to planning and performing intricate reconstructive procedures. Surgeons are able to design accurate patient-specific models for simulating the surgical procedure before it, enabling greater accuracy throughout the actual procedure. Moreover, evolution in biomaterials used for tissue engineering and grafting has the potential for enormous opportunities for designing individually tailored solutions for unique defects. This convergence of technology and surgery not only optimizes healing but also optimizes aesthetic and functional outcomes for patients undergoing tumor resection (de Bree et al., 2017). As science continues to evolve, future research will likely provide increasingly advanced methods for addressing facial reconstruction challenges (Figure 14.9).

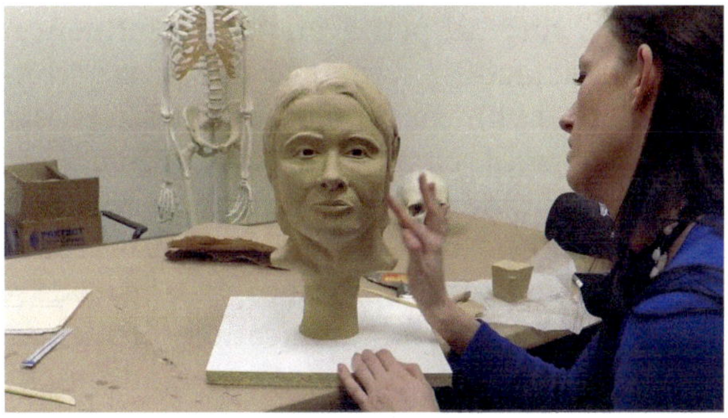

Figure 14.9. Techniques used in facial reconstruction.

Source: https://i.ytimg.com/vi/tQ95nVPJvEE/maxresdefault.jpg.

14.2.3. Psychological Impact of Facial Reconstruction on Patients

The psychological effect of facial reconstruction on oncologic patients is intense and complex. Patients with facial disfigurement from tumors typically experience deep emotional distress, which impacts their self-esteem and social conduct. Appearance of the face automatically equates with individual identity and social acceptance, and reconstructive surgery can be a catalyst for recovery of appearance and psychological well-being. Anticipation of surgical outcome, especially restoration of facial appearance, can influence patients' psychological state because the majority anticipate that improved appearances will be followed by reintegration with society and enhanced quality of life. Noted, facial dynamics restoration is not merely cosmetic rehabilitation but was deeply entangled with mental health, wherein successful reconstruction could restore a sense of normalcy and confidence among facial trauma victims. And the success of reconstructive surgeries also largely lies in the surgical techniques themselves, which can vary in their effectiveness depending on circumstances. The communication among the patient, oncologist, and surgeon is most important in achieving maximum outcome through potential pre-prosthetic surgical preparation that influences global satisfaction with the reconstruction. According to clinical reports, when integrated treatment with comprehensive pre-surgical planning is provided to the patient, the resultant improvement in function and form can greatly reduce anxiety and optimize post-procedure satisfaction. Proper communication throughout the process enables patients to understand their options, get their concerns addressed, and participate actively in their own healing. Not only does this interaction improve surgical results, but also has long-term impacts on patients' psychological health, affirming again the importance of shared medical care in the process of recovery. Moreover, following reconstruction, ongoing care by healthcare providers is essential in developing psychological resilience in patients. The majority of individuals face an intricate process of adjustment as they strive to deal with their new identity after undergoing surgery, grappling with both physical changes and the emotional consequences that result from them. The process of coping with societal attitudes and self-concept issues can lead them to become anxious or depressed, particularly where outcomes are less expected. Therefore, psychological counseling following surgery becomes essential in solving such issues, assisting patients in coping and enhancing their self-concept. Positive outcomes in facial reconstruction ultimately result in increased social interaction and readaptation, as patients slowly begin viewing their reconstructed faces as symbols of resilience rather than reminders of their past, validating the role of psychological support after facial cosmetic surgery (Anderson et al., 2012; Fattah et al., 2012) (Figure 14.10).

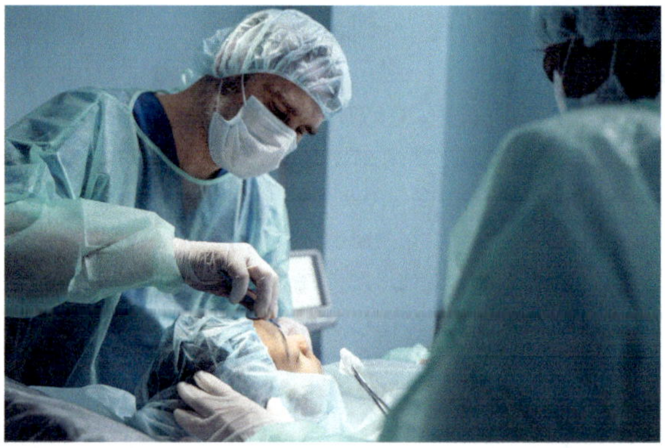

Figure 14.10. Psychological impact of facial reconstruction on patients.

Source: https://nevadaoms.com/wp-content/uploads/2024/04/2149352203.jpg.

Test Your Knowledge

1. What is the primary purpose of reconstructive surgery in restoring both function and aesthetics after facial trauma, disease, or congenital deformities?
2. What key techniques are commonly used in facial reconstruction, and how do they help achieve natural and functional outcomes?

14.3. Preoperative Considerations

Learning Outcome

1. Explain the Patient Assessment and Evaluation
2. Discuss the Importance of Multidisciplinary Teams
3. Focus on Planning for Aesthetic Outcomes

Preoperative considerations are the limelight in oncologic and post-tumor reconstruction in facial cosmetic surgery for the best operating outcomes. High on the list is multidisciplinary coordination among oncologists, surgeons, and prosthodontists. Preoperative planning secures that surgical technique is tailored to the patient's specific needs, particularly after procedures such as maxillectomy. The research highlights the importance of pre-prosthetic surgical preparation that can significantly enhance the prognosis of oral cancer patients by preserving key structures, i.e., alveolar bone or adjacent teeth, which are vital for successful prosthetic management. Preoperative planning with such attention to detail enables not just the rehabilitation of functional capacity but also the aesthetic form, thereby enhancing the quality of life in patients post-surgery (Fattah et al., 2012). Another highly significant consideration is assessment of the patient's psychological status pre-surgery. Patients undergoing oncologic interventions can be discovered to be extremely anxious and emotionally upset, both on account of the diagnosis per se and on account of the alterations they expect in their appearance. Addressing these psychological factors is paramount in ensuring compliance and satisfaction by the patient post-surgery. Preoperative counseling can help patients establish realistic expectations of the reconstructive outcome and adopt coping strategies to nurture their mental and emotional well-being during recovery. Involving the patients in decision-making also confers on them a sense of autonomy and control that can significantly improve the global satisfaction with the surgical outcome (Cortese et al., 2021). In addition, the incorporation of contemporary technology and methods of preoperative planning has revolutionized facial cosmetic surgery following tumor removal. Preoperative imaging and 3D modeling can facilitate visualization by surgeons of the particular anatomical hurdles presented by defects from tumor removal. This sophisticated preparation enables more accurate surgical interventions and assists in the success of postoperative cosmetic and functional restorations. Furthermore, technologies such as the use of hyaluronic acid fillers are now valuable adjuvants in treating surgical sequelae, presenting a minimally invasive technique that contributes to aesthetic results after reconstruction. Surgical teams can decrease disability and enhance cosmetic outcome with these new methods, which is finally the greatest aim of rehabilitating patients' social relationships and self-confidence (Cortese et al., 2021) (Figure 14.11).

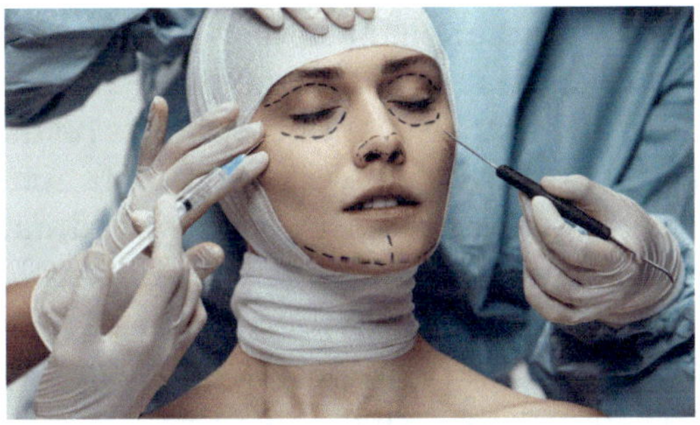

Figure 14.11. Oncologic and post-tumor reconstruction in facial cosmetic surgery.

Source: https://www.vaidam.com/sites/default/files/tests-before-cosmetic-surgery-intro-image-09-23.png.

14.3.1. Patient Assessment and Evaluation

Successful oncologic and post-tumor reconstruction in facial cosmetic surgery is founded on good patient assessment and evaluation. This comprehensive process begins with meticulous clinical history that includes not just the patient's cancer diagnosis and treatment but their psychosocial status and functional issues as well. Considerations such as tumor invasion extent and aesthetic impact are carefully weighed. By incorporating multidisciplinary consultation involving oncologists, surgeons, and counseling support staff, the entire holistic picture is considered so that all elements of patient health and welfare are taken into account in order to plan individualized reconstructive measures. The purpose of this thorough examination is to establish an individualized plan of treatment for the physical as well as psychological stresses of cancer therapy, ultimately resulting in improved patient outcomes and satisfaction. Physical examination is another salient feature of patient examination, with a focus on the specific anatomical region being reconstructed. Careful evaluations of facial balance, vascularization, and tissue integrity are significant as they direct the choice of surgical interventions and prosthetic appliances. For instance, after surgeries such as maxillectomy, the evaluation needs to take into account how defects resulting from such surgeries will impact functions such as speech and mastication. Coordination of reconstructive specialists and oncologic surgeons is required here in order to ensure that pre-prosthetic preparations, such as the preservation of overlying structures, support the patient's potential for successful rehabilitation. This caution is imperative in optimizing not just functional results of the surgery but also cosmetic results that significantly affect the patients quality of life, and which underscores the importance of a careful process of assessment. In addition, psychological testing is a part of patient assessment in oncologic and post-tumor reconstruction cases. Psycho-emotional impact from cancer and its treatments is usually debilitating in nature and results in body image disturbance, anxiety, and depression. These psycho-emotional factors should be evaluated as part of the overall plan of treatment since they play an important role in recuperation as well as in the patient's willingness to undertake reconstructive surgeries. Understanding the emotional and mental state of a patient allows health care professionals to give individualized care and support that may be needed in effective rehabilitation. In organizing reconstructive treatment, as suggested by literature, consideration of possible psychosocial impacts can improve not only aesthetic results but also allow for more satisfactory and holistic recovery, as reported by studies evaluating the significance of pre-prosthetic surgical interventions and their effect on patient rehabilitation (Fattah et al., 2012) (Figure 14.12).

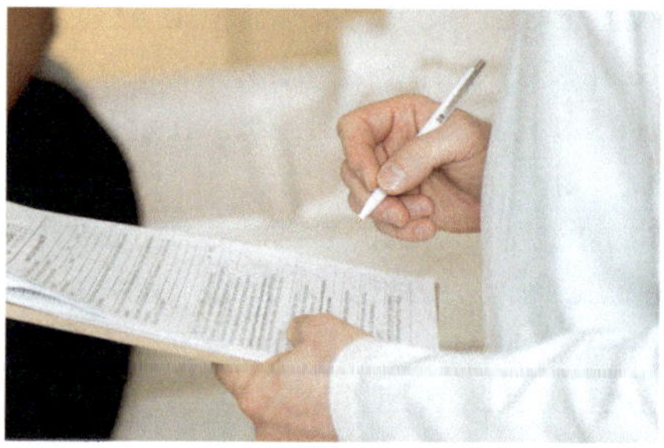

Figure 14.12. Patient assessment and evaluation.

Source: https://external-content.duckduckgo.com/iu/?u=https%3A%2F%2Fi0.wp.com%2Fstudent-nurse-life.com%2Fwp-content%2Fuploads%2F2023%2F03%2Fintroduction-to-assessing-and-implementing-care.jpg%3Ffit%3D1024%252C683&f=1&nofb=1&ipt=4c5422de406e21ec18239f6d1b9328f3d5f0c91e4892276b1ff60eb14ddd4645.

14.3.2. Importance of Multidisciplinary Teams

The complexity of oncologic and post-tumor reconstruction of facial cosmetic surgery demands the formation of multidisciplinary teams, with a balance of various expertise and specializations. This collaboration brings together oncologists, plastic surgeons, dermatologists, radiologists, and even mental health professionals, all with their unique expertise and skills. This cooperative approach is at the core of designing complete treatment plans based on specific patient needs. For instance, integration of oncological knowledge into surgical decisions ensures full understanding of the tumors behavior and associated risks of recurrence. One article emphasized how the use of advanced technology like Piezosurgery has the capacity to enhance surgical precision to a very significant degree while preserving valuable surrounding tissues, thus ensuring that collaboration between team members is necessary to ensure maximum results in complex reconstructive surgeries (Anesi et al., 2014). Secondly, multidisciplinary teams play a crucial role in managing patients following reconstruction to address their holistic needs. Psychological counseling is as essential in facial cosmetic surgery as in the correction of the physical deformity in the patient's appearance, particularly following oncological disfigurement. This interaction with mental health professionals ensures that the psychological and emotional effects of cancer treatment and reconstruction are optimally addressed, thus enhancing the overall recovery of patients. The successful reconstruction of scalp defects, as exemplified in recent case series using autologous grafts and dermal matrices, shows how interdisciplinary collaboration within specialties yields improved operating results and greater patient satisfaction (Gonzaga et al., 2019). The same support system in various aspects is needed in dealing with the intricate process of healing and reintegrating into society after surgery. The advantages of multidisciplinary practice extend beyond clinical effectiveness; they also promote a culture of cross-learning and innovation among medical practitioners. Collaboration of various expertise pushes practitioners to remain updated with the latest developments in methodologies and technology, which is a must in an increasingly evolving specialty like facial cosmetic surgery. By sharing knowledge and experiences, team members can identify best practices and refine protocols, leading to continuous improvement in patient care. Furthermore, such collaboration cultivates a strong professional network that can facilitate research and development initiatives, ultimately pushing boundaries in oncologic reconstruction methodologies. In summary, interaction among various specialties not only benefits but is essential for advancing oncologic and post-tumor reconstruction in facial aesthetic surgery (Figure 14.13).

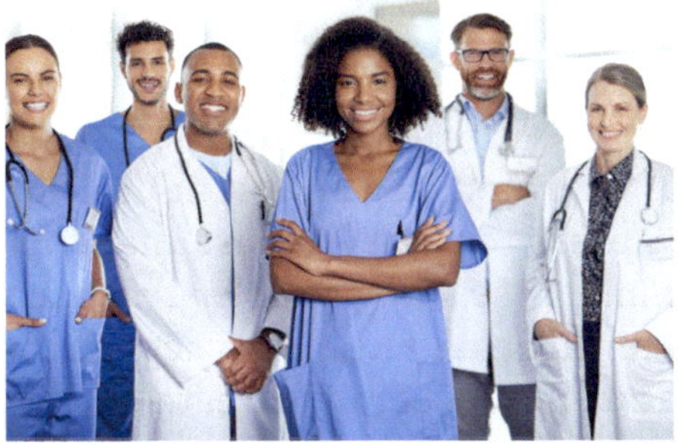

Figure 14.13. Importance of multidisciplinary teams.

Source: https://external-content.duckduckgo.com/iu/?u=https%3A%2F%2Fgettraumainformed.com%2Fwp-content%2Fuploads%2F2022%2F03%2FUntitled-design-e1647928342547-1024x744.png&f=1&nofb=1&ipt=3df54e0f9ebf6af805c237b956853e701afcc53c33a0bf64ae44ebc6fa469596.

14.3.3. Planning for Aesthetic Outcomes

Planning for aesthetic results in oncologic and post-tumor reconstruction of the facial structures is directly associated with the interdisciplinary interaction between oncologists and reconstructive surgeons. This collaboration is particularly crucial in procedures such as maxillectomy, whose size and site of resection significantly influence the possibility of an aesthetically pleasing result. The combination of measures directed at the preservation of adjacent structures, such as premaxilla or alveolar bone, holds the potential to enhance functional and cosmetic results for patients undergoing prosthetic rehabilitation. Pre-prosthetic surgical preps like these allow for an ideal platform for prostheses to be secured on, which further results in successful aesthetic rehabilitation. Efficient communication and planning can therefore not only enhance the prosthetic outcome but also the patient's psychosocial rehabilitation following surgery, underlining the importance of aesthetic components in the overall treatment plan (Fattah et al., 2012). In oncologic breast reconstruction, careful consideration of aesthetic outcomes has a groundbreaking effect on patient recovery and the quality of life. Use of techniques such as pedicled perforator flaps allows for an accurately recreated breast shape and size with minimal scarring visible. The success of such reconstructive techniques depends on their application in preoperative treatment planning, thereby obliterating symmetry and aesthetic issues prior to proceeding. With the achievement of acceptable restoration of size and shape, reconstructive surgeons can mitigate loss and disfigurement feelings normally experienced by patients after mastectomy. Also, since donor site scars are well-placed, they remain concealed, hence contributing to the ultimate aesthetic result. Such planning in totality accentuates reconstruction as more than a functional necessity; it is reconstructing identity and womanhood after cancer treatment (Cillino et al., 2010). Furthermore, patient education regarding expectations and the cosmetic nature of reconstructive surgery is important for achieving desired results. The presentation of patients with an in-depth discussion of potential outcomes and the limitations of reconstruction has the ability to empower them and synchronize their expectations with reasonable ones. These are informed consent, where patients learn about the techniques used and the effects on appearance as a result. Facial symmetry and normal contour correction should be highlighted as features, which will enable the patients to see the end result of their treatment. Support systems psychological should also be incorporated into preoperative care to deal with physical alteration anxieties after surgery. Lastly, concern being shown towards aesthetic outcomes in oncologic reconstruction not only increases physical results but also emotional recovery and patient satisfaction with their recovery process (Figure 14.14).

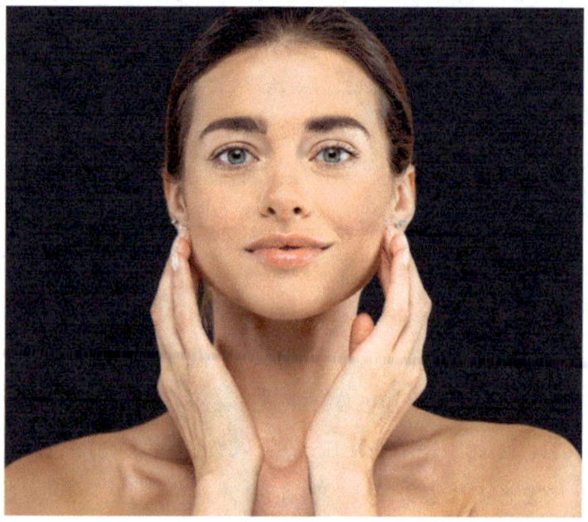

Figure 14.14. Planning for aesthetic outcomes.

Source: https://external-content.duckduckgo.com/iu/?u=https%3A%2F%2Fempireondemand.com%2Fcdn%2Fshop%2Ffiles%2FUnlockingAdvancedAestheticOutcomesCombinationTherapywiththeV-SeriesPlatform-horizontal.webp%3Fv%3D1726258974&f=1&nofb=1&ipt=fdb2fc76441eba71facef7b5c1255a48aa6642fb8088cfb1976a7222eb921bb8.

Test Your Knowledge

1. What key factors should be evaluated during a comprehensive patient assessment before planning facial reconstructive or cosmetic surgery?
2. Why is the involvement of a multidisciplinary team important in ensuring safe, effective, and holistic preoperative planning?

14.4. Surgical Techniques in Reconstruction

Learning Outcome

1. Discuss the Flap Techniques and Their Applications
2. Explain the Grafting Methods in Facial Reconstruction
3. Focus on Innovations in Surgical Technology

Surgical methods in reconstruction following oncologic surgery are heavily responsible for the restoration of function and aesthetics of the facial region. The complexity of reconstructive processes is highlighted by the need to overcome unique issues caused by the removal of cancerous tissues, particularly in areas with intricate anatomical structures such as nerves and vascular systems. Surgeons must skillfully assess the extent of tissue damage and formulate treatments that allow optimal healing with minimal scarring and loss of function. Free tissue transfer and local flap procedures, for instance, allow repositioning of adjacent tissues or transplantation of tissue from a distant part and thus bridge defects caused by the removal of a tumor. This wise selection of techniques is essential in restoring the patients to as much of their preoperative form and function, and therefore the quality of life. Paralysis of the face due to oncologic surgery complicates the reconstructive process further. Surgical techniques need to be adapted not only to restore the physical deformity, but also to restore facial symmetry and expression. Therapies may be directed toward grafting or repair of nerves, local muscle transfer, and static or dynamic sling placement for support of injured facial structures. When reinnervation is feasible, reconnections within the current musculature lead to more natural and functional outcomes. Nonetheless, the intricate facial nerve anatomy typically poses problems for complete rehabilitation. Thus, the synergy of newer surgical methods and a sound understanding of facial dynamics is needed to address the dual requirements of aesthetics and function following tumor removal (Anderson et al., 2012). Reconstruction after oncologic surgery is not only concerned with achieving the short-term aesthetic outcome, but also with considering the long-term factors influencing the patient's psychosocial status. An understanding of the interplay between physical appearance and self-image is essential for reconstruction success. The employment of modern adaptations of established surgical methods may offer optimal results in restoring facial appearance with maintenance of functional integrity. Knowledge of basic surgical principles is relevant, as the reconstructive techniques must be adapted to meet the individual patient's needs, particularly with large tumor resections (Garey et al., 2018). By including these factors in the reconstructive plan, surgeons can optimize overall success of oncologic and tumor-post reconstruction in removing both the physical and psychological scars of surgery (Figure 14.15).

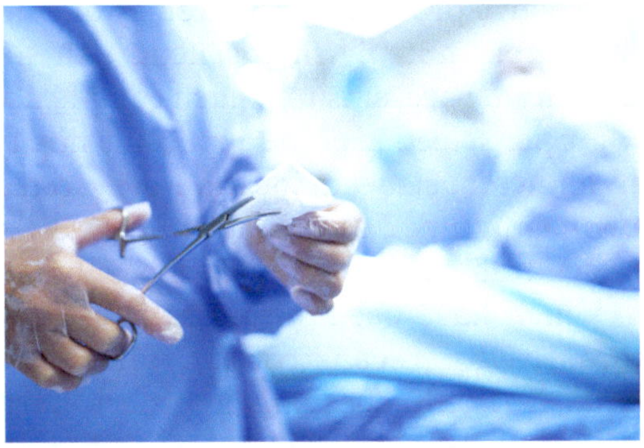

Figure 14.15. Surgical techniques in reconstruction.

Source: https://external-content.duckduckgo.com/iu/?u=https%3A%2F%2Fi0.wp.com%2Ffabknowledge.com%2Fwp-content%2Fuploads%2F2020%2F05%2F2240-scaled.jpg%3Fzoom%3D3%26resize%3D700%252C480%26ssl%3D1&f=1&nofb=1&ipt=31b72e76c89b7ee7a404dc3398fb372cb5323310735c2e77fb4472613fdee480.

14.4.1. Flap Techniques and Their Applications

Flap techniques are the most important technique in oncologic and post-tumor reconstruction, in the restoration of tissue function, aesthetics, and integrity. Flap techniques are used for the transfer of skin, muscle, and fat from one body area to another and the creation of a flap that is nourished by its own blood supply. Flap procedures are particularly relevant in the context of tumor resection for facial cosmetic surgery, where loss of tissue is highly impactful upon both shape and functional capacity, such as speech and swallowing. Recent studies have demonstrated the usefulness of the pedicled perforator flap application in successful volume and envelope skin restoration, particularly in partial breast reconstruction following tumor excision, thereby indicating the versatility of flap procedures in other facial and breast reconstructive operations (Cillino et al., 2010). One additional interesting aspect of flap techniques is the manner in which these procedures can be adapted to confront other reconstructive problems presented by oncologic surgery, most notably in the head and neck. Facial anatomy presents too much complexity to allow proper selection of the applicable flap type based on defect size and location. A systematic review has outlined several locoregional flaps, i.e., the infrahyoid, nasolabial, and submental flaps, which have been successfully employed for oral cavity reconstruction after tumor removal. Not only does this approach correct the immediate anatomical deficits, but it also enhances aesthetically better outcomes, so that the patients have not only functional rehabilitation but also the return to a more normal appearance. Complications of flap procedures are generally low and in reports of flap necrosis in a minimal percentage of procedures, further confirming the reliability of the technique (Accoronna et al., 2024). Moreover, studies using flap techniques in the follow-up of tumor resection have increased over time with advancements in surgical procedures and patient care. Surgeons now make use of cutting-edge imaging technologies and innovative surgical planning to optimize flap design and improve operative results. This patient-specific system allows for more precise reconstructions that meet the special demands of each patient, thereby increasing the satisfaction with both the aesthetic and functional results. Although flap techniques continue to expand in scope of popularity in oncologic and post-tumor reconstruction, clinical trials and research will certainly aid in further evolving these techniques, expediting recovery times, and minimizing complications wherever possible, overall enhancing patient outcomes in the domain of facial cosmetic surgery.

14.4.2. Grafting Methods in Facial Reconstruction

The grafting technique of methods of facial reconstruction is key to successful facial aesthetics and function restoration following oncologic surgery. Skin grafting, normally applied for facial defect resulting from the removal of a tumor, can be classified into various types including split-thickness and full-thickness grafts. Split-thickness grafts, which include the epidermis and part of the dermis, are most often employed for larger defects since they are convenient and cause less donor site morbidity. Both layers of the skin, full-thickness grafts, however, give better cosmetic results and should be utilized on small, more visible sites like the mouth and nose. The literature reports that appropriate grafting technique choice significantly influences healing time and surgical outcome, particularly requiring surgeons to customize their technique to the specific patient needs and individual presentations of the tumor. In the event of major loss of face tissue from oncologic resections, the reconstructive alternatives extend beyond merely skin grafts to more complex techniques that include local flaps and free tissue transfer. Local flaps are useful in that they utilize adjacent tissues to fill in the defects without disrupting vascular supply and typically yield better functional results. For instance, the modified crescentic flap procedure has been successful in correcting defects in the area around the nose to facilitate both functional reconstruction and cosmetic enhancement through adequately camouflaging scars within natural contours. Research has established that such regional methods prefer faster recovery and less postoperative complications, emphasizing their importance in oncologic reconstruction (Arginelli et al., 2016). With accurate planning of these procedures, surgeons can develop the best aesthetic results with fewer psychological disturbances to patients recovered from facial anomalies caused by cancer. Apart from the cosmetic nature, the functional implications of facial grafting methods in tumor post-reconstruction cannot be overstated. Paralysis of the facial nerve is a common complication of head and neck surgery, and individualized rehabilitation programs are needed to establish innervation and musculature for an optimal functional outcome. Grafting techniques involving a combination of nerve repair and tissue reconstruction can provide patients with significant improvement in mobility and expression for a more natural appearance and enhanced quality of life. Secondly, the selection of the method of grafting needs to consider not only aesthetic, but functional outcomes, as some methods will be more accommodating to achieving both objectives. Lastly, the use of grafting in facial reconstruction is critical, as both the physical and psychological dimensions of healing from oncologic surgery are being attended to (Anderson et al., 2012).

14.4.3. Innovations in Surgical Technology

The cosmetic surgery world, particularly in the areas of oncologic and post-tumor reconstruction, is being significantly revolutionized by advances in surgical technology. Contemporary practices are revolutionizing how surgeons approach complex defects, primarily by facilitating enhanced functional and aesthetic outcomes. Much of this paradigmatic change can be attributed to advancements in flap surgery and regenerative medicine, which offer alternative avenues for reconstructive issues. For instance, perforator flap techniques have also achieved an astonishing 96.5% success rate, which has been significantly improved in relation to functional restoration over traditional pedicled flaps. Given that aesthetic satisfaction is highest in facial surgery, these developments are of great promise to enhance patient recovery with reduced complications, further showing the importance of iterative technological developments in surgical techniques (Bernal et al., 2024). An essential component of these advancements is the application of virtual surgical planning (VSP) and computer-aided design/manufacturing (CAD/CAM) systems. These technologies aid in precise anatomical reconstructions, especially important in complex situations such as maxillectomy, where critical defects require meticulous restoration of form and function. Evidence proves that the addition of VSP may streamline operational efficiency, reducing the duration of surgeries while improving the precision of osseous reconstructions. As a result, patient outcomes are greatly enhanced, both aesthetically and in terms of rehabilitation. Furthermore, the aforementioned technologies minimize the risk of complications associated with traditional techniques, presenting a compelling case for the adoption of sophisticated technology in facial reconstructive surgery (Datarkar et al., 2024). Surgical procedures using regenerative medicine are transforming healing processes and realizing optimal recovery results in oncologic patients. Techniques such as the use of platelet-rich plasma (PRP) and bioengineered scaffolds are now viable adjuncts, facilitating wound healing at a rapid rate and drastically lowering the rates of infection. Experiments have also proven that application of these regenerative methods can improve graft survival to up to 90%, a significant improvement over conventional methods. Also, the combination of advanced flap methods with regenerative therapy greatly minimizes complications while providing robust functional and cosmetic results. These developments underscore the necessity for ongoing research and development in surgical technology, with emphasis on their role in the future of oncologic and post-tumor reconstruction in facial cosmetic surgery (Bernal et al., 2024).

Test Your Knowledge

1. How do different flap techniques (local, regional, and free flaps) support tissue repair in facial reconstruction, and what determines the choice of flap?
2. What types of grafting methods are commonly used in facial reconstruction, and how do they contribute to restoring structure and function?

14.5. Postoperative Care and Recovery

Learning Outcome

1. Discuss the Importance of Follow-up Care
2. Explain Managing Complications and Risks
3. Focus on Rehabilitation And Support For Patients

The postoperative recovery following oncologic and post-tumor reconstruction in facial cosmetic surgery is paramount, as it plays a vital role both in the immediate recovery and long-term outcomes. Appropriate care at this stage can avoid complications, minimize discomfort, and improve rehabilitation. Appropriate pain control is a cornerstone of postoperative care, generally dealt with by a combination of pharmacological and non-pharmacological interventions. Individualized management of pain requires frequent assessment of the surgical field and general condition, so patients can carry out necessary activities such as eating and speaking with minimal distress. Closely monitoring for infection, dehiscence, or complications is crucial since these variables can disrupt healing and negatively affect cosmetic results. Postoperative care includes supportive management that facilitates recovery. In maxillary reconstructive surgery, for instance, the employment of a multimodality team of oncologists, plastic surgeons, prosthodontists, and rehabilitation specialists ensures patients receive comprehensive care tailored to their specific surgical experiences. Pre-prosthetic surgical alterations have the potential to enhance prosthetic fit conditions, which subsequently influence functionality and aesthetics after maxillectomy. There is evidence that suggests that there is a significant role contributed by surgeon-prosthodontist interaction toward post-surgical rehabilitation success, for example, research emphasizing the role of preoperative planning and collaborative action in ensuring a satisfactory outcome (Fattah et al., 2012). Such an approach of a team ensures not only current medical needs but also continuity of care along the course of recovery. Modalities and timing of rehabilitation are most crucial in setting the postoperative course of recovery. Newer methods, such as the use of ultrasonic osteotomes, have emerged as useful options for craniofacial surgery and have advantages in bone healing due to accuracy and less injury to surrounding tissues (Anesi et al., 2014). The ability of such equipment to cut smoothly supports better maintenance of important structures, which supports better surgical outcomes and, possibly, better aesthetics. Along with postoperative care, this technique underscores the necessity for the adoption of modern surgical practices that allow for faster recovery and enhanced cosmetic outcomes. Through an emphasis on innovative practice and whole patient care, healthcare professionals can help patients who have had oncologic and facial reconstruction surgery regain function and confidence as they continue down their path to recovery.

14.5.1. Importance of Follow-up Care

For oncologic and post-tumor reconstruction in facial cosmetic surgery, follow-up care cannot be overstated. Post-op management is important to monitor possible complications and ensure optimal recovery. For reconstructive surgery, patients are faced with numerous issues, including handling pain, surgical site infections, and the psychological impact of their appearance. Regular follow-up allows medical specialists to timely address and resolve such issues, which can significantly affect the quality of life of a patient and overall contentment with the outcome of the surgery. Periodic visits provide an opportunity for patients to share their doubts, receive support, and become capable of accessing necessary help, thereby making the rehabilitation process easier after tumor resection and reconstruction. Moreover, follow-up care is necessary to ensure maximum success of prosthetic rehabilitation following maxillectomy or similar surgery. As seen through research, pre-prosthetic surgical preparation substantially optimizes the success of prosthetic treatment among patients of maxillary reconstruction. Interdisciplinary collaboration between oncologists and maxillofacial surgeons during preparatory procedures can optimize sites for prosthetic placement, as described in Fattah et al. (2012). When follow-up care is integrated into this system, it establishes the foundation for adjustments that respond to evolving patient needs, ensuring that what is delivered as prosthetic restoration satisfies functional requirements as well as visual and aesthetic satisfaction. Regular inspections present a chance to make timely adjustments and refinements, which are key to maintaining patient confidence and social adjustment. In addition, the follow-up care function also entails monitoring the physiological impact of the surgical intervention on tissue viability and bone regeneration. The use of advanced technology, such as Piezosurgery, has been observed to have the capability of minimizing trauma to surrounding structures, thereby affecting post-operative recovery. Evaluating the outcome of different osteotomy techniques, as reported in Anesi et al. (2014), is important in deciding the most effective method to facilitate proper recovery and healing after facial reconstructive operations. Postoperative follow-up sessions provide significant insights about healing patterns of bone and soft tissues so that surgeons can analyze whether chosen techniques provide the best results in terms of recovery rate and quality. This unified assessment can have a profound impact on long-term cosmetic results and functional rehabilitation, verifying the position of follow-up management as an integral component of oncologic facial reconstructive practice.

14.5.2. Managing Complications and Risks

Effective management of complications and risks is necessary in oncologic and post-tumor reconstruction in facial cosmetic surgery. The treating surgeons should anticipate potential problems such as infection, wound dehiscence, and necrosis to enhance patient results. Technological innovation, particularly ultrasonic osteotomes, has been found to assist in minimizing bone trauma during surgical procedures. Comparisons of various osteotomy devices discovered that ultrasound-guided equipment, such as Piezosurgery®, produces surfaces with advantageous micromorphologies that can promote bone healing and reossification. These technologies not only address the physical aspect of reconstruction but also minimize risks associated with traditional methods, including rotating or sawing instruments, that lead to increased complications (Anesi et al., 2014). Through their integration, surgeons can optimize the safety and efficacy of facial cosmetic procedures, leading to an overall improvement in the quality of life among cancer survivors. Post-operative complications can potentially change the course of recovery for patients following oncologic reconstruction. Age, pre-existing health conditions, and the size of the original tumor are risk factors that should be evaluated in an attempt to plan surgical procedures accordingly. Certain patients may be at greater risk for complications if they have extensive tissue loss or require high reconstructive procedures, for instance. Surgery teams are stimulated to utilize comprehensive preoperative assessment to determine subjects with high risk and therefore, utilize personalized protocols to minimize post-surgical complications. Furthermore, ongoing education on the latest surgical techniques and materials can improve the capacity of health professionals to manage probable complications confidently. Such practices are instrumental in building a safer operating room and boosting recovery rates among patients undergoing facial reconstruction after tumor resection (Ndongo et al., 2010). Post-operative care and complication management are also important, as early detection encourages timely intervention to improve outcomes from the operation. Postoperative checkups and follow-up make the detection of signs of complications early on possible, allowing them to be treated in due time. Patient education regarding potential signs of infection or other side effects also empowers them to actively seek medical care. Adoption of a standard follow-up schedule, coupled with a patient-centered care approach, is crucial in ensuring the effective management of complications without compromising the overall well-being and satisfaction of the patient and the reconstructive result. With facial cosmetic surgery continuing to advance, emphasis on balanced risk management approaches is pivotal in achieving optimal results in patients who are undergoing oncologic surgery (Anesi et al., 2014).

14.5.3. Rehabilitation And Support For Patients

The rehabilitation and support of oncologic and post-tumor reconstruction patients are multifaceted and include both functional and psychological concerns. The patient, following facial surgery for tumor removal or reconstruction, will often have an extreme change in appearance and function. Such changes are distressing psychologically and potentially impacting self-esteem and quality of life. Therefore, an effective rehabilitation program will include psychological support services so that patients can cope with their new realities. Counseling or support groups, for instance, can offer a forum in which patients can share experiences and strategies, accelerate emotional healing as well as physical recovery. It is significant to note the psychological components of recovery since this can significantly enhance compliance with rehabilitation routines, lead to optimal outcomes, and build resilience during recovery. For patients with facial paralysis secondary to cancer therapies, individualized rehabilitation protocols help ensure maximum recovery of function. Facilitation of the recovery process is most often impeded by the complexity of facial innervation; individualized evaluation takes precedence. As varied as therapy to restore the function of the muscles or surgery for nerve repair and reinnervation, treatment is outlined in Anderson et al. (2012). These approaches not only address cosmetic concerns but also focus on improving functional abilities such as speech, swallowing, and facial expression. Additionally, the integration of new technologies, such as biofeedback systems or electrical stimulation units, can offer alternative avenues for treatment, hence boosting patient motivation and involvement in their rehabilitation. By prioritizing functional recovery as the first step in overall patient care, healthcare practitioners are able to put patients on the path to greater independence and improved quality of life. Pre-prosthetic surgical preparation as a component for realizing best rehabilitation outcomes cannot be overstated. Following operations like maxillectomy, the resulting defects need successful prosthetic replacement to facilitate restoration of function and aesthetics, and this is crucial for the reintegration of patients into social settings. Such success hinges on collaborative efforts between oncologists and maxillofacial surgeons to help ensure effective preservation of the remaining anatomy during primary surgery, as emphasized in Fattah et al. (2012). Such collaboration aids in formulating a pre-prosthetic plan that may include the preservation of significant anatomical structures to maximize function of the prosthetic devices as a whole. An in-depth knowledge of prosthetic and surgical principles can enhance patient outcomes, addressing key areas like speech intelligibility and social interaction after reconstruction. An integrated rehabilitation and support program, thus, is essential in order to optimize physical and psychosocial aspects of rehabilitation for patients undergoing facial cosmetic surgery due to cancer therapy.

Test Your Knowledge

1. Why is consistent follow-up care essential after facial reconstructive surgery, and what aspects of healing are typically monitored?
2. What common complications may occur postoperatively, and how can early detection and management reduce long-term risks?

14.6. Ethical Considerations in Oncologic and Reconstructive Surgery

Learning Outcome

1. Explain the Informed Consent and Patient Autonomy
2. Focus on Balancing Aesthetics with Medical Necessity
3. Discuss Addressing Disparities in Access to Care

In the practice of oncologic and reconstructive surgery, moral principles should come first in surgeons' decision-making. The confrontation between the demand for life-saving procedures and the intention to preserve beauty is embedded in complex dilemmas. Doctors must navigate the ethical landscape between the urgency of patients' health and the accommodation of the psychosocial impacts of disfiguration by tumors. The process generally entices a high level of subtlety in obtaining informed consent for high-pressure treatments that may sacrifice on appearance and balancing realistic patient expectations regarding the end result of reconstructive surgeries. This is compounded when resource availability, patient-informed consent, and the potential for unequal access to high-technology reconstructive modalities are considered, ultimately confronting surgeons with their ethical responsibilities beyond the solution of the immediate clinical challenges of oncologic disease. Furthermore, ethics in reconstructive and oncologic surgery extend to postoperative rehabilitation and aesthetic requirements. The use of new techniques, such as the use of HA fillers as adjuvants in reconstructive surgery, illustrates an even greater ethical concern when it comes to patient satisfaction and quality of life. These methods, previously used for cosmetic reasons, can bring about significant functional and aesthetic gains following surgery, thus improving patient confidence. Still, their introduction challenges the issue of potential over-treatment and the commodification of surgical outcomes, where the outcome becomes more focused on aesthetics than on clinical necessity.

The surgeons will need to consider the implications of using such methods, particularly in sensitive cases where a patient's psychological and emotional healing is interwoven with his or her physical appearance. The ethical responsibility is to make these processes work responsibly, weighing patient safety and satisfaction without compromising the limits of professional medical practice (Cortese et al., 2021).

In addition, the social and cultural components of patient decision-making in reconstructive and oncologic surgery call for an ethical approach that is more nuanced. Personal convictions, cultural norms of beauty, and how accessible the reconstructive procedures are, all come into play in a patient's thought processes regarding what they wish to have done.

The multi-faceted scenario necessitates surgeons to confront their own prejudices and be attuned to body image and personal identity cultural subtleties. Open dialogue with patients regarding what they desire, expect, and fear becomes important in developing an open way of doing things concerning treatment planning. Ethically, surgeons have a responsibility to equip patients with a complete set of information to allow them to make appropriate decisions regarding their treatment in alignment with their own values and conception of healing. These discussions become essential in bridging the gap between surgical technicality and the very personalized process of healing after oncologic operations (Accorona et al., 2024).

14.6.1. Informed Consent and Patient Autonomy

The importance of informed consent in the situation of oncologic and post-tumor reconstruction of facial cosmetic surgery cannot be overstressed. Informed consent is a fundamental principle that allows patients to make autonomous decisions regarding their medical treatment. This practice raises the patient from the status of a passive recipient of medical attention to that of an active participant in their own medical attention. In reconstructive facial procedures, particularly following oncologic surgery, patients are faced with complex decisions that are usually charged with emotional, psychological, and physical implications. Ethical practice necessitates health professionals to communicate risks, benefits, and potential outcomes of accessible surgical options in depth, not only upholding medical practice ethical standards but also respecting the autonomy and personal beliefs of the patient. The formation of informed consent is in harmony with the overall principles of patient autonomy, which becomes particularly important in the field of cancer following reconstructive surgery. Autonomy is an individuals' capacity to exercise control over their decision-making, based on values and wants, particularly in an exceedingly personal and life-changing circumstance such as facial cosmetic surgery. Surgeons should make sure that patients know about the different procedures that can be undertaken, their implications, and what recovery paths to expect. By allowing patients to comprehend the subtleties of their surgical choices, surgeons give them the power to fully participate in the decision-making process. This becomes important to facilitating their emotional recovery and constructive self-concept upon treatment, because patient autonomy can positively enhance overall satisfaction with surgical outcomes, thereby solidifying the importance of informed consent in facilitating patient-centered care. Healthcare providers' responsibility for facilitating informed consent is not merely to convey information but also to create a supportive therapeutic relationship. As a dynamic blend of humanism and science, clinical practice demands practitioners not just to transmit technical information but also to talk to the emotional domain of patient care (Kalaskar et al., 2016). Building trust between the health care team and the patient is crucial in getting patients to relax and open up about their concerns and reconstruction preferences. These relationships also play a significant role in managing the complex terrains of cosmetic surgery decision-making, since patients may seek to balance their individual choices with broader social expectations. In the end, a holistic approach to informed consent prioritizing patient autonomy, emotional support, and honest communication guarantees that the health care process is holistic, dignified, and consonant with the values and projected outcomes of the patients.

14.6.2. Balancing Aesthetics with Medical Necessity

In the context of oncologic and post-tumor reconstruction, the intersection between aesthetics and medical necessity becomes a critical factor for consideration among both surgeons and patients. The physical and psychological impact of facial disfigurement necessitates consideration of both functional recovery and aesthetic restoration. In the majority of patients, particularly those recovering from procedures like mastectomy or radical tumor resections, a natural appearance is a significant part of their psychological well-being and readjustment to society. Reconstructive surgery therefore, must focus not only on restoring anatomical continuity but also on maximizing the aesthetic outcome, as reflected in the many strategies used by reconstructive surgeons. The prevalence of psychological distress following facial surgery renders this balance essential to patient satisfaction and thereby substantiates the intuition that reconstructive activity transcends medical necessity alone to encompass aesthetic desire. The conflicts of balancing aesthetic desires against clinical realities predominantly arise in preoperative consultations, wherein communication between healthcare providers and patients is of paramount importance. Identification of determinants influencing decision-making is of critical concern, particularly in patients undergoing significant reconstruction of their facial appearance. Evidence has shown that breast cancer patients tend to look at cosmetic considerations when deciding on reconstructive operations, similar to the behaviors of facial reconstructive surgery patients (Ndongo et al., 2010).

Surgeons must navigate this ground with sensitivity, acknowledging the differing emotional responses of patients to disfigurement while presenting the medical justification for some operations. This serves to emphasize the need for an individualized approach, acknowledging that patients' notions of success of reconstruction can be extremely individualized and intertwining their body shape with their self-concept. With continually evolving surgical techniques and technology, the possibilities for innovative solutions in the marriage of form and functional necessity only expand. Surgeons are driven to integrate new technologies, such as 3D modeling and bioprinting, into practice, allowing increased degrees of customization of reconstruction and increased ability to address aesthetic issues without compromising medical success. This crossing alludes to an avant-garde trend in the field, whereby technologies facilitate the creation of naturally occurring-looking results that promote healing as well as contentment. These advancements bring with them, however, ethics related to access and equity of care, meaning that surgeons must be sensitive to disparities in patient access to reconstructive options (Ndongo et al., 2010).

Hence, the balance between aesthetic and medical needs is not just a clinical objective but is also a reflection of the evolution of patient treatment in oncology and aesthetic surgery.

14.6.3. Addressing Disparities in Access to Care

Gaps in access to care have an important influence on the outcomes of oncologic and post-tumor reconstruction facial cosmetic surgery patients. Social determinants of health, such as socioeconomic status, location, and insurance coverage, usually determine patients' capacity to receive timely and appropriate care. For instance, patients in economically backward communities will have issues pertaining to transportation, which leads to delayed consultations and treatments. Delaying the process not only lowers the success rate of initial oncologic procedures but also complicates further reconstructive procedures. Addressing these disparities is crucial to ensuring equal access to care, which ultimately improves prognosis and quality of life for the suffering patients. Overall, policies aimed at addressing awareness and access to medical care are necessary in bridging the gap in healthcare availability, particularly for disadvantaged communities disproportionately affected by facial tumors and the resultant reconstruction needs. Besides these disparities in care and accessibility, biases among healthcare practitioners can similarly hinder equal access to oncologic and reconstructive care. Studies have demonstrated that racial and ethnic minorities are most likely to receive levels of care consistent with presumed abilities to tolerate pain or compliance with treatment recommendations. These biases may lead to suboptimal control of pain, decreased referrals for reconstructive surgery, and ultimately, poorer cosmetic results. The addition of cultural competency education to medical school curricula may be the bridge to crossing these biases. Through the provision of a healthcare environment that respects and honors various backgrounds, practitioners can enhance communication, build trust, and promote better care for all patients regardless of demographics. Meticulous training and sensitization can enable practitioners to break through their presuppositions, ultimately enhancing the provision of oncologic and post-tumor reconstructive surgeries for the underrepresented populations. In addition, community outreach programs play a key role in addressing disproportionate access to care in the areas of oncologic and post-tumor reconstruction. Through their direct engagement with communities, medical centers can better identify common hurdles in obtaining care. Educational programs can demystify reconstructive procedures and position them at the forefront of the cancer care process. Secondarily, partnerships with local organizations can promote advocacy for underinsured patient coverage and reimbursement for reconstructive treatment. Outcomes reveal that outreach programs will similarly encourage awareness and utilization of surgical therapy. In anticipation of the growing tumor-related deformity burden, active community outreach is necessary. Investment in such outreach is not only altruistic; it is required to create a more equitable model of healthcare that provides all patients with the ability to access reconstructive care that they need and deserve (Ndongo et al., 2010; Kalaskar et al., 2016).

Test Your Knowledge

1. Why is informed consent essential in oncologic and reconstructive surgery, and how does it support patient autonomy during decision-making?
2. How should surgeons balance a patient's aesthetic preferences with the medical necessity of removing cancerous tissue or restoring essential function?

SUMMARY

In oncologic and post-tumor reconstruction in facial cosmetic surgery, the key is to integrate high-tech surgical expertise and personalized patient care. As demonstrated in this essay, effective outcomes for facial reconstruction following oncological surgery rely on a combined vision of both aesthetic and functional needs. Facial anatomy's inherent complexities render the process more individualized, particularly in the case of addressing issues such as facial nerve paralysis due to cancer treatment. Careful assessment of residual nerve segments and musculature can lead to successful reinnervation methods, ultimately restoring patients closer to their original form and higher mobility. This complementarity of oncologic control and reconstructive surgery emphasizes the necessity of a multidisciplinary treatment, involving surgeons, oncologists, and rehabilitation specialists (Anderson et al., 2012). Furthermore, the pursuit of aesthetic reconstruction after oncological intervention presents unique challenges and opportunities for innovation in surgical techniques. The pedicled perforator flap is now considered a choice for breast reconstruction following tumor removal and is a suitable metaphor for facial reconstruction. Just as in breast reconstruction, the addition of tissue can reconstructively restore contour and volume, so too can these concepts be used in facial reconstruction, restoring both function and appearance following surgery. The early outcomes present promising results, with complete flap survival and satisfactory restoration of size and form, toward the possibility of improving patient satisfaction and global quality of life in this region (Cillino et al., 2010). In the end, the conclusion reached by this discussion of oncologic and post-tumor reconstruction in facial cosmetic surgery is that the future lies in continued refinement of the technique and the fostering of an empathic appreciation of patient experience. The gains achieved in terms of function and appearance can have a very powerful impact on the psychological and emotional well-being of patients subsequently. Thus, embracing a patient-centered approach that guarantees personalized treatment protocols will not only advance surgical outcomes but also the quality of care provided to oncologic surgery and subsequent reconstruction candidates. Engaging patients in their reconstructive process guarantees long-term satisfaction and improved quality of life after oncological complications.

The oncologic principles applied to facial cosmetic surgery signify the significance of addressing the aesthetic as well as functional issues of post-tumor reconstruction. Advances in technology and surgery have significantly enhanced the outcomes of patients with facial reconstruction after oncologic treatment. A key factor is selecting proper osteotomes, which have been altered with the development of ultrasonic tools such as Piezosurgery® and the newer models. These instruments have shown improved micromorphology and reduced osteotomized bone surface roughness compared to the standard rotating and sawing instruments. The implications of these findings are enormous; not just do they highlight the importance of precision in surgical procedures, but they also reflect improved bone healing and reossification, thereby maximizing the reconstructive process in cranio-facial surgery (Anesi et al., 2014). In addition to the reconstructive aspects, the application of fat grafting has emerged as a significant field of interest for enhancing aesthetic results following tumor removal. Autologous adipose tissue serves various purposes, including restoration of contour and volumetric support. However, challenges such as variability in long-term volume retention necessitate optimal knowledge of the factors controlling fat graft survival. Research on adipose tissue-derived stem cells (ASCs) has led to new techniques to improve outcomes. Enrichment of lipoaspirate with ASCs has been reported by studies to increase angiogenesis and viability of adipocytes, addressing the universal issue of graft resorption. With regard to these techniques, in addition to issues of oncological safety, a complex setting in which fat grafting can improve or complicate reconstruction (Vyas, 2016) is raised. It is important to address the subtleties of oncologic and cosmetic surgery simultaneously in order to provide the optimal patient outcome. Aesthetic enhancement versus oncologic safety is a compromise that must be made a priority, as evidenced by research and regulatory interest in the significance of ASCs for fat grafting. An integrated understanding of the interactions between cancer biology, surgical techniques, and tissue engineering techniques will guarantee future improvements in facial cosmetic surgery after a tumor. Therefore, the new paradigms in the specialty emphasize multidisciplinary approaches, integrating surgical innovation and oncologic precision to enhance quality of life in patients undergoing reconstructive surgery (Vyas, 2016).

KEY TERMS FROM THIS CHAPTER

- Tumor Resection
- Mohs Surgery
- Basal Cell Carcinoma
- Melanoma
- Local Flap
- Free Flap
- Skin Grafting
- Bone Reconstruction
- Margins of Excision
- Cutaneous Malignancy
- Squamous Cell Carcinoma
- Defect Reconstruction
- Regional Flap
- Microvascular Anastomosis
- Soft Tissue Reconstruction
- Functional Restoration

CRITICAL THINKING QUESTIONS

1. **The most common malignant tumor of the facial skin is:**
   a. Melanoma
   b. Basal cell carcinoma
   c. Squamous cell carcinoma
   d. Merkel cell carcinoma
2. **What is the most important consideration in reconstruction of nasal ala defects?**
   a. Skin color match
   b. Structural support restoration
   c. Scar position
   d. Donor site morbidity
3. **Which technique is considered the gold standard for margin control in facial skin cancer?**
   a. Wide excision
   b. Cryotherapy
   c. Mohs micrographic surgery
   d. Laser excision
4. **The primary goal of oncologic facial reconstruction is:**
   a. Aesthetic enhancement
   b. Functional restoration and cosmesis
   c. Immediate scar reduction
   d. Symmetry correction only
5. **A full-thickness defect of the lower eyelid is best reconstructed using:**
   a. Advancement flap
   b. Mustardé flap
   c. Hughes tarsoconjunctival flap
   d. Skin graft

Short Answer Questions

1. What are the primary goals of oncologic reconstruction in facial surgery?
2. Why is achieving clear surgical margins essential in facial tumor excision?
3. What makes Mohs micrographic surgery particularly suitable for facial skin cancers?
4. How does the location of a tumor influence the choice of reconstruction technique?
5. What factors determine whether a skin graft or a local flap is used after tumor removal?
6. What is the role of sentinel lymph node biopsy in the management of facial melanoma?
7. How does defect size affect reconstruction planning following tumor excision?

Answers to Critical Thinking Questions

1. (b) 2. (b) 3. (c) 4. (b) 5. (c)

REFERENCES

1. Accorona, R., Achena, A., Awny, S., Cremasco, et al. (2024). *Oral reconstruction with locoregional flaps after cancer ablation: A systematic review of the literature.* https://core.ac.uk/download/638813116.pdf (accessed on 14th July 2025).
2. Adams, N. J., Adrián, T. M., Allen, L. R., Arcelus, et al. (2022). *Standards of care for the health of transgender and gender diverse people, Version 8.* http://diposit.ub.edu/dspace/bitstream/2445/189561/1/Standards%20of%20Care%20for%20the%20Health%20of%20Transgender%20and%20Gender%20Diverse%20People%20Version%208.pdf (accessed on 14th July 2025).
3. Anderson, Asaoka, Berghaus, Booth, Coulson, Cross, Croxson, et al. (2012). *Re-animation and rehabilitation of the paralyzed face in head and neck cancer patients.* https://deepblue.lib.umich.edu/bitstream/2027.42/89486/1/21286_ftp.pdf (accessed on 14th July 2025).
4. Anesi, A., Cavani, F., Chiarini, L., Ferretti, et al. (2014). *Preliminary findings of a potenziated piezosurgical device at the rabbit skull.* https://core.ac.uk/download/80171725.pdf (accessed on 14th July 2025).
5. Arginelli, F., Bellini, P., Ferrari, B., Losi, et al. (2016). *Crescentic flap for the reconstruction of the nose after skin cancer resection.* https://core.ac.uk/download/84495439.pdf (accessed on 14th July 2025).
6. Bernal, J. G. T., Galindo, A. S., García, M. F. R., Javier, et al. (2024). *Advances in flap surgical techniques and regenerative approaches for reconstruction of extensive defects in cutaneous squamous cell carcinoma: A systematic review of functional and aesthetic outcomes.* https://core.ac.uk/download/635338710.pdf (accessed on 14th July 2025).
7. Cillino, M., Cordova, A., D'Arpa, S., Liuzza, et al. (2010). *Algorithm of partial breast reconstruction with pedicled perforator flaps.*2nd ITALIAN MEETING ON PERFORATOR FLAPS – Bologna, 26th-27th November 2010. ASTRACT BOOK Cured by: Dott.ssa Rossella Sgarzani Dott. Luca Negosanti brought to you by COREView metadata, citation and similar papers at core.ac.ukprovided by Archivio istituzionale della ricerca - Università di Palermo https://core.ac.uk/download/53293997.pdf (accessed on 14th July 2025).
8. Cortese, A., Chirico, F., Tartaro, G., Audino, G., Colella, G., Rugge, L., Sgaramella, N., et al. (2021). *Non-surgical touch-up with hyaluronic acid fillers following facial reconstructive surgery.* https://core.ac.uk/download/599516555.pdf (accessed on 14th July 2025).
9. Datarkar, A., Daware, S., & Khruomo, A. (2024). *Methods for functional and aesthetic rehabilitation of maxillectomy defect: A systematic review.* https://core.ac.uk/download/620836611.pdf (accessed on 14th July 2025).
10. de Bree, R., Ferlito, A., Olsen, K. D., Quer, et al. (2017). *Deep Lobe Parotidectomy—Why, When, and How?* https://core.ac.uk/download/604637332.pdf (accessed on 14th July 2025).
11. Garey, L., & Maillard, G. F. (2018). *Plastic Surgery After Ablative Cancer Surgery.* https://core.ac.uk/download/159156664.pdf (accessed on 14th July 2025).
12. Goldhirsch, A., Curigliano, G., Petit, J. Y., Rietjens, M., & Lohsiriwat, V. (2011). *Autologous fat transplantation in patients with breast cancer: Silencing or fueling cancer recurrence.* https://core.ac.uk/download/572847921.pdf (accessed on 14th July 2025).

13. Gonzaga, C. B., Glória Filho, E., Miqueloti, M. B., Freire, R. A. V., & Ribeiro, V. da S. A. (2019). *Scalp reconstruction after wide resection of an angiosarcoma*. https://core.ac.uk/download/587685526.pdf (accessed on 14th July 2025).

14. Lankage, D. L. M. (2023). *Factors influencing patient choice in type of breast reconstruction: A qualitative study*. https://core.ac.uk/download/571214680.pdf (accessed on 14th July 2025).

15. Deepak M. Kalaskar, Peter E. Butler, Shadi Ghali. (2016). *Textbook of Plastic and Reconstructive Surgery*. ISBN: 978-1-910634-37-0 (Hbk.) https://core.ac.uk/download/79526588.pdf

16. (accessed on 14th July 2025).

17. Ndongo, B. N., Mballa, G. A. E., Hyder, A. A., Juillard, et al. (2010). *Patterns of injury and violence in Yaoundé Cameroon: An analysis of hospital data*. https://core.ac.uk/download/323075033.pdf (accessed on 14th July 2025).

18. Vyas, K. S. (2016). *The role of fat grafting and adipose-derived stem cells in breast reconstruction*. https://core.ac.uk/download/232574356.pdf (accessed on 14th July 2025).

ADVANCES, TECHNOLOGIES, AND PRACTICE MANAGEMENT IN FACIAL COSMETIC

15

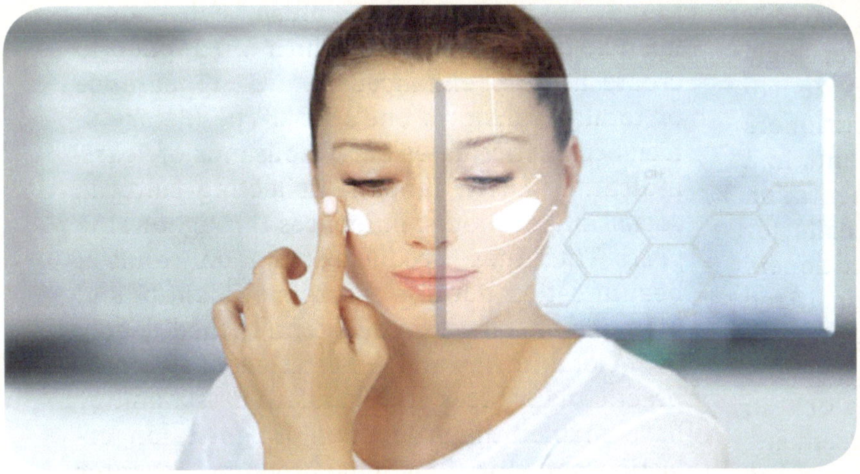

LEARNING OBJECTIVES

After studying this chapter, you will be able to:

1. Describe the historical perspective of facial cosmetics;
2. Highlight the latest technologies in facial cosmetics;
3. Define the non-surgical cosmetic treatments;
4. Discuss the surgical technological advances in facial cosmetics;
5. Comprehend practice management in cosmetic clinics;
6. Be familiar with regulatory and ethical considerations.

Introduction

Over the past decade, facial cosmetics have witnessed revolutionary advances fueled by the wave of technology innovation as well as changing consumer expectations. The use of cutting-edge technologies is transforming many facets of cosmetic procedures, from the formulation and application to overall effectiveness. From advanced imaging systems to nanotechnology, clinicians now have available to them technology that not only enhances the application process but also results in more targeted and effective outcomes. An important tendency in this area is the greater application of nanomaterials, which have emerged as the most important tools to prepare cosmetics and skincare products with improved penetration into the skin and with improved therapeutic effects. With the industry increasingly embracing such advancements, a certain understanding of their implications on practice management remains the utmost priority, so that practitioners can utilize such technologies effectively to meet the needs of their clients according to safety and efficacy parameters (Joseph et al., 2023). Furthermore, with the continuous advancements in facial cosmetics, practitioners are compelled to reconsider their management strategies in order to best capitalize on these developments. Effective practice management in today's world is necessitated by a comprehension of the technology landscape as well as consumer patterns. While minimally invasive facial treatments and personalized skincare regimes are on the rise, practitioners are presented with a complex landscape where exposure to newer technologies, including machine learning and artificial intelligence, becomes increasingly vital. These technologies facilitate evidence-based decision-making, allowing practitioners to tailor treatments to individual patients in a relevant manner. However, the implementation of such advanced technologies also calls for ongoing training and education for practitioners to ensure there is a dynamic and sensitized workforce that is capable of optimizing practice outcomes. With increasingly complex cosmetic treatments, practice management work in facilitating the integration of such advancements is fundamental to ensure patients receive the optimal quality of care (de Vries & Schallig, 2022). The destiny of facial cosmetics is also shaped by technological progress, as well as the importance of ethical practice and care for patients. With more access to aesthetic treatments, concerns over safety, effectiveness, and ethical marketing practices come into the limelight. Practitioners are faced with the dilemma of balancing ethical standards when promoting effective technology that benefits patients. This kind of approach requires constant dialogue among stakeholders, including researchers, practitioners, and regulatory bodies, to govern the changing landscape of cosmetic enhancement judiciously. Focusing on technological advancement and ethics, the application of facial cosmetics can continue in such a manner as to attain greater patient confidence and satisfaction. Ultimately, the combination of technology, practice management, and regulation in an ethical framework will guide the pace of innovation in this rapidly evolving domain towards sustained growth and advancement in the years to come.

Definition of Facial Cosmetics

Facial cosmetics form a broad range of cosmetic products and treatments intended to enhance or modify the appearance of an individual, primarily in the cosmetic definition of the face. This category includes items such as foundations, concealers, blush, eyeshadow, lipstick, and highlighters, which are applied to create a more enhanced natural appearance or totally transform one's look. The history of facial cosmetics dates back thousands of years, indicating a rich timeline reflecting cultural, social, and economic influences throughout the years. Thus, these products are not only tools of beautification but also symbols of identity and methods of self-expression, entrenched deeply in societal norms and expectations. In current practice, advances in formulation technology have enabled the production of lighter, longer-lasting, and more functional products that cater to diverse skin types and personal desires. The significance of face makeup extends far beyond simple enhancement; it plays a crucial role in one's self-esteem and social interactions. The psychological impact of cosmetics has long been established, linking the use of such products to enhanced confidence and self-image. Such is an indication of the intersection of individual identity and cultural norms of beauty standards. In an era where mass media and instantaneous visual information dominate the public sphere, the need for creative solutions in facial cosmetics has skyrocketed. Practitioners finding themselves in this environment need to comprehend the multiple layers of customer motivation to develop effective practice management techniques in the area of facial cosmetics. The responsiveness of the industry to customers' needs fuels constant innovation in product lines and educational initiatives, emphasizing the need for a balanced approach towards satisfaction and loyalty in customers. Advances in the IoT space have also witnessed the infusion of technology in the domain of facial cosmetics, making it not just easier to develop products but also providing for bespoke experiences for customers. Technologies such as augmented reality applications allow consumers to experiment with products virtually prior to purchase, thus transforming the shopping experience.

Moreover, the sustainability and clean beauty trend has compelled cosmetic businesses to rethink ingredients and production, emphasizing safe, eco-friendly products that cater to enlightened consumers (Boyen et al., 2025). With a changing market, professionals must be adaptable and aware of these trends to maintain competitiveness. Through exposure to scientific research and consumer feedback, professionals will not only be enriching their product knowledge but will also become contributory forces for shaping the future of facial cosmetics and creating a more embracing and innovative industry landscape (Kivnick et al., 2014) (Figure 15.1).

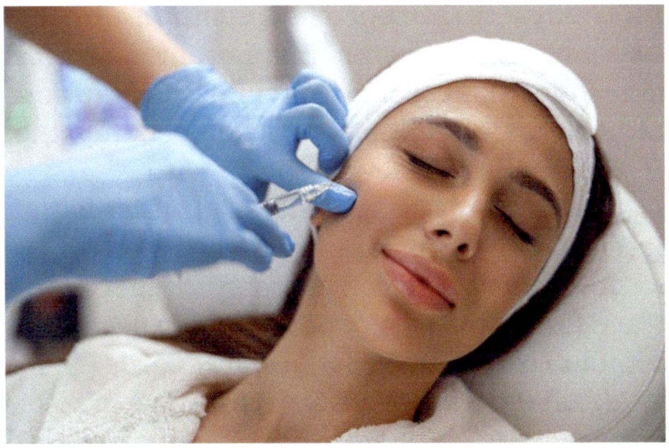

Figure 15.1. Woman getting injection in her face at plastic surgery.

Source: https://virginiaoralsurgeryspecialists.com/wp-content/uploads/2022/07/woman-getting-injection-in-her-face-at-plastic-sur-2022-04-05-15-41-43-utc-scaled.jpg.

Importance of Advances in Technology

The rapid speed of technology has a determining role in reshaping the facial cosmetic scene, both by making treatment more efficient and the information more accessible to the consumer. Advances in non-surgical cosmetic treatments, such as laser therapy and injectable fillers, are an incredible shift towards safer, more effective alternatives to traditional surgery. The integration of advanced technologies has decreased recovery times and lowered risks, appealing to increasingly educated patient groups that value efficacy and safety. Further, patients utilizing extensive information resources on cosmetic procedures have a greater satisfaction rate and increased self-confidence following treatment, emphasizing the value of educated decision-making within this evolving environment (Reisenwitz & Fowler, 2021). This access fuels not only consumer trust but also a competitive marketplace, placing technological advancement as a central component among practice management strategies for cosmetic practitioners. Technological advancements also provide invaluable tools for marketing and patient engagement in the facial cosmetics marketplace. Creating platforms for social media marketing and virtual consultations enables an instant line of contact between practitioners and potential clients, promoting new procedures and in-the-moment results. This shift toward web engagement is reflective of changing consumer sentiment, particularly among newer generations that are inherently predisposed toward online information and visual content. Notably, patients who embrace the full continuum of accessible cosmetic information have proven to possess a reduced cognitive age and greater response to targeted marketing efforts, further highlighting the importance of technology strategy implementation (Reisenwitz & Fowler., 2021). The combined use of technology and aesthetics brings to life a colorful marketing world, where offices are in a position to effectively establish brand loyalty and have a steady stream of clients. Moreover, the interplay of developments in artificial intelligence (AI) and the visualization of aesthetic treatments has become a revolutionary aspect of office management. Immersive systems utilizing AI-generated images produce tailor-made experiences for prospective patients, allowing decision-making to be streamlined from a previously uncertain process. Considering AI-generated images portrays how these technologies can reaffirm or complicate gender stereotypes and norms in the beauty industry. This advanced sensitivity to the visual representation is in harmony with broader social trends and facilitates the practitioner's role in promoting varied and inclusive concepts of beauty. As technology further improves, its impact on practice management in facial cosmetics will increasingly become more profound, allowing more individualized and efficient care while adapting to the more diverse source base of client populations (Figure 15.2).

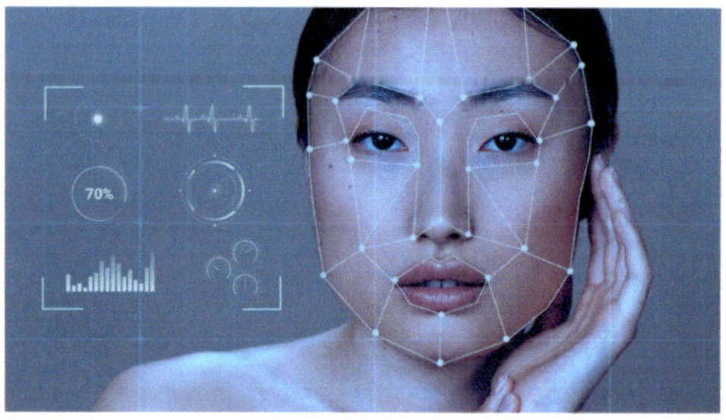

Figure 15.2. Evolution of technology in reshaping the landscape of facial cosmetics.

Source: https://sprivil.com/wp-content/uploads/2025/01/2150038888-1.webp.

Overview of Practice Management in the Industry

Successful practice management in the facial cosmetics sector is more necessary than ever with technology and innovation development altering consumer needs and industry standards. The integration of management strategies within practices in the cosmetic field is closely connected to the enhanced quality of services provided. With the competition that now exists in clinics, the implementation of holistic systems of practice management that include scheduling appointments, patient communication, and data management has become unavoidable. By streamlining operations as well as adopting patient-centered approaches, practitioners can enhance client relationships, hence achieving maximum patient satisfaction and loyalty. On foundations established within other sectors, for instance, marine research as defined by the Marine Board, the cosmetic sector can borrow such common ground to identify best practices that eventually enhance both clinical efficacy and business acumen (Boyen et al., 2025). Furthermore, evolving perspectives of aesthetic treatments compel practitioners to adapt to technological advancements to ensure effective management. Technologies such as telemedicine, emerging imaging technology, and online marketing technology make up invaluable devices to enhance cosmetic practice operational capability. With the application of these technologies, practitioners are in a position to offer bespoke solutions that meet unique client needs, establishing a new platform for client engagement and retention. But the test comes in reconciling potential ethical challenges concerning consumer perceptions and commercialization, most importantly, that of reconciling best practices with the way brand identity is represented. This is all within broader corporate branding concerns where corporations must considerably connect their practices to community norms and expectations without compromising ethical standards (Avery et al., 2007). Lastly, facial cosmetic practice management is an intricate ballet of clinical excellence, technology integration, and moral practice. On one hand, practitioners hone their technique through comments received from consumers and industry norms, yet they must also stay abreast of the swift rate of aesthetic advancement by virtue of continuous education and workforce development. Their success is not just dependent on clinical skill but also on the synergistic application of management theory that builds a positive work environment and enhances the patient experience. As we examine the intersection of technology innovation with successful practice management, it is certain that the future of the business will be shaped by those who prioritize a balanced and ethical strategy for the provision of cosmetic care.

15.1. Historical Context of Facial Cosmetics

Learning Outcome

1. Evolution of Cosmetic Practices
2. Key Milestones in Cosmetic Technology
3. Focus on Cultural Influences on Cosmetic Use

The history of facial cosmetics starts way back in ancient times, when the use of paraphernalia was not merely for beauty but also took on cultural and social functions. In Ancient Egypt, for instance, cosmetics were applied by both men and women as a protection against the intense sun, as well as for ritual purposes. Khol and face paints were common, symbolizing status and a deity figure. As societies progressed towards the Greco-Roman era, cosmetic applications rose because of the influence of class divisions. The elite would depict elaborate face makeup, whereas societal opinions started blending beauty with morality. Thus, the history of cosmetics reflects the positive tension between utilitarian functionality and cultural values and results in modern practices of facial cosmetics that are prompted by aesthetic necessity and deep societal consequences. The Renaissance was a turning point in beauty's understanding with the development of art and philosophy, defining the finer points of cosmetic use. It was also during this time that the beautified image of womanhood arose, and with it, facial cosmetics multiplied within the affluent classes. Ingredients like lead powders and vivid pigments came to symbolize beauty, though at a cost to health. This was a time of opulent depictions of beauty within works of art, and it strengthened the view that cosmetics were used to express social standing and identity. These historical changes highlight the inherent richness of cosmetic practices and herald an evolution that continued through into the Enlightenment, eventually providing the foundations for the commodified beauty industry that exists today. As the modern period progressed, advances in industry created major changes in the production and availability of cosmetics. The late 19th and early 20th centuries saw the emergence of brands that capitalized on the beauty revolution, transitioning cosmetics from homemade concoctions to mass-produced goods.

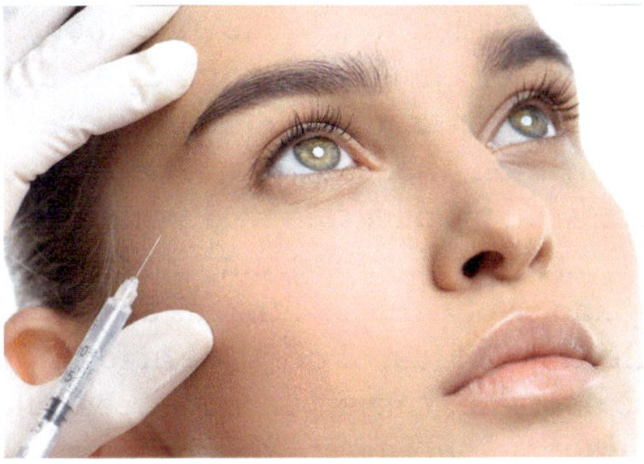

Figure 15.3. Historical evolution of facial cosmetics.

Source: https://hedoxclinic.co.uk/wp-content/uploads/2021/02/botox-1024x680.jpg.

Innovations in marketing, inclusive of widely circulated advertisements, began linking cosmetics to notions of modernity and empowerment, thus reshaping societal standards. Furthermore, movements advocating for women's rights intertwined with beauty norms, revealing a unique relationship between empowerment and appearance. The rich negotiation of such themes, coupled with the commercialization of beauty, directs consideration toward how long-standing facial cosmetics history continues to be underpinned by changing historical context, reflecting complex social narratives and shaping practice management in the field today (Avery et al., 2007; Garrisi et al., 2018) (Figure 15.3).

15.1.1. Evolution of Cosmetic Practices

The evolutionary history of cosmetic practices has witnessed substantial changes, particularly since the advent of advanced technologies and techniques. Conventional cosmetics comprised mostly natural substances, such as minerals and plant extracts, applied for beautification and social communication. With the progress of societies, so evolved the cosmetic techniques and ingredients, culminating in synthetic products. This shift was driven by a demand for range, affordability, and durability, allowing cosmetic corporations to sell to a broader segment. The introduction of chemical technologies during the latter 20th century, as well as the worldwide homogenization of beauty standards, triggered the increase in product complexity and diversity that eventually reshaped assumptions regarding efficacy and safety. This continuous development is a reflection not just of progress in technology but also of greater convergence between culture and personal identity in shaping cosmetics, marking a distinct watershed in the art of facial aesthetics. Practice of cosmetic procedures has expanded dramatically in recent years with impetus coming from advances in non-surgical aesthetics (NSA). The growing popularity of minimally invasive procedures, such as dermal fillers and Botox, is symptomatic of a consumer preference for subtle enhancement over mainstream surgery. All of these developments allow for tailored alterations with less downtime, and prioritize above all safety and convenience. But the rapid growth of NSA procedures has raised training and standardization concerns across the industry. As described in research dedicated to the necessity for a well-structured postgraduate program in NSA, there is a strong need for complex education and training systems to equip practitioners with skills and knowledge to deliver these techniques correctly. The growth of such educational platforms is a reflection of the dynamic nature of cosmetic procedures and the importance of evidence-based education in delivering quality patient outcomes amidst this dynamism (Kumar, 2021). Along with procedural development, technology infusion in cosmetic procedures also encompasses marketing and patient management. Social media has transformed consumer engagement, with individuals being able to influence trends and make products popular. This shift demands that cosmetic professionals embrace electronic tools not only for marketing but also to educate patients and manage post-treatment. Additionally, using data analytics in practice management simplifies clinical operations, leading to better patient outcomes through individualized treatment protocols. With the rising need for cosmetic treatments, it is important that one addresses cosmetic practice management with a strategic plan encompassing clinical competency and effective communication skills. With such an interdisciplinary approach , practitioners are well-positioned to address the challenges in the current cosmetic age, rendering patient satisfaction and safety as the utmost concern of practice (Boyen et al., 2025) (Figure 15.4).

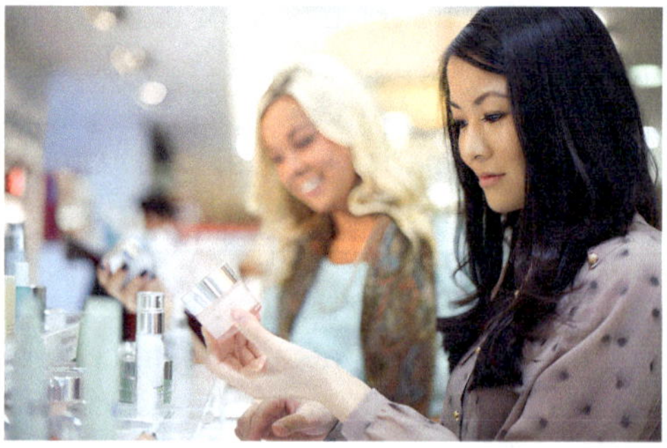

Figure 15.4. Cosmetic practices.

Source: https://mscosmeticslab.com/wp-content/uploads/2024/07/gettyimages-171278045-170667a-1-2.jpg.

15.1.2. Key Milestones in Cosmetic Technology

Evolution in cosmetic technology has been marked by some significant milestones that have had an overwhelming influence on facial cosmetics. One of the most significant has been the coming of minimally invasive treatment, which promoted a shift in public perception towards aesthetic treatments. This has been particularly realized in the popularity of injectable treatments like Botox and dermal fillers. Not only do these treatments provide instant gratification, but they also offer faster recovery times, making cosmetic treatments more affordable to more individuals. Further, advances in the formulation and delivery of cosmetic active ingredients enabled a better understanding of how the product would interact with skin appearance and health. These advancements have hastened consumer buying of products that provide transformational effects while, at the same time, enhancing overall skin health, thus merging beauty and health in new ways. Another trend in the cosmetic industry is the formulation of non-surgical aesthetic (NSA) treatments, which mark a dramatic shift away from traditional surgical alternatives towards less intrusive solutions. The increasing popularity of NSA treatments has required the development of official training and education programs tailored specifically to these technologies. While the integration of NSA training within postgraduate clinical education has been challenging, efforts to develop an evidence-based curriculum have been robust. This move toward formal education is a sign of the mounting appreciation for NSAs role within the cosmetic industry. Programs that focus on standardized assessment techniques, such as the objective structured practical examination (OSPE) and the objective structured clinical examination (OSCE), have been effective in improving practitioners' training. Such models of learning provide necessary skills and knowledge that are relevant in a dynamically changing industry, ensuring safe and effective practices for patients. The use of digital technologies in cosmetic practice is a sea change that shifts the manner in which practitioners engage with patients and provide their services. The arrival of virtual and augmented reality in the cosmetic consultation field allows patients to preview how they might appear post-treatment, leading to better-informed choices. Simulations of procedures in real time reduce fear and enhance satisfaction with the chosen treatment. Furthermore, advancements in data analysis contribute to the robustness of practice management, enabling clinics to learn better about treatment effectiveness, patient needs, and market trends. Through this method of analysis, customized treatment plans are achieved, with services being adjusted to suit patients' needs and maximize success rates. As thus cosmetic technology continues to evolve, the inclusion of new treatments and efficient practice management becomes increasingly important in adapting to changes in the industry (Figure 15.5).

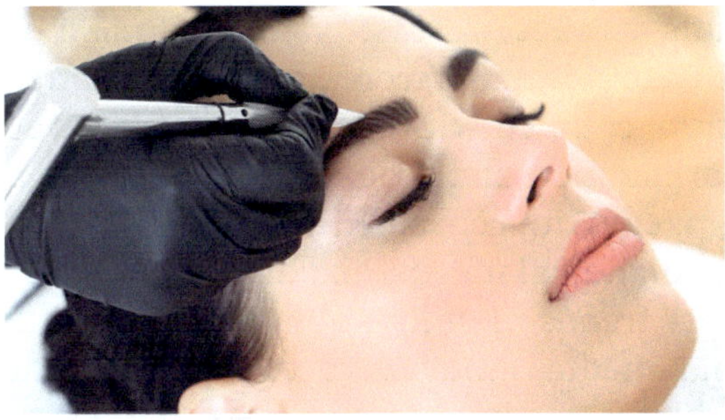

Figure 15.5. Cosmetic technology.

Source: https://soulskinclinic.com/wp-content/uploads/2022/11/Micro-Blading-2.webp.

15.1.3. Cultural Influences on Cosmetic Use

Cultural influences significantly affect the use and perception of cosmetic products, and they become an integral part of societal norms and identity. Beauty standards in other societies are typically dictated by economics, history, and society. For instance, in the majority of Western nations, youthfulness is the preferred norm, and due to this, there has been an increase in the demand for anti-aging treatments and products. Contrastingly, there have been Asian cultures where the desire for light skin has continued the use of whitening creams and sunblock. These are not shallow beauty standards; they affect individuals' self-esteem and can drive their choice concerning the use of cosmetics. Knowing the cultural dimensions is of utmost importance to facial cosmetic practitioners because it forms the basis of effective marketing and the development of suitable products for target consumer groups. The cosmetic industry has come to further realize the importance of cultural narratives, and this has witnessed an explosion of products that cater to diverse beauty standards. Such an adaptation stems from a recognition of diverse cultural worldviews regarding aesthetics, which can drive purchasing habits strongly. For example, increased campaigns for inclusive beauty have led to the diversification of product lines by brands to reflect a greater variation in skin types and colors. It underscores how appreciation of culture, coupled with technological innovation in formulation and production, enables clearer alignment with consumer demands. In addition, with digital platforms making it possible for beauty trends to diffuse quickly—ranging from social media influencers to virtual makeup products in the metaverse—such cultural influences continue to change. Practitioners, have to remain vigilant to such changes to be able to manage product innovation and marketing strategies capable of communicating effectively with current consumer emotions (Damar, 2022). The intersection of such cultural influences with modern technology also offers new possibilities for the cosmetic industry. Artificial intelligence advancements, for example, enable the offering of tailored experiences in cosmetic use, tailoring products to individual preferences based on culture. AI can identify consumer trends and tastes across various populations and thereby inform product innovation and niche marketing. Coupling augmented reality capability enables consumers to try cosmetic products virtually, enhancing their shopping experience and inducing trial over cultural divides. These technologies are particularly relevant when it comes to globalization, where cultural exchanges introduce new standards and practices of beauty. Cosmetic practitioners, therefore, must engage with such technologies in mind while being sensitive to culture, so that the products and services they offer resonate closely with their multicultural clientele (Kazimierczak et al., 2024) (Figure 15.6).

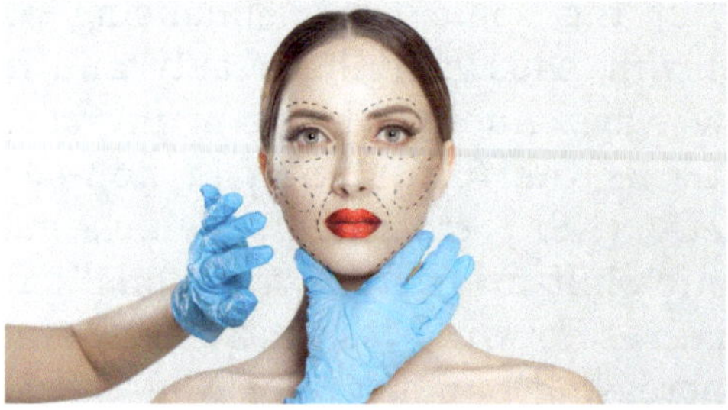

Figure 15.6. Cultural influences on cosmetic use.

Source: https://external-content.duckduckgo.com/iu/?u=https%3A%2F%2Fbioscops.com%2Fwp-content%2Fuploads%2F2024%2F10%2FCultural-Influences-on-Modern-Cosmetic-Surgery-Trends.webp&f=1&nofb=1&ipt=c8b9075f2a2ae00c402d04bda3a937826a94438754ae11d0b151aa79c8293922.

Test Your Knowledge

1. What are some key milestones in the evolution of cosmetic technology throughout history?
2. How have cultural and societal influences shaped the use of facial cosmetics in different regions?
3. Describe the major historical developments that contributed to modern facial cosmetic practices.

15.2. Current Technologies in Facial Cosmetics

Learning Outcome

1. Understand Innovations in Cosmetic Formulations
2. Focus on Advances in Application Techniques
3. Discuss the Role of Digital Technology in Cosmetic Design

The development of current technologies in facial makeup has allowed a transformation of the way consumers perceive and consume these products. Through the integration of artificial intelligence and machine learning, companies in the beauty industry are now able to personalize their suggestions based on the individual's skin tone, skin type, and personal preferences. Such a customized approach not only enhances the level of user satisfaction but also promotes a self-interactive consumption. Such technologies encompass augmented reality (AR) technology, whereby customers are able to try out products virtually prior to buying them, bridging the gap between physical and web stores.

Uptake of such leading-edge tools is part of a broader trend among the cosmetic industry toward personalization to meet the range of needs consumers have, so the products resonate on a deeper level, resulting in increased sales and brand loyalty. Moreover, nanotechnology application in skin cosmetics has provided new avenues of product performance and safety. Nanoparticles are used in products more frequently to enable increased penetration and absorption that lead to more effective delivery of active ingredients to the skin. It allows the development of light, fast-absorbing products that provide amazing results without interfering with the health of the skin. However, as paramount in recent studies, the use of nanoparticles also necessitates a thorough understanding of their possible toxicity and environmental impact, thus sparking ongoing research in their long-term effects on human health and the environment (Joseph et al., 2023). As the industry progresses, the prudent balancing of innovation and safety will be crucial in guaranteeing consumer trust and sustainable growth. Furthermore, with the development of biotechnological advancements, the formulation of cosmetic products has also evolved, with much focus on ethicality and sustainability.

The majority of brands today utilize bioengineered ingredients that are able to mimic the performance of traditional cosmetics while reducing reliance on non-renewable sources. This not only responds to the consumer's demand for green products but also demonstrates the growing concern regarding the ecological impact of the cosmetics sector. Advances such as gene editing and cellular agriculture are unveiling possibilities for sustainable manufacturing, aligning with global sustainability goals. With continuous innovation in the sector, such technological advancements have the potential to reorient standards and shift norms within the realm of cosmetic formulation (de Vries & Schallig, 2022) (Figure 15.7).

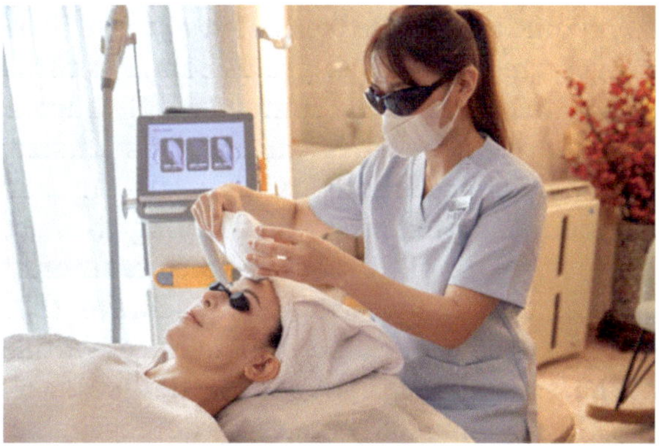

Figure 15.7. Current technologies in facial cosmetics.

Source: https://kellyoriental.com/wp-content/uploads/2022/05/Facial-600x400.jpg.

15.2.1. Innovations in Cosmetic Formulations

The cosmetic formulation history has been strongly impacted by the introduction of nonsurgical facial rejuvenation treatments. Increased public demand for these noninvasive procedures has led to revolutionary breakthroughs in product development and technological advancement. In the past decade, there has been an increase in treatment modalities for cosmetic professionals, in large part due to the inception of botulinum toxin and a variety of dermal fillers. As referenced in Bowler et al. (2009), the facial rejuvenation market has altered with increased physicians providing these treatments to address rising demand. This evolution has also impacted the behavior of consumers and compelled the medical community to embrace and advance their methods of cosmetic improvement, with the ultimate result being an enhanced understanding of the subtleties in facial appearance. Among the cosmetic innovations, the most prevalent and successful method for managing facial aging has been hyaluronic acid (HA) dermal fillers. Time impacts the aging process by inducing various cellular and anatomical changes that lead to a reduction in soft tissue volume, as elaborated in Brandt et al. (2008). HA filler development has revolutionized the treatment of these aging changes among medical professionals, shifting the way they craft facial contouring. Hyaluronic acid's unique properties, including its amazing water-binding ability, make it an amazing treatment for plumping and shaping the face. These types of fillers are a safe, temporary solution that allows clients to achieve their desired aesthetic outcome without the downtime and hassles of surgery. To this, the use of HA fillers has been majorly fueled by demographics, namely the baby-boomer generation. This group has a desperate desire to appear "young" and yet still live an active life; thus, safe and effective cosmetic products are more desirable than ever. Eight HA dermal fillers are now approved by the Food and Drug Administration for sale in the United States, and this represents growing acceptance and use of these new products in facial aesthetics. As noted by Brandt et al. (2008), HA product futures look promising, and research on further improving their performance and expanding their applications for facial rejuvenation continues. Practice management and client expectations, therefore, will be affected by advances in cosmetic formulations in the ever-evolving realm of facial cosmetics (Figure 15.8).

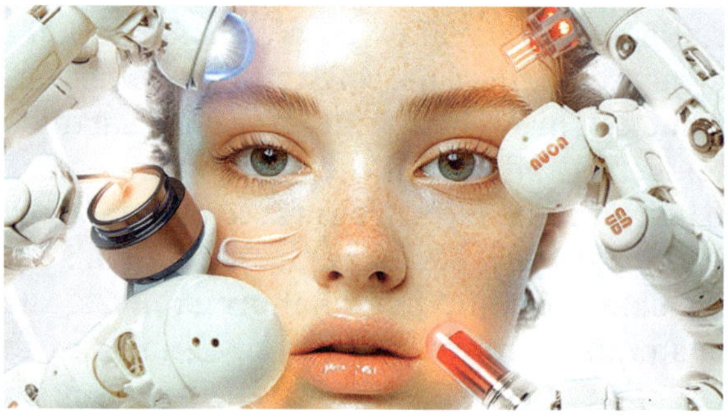

Figure 15.8. Cosmetic formulations.

Source: https://img.gcimagazine.com/files/base/allured/all/image/2025/01/Head_Banner_Pic.677c19bd73e8d.png?auto=format%2Ccompress&q=70&w=700.

15.2.2. Advances in Application Techniques

The evolution of application techniques in facial cosmetics has revolutionarily transformed the industry, enhancing product functionality and presentation. Previously, application techniques were rudimentary, resulting in uneven results or a weird look. Nowadays, advanced developments have initiated a variety of new tools and techniques that not only enhance user experience but also support a variety of skin types and preferences. For instance, technological improvements in airbrushes now allow for a smooth finish that simulates natural skin texture and also buildable coverage. Furthermore, application methods such as baking and strobing are now popular, allowing individuals to achieve radiant skin or long-lasting makeup, respectively. Such innovations encourage an independent approach to beauty, allowing individuals to embrace their unique features while at the same time enhancing their overall look. Moreover, where cosmetics have converged with technology, a new age of application methods has arisen in the form of online platforms. Augmented reality (AR) technology and Android apps allow consumers to test products virtually prior to purchasing, making product selection efficient without causing dissatisfaction. Not only does this technological advance revolutionize the buying process of consumers but also provides brands with more efficient means of engaging with consumers. By providing detailed lessons and instant feedback, these apps foster a culture of self-enablement and makeup application skill development. Moreover, business houses have started using data analytics to refine their offerings and fine-tune marketing to make them more targeted, ensuring they are aligned with shifting consumer preferences and tastes. More sustainable practice in the business has also influenced application trends, compelling brands to become innovative for the eco-conscious consumer. Waste-reducing methods—reusable applicators and refillable containers—are on the rise. This not only addresses the environmental concern, but it also encourages a more mindful approach to beauty treatments. While companies are striving to decrease their impact, eco-friendly application methods take center stage, creating a sense of responsibility among consumers, now better informed about the impact of their actions. In addition, the use of educational content on sustainable use in product advertising raises responsible consumption significance, therefore brand loyalty and consumer accountability. With these new ways, the facial cosmetic industry is technical as well as ethical in orientation, with a thorough change in practice management (Figure 15.9).

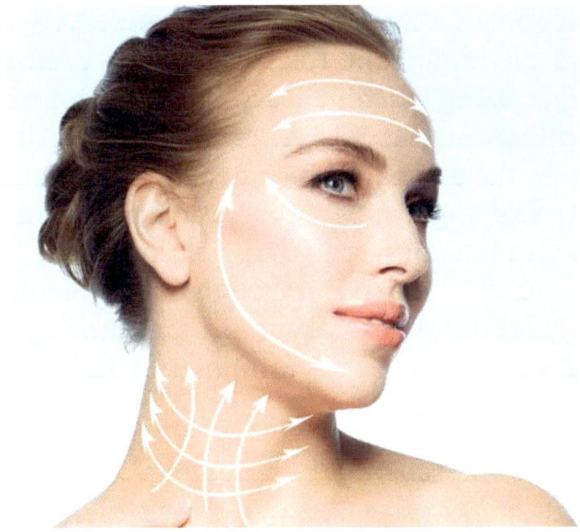

Figure 15.9. Application techniques in facial cosmetics.

Source: https://iicad.org/wp-content/uploads/2024/06/IICAD-Mumbai-1-1200x600.png.

15.2.3. Role of Digital Technology in Cosmetic Design

In the practice of cosmetic design, the application of technology is transforming traditional methods into vibrant, precise ones. One of the technologies that has empowered cosmetic artists to create very detailed and personalized designs to a high degree of precision is computer-aided design (CAD). This allows for a smooth synthesis of creative imagination and technological innovation, elevating the practice within facial cosmetics. Furthermore, augmented reality (AR) technologies enable clients to visualize possible outcomes before actually undergoing procedures. Through the simulation of various cosmetic procedures in a virtual environment, clients are more confident in their choices, resulting in a generally improved experience. The use of digital technologies not only streamlines the design process but also allows practitioners to refine their skills, offering customized solutions that respond to the diverse needs of their patients, a reflection of the evolving world of facial cosmetic treatments. The use of developments in artificial intelligence (AI) also plays an important role in shaping cosmetic design. Using machine learning algorithms and deep learning models, AI can learn from large sets of facial images and derive personalized traits and suggest best cosmetic treatments. In oral and maxillofacial (OMF) cosmetic surgery, specifically, AI assists in preoperative planning and prediction of outcomes, optimizing the surgeon's ability and minimizing risks with human analysis.

The increasing reliance on AI readies practitioners for making informed therapeutic decisions, thus ensuring the aesthetic ideals are in congruence with the anatomical features of each patient. This shift towards digital intelligence is typical of a broader paradigm within the cosmetic industry, where technology is not only expected to enhance procedural efficacy but also has a primary role to play in issues of ethical importance about patient information and treatment transparency, such as in emerging technologies applied in medical practice (Rokhshad et al., 2023). Of greater significance is that the development of the metaverse represents an epoch-changing platform for the integration of digital technology and cosmetic design. With the application of virtual reality (VR) and augmented reality (AR), the metaverse offers unprecedented opportunities for immersive client consultations and interactive learning opportunities for professionals. With clients engaging with avatars that display their potential cosmetic outcomes within an imaginary space, they are able to explore many design options in real time, thus helping them make more informed decisions on their cosmetic journey. This innovation extends beyond client consultation, with metaverse platforms being used by health practitioners to simulate training, refining their techniques in a risk-free environment. With recent technological advances, incorporating metaverse elements into the cosmetic design process represents a significant shift in practice management, with increased client satisfaction and improved surgical outcomes on the horizon (Damar, 2022) (Figure 15.10).

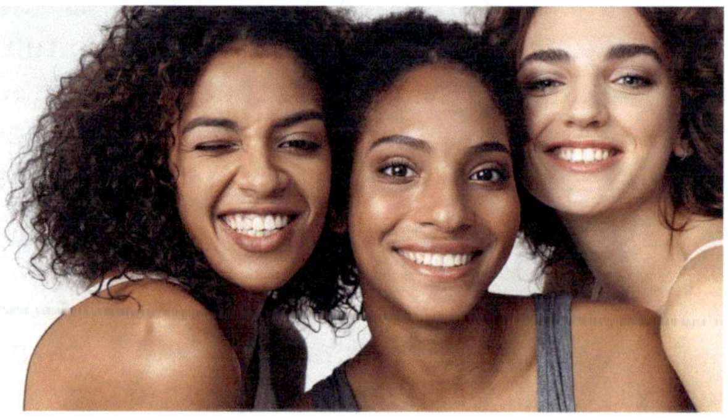

Figure 15.10. Role of digital technology in cosmetic design.

Source: https://www.thequeenzone.com/wp-content/uploads/2024/11/gorgeous-woman.-Dean-Drobot-via-Shutterstock.jpg.

Test Your Knowledge

1. What recent innovations in cosmetic formulations have improved efficacy and safety in facial cosmetics?
2. How have advances in application techniques enhanced precision and outcomes in cosmetic procedures?
3. What role does digital technology play in modern cosmetic design and treatment planning?

15.3. Non-Surgical Cosmetic Procedures

Learning Outcome

1. Overview of Popular Non-Surgical Treatments
2. Focus on Safety and Efficacy of Non-Surgical Options
3. Explain Patient Satisfaction and Outcomes

The rising popularity of non-surgical cosmetic treatments is an overall trend toward beautification with minimal recovery time and risk. Treatments such as dermal fillers, Botox injections, and chemical peels are now routine, as individuals desire subtle but noticeable changes. The treatments have many benefits, including immediate results, less risk than surgical procedures, and relatively low costs. Consequently, practitioners in the main are faced with more demand from patients starved for rejuvenation but not with the burden of traditional surgical interventions. Besides, faster developments in formulations of products, methods of application, and delivery systems have entrenched non-surgical options firmly as viable alternatives, thereby altering the landscape of facial aesthetics entirely. Increased availability and popularity of such treatments reflect their pivotal role in the beauty standards today, in support of the contention that patients are able to achieve desired outcomes more easily than ever before. In addition to their functional uses, technological improvements have spawned enormous innovation in the field of non-surgical cosmetic therapy. Non-invasive treatments like laser treatment and ultrasound treatments use innovative mechanisms to enhance the quality of skin, reduce the perceptibility of wrinkles, and stimulate collagen production. These techniques take advantage of innovations like nanotechnology to target drugs at the intended locations and maximize therapeutic impacts, thereby enhancing the effectiveness of interventions (Joseph et al., 2023). Furthermore, the incorporation of 3D printing technologies has already begun transforming practice management through the capability for printing patient-specific models for pre-procedure simulation and planning. This incorporation enhances efficiency and outcome while showing remarkable synergy between technology and non-surgical care. With professionals embracing such advances, patients benefit from enhanced procedural tailoring, which equates to improved satisfaction as well as superior aesthetic results. Despite the rapid expansion and demand for non-surgical cosmetic treatments, there are still a few issues within the practice management space. Some of the practitioners hurrying to be in the business might be unaware of regulating and ethics requirements, which are indispensable to ensure patient safety and satisfaction as well.

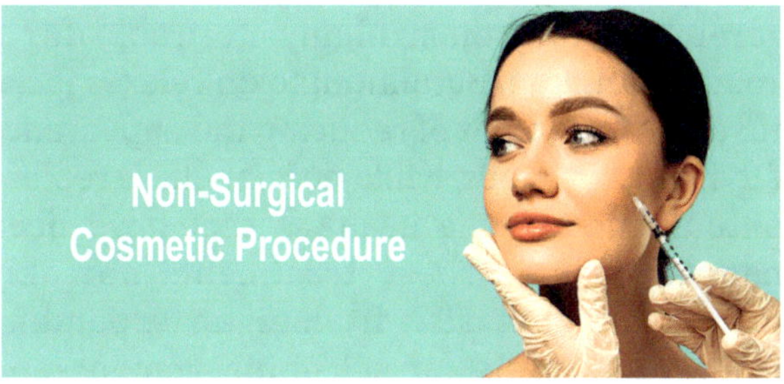

Figure 15.11. Non-surgical cosmetic procedures.

Source: https://drlouisedelange.com/wp-content/uploads/2025/03/BLOG-DE-LANGE-1.png.

Additional training in the existing technologies, techniques, and materials required to maintain high-quality care is the success factor. As new emerging solutions and technologies arise, healthcare practitioners will be required to catch up with trends that might affect the outcome of procedures, such as the expansion of personalized treatments, driven by advancements in 3D printing and enhanced imaging (Meyer-Szary et al., 2022). Developing an ethic of continuous learning and adaptation is therefore necessary for practitioners who will be capable of effectively handling the complexities in non-surgical cosmetic practice. This focused approach will not only improve the safety and satisfaction of patients but will also maintain the professionalism and credibility of the aesthetics field (Figure 15.11).

15.3.1. Overview of Popular Non-Surgical Treatments

In the practice of facial cosmetics, non-surgical treatments have become extremely popular, allowing patients to avail themselves of techniques to enhance their appearance without going through invasive surgeries. Among the most popular treatments are injectable applications, such as botulinum toxin and dermal fillers. Minimal and brief in application, these procedures take little to no downtime, thereby making them highly desirable for a broad population. Botulinum toxin relaxes facial muscles to the point of reducing the appearance of dynamic wrinkles, while dermal fillers replace contour and volume in areas that have been changed by age. These treatments not only treat beauty but also fit into an expanding societal emphasis on self-improvement and maintenance, validating the role of non-surgical interventions in contemporary cosmetic care. Another novel non-surgical facial rejuvenation method is photodynamic therapy (PDT), which takes advantage of the interaction between light and photosensitizers to treat a range of skin disorders. PDT is increasingly known for its utility in the treatment of precancerous cells, sun-damaged skin, and even acne, demonstrating its versatility. With its ability to facilitate targeted cell destruction while modulating the immune response, PDT has become a holistic therapeutic avenue in dermatology. As the ease of delivery of treatment increases, so too can the dermatologist easily offer PDT as an option, thereby facilitating the patient experience by means of non-invasive treatment. This greater acceptance of PDT by the cosmetic industry is reflective of a shift towards the introduction of advanced applications of technology to face treatments, emphasizing the demand for non-surgical methods of present-day care. In addition, LED-red light therapy is also attracting interest for its ability to modulate cellular activity in skin fibrosis, a source of concern for most patients who receive facial cosmetic procedures.

The efficacy of LED-RL has already been depicted in preliminary clinical trials of minimizing post-surgical scarring, which indicates its promise as an adjuvant treatment in cosmetic care. Harnessing specific wavelengths of light to control fibroblast activity and collagen production, LED-RL provides a new, non-invasive therapeutic modality for enhancing the quality of postoperative outcomes. Beyond cosmetics, its potential is to improve skin quality in general as well as the healing process. As is confirmed in studies, integration of LED-RL into cosmetic treatment regimens can potentially pave the way for setting the trend for elevated standards of facial appearance, affirming the paradigm shift towards non-surgical, safer procedures while focusing on both outcome and patient well-being (Heilman et al., 2019; Lin et al., 2014) (Figure 15.12).

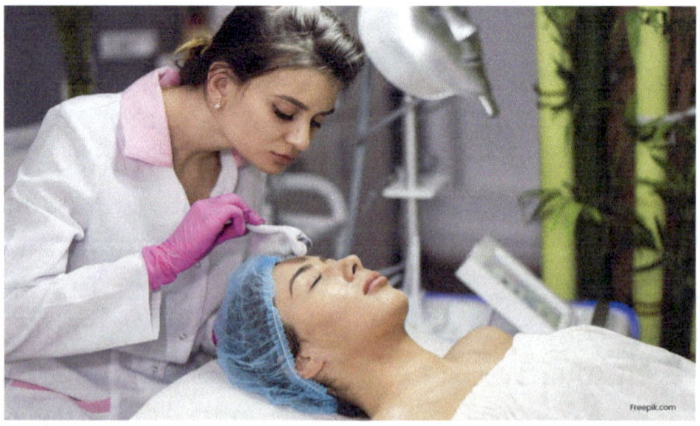

Figure 15.12. Popular non-surgical treatments.

Source: https://www.osvidermatology.com/wp-content/uploads/2023/11/advance-treatment.jpg.

15.3.2. Safety and Efficacy of Non-Surgical Options

The revelation of non-surgical modalities in facial cosmetics has gained popularity on a wide scale due to their safety and efficiency in enhancing quality without the dangers associated with surgery. Techniques such as dermal fillers, neurotoxin injections, and platelet-rich plasma (PRP) therapy are now highly demanded alternatives that promise rejuvenation with less downtime. The efficacy of treatments like these is pointed out by their ability to create focused results, such as wrinkle relaxation and volume increase, while reducing recovery times traditionally required by surgical interventions. As observed in recent studies, non-surgical interventions have been shown to have a significant impact on patient satisfaction and aesthetic results, thus being valid choices in modern-day facial cosmetic treatment, where client safety and natural results remain priorities. Particularly, PRP therapy is gaining popularity for its diverse applications in cosmetic dermatology. With the application of the body's own inherent healing process, PRP enhances the skin texture, promotes hair growth, and accelerates the wound healing process. Because PRP employs the patient's own plasma, it is less likely to cause any harmful reactions, thus possessing a good safety profile. Current literature points to its application not just in improving the appearance of the skin but also in treating chronic wounds and reversing aging skin. With an understanding of the mechanism of PRP being augmented, its utilization in aesthetics has continued to rise, underlining the importance of evidence-based practices in ensuring safety and efficacy in non-surgical aesthetic interventions (Patel et al., 2023). Although generally there is less danger of complications linked with non-surgical treatments than with surgery, it is nonetheless required to answer to the regulatory and technological frameworks that govern their administration. The Food and Drug Administration (FDA) has established stringent standards for medical treatments and devices, developing a whole process for the regulation and approval of non-surgical cosmetic therapies. This rule seeks to guarantee that the devices used in such therapies are effective and safe. In addition, with emerging technology, innovations such as artificial intelligence and Internet of Things (IoT) are revolutionizing practice management by allowing practitioners to use data-driven intelligence to advance patient care (Tettey et al., 2023). By keeping an eye on the regulatory framework and adopting innovation, practitioners can significantly enhance the safety and efficacy of non-surgical procedures in facial cosmetology (Figure 15.13).

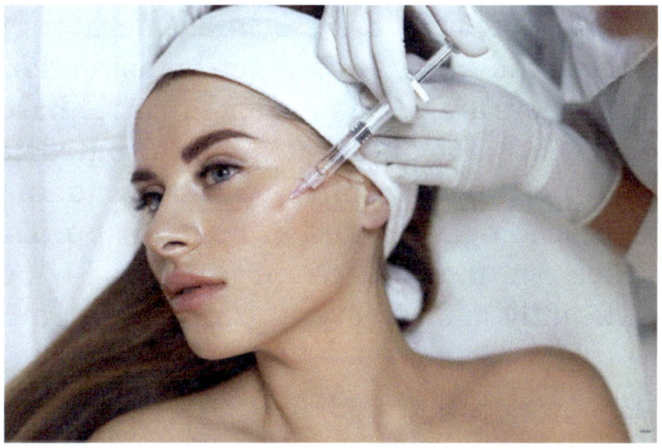

Figure 15.13. Safety and efficacy of non-surgical options.

Source: https://cdn.jasonbdiamond.com/wp-content/uploads/2023/12/14155942/Shutterstock_1724712010.jpg.

15.3.3. Patient Satisfaction and Outcomes

Given the extremely competitive facial cosmetics market in today's world, patient satisfaction is a key indicator of success for both the practitioner and the quality of procedure carried out. Recent advances in technology and methodology in aesthetic medicine have transformed the industry to a great extent, making treatments more personalized. Patients today expect customized approaches to treating their particular concerns, which is key to providing favorable outcomes. Emerging studies have emphasized the pivotal relationship between appropriately created training for non-surgical aesthetic (NSA) treatments and improved patient experiences. These procedures, many of which are carried out in private clinics, call for an elaborate model of training to guarantee practitioners possess the technical ability as well as people skills required to optimize patient interactions and, in the process, create more satisfaction (Kumar, 2021). The integration of feedback from patients into practice management has been increasingly important in guaranteeing facial cosmetic treatments yield positive results. Growing literature supports the assertion that patient-reported outcomes are essential indicators in assessing the success of aesthetic interventions. Practitioners are urged to adopt evidence-based models that not only track clinical outcomes but also carefully monitor patients' emotional and psychological states. A holistic approach focuses on the client's perspective, which significantly adds to overall satisfaction rates. As the somatology profession evolves, the blending of systematic training, as portrayed in overviews of the practice area, works to accentuate the importance of comprehending the technical and emotional aspects of caring for patients (Vosloo, 2025). Consequently, education and skill acquisition cannot be overstressed in facial cosmetic practice. Continuing professional education via a robust curriculum is the impetus for enhanced patient outcomes and satisfaction rates. There is evidence to show that organized courses of education, such as those built via the Delphi method, can foster critical thinking and practical skills needed within this very complex area of practice. Also, developing effective rapport between somatologists and patients raises the prospects of compliance by patients with post-treatment instructions and follow-ups, eventually leading to better aesthetic results. The practitioners must thus be responsive to both technological advancements and educational needs to ensure that they are adequately equipped to counter evolving patient expectations while promoting long-term satisfaction (Kumar, 2021; Vosloo, 2025)

Test Your Knowledge

1. How is the safety and efficacy of non-surgical cosmetic procedures evaluated?
2. What factors influence patient satisfaction and outcomes following non-surgical cosmetic treatments?

15.4. Surgical Advances in Facial Cosmetics

Learning Outcome

1. Discuss Latest Techniques in Facial Surgery
2. Focus on Minimally Invasive Surgical Options
3. Explain the Ethical Considerations in Surgical Practices

Recent surgical advancements in facial cosmetics have revolutionized procedures that plastic surgeons and other specialists employ. Previously, procedures were considered invasive and complex. However, due to technological improvements, there has been apparent procedural simplification. For instance, the application of minimally invasive techniques such as endoscopic brow lifts and transconjunctival blepharoplasty has minimized downtime while enhancing aesthetic outcomes. Surgeons can now utilize procedures that minimize scarring and bruising, thus making aesthetic surgery less intimidating for patients. Additionally, the new technology of 3D imaging systems offers precise pre-surgical assessments, optimizing surgical planning and allowing more accurate post-surgical result predictions, thus enhancing patient satisfaction. As cosmetic surgery advances, patient-centric and accuracy-focused approaches are likely to impact further development within the specialty so that surgery remains at the center of enhancing facial attractiveness as per the patient's wish. Another improvement in surgical technology is the increasing use of fat grafting as a means of facial rejuvenation. This technique has volumetric augmentation with natural results through the utilization of the patient's adipose tissue and has superior results compared to traditional filler injections. The recent innovations have improved the procedure, such as the development of advanced harvesting and purifying techniques, which enhance the survival of the graft and reduce complications. Physicians now have sophisticated liposuction techniques through which they can harvest good-quality grafts that yield esthetically pleasing facial contour refinement. In addition, the suggested surge in minimally invasive procedures can also be interpreted in terms of the trend towards preserving the natural appearance of the face. Therefore, not only does the procedure indicate a tendency towards natural outcomes, but also a broader trend for cosmetic procedures that is concerned with safety and long-term satisfaction for patients who receive facial enhancement. The addition of interdisciplinary collaboration has also taken center stage as one of the most important trends in surgical facial cosmetics. With further developed comprehension of the intricacy of facial anatomy, practitioners from all fields, such as dermatology, maxillofacial surgery, and oculoplastic surgery, are coming together to offer whole-brained care to patients. This collaborative practice is also observed by joint procedures, wherein surgeons address multiple cosmetic concerns simultaneously, resulting in effective treatment schedules and higher overall patient satisfaction. Moreover, the adoption of new standards of direction, as realized within the cosmetic practice, enhances the significance of an integrated approach to handling facial cosmetic treatment, enabling experts to share information and enhance the quality of patient treatment. Finally, the cosmetic surgical future lies at the nexus of collaboration and innovation, leading to more streamlined treatment paradigms and happier patients in the field of cosmetics (Figure 15.14).

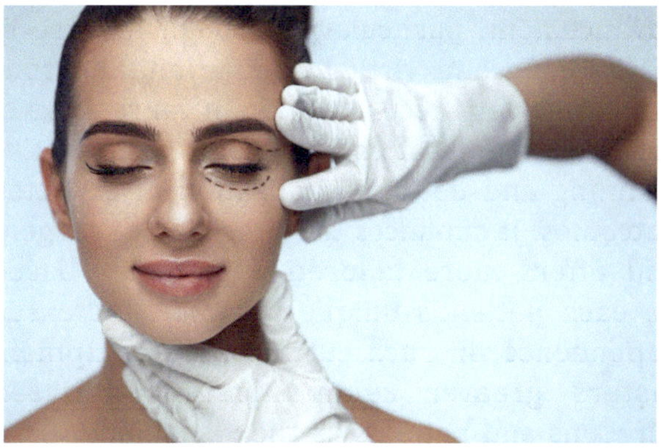

Figure 15.14. Surgical advances in facial cosmetics.

Source: https://external-content.duckduckgo.com/iu/?u=https%3A%2F%2Fpoppcosmeticsurgery.com%2Fwp-content%2Fuploads%2F2021%2F12%2FCosmetic-Surgery.jpg&f=1&nofb=1&ipt=3ebf983c95a023a892981ea711f48b483996e3cb7c8408433e597b1067838bca.

15.4.1. Latest Techniques in Facial Surgery

The rapid progress in facial surgery over the past few years has been highlighted through the use of minimally invasive techniques, which have changed patient care and outcomes dramatically. Surgeons increasingly employ endoscopic surgery, which allows for smaller incisions and minimal tissue destruction, and thus rapid recoveries and reduced scarring. This method has proven particularly valuable in operations such as brow lifts and facelifts, which once generated a lot of downtime. Growing expertise with these operations is part of a broader movement toward patient satisfaction and safety, in which individuals can achieve their cosmetic objectives with less physical and psychological cost. Such innovation not only enhances the surgery process but also demonstrates the capability of the medical sector to react and adapt to the increasing demand for effective but minimally invasive facial cosmetic surgeries. Moreover, the role of technology in facial surgery has seen spectacular advancement, particularly through the use of 3D imaging and virtual simulation. Surgeons can create very accurate anatomical replicas of patients' faces that enable easier preoperative planning and better visualization of expected outcomes. It enhances the precision of surgery and offers more tailored approaches based on each patient's unique anatomy. Increased dependence on such cutting-edge equipment fosters greater communication between surgeons and patients as the visual aids assist in creating proper patient expectations. Besides, the advancement of surgical procedures through improved imaging assists in continuous learning and professional development in the profession to enable practitioners to maintain efficiency in carrying out contemporary approaches. With these advancements in technology, they too can continue to revolutionize facial surgery procedures in the field of cosmetics. The record-breaking need for facial cosmetic procedures has also been driven by the call for holistic education and training in non-surgical aesthetics. In order to fill the knowledge gap, evidence-based postgraduate programs are being designed, emphasizing the newest non-surgical techniques like fillers and botulinum toxin therapy. Development of formal training systems is important to ensure that the standards of care are upheld, as there are increased professionals entering the field by virtue of public interest in the noninvasive treatments (Bowler, 2009). This educational focus is paramount, given that an educated practitioner can significantly influence patient satisfaction and safety. Furthermore, the incorporation of approaches such as objective structured clinical examinations (OSCE) allows for testing of fundamental competencies in aesthetic practice (Kumar, 2021). As facial cosmetics evolve with newer techniques and technology, the movement towards structured education paths is vital for long-term growth in the industry (Figure 15.15).

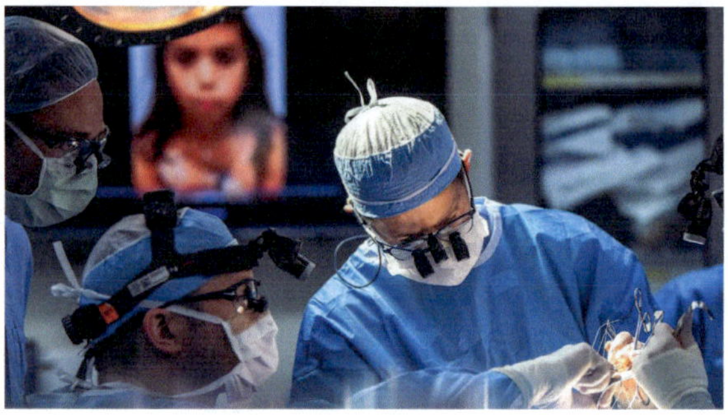

Figure 15.15. Advances in facial surgery.

Source: https://assets.clevelandclinic.org/transform/LargeFeatureImage/69603611-5eca-4061-9dde-ecb8b5c86bfc/CCC_2191938_06-08-21_349_AMO.

15.4.2. Minimally Invasive Surgical Options

Minimally invasive surgical options have significantly transformed the face of facial cosmetic procedures, giving patients efficient options over traditional surgeries. These innovative techniques are characterized by small incisions, less trauma to the surrounding tissues, and shorter recovery times, and as such, more patients are turning to them to attain their desired aesthetic enhancements. Given facial aging's complex interaction of intrinsic and extrinsic forces, the combination of surgical and non-invasive methods provides a holistic approach to treatment. Therapies such as Ultherapy and fat grafting exemplify the trend as they achieve remarkable outcomes in rejuvenation without long recoveries typical of more invasive treatments. This shift towards refinement in surgical intervention is a growing recognition of taste in aesthetics and a desire for naturally appearing outcomes, and hence minimally invasive treatments form a major part in practice management strategies (Portilla et al., 2024). In addition to lifts and tightening, the growing popularity of neurotoxin injections and fillers has transformed the landscape of minimally invasive cosmetics. All of these non-surgical therapies ease the anxieties of risk and cost that otherwise accompany traditional surgical procedures. With therapies like Botox and dermal fillers, doctors can create significant facial enhancements with minimal downtime, corresponding to the expanding need for convenient and effective cosmetic treatments. These therapies, in turn, provide a lower-risk profile, with complications being rare and generally temporary. According to existing evidence, the rates of patient satisfaction with such minimally invasive techniques are remarkably high, further validating their efficacy and widespread use in contemporary practice. This dual technique, applying both minimally invasive surgical and non-surgical treatments, allows practitioners to provide a diverse array of interventions tailored to every patient's interests and requirements (Timraz et al., 2025). The use of newer technology in minimally invasive surgery has raised procedural precision and patient outcomes, a great advancement of facial cosmetic surgery. Procedures such as thread lifts, where polydioxanone (PDO) and polylactic acid (PLA) materials are used, are great examples of how this branch has evolved to provide effective lifting and contouring with minimal downtime. These treatments stimulate collagen generation, giving patients not just immediate aesthetic gains but also long-term rejuvenating effects in the future. Moreover, technologies like high-intensity focused ultrasound (HIFU) and radiofrequency procedures have further expanded the scope of non-invasive treatments, enabling practitioners to tailor treatments based on individual patient needs. With the help of these technological developments, practitioners are able to increase their service, enhance patient satisfaction, and manage the practice efficiently in a competitive market. Synergistic application of minimally invasive approaches and new technologies emphasizes the evolving dynamics in facial cosmetic surgery (Portilla et al., 2024) (Figure 15.16).

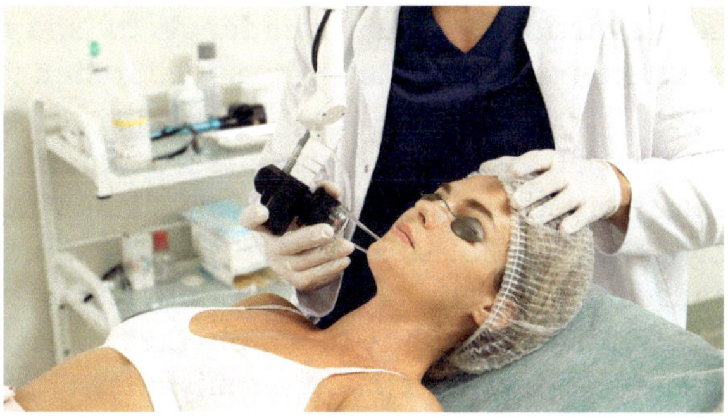

Figure 15.16. Minimally invasive surgical options.

Source: https://symbiosishospital.com/wp-content/uploads/2022/03/Symbiosis-Invasive-Surgeries.jpg.

15.4.3. Ethical Considerations in Surgical Practices

With the rapidly evolving age of facial cosmetics, ethical considerations in surgical practices acquire further significance. With procedure availability being ever more enabled by technology, the specter of inapt training among practitioners can lead to serious patient injury. The absence of formal training schemes within non-surgical aesthetics has highlighted the imperative for an evidence-based curriculum, as evidenced recently in a study that identified current knowledge gaps in the specialty (Kumar, 2021). This points to the ethical obligation of medical staff to not just take up continuous learning but also engage in comprehensive learning programs that ensure proficiency with new technologies. The necessity of maintaining patient safety and joy still remains topmost, since any lapse in ethics would result in bodily and psychological harm to patients undergoing cosmetic enhancement. Another pressing ethical concern of surgical practice is that of the process of informed consent, which underlies patient autonomy. Surgeons and practitioners have a duty to ensure that patients understand risks, benefits, and achievable outcomes of cosmetic procedures, particularly because social media and advertising have a tendency to shape expectations in misleading ways (Fedorchenko, 2024). This poses a threat of misalignment between patient expectations and surgical reality. Ethical practice demands that physicians not only provide full disclosure but also sympathetic counseling that accepts patients' motivations for such treatments. Failure to uphold these ethical standards creates a climate of misinformation and exploitation, which ultimately undermines the trust so essential to the doctor-patient relationship. Last, the social implications of aesthetic enhancement deserve ethical scrutiny, particularly the perpetuation of unrealistic beauty ideals. The increasing volume of cosmetic surgeries can promote a culture with a higher value of physical appeal than other attributes, further increasing body dysmorphic disorder and low self-worth in vulnerable groups. As trends currently indicate, the increase in procedures is often accompanied by social pressures, thus making the ethical climate for practitioners even more difficult (Fedorchenko, 2024). It is incumbent upon practicing professionals not only to be responsive to these pressures but also to labor on behalf of patient-centered care that supports healthy body image and psychological well-being. Knowledge of the broader social context in which these ethical concerns operate is essential in traversing the sensitive terrain of surgical practice in facial aesthetics.

Test Your Knowledge

1. What are the latest techniques in facial cosmetic surgery that have improved surgical outcomes?
2. How have minimally invasive surgical options changed the approach to facial cosmetic procedures?
3. What ethical considerations must surgeons keep in mind when performing facial cosmetic surgeries?

15.5. Practice Management in Cosmetic Clinics

Learning Outcome

1. Importance of Effective Management Strategies
2. Staff Training and Development
3. Patient Relationship Management

Practice management in aesthetic clinics has also become more complex as the changes brought about by advancing technology reshape the landscape of cosmetic medicine. Modern practices are confronted not only with traditional business protocol but also with the procedures of integrating new procedures that address the client's demand for outcome-based treatments. As the cosmetic surgery market continues to grow, professionals are tasked with adopting multidimensional management processes including patient education, operational efficiency, and financial prudence. The inclusion of new methods, such as dorsal augmentation (DA) rhinoplasty, calls for advanced training and ongoing professional development to remain up-to-date with this competitive market. By implementing effective practice management systems, clinics are able to enhance patient satisfaction, provide superior treatment results, and ultimately develop a sustainable practice that answers changing consumer demands and the rapid rate of technological advances (Nikparto et al., 2024). In addition to safeguarding patient safety and quality of care, which are foremost concerns in the field of cosmetic procedures, effective practice management becomes imperative. The incorporation of regenerative medicine techniques, such as the use of platelet-rich plasma (PRP) for wound healing, underscores the need to have stringent procedure protocols instituted by cosmetic clinics. Management strategies that prioritize safety can reduce the possibility of new technology pitfalls, thus creating a culture of trust among consumers. Monitoring clinical practice and vigilant observation of patient outcomes over time can form the foundation of quality improvement initiatives.

Having adequate guidelines and staff training adds an overall enhancement in patient experience through an informed and compassionate setting that favors the long-term operation of the clinic in the highly regulated setting of cosmetic services (Patel et al., 2023). Finally, the financial sustainability of cosmetic clinics is reliant on a good practice management plan that considers operational costs as well as generating revenues. With the increasing popularity of beauty treatments, clinics must develop a strong grasp of consumer behavior and market trends in order to devise appropriate pricing mechanisms based on the value of service. Leveraging the most up-to-date technology in marketing campaigns, such as social media interaction and online consultation, can enhance client acquisition and retention activities. In addition, effective financial planning steps like cost-benefit analysis and resource allocation allow clinics to be competitive without sacrificing sustainable development. Through a mix of the latest advances in cosmetic treatments and effective management of practice, clinics can position themselves in an increasingly dynamic and evolving business sector in facial aesthetics (Figure 15.17).

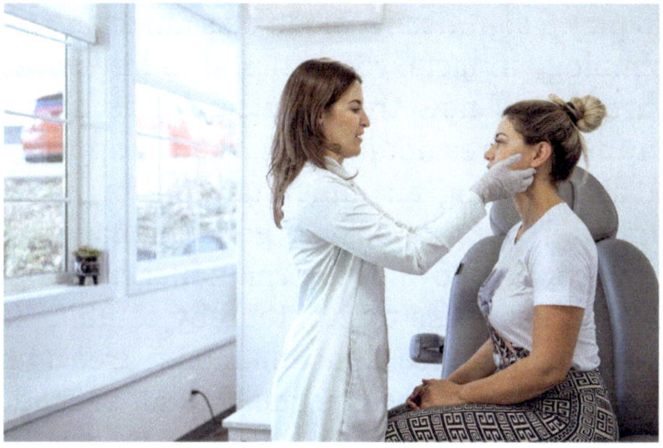

Figure 15.17. Practice management in cosmetic clinics.

Source: https://medizinonline.com/wp-content/uploads/2018/09/iStock-1359714290.jpg.

15.5.1. Importance of Effective Management Strategies

Effective management of facial cosmetic treatment advancements is essential in ensuring patient safety and satisfaction. With technologies evolving constantly, practitioners must develop effective management strategies in order to handle the changes. The strategies involve an extensive array of business practices, including staff training, patient engagement, and health regulation compliance. An example is the application of light-emitting diode-red light (LED-RL) technology, which offers new therapeutic avenues, but its usage requires best-practice comprehension of the protocol in order to gain maximum benefits of treatment and avoid side effects. Evidence indicates that excessive procedural transgressions may lead to suboptimal consequences in their application for the management of skin fibrosis, which highlights the mutualistic relationship between technology, practice management, and clinical results (Heilman et al., 2019). Considering these facts, the importance of strategic management in practice cannot be exaggerated, as it has a direct impact on enhanced patient outcomes and service quality. Apart from operational management, effective marketing and education also play a significant role in disseminating new technology in facial cosmetics. Building patient awareness of new treatments such as LED-RL therapy requires not just a marketing approach, but also gaining an understanding of patient fears and perceptions. A good management approach can allow for informational campaigns that address these topics, thereby establishing patient confidence and enhancing treatment uptake rates. Equally important is staff education to ensure all staff deliver uniform, credible information on procedures and outcomes. Since education and marketing have priority in effective sound management strategies, practice can excel in a competitive marketplace, resulting in increased patient engagement and loyalty (Nova Southeastern University, 2014).

The intersection of education and management, thus, offers windows of opportunity for effective integration of state-of-the-art technologies in practice. Lastly, the impact of flawed management strategies directly affects clinical success and patient health In the rapidly changing field of facial cosmetics. Incompetent management may not only risk the efficacy of treatment but also cause patient dissatisfaction and safety risks. For example, incompetent standardized practices when applying LED-RL can produce inaccurate results and potential complications. Therefore, developing management guidelines that maintain the guidelines for treatment and safety standards is necessary. This includes regular checks on procedure and results to enable consistent improvement. Emphasizing management's adoption of technology is crucial in order to promote patient safety, enhance treatment outcomes, and maintain practice in cosmetic practice. While forward steps continue to redefine the arena, good management practice will remain crucial in bridging challenges and maximizing gains in facial cosmetics (Heilman et al., 2019).

15.5.2. Staff Training and Development

Staff training and development in the field of facial cosmetics cannot be overstated, particularly in a company that keeps changing with new technologies and evolving customer preferences. Continuous education courses, as pointed out by recent studies, are required to equip employees with the information and skills necessary to cope with the complexities of cosmetic products and treatments. As observed in a cosmetic and dermatologic sciences continuing medical education (CME) initiative launched in 2008, the training significantly enhanced practitioners' understanding of cosmetic formulations, dermatologic sciences, and legal requirements. This knowledge gap, as typically experienced by practitioners and consumers, may generate misperceptions on product efficacy and safety, which ultimately impacts client confidence and satisfaction (Huo et al., 2023). Hence, expert training programs are necessary to equip employees not just with theoretical expertise but also with real-world expertise that enhances professional abilities. Furthermore, the integration of advanced technology within training programs will further strengthen the learning experience of the staff in the face cosmetic industry. For example, the utilization of digital platforms for the delivery of training videos, virtual simulations, and interactive sessions can facilitate staff in comprehending complex ideas more effectively. These methodologies not only bridge the gap between traditional education and modern learning patterns but also address different styles of employees to learn. By unveiling the positive comments from the CME program trainees, the incorporation of practical sessions and recent developments in cosmetic science assists in enhancing their knowledge and enthusiasm for their work. This strategy not only acquaints the workers with the delivery of maximum service to customers but also gives them the confidence to deal with the evolving problems in an intensely competitive marketplace (Huo et al., 2023). Ultimately, well-framed training modules can lead to improved employee performance and customer satisfaction with facial cosmetics. Besides, creating a corporate culture of highest regard for employee training and development is consistent with general industry goals of maintaining public trust and skin well-being. Subject to pressure from community standards and consumer demands, businesses are compelled to tread carefully on branding and employee conduct to avoid conflicts over workplace discrimination and harassment, as most labor and legal studies have noted. By ensuring employees are effectively trained to understand and implement ethical branding practices, companies can assist in avoiding risks for deceptive advertising and enhance their reputations. Training should not only include cosmetic science but also customer interaction facets and corporate social responsibility so employees can advocate accurate information and client well-being. By doing so, ongoing training reinforces the innate correlation between staff development and overall company success within the ever-changing universe of facial cosmetics.

15.5.3. Patient Relationship Management

With the rapidly changing universe of facial cosmetics, effective patient relationship management (PRM) has become an intrinsic part of practice management. The nature of cosmetic procedures demands not just technical competence but also a mature understanding of patient expectations and emotional needs. Developing a robust PRM strategy ensures effective communication and enhancing confidence, which is vital in addressing patients' complaints regarding treatment outcomes. As practitioners adopt advanced equipment to enhance the delivery of services, integrating such gadgets within a formalized PRM system ensures constant engagement with the patients, thus allowing them to make informed decisions. The emphasis on building relationships in such an environment is of top priority, since patient satisfaction depends largely on trust, with follow-up visits and recommendations that are key to business growth.

The setup of evidence-based training has also transformed the dynamics of patient care in non-surgical aesthetics (NSA), putting further focus on the work of PRM in a niche sector. Modern training programs, findings of current studies now indicate, emphasize the practitioner's requirement to not only be technical experts but also to possess interpersonal skills that will allow them to practice PRM effectively. By fostering a curriculum grounded in extensive literature reviews and global needs analysis, educational institutions can better prepare their aesthetic practitioners to appropriately engage with their patients.

This approach is with the growing realization that high-quality patient experience increasingly hinges on personalized interactions that are susceptible to being augmented by media that enable continuous interaction and feedback between the practitioner and patient and are hence in line with the core tenets of patient relationship management (Kumar, 2021). Corporate branding and patient experience cross-linking makes the landscape of PRM in facial cosmetics even more complex. As practices develop marketing strategies that are sensitive to community values, they must guard against the use of branding that would subtly reinforce stereotypes or be harmful to patient interactions. The challenge is finding a balance between aesthetics and professional norms so that marketing does not detract from the quality of services provided. The practitioners must institute a PRM approach that not only highlights their skills but also addresses any body image and personal identity issues that are present in the community, as these are directly tied to patient loyalty and satisfaction. Effective PRM in branding can enhance the overall patient experience, ultimately locking in the practitioner's reputation in a competitive market (Avery et al., 2007).

Test Your Knowledge

1. Why are effective management strategies important for the success of a cosmetic clinic?
2. How does staff training and development contribute to quality patient care in cosmetic practices?
3. What are key approaches to building and maintaining strong patient relationships in cosmetic clinics?

15.6. Regulatory and Ethical Considerations

Learning Outcome

1. Focus on Importance of Effective Management Strategies
2. Explain the Staff Training and Development
3. Discuss the Patient Relationship Management

The world is more regulated and guided by ethical factors that are pivotal in ensuring consumer safety, as well as industry integrity. With technological advances breeding novel cosmetic treatments and products, regulatory authorities must lay out detailed guidelines. The regulations must ensure not only product safety and efficacy but also the ethical aspects of this marketing practice that can deceive consumers. For instance, cosmetic misuse as a result of misinformation may result in ill effects, necessitating a regulatory mechanism that bridges the existing gap in knowledge among users and cosmetic practitioners, as facilitated by the evidence of ongoing continuing medical education (CME) programs tailored for cosmetic practitioners (Huo et al., 2023). Such a convergence of education and regulation builds good practice and promotes public trust in cosmetic sciences. Besides regulatory stipulations, ethical considerations are the basis for practice management for the facial cosmetics business. Practitioners must adhere to ethical principles such as beneficence, where clients' well-being is the principal concern. An ethical informed consent and avoidance of deceptive advertising claims are highly critical factors that clinicians should not forget during their encounters with patients. Industry players' focus on professionalism is supplemented by education efforts; training courses in cosmetic and dermatologic sciences have demonstrated a remarkable increase in clinicians' understanding of the scientific as well as ethical aspects of practice (Huo et al., 2023). This unification of ethical principles into everyday practice not only enhances the quality of care that is being delivered but also works to enhance the image of the cosmetic industry as a whole, thereby creating a climate where consumers have confidence in their choices. In addition, the interdisciplinary discussion facilitated by regulatory bodies can go a long way to enhance the overall ethical discussion within the cosmetic industry. By facilitating discourse among researchers, clinicians, and policy makers, organizations can work towards having more responsive and coherent policies that encompass the high pace of technological developments. Marine science organizations' efforts, as noted in the Marine Board-ESF work, highlight that efforts should be made to foster an interdisciplinary platform to address complex scientific as well as ethical issues. A similar approach in the cosmetic field would have regulators and practitioners joining together to develop regulations protecting consumers and professional standards alike. Thus, embracing an all-encompassing approach incorporating regulatory oversight, continued education, and ethical practice is crucial in regulating the emerging face of facial cosmetics.

15.6.1. Overview of Regulations Governing Cosmetic Practices

The regulation governing cosmetic practice is also multifaceted, encompassing numerous considerations from efficacy and safety to marketing and distribution. In the USA, the Food and Drug Administration (FDA) is the primary regulator of the cosmetics industry. Unlike pharmaceuticals, which are subjected to rigorous pre-market approval, cosmetic products in themselves are not subject to such a high degree of assessment before being placed on the market. This regulatory climate is a potential danger to the consumer because the products may contain poisonous substances or lack the advertised benefits. With the technology of cosmetics evolving through new processes and technologies, the need for updated rules that take into consideration current innovations is more pressing. A comprehensive organization covering the educational and operating skills of the practitioners and consumer protection is essential in managing the challenges and advancements of facial cosmetics. Increased popularity for non-surgical aesthetic treatments has raised demands for improved training and regulation within the cosmetic industry. Although non-surgical aesthetic (NSA) procedures are becoming increasingly popular, their dominance within private clinics, as opposed to academic medical centers, has resulted in a void of vigilance and education. To close this gap, the establishment of evidence-based postgraduate curricula for NSA has emerged as a necessary requirement for guaranteeing that practitioners not only meet ethical standards but also clinical competencies. Evidence has been discovered regarding how literature systematic reviews and Delphi studies can inform curriculum development, thereby forming a solid basis that integrates critical thinking and enquiry-based learning in NSA training (Kumar, 2021). This systematic method can enhance the level of care given in facial cosmetic treatment by professionalizing education. The intersection of race and gender in cosmetic control has an additional complexity that needs to be thoroughly interrogated. The control of skin-lightening cosmetics provides a useful case study, with the extensive racial and gender assumptions included in cosmetic law. Women of color, who are disproportionately targeted by these products through hostile marketing and toxic chemicals, are in grave danger of health complications due to the absence of regulatory intervention. The legacy exclusion of women from trials has contributed to such issues, rendering an intersectional framework for analysis indispensable in guiding policy reforms (Campbell et al., 2024). Such an analytic focus not only assists in understanding the unique health impacts felt by minority groups but also emphasizes the necessity of inclusive regulatory frameworks, placing emphasis on the well-being and protection of all as consumers. The construction of cosmetic regulation must therefore be attentive to plural experiences to create equitable standards regarding health and safety.

15.6.2. Ethical Dilemmas in Cosmetic Procedures

More cosmetic surgery over the last few years has garnered serious ethical issues, particularly with the fast pace of technology that has enabled such procedures to become more accessible. The main issue is the risk of the medical profession indulging in cosmetic desires over genuine healthcare requirements. This shift of focus raises serious issues regarding informed consent since the patients are not going to be given proper insight into what the implications of such elective procedures will be. Dermatosurgery is now walking the thin line between medical and cosmetic intentions, befuddling physicians' ethical requirements. The task of harmonizing patient satisfaction and medical ethics has increased as social norms of beauty evolve (Ekomwereren et al., 2023). As the demand for cosmetic surgery increases, practitioners must carefully work on these ethical issues to ensure patients' safety and well-being and preserve standards of care. Furthermore, the commercialization of cosmetic surgery presents added ethical challenges. The market dynamics of the cosmetic industry foster aggressive marketing practices tending to deceive about the nature of these surgical procedures. Patients can be under pressure to achieve unrealistic beauty ideals, which worsens the ethical challenge that is encountered by practitioners. Profit may be achieved at the expense of clinical judgment, and this can result in over-treatment or ignoring the patient's mental health. Mental wellness is particularly important to address, as people are getting cosmetic treatments to correct underlying psychological issues instead of for aesthetic needs that are genuine. As is observed by Ekomwereren et al. (2023), open communication between medical professionals and patients is important in averting such risks. It is the role of health practitioners to uphold professional ethics while meeting the growing demand for cosmetic surgery within a society that only continues to place more emphasis on looks. As a result of technological advancement, ethical questions are also complicated by the integration of artificial intelligence (AI) within the management and execution of procedures. As AI becomes more engagement by AI in forming patient experience and outcomes, there are pressing issues about data privacy and security. Misuse of personal information is a concerning issue around consent and transparency. Incorporation of AI into cosmetic practice must be undertaken with vigilance to ensure that patient rights are not violated. The performance of AI in translating patient desires over medical needs continues to evolve. As theorized in, human-AI cooperation may revolutionize ethical frameworks in healthcare, with careful observation being needed to prevent exploitation or harm. It will be essential to strike a delicate balance between ethics and innovation in creating a system that ensures patient autonomy without stifling accountable practice in an evolving environment.

15.6.3. Impact of Regulations on Practice Management

The impact of regulation on practice management in the facial cosmetics industry has come more sharply into focus as the industry continues to evolve. As technology and methods of treatment evolve, practices are forced to deal with a highly regulated climate that monitors their actions. Regulation systems intended to ensure patient safety and practitioner responsibility can also pose significant challenges for practice management. For instance, compliance with certification requirements and health standards necessitates ongoing training and investment. Hence, practitioners are compelled to make investments in terms of keeping abreast with these regulations, detracting from time and investment that otherwise could be spent on enhancing services and being creative within practice. Lastly, the interplay between regulatory standards and corporate branding makes it problematic to strategize practice management in facial cosmetics. Businesses typically seek to establish a specific brand image so that they can compete better, but this must go hand in hand with legal compliance. Marketing procedures and the advertisement of plastic surgery are subject to laws that demand a balancing act between effective branding and adherence to ethical standards. As mentioned, in environments where sexualized branding does not align with what is accepted by society, laws may intervene and ban practices leading to unwanted working environments. This dynamic also shows the importance of having an understanding of local community norms, the ethical implications of branding in the regulated space, and thereby influencing practice decision-making processes. Finally, the influence of regulations on practice management also reaches into establishing certain professional standards and guidelines that must be followed by practitioners. Regulating authorities provide useful frameworks that can enhance practice quality through structured guidelines and recommendations. However, simultaneously, these regulations can suppress innovation when they are overly restrictive. Clarity and flexibility of regulations are crucial so that there is an appropriate setting for embracing technological advances in clinical practices. Facial cosmetic professionals struggle to maintain the vagueness of adhering to regulations and the need to deal with new practices that take care of patients' needs and expectations. Lastly, the intersection of practice management and regulation is an ideal area for continued study, as how successfully one can accommodate these forces will influence the future course of the facial cosmetics industry.

Test Your Knowledge

1. How does staff training and development ensure compliance with ethical and legal standards?
2. What ethical principles should guide patient relationship management in cosmetic clinics?

SUMMARY

It should be evident that the advancement of this career is highly influenced by scientific discovery and technological integration. Within the past few decades, practitioners have witnessed a drastic shift in patient expectations as well as treatment methods. With the development of new technologies and materials, they have transformed the landscape of aesthetic treatments so that practitioners are able to offer more effective and safer treatments that can treat a large population of patients. Utilization of advanced technologies such as nanotechnology and biocompatible fillers not only enhanced results but also promoted more interest in the study of aesthetic medicine underway. This trend underscores the necessity of continuous professional education and a responsive nature in practitioners to offset the dynamic nature of the practice. The facial cosmetics revolution is also underscored by heightened emphasis on individually tailored treatment protocols, driven by a viewpoint of unique anatomy and aesthetic goals. With diagnostic methods and materials still being developed, practitioners are now in a position to individualize treatment more effectively according to patient requirements, thus raising satisfaction and efficacy. In the recent past, minimally invasive treatments have also made facial cosmetic treatments more and more accessible, more so in an attractive and viable way for a wider populace. This democratization of cosmetic care is a cultural revolution, in which beauty and self-care are not only material aspirations, but essential components of healthful living. Such demographic advancement mandates that there be ongoing discussion regarding ethical practice, best practices, and patient education, so that the expansion of access is accompanied by commitment to safety and efficacy. Lastly, the conclusion drawn via evaluation of facial cosmetics innovation is that an integrated approach that merges technology, patient care, and severe management practices is required. As the industry innovates, practitioners need to remain informed about emerging technologies and their applications, such as innovations of Joseph et al. (2023), which stated the significance of nanotechnology in advancing medical treatments. Moreover, with specialties such as cutaneous conditions being addressed in the domain of cosmetics, marrying aesthetic practice with knowledge from other medical specialties, as envisioned in de Vries & Schallig (2022), paves the way for future innovations. The future demands adherence to the ethics of practice, lifelong learning, and adherence to standards of care for the achievement of both aesthetic and patient safety.

The facial cosmetic environment is undergoing a dramatic change due to the advancement of technology, enhancing patient experience and practitioner capabilities. Central to this change is the integration of the latest modalities, which not only maximize aesthetic enhancement but also patient safety and satisfaction. Intelligent devices have transformed practice management, allowing practitioners to become more bespoke in their engagements with clients. For instance, the application of artificial intelligence in cosmetic treatments for the face assists with predictive analysis to ensure treatment plans are optimized to meet individual needs. Such a paradigm shift is a representation of embracing innovative technologies that are in agreement with ethical standards and professional practices, leading to better patient outcomes as well as enhanced industry relations. The role of social media and forums in facial cosmetic treatment has become increasingly influential, shaping public perception and patient demand. Particularly, the beauty blogging phenomenon enables individuals with facial disfigurement to narrate their experiences and rebuild their identity. These self-narrative accounts, as opposed to normalized journalistic accounts, bear witness to the complexity with respect to disability and beauty. By examining the narrative exchanged between beauty bloggers and traditional journalism, it becomes evident that these platforms can coexist to enrich societal understanding of disfigurement and challenge conventional representations. As practitioners keenly observe these communications, they are better equipped to engage with diverse patient narratives, fostering an inclusive approach to cosmetic enhancement that respects individual stories and experiences (Garrisi et al., 2018). Moreover, progress in artificial intelligence and smart technologies brings forth prospects and issues for the cosmetics industry. Personalized experiences have increasingly become popular, necessitating the development of convergence platforms that will be capable of fulfilling varied consumer demands in addition to guaranteeing accessibility. Innovations such as the Internet-of-Mirrors (IoM), encompassing networked smart mirrors, register this prospect as it offers interactive and tailored consultations for beauty and health routines. Nonetheless, gaping holes in the existing portfolios still remain, especially in relation to their mass adoption and uptake into day-to-day practice. To be able to maximize these developments, the sector has to place greater importance on research and development activities designed to bridge these loopholes as well as further improve the functionality of autonomous solutions. In this way, practitioners are able to improve service provision, better bringing it in line with modern-day consumer expectations (Fatima et al., 2023).

KEY TERMS FROM THIS CHAPTER

- 3D Imaging
- Virtual Surgical Simulation
- Intraoperative Navigation
- Laser Technology
- Ultrasound-Guided Procedures
- Injectable Therapies
- Electronic Medical Records (EMR)
- Quality Assurance
- Computer-Aided Surgical Planning
- CAD/CAM Technology
- Endoscopic Techniques
- Radiofrequency Devices
- Robotic-Assisted Surgery
- Patient Workflow Optimization
- Teleconsultation
- Regulatory Compliance

CRITICAL THINKING QUESTIONS

1. **Which technology has greatly improved preoperative planning in facial cosmetic surgery?**
   a. Laser Doppler
   b. 3D imaging and simulation
   c. Ultrasound
   d. Traditional photography
2. **Computer-assisted surgical guides are primarily used for:**
   a. Minimizing anesthesia
   b. Accurate implant placement and bone reconstruction
   c. Skin resurfacing
   d. Hair transplantation
3. **Which energy-based device is commonly used for non-invasive skin tightening?**
   a. Radiofrequency
   b. Scalpel
   c. Cryotherapy
   d. Electrocautery
4. **What is a major advantage of minimally invasive facial cosmetic procedures?**
   a. Permanent results
   b. Reduced downtime and faster recovery
   c. No anesthesia needed
   d. No follow-up required
5. **Fractional lasers are primarily used for:**
   a. Hair removal only
   b. Skin resurfacing and rejuvenation
   c. Deep bone contouring
   d. Fat reduction

Short Answer Questions

1. How has 3D imaging and simulation improved preoperative planning in facial aesthetics?
2. What role do computer-assisted surgical guides play in facial reconstruction and implant placement?
3. Describe the advantages of using laser and energy-based devices in modern facial rejuvenation.
4. How has the development of minimally invasive techniques changed patient recovery and outcomes?
5. What are the key considerations in maintaining patient safety while adopting new cosmetic technologies?
6. Explain the importance of digital documentation and patient record management in facial cosmetic practice.

Answers to Critical Thinking Questions

1. (b) 2. (b) 3. (a) 4. (b) 5. (b)

REFERENCES

1. Timraz, J. H., Bakour, H. A., Samman, R. R., Alawi, K. M., Bava, F. S. M., Alkhdaidi, F. A., AlGhorab, M. A., Alabbassi, M. A., Thalib, H. I., Khan, S., Makki, F., & Alsolamy, A. (2025). Advancements in Non-Invasive Plastic Surgery Techniques: Evaluating Efficacy, Safety, Patient Outcomes and Potential Complications. *South Eastern European Journal of Public Health*, 4078–4099. https://doi.org/10.70135/seejph.vi.5983(accessed on 14th July 2025).
2. Araya, D., & Marber, P. (2023). *Augmented Education in the Global Age*. Routledge eBooks. https://doi.org/10.4324/9781003230762.
3. Avery, D., & Crain, M. (2007). *Branded: Corporate image, sexual stereotyping, and the new face of capitalism*. https://core.ac.uk/download/62548098.pdf (accessed on 14th July 2025).
4. Bowler P. J. (2009). Impact on facial rejuvenation with dermatological preparations. *Clinical interventions in aging*, *4*, 81–89. https://doi.org/10.2147/cia.s3524(accessed on 14th July 2025).
5. Boyen, C., Børresen, T., Dobson, A., Höfle, et al. (2025). *Marine biotechnology: A new vision and strategy for Europe*. https://core.ac.uk/download/pdf/29241634.pdf (accessed on 14th July 2025).
6. Brandt, F. S., & Cazzaniga, A. (2008). *Hyaluronic acid gel fillers in the management of facial aging*. https://core.ac.uk/download/pdf/8185430.pdf (accessed on 14th July 2025).
7. Campbell, C. (2024). *Intersectionality Matters in Food and Drug Law*. https://core.ac.uk/download/647851141.pdf (accessed on 14th July 2025).
8. Portilla, A. S. P., Portilla, C. S. P., Palacios, G. S. G., Rodríguez, B. S. P., Castillo, S. G. A., Espin, N. E. P., & Pita, G. P. M. (2024). The integration of surgical and dermatological techniques in the treatment of cutaneous aging: multidisciplinary approaches and clinical outcomes - a comprehensive systematic review of current literature. *International Journal of Research in Medical Sciences*, *12*(5), 1659–1667. https://doi.org/10.18203/2320-6012.ijrms20240943(accessed on 14th July 2025).
9. Damar, M. (2022). What the literature on medicine, nursing, public health, midwifery, and dentistry reveals: An overview of the rapidly approaching metaverse. *Journal of Metaverse*, *2*, 62–70. https://doi.org/10.57019/jmv.1132962.
10. de Vries, H. J. C., & Schallig, H. D. F. H. (2022). Cutaneous leishmaniasis: A 2022 updated narrative review into diagnosis and management developments. *American Journal of Clinical Dermatology*, *23*, 823–840. https://doi.org/10.1007/s40257-022-00726-8.
11. Edmonds, A. (2014). *Surgery-for-life: Aging, sexual fitness and self-management in Brazil*. Anthropology & Aging Quarterly 2014: 34 (4) https://core.ac.uk/download/28979727.pdf (accessed on 14th July 2025).
12. Ekomwereren, O., Shehryar, A., Yahya, N. A., Rehman, A., Affaf, M., Chilla, S. P., Kumar, U., et al. (2023). Mastering the art of dermatosurgery: Aesthetic alchemy in medical excellence. *Cureus*. https://doi.org/10.7759/cureus.49659.
13. Fatima, H., Imran, M. A., Mohjazi, L., Taha, et al. (2023). *Internet of mirrors for connected healthcare and beauty: A prospective vision*. http://arxiv.org/abs/2311.14734 (accessed on 14th July 2025).

14. Fedorchenko, Y. (2024). ANTI-AGING COSMETIC PROCEDURES: BENEFITS AND RISKS. *Anti-Aging Eastern Europe, 3*(3), 135-140. https://doi.org/10.56543/aaeeu.2024.3.3.04(accessed on 14th July 2025).

15. Reisenwitz, Timothy and Fowler, Jie G. (2021) "An Analysis on Engaging "Beauty Work"," Atlantic Marketing Journal: Vol. 10 : No. 2 , Article 6. Available at: https://digitalcommons.kennesaw.edu/amj/vol10/iss2/6 (accessed on 14th July 2025).

16. Garrisi, D., Johanssen, J., Johanssen, et al. (2018). *Competing narratives in framing disability in the UK media: A comparative analysis of journalistic representations of facial disfigurement versus practices of self-representations online.* https://core.ac.uk/download/161104198.pdf (accessed on 14th July 2025).

17. Heilman, E., Isseroff, R. R., Jagdeo, J. R., Jakus, et al. (2019). *A dose-ranging, parallel group, split-face, single-blind phase II study of light emitting diode-red light (LED-RL) for skin scarring prevention: Study protocol for a randomized controlled trial.* https://core.ac.uk/download/323070347.pdf (accessed on 14th July 2025).

18. Huo, W., Wang, X., Wang, X., Wang, X., Shu, X., & Li, Y. (2023). *Promoting public skin health through a national continuing medical education project on cosmetic and dermatologic sciences: A 15-year experience.* https://core.ac.uk/download/593349901.pdf (accessed on 14th July 2025).

19. Joseph, T. M., Mahapatra, D. K., Esmaeili, A., Piszczyk, Ł., Hasanin, M. S., Kattali, M., Haponiuk, J. T., et al. (2023). Nanoparticles: Taking a unique position in medicine. *Nanomaterials, 13*, 574–574. https://doi.org/10.3390/nano13030574.

20. Kazimierczak, N., Kazimierczak, W., Serafin, Z., Nowicki, P., Nożewski, J., & Janiszewska-Olszowska, J. (2024). AI in orthodontics: Revolutionizing diagnostics and treatment planning—A comprehensive review. *Journal of Clinical Medicine, 13*, 344–344. https://doi.org/10.3390/jcm13020344.

21. Kivnick, H. Q., Twigg, J., & Martin, W. (2014). *The Challenge of Cultural Gerontology.* https://core.ac.uk/download/30339730.pdf (accessed on 14th July 2025).

22. Kumar, Narendra; (2021) Design, Development and Implementation Framework for a Postgraduate Non-Surgical Aesthetics Curriculum. Doctoral thesis (Ph.D), UCL (University College London).(accessed on 14th July 2025).

23. Lin, J. Y., & Wan, M. T. (2014). *Current evidence and applications of photodynamic therapy in dermatology.* https://core.ac.uk/download/28949556.pdf (accessed on 14th July 2025).

24. Meyer-Szary, J., Luis, M. S., Mikulski, S., Patel, A., Schulz, F., Tretiakow, D., Fercho, J., et al. (2022). The role of 3D printing in planning complex medical procedures and training of medical professionals—Cross-sectional multispecialty review. *International Journal of Environmental Research and Public Health, 19*, 3331–3331. https://doi.org/10.3390/ijerph19063331.

25. Mubashir, M. (2024). *The gendered dress of DALL-E 2: Exploring profession-based images in the Indian context.* https://core.ac.uk/download/616689178.pdf (accessed on 14th July 2025).

26. Naik, M. (2015). Donate eyes, not patients!. *Indian Journal of Ophthalmology, 63*, 564, 565. https://www.semanticscholar.org/paper/725523a9575cbdbb3e3af205ca0a8d83e9856093.

27. Nikparto, N., Yari, A., Mehraban, S. H., Bigdelou, M., Asadi, A., Darehdor, A. A., Nezaminia, S., et al. (2024). The current techniques in dorsal augmentation rhinoplasty: A comprehensive

review. *Maxillofacial Plastic and Reconstructive Surgery, 46.* https://doi.org/10.1186/s40902-024-00418-9.

28. Nova Southeastern University. (2014). *Academic Impressions, 2014.* https://core.ac.uk/download/51073269.pdf (accessed on 14th July 2025).

29. Patel, H., Pundkar, A., Shrivastava, S., Chandanwale, R., & Jaiswal, A. M. (2023). A comprehensive review on platelet-rich plasma activation: A key player in accelerating skin wound healing. *Cureus.* https://doi.org/10.7759/cureus.48943.

30. Rokhshad, R., Keyhan, S. O., & Yousefi, P. (2023). *Artificial intelligence applications and ethical challenges in oral and maxillo-facial cosmetic surgery: A narrative review. Maxillofacial Plastic and Reconstructive Surgery, 45.* https://doi.org/10.1186/s40902-023-00382-w.

31. Tettey, F., Parupelli, S. K., & Desai, S. (2023). A review of biomedical devices: Classification, regulatory guidelines, human factors, software as a medical device, and cybersecurity. *Deleted Journal, 2,* 316–341. https://doi.org/10.1007/s44174-023-00113-9.

32. Vosloo, M. (2025). *A framework to position the somatology profession in South Africa.* https://core.ac.uk/download/222966444.pdf (accessed on 14th July 2025).

INDEX

A

Ablative Laser 332
Abnormalities 402, 403, 404, 405, 411, 413, 414, 416, 418, 421, 425
Acetylcholine 274, 281, 282, 288
Adherence 38, 51
Adipose-derived stem cells (ASCs) 435
Adipose tissue 244, 254, 260, 270
Adjunctive treatments 371
Aesthetic 107, 108, 109, 110, 111, 112, 113, 114, 115, 116, 117, 118, 119, 120, 122, 123, 126, 127, 128, 129, 130, 131, 132, 133, 134, 135, 136, 137, 138, 142, 143, 144, 145, 146, 147, 148, 149, 150, 152, 153, 154, 156, 157, 158, 159, 160, 162, 164, 165, 166, 167, 168, 169, 170, 171
Aesthetic Analysis 101
Aesthetic appearance 37, 38
Aesthetic applications 245, 258, 270
Aesthetic Balance 66
Aesthetic beautification 245, 270
Aesthetic beauty 401
Aesthetic goals 217, 221, 231, 232
Aesthetic improvements 243, 245, 267, 270
Aesthetic integrity 341
Aesthetics 1, 2, 3, 4, 5, 6, 7, 8, 9, 10, 11, 12, 13, 14, 15, 17, 18, 19, 20, 21, 22, 23, 24, 25, 26, 27, 30, 31, 33, 34
Aesthetics entwines 110
Aesthetic Subunits 364
Aesthetic therapy 11, 15
Aesthetic treatments 466, 468, 471, 489, 492
Afflicted body 434
Anatomical knowledge 144
Anatomical measurements 39
Anatomical structures 211
Anatomical variations 176
Anatomic configuration 341
Anesthesia 144, 151, 159, 167
Anti-aging procedures 109
anti-aging treatments 472
Antibiotics 16
Anticoagulant medication 108
Appearance post-surgery 142
Artificial intelligence (AI) 468, 476, 490
Artistic skill 338, 342
Assessment 434, 445, 446, 452, 453, 454, 459
Assessment process 74, 80, 83, 84, 85, 89
Association of Plastic Aesthetic Surgery (AICPE) 109, 128, 132, 136
Asymmetry 372
Atmosphere 76
Attractiveness 143
Augmentation 244, 245, 247, 248, 250, 251, 253, 260, 262, 263, 267, 269, 270, 271
Augmented reality (AR) 473, 475, 476
Autologous bone 370, 376, 380, 390, 395

Avulsion Injuries 396

B

Balance crucial 434
Basal cell carcinoma (BCC) 438
Bespoke techniques 364
Bioactive materials 370
Biocompatibility 246, 250
Biocompatible materials 249, 275
Biological 2, 4, 5, 15, 19, 20, 30, 401
Biometrics 338
Blepharoplasty 107, 108, 109, 110, 111, 112, 113, 114, 115, 116, 117, 118, 119, 120, 121, 122, 123, 124, 125, 126, 127, 128, 129, 130, 131, 132, 133, 134, 135, 136, 137, 138, 139, 140
Body Contouring 66
Bone Grafting 396
Bone morphogenetic proteins (BMPs) 370
Bone Reconstruction 364, 460
Bone structure 246, 270
Botulinum neurotoxin type A (BoNTA) 9
Botulinum toxin 273, 274, 275, 276, 277, 278, 279, 280, 281, 282, 283, 285, 289, 290, 291, 292, 293, 294, 295, 296, 297, 298, 300, 301, 302, 303
Botulinum toxin injection 13, 24
Botulinum Toxin Type A 301
Brachycephalic Obstructive Airway Syndrome (BOAS) 5
Brand identity 468
Breast augmentation 38, 50, 63
Broader population 107
Brow Ptosis 239
Brow ridges 218
Buccal fat pad 31

C

CAD/CAM Technology 493
Cancer microenvironments 435
Candidacy Criteria 101
Cannula Technique 301
Carbon dioxide (CO2) 306, 309
Cervicofacial liposuction 244, 262, 269, 270
Cervicofacial Rhytidectomy 168
Cheekboneness 5
Chemical Peels 310, 332
Chemical peels constitute 310
Circumstances 444
Cleft Lip 404, 405, 428
Cleft Palate 428
Client engagement 468
Clinical competency 470
Clinical efficacy 468
Clinical operation 470
Clinical skill 469
Closed Approach 204
Clostridium botulinum 274, 277, 278, 282
CO_2 Laser 332
Cognitive development 403
Collagen Stimulation 332
Combination therapy 244, 270
Communication 440, 442, 444, 448, 457, 458
Community engagement 354
Complex deformities 402
Complexity 176, 177
Comprehension 370
Comprehensive treatment protocols 402
Computer-Aided Surgical Planning 493
Congenital adrenal hyperplasia (CAH) 54
Congenital malformation 402, 411
Consistency 370
Consumer engagement 470
Consumerism 176
Consumer patterns 466
Consumer protection 277
Contemporary 142, 144, 145, 163
Contemporary medicine 175, 178
Contemporary society 245
Contributes 244, 267, 270
Contusion Management 396
Conversation 75, 87
Convolutional neural networks (CNNs) 344
Coronal Brow Lift 239
Corrugator Supercilii 239
Cosmetic 37, 38, 39, 40, 41, 42, 43, 44, 45, 46, 47, 48, 49, 50, 51, 52, 53, 54, 55, 56, 57, 58, 59, 60, 61, 62, 63, 64, 65, 66, 67, 69, 70, 71
Cosmetic alterations 158, 159

Cosmetic augmentation 275
Cosmetic dentistry 280
Cosmetic design 475, 476
Cosmetic desires 177, 189
Cosmetic enhancement 244, 266
Cosmetic face 75, 99
Cosmetic facial environment 212
Cosmetic facial surgery 73, 74, 75, 76, 77, 78, 79, 80, 81, 82, 83, 84, 85, 86, 87, 88, 89, 90, 91, 92, 93, 94, 95, 97, 98, 100, 101, 102, 105, 141
Cosmetic indication 115
Cosmetic industry 306, 471, 472, 473, 475, 476, 478, 486, 488, 489, 490
Cosmetic practices 469, 470, 472, 488
Cosmetic procedures 75, 80, 87, 142, 145, 157, 162, 167, 211, 212, 213, 217, 218, 219, 223, 224, 226, 242
Cosmetic professionals 437
Cosmetic surgeons 110
Cosmetic surgery 141, 142, 144, 145, 146, 159, 160, 161, 162, 167
Cosmetic technology 471, 472
Cosmetic therapy 477
Cosmetic treatments 273, 275, 276, 278, 283, 285, 287, 290, 291, 292, 296, 297, 298
Craniofacial Anomalies 428
Craniofacial procedures 8
Craniofacial reconstruction 371, 390, 442
Craniofacial tissue 8
Craniosynostosis 406, 428, 429
Cross-Linking 301
Cultural influences 471, 472
Curriculum design 277
Cutaneous integrity 434
Cutaneous Malignancy 460
Cutting-edge technologies 465
Cybersecurity 338

D

Databases 244
Deep learning 476
Deep plane facelifts 142, 167
Defect Reconstruction 460
Dermal Fillers 273, 275, 284, 288, 301
Dermal Remodeling 332
Dermatochalasis 136
Dermatological surgery 306
Dermatological treatments 273, 281
Dermatologic treatment 17
Dermatology 305, 306, 310, 311, 312, 313, 314, 315, 316, 318, 319, 320, 321, 329, 331, 335
Dermis 31, 32
Diagnostic accuracy 74
Dialogues 38
Diffusion 301
Digital technologies 471, 475
Direct Brow Lift 239
Disease 176, 435, 438, 442, 455
Disfigurement 434, 437, 442, 443, 447, 448, 457
Donor Site Morbidity 364
Dorsal Hump 204
Dorsal Preservation 176, 204
Dramatic alterations 246, 270
Dry eye syndrome 108, 113, 123, 126
Dynamic Wrinkles 301
Dyschromia 319
Dysmorphisms 404

E

Effective communication 76, 87
Effective communication skills 470
Effective cosmetic treatment 280
Effective management 468, 485, 488
Effective risk assessment 88
Efficacy 306, 308, 309, 311, 312, 313, 314, 316, 317, 319, 321, 323, 325, 326, 329, 330, 331, 435, 436, 454
Electromyography (EMG) 12
Electronic Medical Records (EMR) 493
Emotional impact 401, 404
Emphasis 109, 129, 136
Endoscopic Brow Lift 227, 239
Endoscopic Techniques 493
Energy-based devices 244, 251, 258, 262, 269, 270
Ensure effective 244, 270
Environmental exposure 402, 413
Epidermal Ablation 332
Epidermis 13, 14, 31, 32, 438, 450

Equity 39, 45
Erythema 306, 307, 309, 320, 321, 322, 323, 330, 331
Ethical cosmetic surgery 38
Evidence-based guidelines 73
Exclusive esthetic 442
Existence 213
External appearances 39
Eyelid Crease 136
Eyelid Ptosis 136

F

Face phenomenon 213, 217
Facial aesthetic 107, 110, 113, 116, 118, 120, 122
Facial Aging Patterns 101
Facial anatomy complexity 355
Facial anatomy knowledge 9
Facial artery perforator (FAP) 370
Facial attractiveness 143
Facial balance 249, 260, 265, 271
Facial beauty 245, 249, 254, 260, 261, 266, 270
Facial bony skeleton 370
Facial contouring theory 244
Facial cosmetics 465, 466, 467, 468, 469, 471, 472, 473, 474, 475, 476, 478, 479, 480, 481, 482, 483, 486, 487, 488, 489, 490, 491, 492
Facial cosmetology 274
Facial deformities 401, 402, 403, 408, 410, 411, 412, 413, 415, 417, 419, 421, 425, 426, 429
Facial dynamics 143
Facial expression 143, 338, 341
Facial Fractures 396
Facial harmony 213, 223
Facial implants 243, 244, 245, 246, 247, 249, 250, 251, 252, 255, 256, 263, 267, 269, 270, 271
Facial injuries 371, 372, 373, 377, 384
Facial Landmarks 101
Facial Ligaments 168
Facial Nerve Preservation 364
Facial Proportions 101
Facial reconstruction 337, 338, 339, 340, 341, 342, 343, 344, 345, 346, 347, 348, 349, 350, 351, 352, 353, 354, 355, 356, 357, 358, 359, 360, 361, 362, 363, 364, 365, 367
Facial skeleton 1, 3, 5, 6
Facial structure 6, 10, 18, 244, 246, 247, 249, 251, 256, 260
Facial trauma 369, 370, 372, 373, 374, 375, 376, 377, 378, 381, 383, 384, 385, 388, 389, 390, 395, 396, 397
Facial volume 149, 154
Fact-based representation 338
Fat Prolapse 136
Fatty tissue accumulation 244
Flap Reconstruction 66
Flaw correction 244
Flexibility 212, 215, 228, 234
Fluence 332
Forehead Rhytids 239
Forensic science 338, 339, 340, 341, 342, 344, 347, 348, 349, 357, 360, 363, 367
Fractional photothermolysis (FP) 317
Fractional Resurfacing 332
Free Flap 460
Free Tissue Transfer 364
Frequent complication 150
Frontalis muscle 31
Frontalis Muscle 239
Functional Assessment 83
Functional Impairment 428
Functional Restoration 66, 364, 460
Functional Rhinoplasty 181, 204
Function restoration 364, 372

G

Gel injection 263
Genetic defects 402, 411
Genuine 143
Geography 90
Global pandemics 74
Global sustainability 473
Graft Survival 66
Gynecology 278, 279, 281, 293

H

Hairline Incision 168, 239
harmonization 38

Health 305, 308, 311, 312, 317, 318, 321, 323, 324, 326, 327, 329, 330
Health concerns intrinsic 176
Health issues 53, 54
Health professionals 402, 411, 415, 422
Hematoma 122, 129, 149, 152, 155, 159, 161, 171, 172
Hematoma formation 152, 155, 161
Hemifacial Microsomia 407, 428, 430
Heterogeneity 405, 407, 410
Holistic approach 307, 433, 457
Holistic treatment 108
Hormonal imbalances 15
Human anatomy 187, 339, 347, 349
Human experience 245
Human face 211
Human face anatomy 341
Human interpersonal communications 10
Humanity 75
Human papillomavirus (HPV) 438
Human skin 16
Hyaluronic acid fillers 275, 283, 303
Hyaluronic acid (HA) 145, 474
Hyperpigmentation 308, 309, 310, 312, 319, 320, 321, 322, 328, 329, 330
Hypertension 108, 113, 119, 124, 126, 135
Hypodermal adipose tissue 15
Hypodermis 31

I

Identity 211, 213, 218, 224
Ideology 178
Impact beyond cosmetic improvement 310
Implant surgery 247, 248, 254, 260, 267
Infection 108, 122, 123, 124, 125, 127, 129
Informed consent 176, 191, 198
Informed Consent 97
Injection Plane 301
Injection Units 301
Innovation 175, 202, 465, 466, 468, 469, 472, 473, 475, 476, 477, 479, 481, 482, 490, 491, 492
Instructions 108, 126, 128
Interpersonal 176
Intraoperative Navigation 493

J

Jacial rejuvenation 142, 143, 144, 145, 147, 148, 151, 152, 154, 160, 167, 168, 170, 171, 172
Jowl Correction 168

L

Laser energy 306
Laser Parameters 332
Laser Technology 493
Laser therapy 306, 310, 313, 314, 317, 319, 325, 326, 329, 330, 331, 332, 333
Laser treatment 305, 307, 311, 312, 316, 321, 323, 325, 326, 327, 330, 335
Lateral Brow Elevation 239
Lateral Canthopexy 136
Lid Laxity 136
Lip Augmentation 301
Liposculpture 243, 244, 245, 246, 247, 248, 249, 250, 251, 252, 254, 255, 256, 257, 260, 261, 262, 263, 264, 265, 267, 269, 271, 272
Liposuction 243, 263
Lipotransfer techniques 436
Local Flap 460
Lower Eyelid Blepharoplasty 113, 136
Lumpectomy 442

M

Machine learning algorithms 476
Macrognathia 428
Magnitude 437
Malposition 108, 124, 125
Management 149, 152, 163, 166, 172
Mandibular angle 31
Mandibular Fracture Fixation 396
Margins of Excision 460
Marionette lines 31
Market trends 471, 485
Masseter muscle 31
Maxillectomy 435, 438, 441, 445, 446, 447, 451, 452, 453, 455, 462

Maxillofacial 379, 387, 390, 400
Mechanisms 273, 279, 305, 311, 312, 315, 324, 334
Medial Brow Elevation 239
Medial Canthal Tendon 136
Medical ability 39
Medical advisers 39
Medical History 78, 101
Medical innovation 245
Medical practice 109
Medical technology 372
Melanoma 438, 460, 461
Mental health 38, 47, 54, 55, 56, 57, 59
Mental wellness 251
Methodology 442
Meticulous approach 179
Meticulous planning 49, 65
Microdermabrasion 311, 332
Microdermabrasion integration 311
Micrognathia 428
Micromorphology 436, 441, 442, 459
Microspot density 309
Microsurgical techniques 49
Microtia 402, 407, 409
Microtia patients 14
Microvascular Anastomosis 460
Midface Hypoplasia 428
Minimal Access Cranial Suspension Lift (MACS) 145
Mixed Reality (MR) 440
Modern cosmetic 305
Modern society 214, 245, 246
Mohs Surgery 460
Molar-Incisor Hypomineralization (MIH) 405
Morphological aspect 401
Motivations 75, 78, 84, 86, 96, 98
Multicultural society 339
Multi-dimensional approach 249
Multidisciplinary Management 428
Muscle coordination 12
Muscle Relaxation 301
Muscles 1, 2, 3, 5, 9, 10, 11, 12, 13, 15, 30, 34, 35
Muscle transfers 434, 443
Muscular dysfunction 274
Muscular function 434

N

Nanotechnology 465, 473, 477, 492
Nasal Anatomy 204
Nasal Bridge 204
Nasal bumps 181
Nasal integrity 176, 189
Nasal Septum 204
Nasal Valve 204
Nasolabial fold 31
Natural expression 275
Neck lift surgery 152
Nervous system 402, 428, 432
Neuromuscular blockade 282
Neuromuscular junction 274, 282, 302
Neurotization 439, 443
Neurotoxic protein 274
Neurotoxin 212, 230, 234, 235, 238
Neurotoxin Injection 301
Neurotransmitter 281
Non-Ablative Laser 332
Non-cosmetic applications 309
Non-surgical aesthetics 275, 276, 280, 294, 298, 300
Nonsurgical interventions 243
Nonsurgical techniques 212
Non-verbal communication 5
Nutritional 108, 119, 126

O

Objective structured clinical examination (OSCE) 471
Objective structured practical examination (OSPE) 471
Obtain realistic 152
Occlusion management 338
Oncologic 433, 434, 435, 436, 437, 438, 439, 440, 441, 442, 443, 445, 446, 447, 448, 449, 450, 451, 452, 453, 454, 455, 456, 457, 458, 459, 460, 461
Oncologic surgery 433, 434, 435, 437, 439, 440, 441, 449, 450, 451, 454, 455, 456, 459
Ongoing learning 40

Online marketing technology 468
Open Approach 204, 209
Open communication 76, 82, 84, 92, 97, 99
Open Reduction and Internal Fixation (ORIF) 396
Operational capability 468
Optimal balance 145
Oral and maxillofacial (OMF) 476
Oral squamous cell carcinoma (OSCC) 438
Orbicularis oculi 31
Orbicularis oris 31
Orbital Floor Repair 396
Orbital Septum 136
Organization of Scientific Area Committees 338
Orthodontia 18
Orthognathic surgery 7, 401, 412, 419, 420, 425, 426, 432
Osteotomes 7, 24
Osteotomy 204

P

Patient 37, 38, 39, 40, 41, 43, 44, 45, 46, 47, 48, 49, 50, 51, 52, 53, 54, 55, 56, 57, 58, 59, 60, 61, 62, 63, 64, 65, 68
Patient anatomy 177, 190
Patient assessment 74, 75, 76, 78, 79, 81, 83, 85, 86, 87, 89, 91, 97, 100
Patient comfort 178, 188
Patient Expectations 84, 101
Patient experience 278
Patient management 470
Patient safety 142, 145, 146, 147, 160, 165
Patients experience 146
Patient-specific planning 364
Patients' skin 15
Patient Workflow Optimization 493
Periauricular Incision 168
Personal ambitions 212
Personal identity 38, 39, 146
Personalization 338
Phenomenon embodies 3
Philtrum 31
Photographic Documentation 101
Photothermolysis 332, 334
Physical alteration 38
Physical appearance 176, 195, 196, 198, 213
Physical aspect 370
Physical deformity 370
Physical transformation 213
Piezosurgery 7, 24
Plastic surgery 41, 49, 50, 53, 61, 70
Platysmal Bands 168
Platysma Muscle 168
Platysmaplasty 168, 169
Polydioxanone (PDO) 148, 151, 167
Polyethylene 246, 249, 271
Postblepharoplasty healing process 126
Postgraduate program 470
Postoperative 108, 112, 126, 127
Postoperative care 74, 77, 80, 88, 89, 95, 101, 152, 156, 161, 165
Postoperative Care 60
Post-Treatment Care 328
Potential side effects 307, 312, 324, 329, 330, 331
Practice management 465, 466, 467, 468, 469, 470, 471, 475, 476, 477, 479, 480, 483, 484, 485, 487, 488, 490, 491, 492
Practitioners 38, 40, 45, 47, 55, 57, 60, 61, 62, 63, 64, 466, 472, 480, 488
Pregnancy maternal health 413
Preliminary assessment 75
Preoperative consultation 75, 86
Pre-operative counseling 38
Preoperative planning 76, 82, 103
Pre-surgical planning 444
Pretarsal Muscle 136
Pretrichial Incision 239
Primary operation 433
Production 148, 150, 157, 466, 467, 469, 472, 477, 478
Professional consensus 74
Propensity 436
Proportion 2, 3, 4, 5, 6, 7, 17, 20, 21, 34, 66
Psychological 73, 74, 75, 76, 77, 78, 79, 80, 86, 87, 88, 89, 90, 91, 93, 94, 95, 96, 97, 100, 107, 110, 115, 116, 117, 119, 125, 127, 130, 131, 132, 134, 143, 146, 152, 153, 155, 158, 159, 162, 167, 433, 434, 435, 436,

437, 439, 440, 441, 442, 443, 444, 445, 446, 447, 448, 449, 451, 453, 454, 456, 457, 459
Psychological Evaluation 101
Psychological forces 212
Psychological issues 370
Psychological recovery 371, 372, 376
Psychological relevance 317
Psychologists 177
Psychosocial 14, 33, 144
Psychosocial adaptation 403, 408
Psychosocial sequelae 434
Psychosocial well-being 404
Public safety 339, 363
Pulse Duration 332
Pursue surgical correction 38

Q

Quadrantectomy 439
Quality Assurance 493

R

Radiofrequency Devices 493
Radiofrequency Resurfacing 332
Rapid expansion 17
Realistic expectations 249, 255, 264
Reconstructive Ladder 66, 364
Reconstructive procedure 178
Reconstructive rhinoplasty 176, 179
Reconstructive surgeon 434
Reconstructive surgery 37, 38, 39, 40, 41, 42, 43, 44, 45, 47, 49, 51, 52, 53, 54, 55, 56, 57, 58, 59, 60, 61, 62, 63, 65, 66, 67, 69, 70, 71
Redundant skin 107
Regional Flap 460
Regional Flaps 364
Regulatory Compliance 493
Reinforcing 144
Rejuvenation 274, 282, 285, 286, 303
Responsibility 38, 45, 61, 475, 487, 490
Retinoids 16
Retroauricular Incision 168
Rhinoplasty 4, 175, 176, 178, 179, 180, 181, 182, 183, 184, 185, 186, 187, 192, 194, 196, 198, 199, 200, 203, 206, 208, 209
Rhinoplasty Outcome Evaluation (ROE) 181, 196, 203
Rhytidectomies 150, 151, 167, 173
Rhytidectomy 141, 142, 143, 144, 146, 147, 148, 149, 151, 152, 154, 155, 156, 157, 158, 159, 160, 161, 163, 164, 165, 167, 169, 170, 171, 172
Rigid Fixation 396
Risk Assessment 88, 101
Robotic-Assisted Surgery 493
Robust datasets 341

S

Safety protocols 275
Sagging skin 142, 148, 149, 152, 154, 155, 156, 167
Salivary gland tumors 438
Scar Camouflage 364
Scar Formation 66
Scientific community 338
Self-confidence 247, 248, 249, 252
Septum 177, 182, 183, 184, 205
Significant developments 146
Skeletal Framework Analysis 101
Skeletal remains 338, 342, 347, 348, 356
Skeletal structure 5, 7
Skill deficiencies 306
Skin cancer 16
Skin disease 17
Skin Grafting 364, 460
Skin imperfections 306, 310, 319, 331
Skin laxity 149, 151, 154, 155, 167
Skin Quality Assessment 101
Skin Redraping 168
Skin Redundancy 136
Skin resurfacing 305, 306, 307, 308, 309, 310, 311, 313, 314, 315, 316, 317, 318, 319, 320, 321, 322, 323, 324, 325, 326, 327, 328, 329, 330, 331, 332, 333, 334
Skin texture 23, 24, 145, 308, 311, 312, 317, 318
Social acceptance 146
Social context 142
Social existence 245
Social interaction 435, 439, 444, 455
Social judgments 7, 26

Social perception 4, 7
Social preoccupation 152
Social pressures 276
Social prospects 143
Social quality 152
Societal consequences 469
Societal influence 39
Societal opinions 469
Societal values 144
Society 339, 352, 353, 354, 363
Sociocultural functions 38
Soft Tissue Assessment 101
Soft Tissue Augmentation 301
Soft Tissue Coverage 364
Soft Tissue Laceration Repair 396
Soft Tissue Management 66
Soft Tissue Reconstruction 460
Soft tissue vaporization 306
Somatology 306, 309, 311, 313, 329, 334, 336
Sophistication 232
Spreader Graft 204
Squamous cell carcinoma (SCC) 438
Strategic planning 438
Subciliary Incision 136
Subgaleal Dissection 239
Submental Liposuction 168
Subperiosteal Dissection 239
Subplatysmal Fat 168
Suitable surgeon 232
Superficial musculo-aponeurotic system (SMAS) 142
Surgeons 38, 40, 41, 42, 43, 45, 47, 55, 59, 61
Surgery 175, 176, 177, 178, 180, 181, 182, 183, 184, 187, 188, 189, 190, 191, 192, 193, 194, 196, 197, 198, 199, 200, 201, 202, 203, 206, 207, 208
Surgical endeavors 37
Surgical interventions 38, 39, 52, 54, 55
Surgical outcome 476, 484
Surgical planning 73, 74, 75, 76, 77, 78, 80, 81, 82, 83, 84, 85, 86, 87, 90, 91, 92, 96, 98, 99, 100, 101, 102, 218, 226
Surgical procedure 107, 112, 118, 126
Surgical techniques 74, 77, 82, 83, 91, 93, 94, 95, 106, 211, 215, 223, 226, 227, 236, 401, 407, 408, 420, 421, 423, 424, 428
Surgical technology 37, 40, 44, 51, 52
Sustainable growth 473
Symmetry 66, 403, 404, 407, 408, 409, 421, 423, 427
Symmetry Evaluation 101
Syndromic congenital 404
Syndromic Deformities 428
Synthetic implants 244, 259

T

Targets muscle 274
Technological innovations 340
Technology infusion 470
Teleconsultation 493
Temporal Brow Lift 239
Tendency 465, 481, 484
Texture 212, 214, 235, 236, 238
theoretical knowledge 307
Therapeutic potential 306
Tissue Expansion 66
Tissue Matching 364
Tissue Viability 66, 364
Titanium Plates and Screws 396
Toxicity 473
Tranexamic acid (TXA) 159, 161
Transconjunctival Approach 136
Transferring tissue 443
Transformation 155, 159, 167
Transformative advancement 364
Transforming 107
Transmission 143
Trauma 175, 176, 177, 185, 186, 203, 337, 342, 348, 355, 363, 365
Trauma reconstruction 369, 370, 371, 372, 373, 374, 376, 377, 378, 379, 380, 381, 382, 385, 386, 387, 388, 389, 390, 391, 392, 393, 394, 395, 396, 397, 399
Traumatic injuries 370, 373
Traumatic injury 39
Treatment efficacy 13
Tumor Resection 460

U

Ubiquity 213
Ultherapy 150, 167
Ultrasonic-assisted liposuction 261
Ultrasound-Guided Procedures 493
ultraviolet (UV) 438
Unified environment 76
Unique human experience 354
Unrealistic expectations 177, 201
Upper Eyelid Blepharoplasty 112, 136

V

Vascular occlusion 275, 291, 293
Vascular Supply 364
Vehicular accident 370
Virtual Surgical Simulation 493
Viscosity 301
volumetric changes 154
Volumetric restoration 278
Volumization 301

W

Wavelength 332
Wound Bed Preparation 364
Wound Healing 66

Z

Zygomatic arch 31
Zygomatic bones 1, 3, 4, 6
Zygomaticomaxillary Complex (ZMC) 396
Zygomaticus major 31